VOLUME ONE HUNDRED AND THIRTY TWO

INTERNATIONAL REVIEW OF NEUROBIOLOGY

Parkinson's Disease

INTERNATIONAL REVIEW OF NEUROBIOLOGY

VOLUME 132

SERIES EDITOR

PATRICIA JANAK

Janak Lab, Dunning Hall
Baltimore, MD, USA

PETER JENNER

Division of Pharmacology and Therapeutics
GKT School of Biomedical Sciences
King's College, London, UK

VOLUME ONE HUNDRED AND THIRTY TWO

INTERNATIONAL REVIEW OF NEUROBIOLOGY

Parkinson's Disease

Edited by

KAILASH P. BHATIA

Institute of Neurology, UCL, London, United Kingdom

K. RAY CHAUDHURI

National Parkinson Foundation International Centre of Excellence, Kings College and Kings College Hospital; Maurice Wohl Clinical Neuroscience Institute, Kings College; National Institute for Health Research (NIHR) Mental Health Biomedical Research Centre (BRC) and Dementia Unit at South London and Maudsley NHS Foundation Trust, London, United Kingdom

MARIA STAMELOU

University of Athens Medical School, Hospital Attikon; HYGEIA Hospital, Athens, Greece; Philipps University, Marburg, Germany

ELSEVIER

ACADEMIC PRESS

An imprint of Elsevier

Academic Press is an imprint of Elsevier
50 Hampshire Street, 5th Floor, Cambridge, MA 02139, United States
525 B Street, Suite 1800, San Diego, CA 92101-4495, United States
The Boulevard, Langford Lane, Kidlington, Oxford OX5 1GB, United Kingdom
125 London Wall, London, EC2Y 5AS, United Kingdom

First edition 2017

ISBN: 978-0-12-809714-4
ISSN: 0074-7742

For information on all Academic Press publications
visit our website at https://www.elsevier.com/books-and-journals

Publisher: Zoe Kruze
Acquisition Editor: Kirsten Shankland
Editorial Project Manager: Andrea Gallego Ortiz
Production Project Manager: Surya Narayanan Jayachandran
Cover Designer: Alan Studholme

Typeset by SPi Global, India

CONTENTS

CONTRIBUTORS

Dag Aarsland
Institute of Psychiatry, Psychology and Neuroscience, King's College London, London, United Kingdom

Angelo Antonini
University of Padua, Padua, Italy

Daniela Berg
Christian-Albrechts-University of Kiel, Kiel, Germany

Kailash P. Bhatia
Institute of Neurology, UCL, London, United Kingdom

Kalyan B. Bhattacharyya
RG Kar Medical College & Hospital, RG Kar Road, Kolkata, India

Roongroj Bhidayasiri
Chulalongkorn Center of Excellence for Parkinson's Disease & Related Disorders, Faculty of Medicine, Chulalongkorn University and King Chulalongkorn Memorial Hospital, Thai Red Cross Society, Bangkok, Thailand; Juntendo University, Tokyo, Japan

Bas R. Bloem
Radboud University Medical Centre, Donders Institute for Brain, Cognition and Behaviour, Nijmegen, The Netherlands

Raquel Bouça-Machado
Clinical Pharmacology Unit, Instituto de Medicina Molecular, Lisbon; CNS-Campus Neurológico Sénior, Torres Vedras, Portugal

K. Ray Chaudhuri
National Parkinson Foundation International Centre of Excellence, Kings College and Kings College Hospital; Maurice Wohl Clinical Neuroscience Institute, Kings College; National Institute for Health Research (NIHR) Mental Health Biomedical Research Centre (BRC) and Dementia Unit at South London and Maudsley NHS Foundation Trust, London, United Kingdom

Carlo Colosimo
Santa Maria University Hospital, Terni, Italy

Ilaria Cova
Center for Research and Treatment on Cognitive Dysfunctions, Institute of Clinical Neurology, Luigi Sacco' Hospital, University of Milan, Milan, Italy

Veronika Datieva
Russian Medical Academy of Postgraduate Education, Moscow, Russia

Roberto Erro
Center for Neurodegenerative Diseases (CEMAND), University of Salerno, Fisciano, Italy; Institute of Neurology, UCL, London, United Kingdom

Joaquim J. Ferreira
Clinical Pharmacology Unit, Instituto de Medicina Molecular; Laboratory of Clinical Pharmacology and Therapeutics, Faculty of Medicine, University of Lisbon, Lisbon; CNS-Campus Neurológico Sénior, Torres Vedras, Portugal

Emily Frost
National Parkinson Foundation International Centre of Excellence, Kings College and Kings College Hospital; National Institute for Health Research (NIHR) Mental Health Biomedical Research Centre (BRC) and Dementia Unit at South London and Maudsley NHS Foundation Trust, London, United Kingdom

Grace Harington
National Parkinson Foundation International Centre of Excellence, Kings College and Kings College Hospital; National Institute for Health Research (NIHR) Mental Health Biomedical Research Centre (BRC) and Dementia Unit at South London and Maudsley NHS Foundation Trust, London, United Kingdom

Peter Jenner
Institute of Pharmaceutical Science, King's College London, London, United Kingdom

Beom S. Jeon
Parkinson Disease Study Group, Seoul National University Hospital; Movement Disorder Center, Neuroscience Research Institute, College of Medicine, Seoul National University, Seoul, South Korea

Iskandar Johar
Institute of Psychiatry, Psychology and Neuroscience, King's College London, London, United Kingdom

Julia Johnson
National Parkinson Foundation International Centre of Excellence, Kings College and Kings College Hospital; National Institute for Health Research (NIHR) Mental Health Biomedical Research Centre (BRC) and Dementia Unit at South London and Maudsley NHS Foundation Trust, London, United Kingdom

Hee J. Kim
Konkuk University School of Medicine; Parkinson Disease Study Group, Seoul National University Hospital, Seoul, South Korea

Christos Koros
National and Kapodistrian University of Athens Medical School, "Attikon" Hospital, Athens, Greece

Abhishek Lenka
National Institute of Mental Health & Neurosciences, Bangalore, Karnataka, India

Roberto Marconi
Misericordia Hospital, Grosseto, Italy

Luca Marsili
Sapienza University of Rome, Rome; Misericordia Hospital, Grosseto, Italy

Pablo Martinez-Martin
National Center of Epidemiology and CIBERNED, Carlos III Institute of Health, Madrid, Spain

Laurie K. Mischley
Bastyr University Research Institute, Kenmore; UW Graduate Program in Nutritional Sciences; University of Washington (UW), Seattle, WA, United States

Brit Mollenhauer
Paracelsus-Elena-Klinik, Kassel; University Medical Center, Göttingen, Germany

Flavia Niccolini
Neurodegeneration Imaging Group, Institute of Psychiatry, Psychology and Neuroscience (IoPPN), King's College London, London, United Kingdom

Bianca Nitu
Colentina Clinical Hospital, Bucharest, Romania

Per Odin
Faculty of Medicine, Lund University, Lund, Sweden; Central Hospital, Bremerhaven, Germany

Chandrasekharapillai Padmakumar
Parkinson's Disease Service for the Older Person, Rankin Park Centre, John Hunter Hospital, Newcastle, NSW, Australia

Gennaro Pagano
Neurodegeneration Imaging Group, Institute of Psychiatry, Psychology and Neuroscience (IoPPN), King's College London, London, United Kingdom

Pramod K. Pal
National Institute of Mental Health & Neurosciences, Bangalore, Karnataka, India

Marios Politis
Neurodegeneration Imaging Group, Institute of Psychiatry, Psychology and Neuroscience (IoPPN), King's College London, London, United Kingdom

Ronald B. Postuma
L7-305 Montreal General Hospital, Montreal, Canada

Mubasher A. Qamar
National Parkinson Foundation International Centre of Excellence, Kings College and Kings College Hospital; Maurice Wohl Clinical Neuroscience Institute, Kings College; National Institute for Health Research (NIHR) Mental Health Biomedical Research Centre (BRC) and Dementia Unit at South London and Maudsley NHS Foundation Trust, London, United Kingdom

Fiona Roberts
National Parkinson Foundation International Centre of Excellence, Kings College and Kings College Hospital; National Institute for Health Research (NIHR) Mental Health Biomedical Research Centre (BRC) and Dementia Unit at South London and Maudsley NHS Foundation Trust, London, United Kingdom

Miguel Rosa-Grilo
King's College London and King's College Hospital, London, United Kingdom

Anna Sauerbier
King's College London and King's College Hospital, London, United Kingdom

Sebastian R. Schreglmann
Institute of Neurology, UCL, London, United Kingdom

Athina Simitsi
National and Kapodistrian University of Athens Medical School, "Attikon" Hospital, Athens, Greece

Federica Spinnato
University of Palermo, Faculty of Medicine, Palermo, Italy

Maria Stamelou
University of Athens Medical School, Hospital Attikon; HYGEIA Hospital, Athens, Greece; Philipps University, Marburg, Germany

Leonidas Stefanis
National and Kapodistrian University of Athens Medical School, "Attikon" Hospital, Athens, Greece

Raquel N. Taddei
King's College London and King's College Hospital, London, United Kingdom

Jonathan Timpka
Faculty of Medicine, Lund University, Lund, Sweden

Nataliya Titova
Federal State Budgetary Educational Institution of Higher Education "N.I. Pirogov Russian National Research Medical University" of the Ministry of Healthcare of the Russian Federation, Moscow, Russia

Sally Trump
National Parkinson Foundation International Centre of Excellence, Kings College and Kings College Hospital; National Institute for Health Research (NIHR) Mental Health Biomedical Research Centre (BRC) and Dementia Unit at South London and Maudsley NHS Foundation Trust, London, United Kingdom

PREFACE

Two hundred years back, James Parkinson described the condition we now call Parkinson's disease (PD) based on clinical observations of cases he named the "shaking palsy." Much of the seminal observations of Parkinson still remain valid: the core motor features, some nonmotor observations (sleep dysfunction, delirium, constipation), as well as possibly the first description of prodromal pain in PD. Yet much has changed. We now know PD is much more than a simple motor disorder driven by central dopamine deficiency secondary to nigral cell loss. There is now recognition of preprodromal PD with genetic mutations as biomarkers. There is a long prodromal period dominated by nonmotor symptoms, and the motor syndrome of PD has become complex with recognition of a palliative stage as patients live longer. Neuroprotection, a key unmet need, is becoming feasible if treatment is started at the prodromal or preprodromal stage when there are no motor symptoms. Personalized medicine is emerging as the possible future strategy for the management of PD. Yet we also have major hurdles in our quest for progress in understanding, treating, and attempting to "cure" PD. Levodopa dramatically reversed the motor syndrome of PD, bringing a Nobel Prize to Arvid Carlsson; 50 years later it still remains the gold standard of treatment for PD that is cost effective as well as efficacious. No therapies have been successful for neuroprotection or neuromodulation. Nonmotor aspects of PD have remained poorly researched with no robust animal models. Large investments in stem cell, genetic, and other restorative therapies have been unproductive. In part this has been related to our failure to understand the complexity of PD, a complex multineurotransmitter dysfunction-related central and peripheral disorder. This book aims to address these issues which chart the progress, and also unravels the difficulties of understanding PD. Chapters, written by key opinion leaders from across the world, detail all aspects of this condition, from the prodromal stage to the palliative, covering pathophysiology, motor and nonmotor symptoms, diagnosis, biomarkers, and treatment. We hope the contents will help the readers to understand PD in a truly holistic manner and hopefully affect their clinical practice in a positive manner for the people with Parkinson's.

Kailash P. Bhatia
K. Ray Chaudhuri
Maria Stamelou

CHAPTER ONE

Hallmarks of Clinical Aspects of Parkinson's Disease Through Centuries

Kalyan B. Bhattacharyya[1]
RG Kar Medical College & Hospital, RG Kar Road, Kolkata, India
[1]Corresponding author: e-mail address: kalyanbrb@gmail.com

Contents

Abstract

James Parkinson published a treatise *"An Essay on The Shaking Palsy"* in 1817. However, there is historical evidence that there were rudimentary descriptions of the disease long before Parkinson brought it to light. Later day physicians have added to the spectrum of the motor aspects of the disease over the last 200 years and the gamut of its clinical presentation is now known to be more ubiquitous than what was supposed earlier. In the 1960s, atypical Parkinsonism is identified as a distinct and separate entity, and after the introduction of levodopa in clinical practice, a variety of late motor complications have been described. Various stages of disability and motor scales have been devised which have helped in identifying and classifying the degree of severity of the disease. However, such impeccable was the original description that virtually little could be modified and later works have only added to the original text.

1. INTRODUCTION

James Parkinson was born on April 11, 1755, as the first child of Mary and John Parkinson. His father was an apothecary at 1 Hoxton Square, Shoreditch, in the southern part of London where Parkinson lived and practiced for the rest of his life. In the year 1817, he wrote a treatise entitled "*An*

International Review of Neurobiology, Volume 132
ISSN 0074-7742
http://dx.doi.org/10.1016/bs.irn.2017.01.003

Essay on the Shaking Palsy," published by Sherwood, Neely, and Jones, London, which ran into 66 pages. There were five chapters, namely, *(a) definition, history, illustrative cases, (b) pathognomonic symptoms examined, tremor coactus, sclerotyrbe festinans, (c) shaking palsy distinguished from other diseases with which it may be confounded, (d) proximate cases, remote cases, illustrative cases, and (e) considerations respecting the means of* cure (Bhattacharyya, 2011; Jefferson, 1973; Parkinson, 1817; Pearce, 1989; Thorpe-Gardner, 2010). Jefferson from Queen Elizabeth Hospital, Birmingham, and his biographer, wrote, "*It sharply illumined a clinical entity which had been only dimly apprehended before that date*" (Jefferson, 1973), and it seems that in these days, when eponyms are not generally favored, Parkinson's disease is one entity which is likely to stand the ruthless grind of time even if all others are expunged from the medical lexicon. In terms of clarity of thought and picturesque clinical portrayal, this classic description has virtually no peer in the annals of medicine. His description of the signs and symptomatology could hardly be improved upon in later days, and such apt and apposite account bear testimony to his outstanding clinical acumen. WR Sanders wrote, "… *succeeding authors have, in general, simply quoted it, or have … overlooked the disease altogether*" (Sanders, 1865). Jefferson further wrote,

> *"Even now the essay can be read with profit, not only because it is a superb model of lucid clinical description, but because it is written with such lucid mastery of style that it must give pleasure to anyone with taste for English prose. It is also a model of logical use of clinical experience… Considering the limited scope of neurological knowledge in his day, it is astonishing that his deductions were so close to the target zone of the substantia nigra…"*
>
> ***Jefferson (1973)***

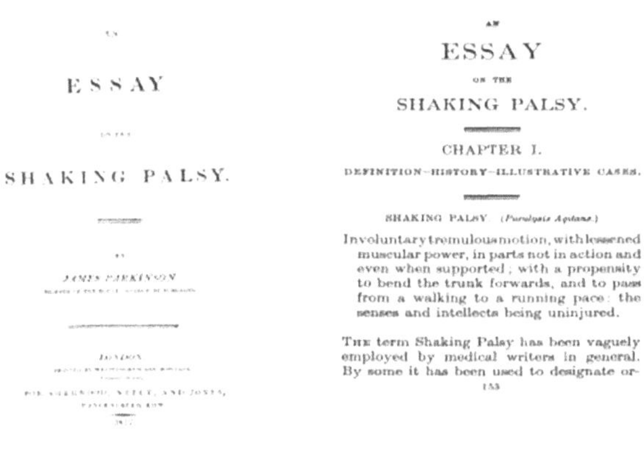
ESSAY
SHAKING PALSY.

AN
ESSAY
ON THE
SHAKING PALSY.

CHAPTER I.
DEFINITION–HISTORY–ILLUSTRATIVE CASES.

SHAKING PALSY. (*Paralysis Agitans.*)

Involuntary tremulous motion, with lessened muscular power, in parts not in action and even when supported; with a propensity to bend the trunk forwards, and to pass from a walking to a running pace: the senses and intellects being uninjured.

The term Shaking Palsy has been vaguely employed by medical writers in general. By some it has been used to designate or-

153

Cover Page and Opening Page of the* 1st *Edition of James Parkinson's Treatise

Source: www.archive.org www.todayinsci.com

There is no verified portrait of James Parkinson, even in the National Art Gallery. Photography was invented decades after his death by Henry Fox Talbot (1800–77) in England in the 1840s (Bhattacharyya, 2011). Three photographs bearing his name can be traced by searching the Internet. The bearded man is in all likelihood, James Cumine Parkinson, a midshipman, who lost his interest in his vocation and later settled in the colonies of New Zealand and Tasmania. The one dressed in garish apparel with a cane stick in hand was a dentist who died in 1889. However, Simon R.W. Scott wrote that the "*Elusive Parkinson*" is possibly represented in a painting in a book, *The Villager's Friend and Physician*, written and sketched by Parkinson himself, and he is seen lecturing before the gathering, though the evidence is scanty (Scott Simon, 2015).

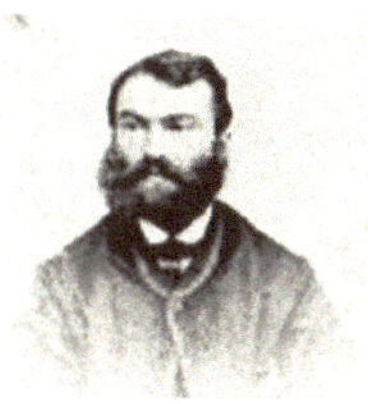

James Cumine Parkinson* *(1832–87)

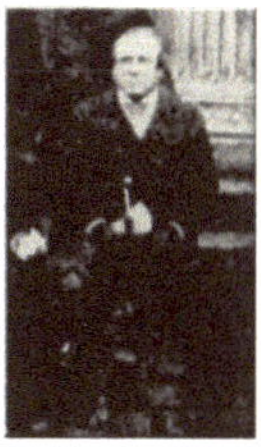

James Parkinson* *(–1895)

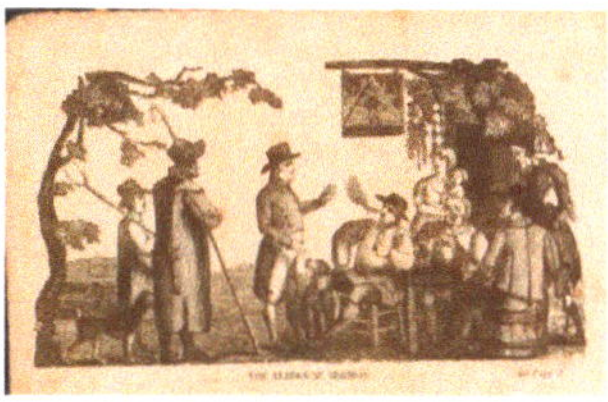

James Parkinson, the Village Physician* *(1755–1824)

Source: www.viartis.net searching4james.files.wordpress.com wellcome images

Parkinson described only six cases in his treatise. He followed one of them till the last stage and encountered two others casually in the streets of London. The fourth patient came to him for treatment of an abscess, while he saw the fifth patient at a distance who had been walking, "*only in a running pace.*" The sixth case is of some historical interest since his tremor was relieved following an attack of cerebrovascular accident, and Parkinson noted, "*as the paralyzed state was removed, the shaking returned*" (Cedarbaum & Gancher, 1992). Later day historians often question whether his first case was one of multiple system atrophy, since he developed incontinence of sphincters (Bhattacharyya, 2011).

In the beginning, Parkinson summarized as follows:

> *"Involuntary tremulous motion, with lessened muscular power, in parts not in action and even when supported; with a propensity to bend the trunk forward, and to pass from a walking to a running pace, the senses and intellect being uninjured."*
>
> ***Pearce (1989)***

Here are some excerpts from the actual text:

> *"So slight and imperceptible are the first inroads of this malady, and so extremely slow its progress, that it rarely happens that the patient can form any recollection of the precise period of its commencement. The first symptoms perceived are a slight sense of weakness, with a proneness to trembling … most commonly in one of the hands and arms. … in less than twelve months or more, the morbid influence is felt in some other part. After a few more months the patient is found to be less strict than usual in preserving an upright posture … in a few months this limb becomes agitated by similar tremblings, and suffers a similar loss of power.*
>
> *…While at meals the fork is not being duly directed frequently fails to raise the morsel from the plate, which, when seized, is with much difficulty conveyed to the mouth. At this period the patient seldom experiences suspension of the agitation of the limbs. Commencing for instance in one arm, the wearisome agitation is borne until beyond sufferance, when by sudden changing the posture it is for a time stopped in that limb, to commence generally, in less than a minute in one of the legs, or in the arm of the other side, … the disease proceeds, … the hands fail to answer the dictates of the will. Walking becomes a task which cannot be performed without considerable attention. … The legs are not raised to that height, … so that utmost care is `necessary to prevent frequent falls … writing can now be hardly accomplished; … propensity to lean forward becomes invincible, and the patient is thereby forced to step on the toes and forepart of the feet, whilst the upper part of the body is thrown so far forward as to render it difficult to avoid falling on the face. … being at the same time, irresistibly impelled to take much quicker and shorter steps, and thereby to adopt unwillingly a running pace. … the bowels… had all along been torpid, the expulsion of faeces requiring mechanical aid. … his words are now scarcely intelligible… no longer able to feed himself … saliva is constantly draining from the mouth, mixed with particles of food he is no longer able to clear from inside of the mouth.*
>
> *… The power of conveying the food to the mouth is at length so much impeded that he is obliged to consent to be fed by others. As the disease proceeds towards its last stage, the trunk is almost permanently bowed, … and the tremulous agitation becomes violent…. The chin is now almost immovably bent down upon the sternum. The slops with which he is attempted to be fed, with the saliva, are constantly trickling from the mouth. The power of articulation is lost. The urine and faeces are passed involuntarily; and at the last, constant sleepiness, with slight delirium and other marks of extreme exhaustion, announce the wished-for release."*
>
> ***Pearce (1989)***

1.1 Before James Parkinson

It should be borne in mind that long before James Parkinson a number of physicians alluded to a similar condition in the past (Cedarbaum &

Gancher, 1992; Currier, 1996; Goetz, 2011; http://www.viartis.net/parkinsons.disease/history.htm; Larner, 2014a; Lees, 2007; Parkinson, 1833; Pearce, 1989; Thorpe-Gardner, 2010; www.wikipedia.com: History of Parkinson's disease). An Egyptian papyrus, as old as 12th century BC, described symptoms in a king with drooling saliva as if "*divine old age has slackened his mouth, he cast his spittle upon the ground and spit it out,*" and in all likelihood, this suggests PD, while certain biblical accounts also attest to the recognition of tremulous illnesses (www.wikipedia.com: History of Parkinson's disease; http://www.viartis.net/parkinsons.disease/history.htm). In ancient India, the Ayurvedic system of medicine used an agent, *Mucuna pruriens* or *Atmagupta*, which is known to contain levodopa and is used even today (Manyam, 1990; Rana, 2016; Vaidya, Rajgopalan, Mankodi, et al., 1978). In India, PD was known as *Kampavata* as far back as 5000 BC and the ancient Chinese medical text, "*Huang di nei jing su wen,*" described some of the symptoms of a malady which read like that of PD (http://www.viartis.net/parkinsons.disease/history.htm). Claudius Galen of Greece (129–200) gave an account of a disease, closely resembling PD with rest tremor, postural changes, and paralysis in 175 AD. He described a patient as, "*… wild, wide open eyes and lying in bed rigid, as if he was made of wood with tremor, constipation and psychiatric symptoms.*" He described tremor as "*an involuntary alternating up and down motion*" (www.wikipedia.com: History of Parkinson's disease; http://www.viartis.net/parkinsons.disease/history.htm).

Parkinson himself referred to the early writings of Galen and Juncker, the German physician (1679–1759), who distinguished tremor as, "*either Active—sudden affections of the mind, terror, anger or Passive – dependent on debilitating causes such as advanced age, palsy, etc.*" (Cedarbaum & Gancher, 1992; Pearce, 1989). Incidentally, Parkinson himself distinguished the entity he described from *tremor tremulentus*, which was due to "*indulgence in the drinking of spirituous liquors … immoderate employment of tea and coffee… or to advanced age*" and regarded it as a "*species of palsy*" (Cedarbaum & Gancher, 1992). Most novel ideas germinate from something past, remote or recent, and Robert Currier from the University of Mississippi raised the question whether it was the great John Hunter who goaded Parkinson to study the problem (Currier, 1996). Hunter used to organize night lecture courses on surgery, and Parkinson at the age of 30 in 1785 attended the classes and kept notes written in shorthand (Currier, 1996). After Parkinson died in 1824, his son J.W.K. Parkinson published his father's writings in 1833 as a commemorative volume entitled "*Hunterian Reminiscences, Being the*

Substance of a Course of Lectures on the Principles and Practice of Surgery, Delivered by the Late Mr. John Hunter" (Currier, 1996; Parkinson, 1833). Parkinson described one case described by Hunter.

> *"... every part shook which was not fully supported ... in sleep the vibratory motions of the muscles ceased ... and it is likely that he was describing a case of essential tremor. However, while describing another case he said, '... muscles which are entirely at the command of the will, ... take on involuntary actions and they never tire. For instance, Lord L's hands are almost perpetually in motion, and he never feels the sensation in them of being tired. When he is asleep his hands... are perfectly at rest; but when he wakes in a little time they begin to move."*
>
> ***Currier (1996)***

Most certainly, this reads like a convincing description of PD, and that Parkinson owed his allegiance to Hunter is quite clear in the last sentence of his classic essay:

> *"... how few can estimate the benefits bestowed on mankind, by the labors of a Morgagni, Hunter, or Baillie."*
>
> ***Parkinson (1817)***

Two authors who cast a spell on Parkinson's mind are Sylvius de la Boë (1614–72) and François Boissier de Sauvages de la Croix (1706–67) (http://www.viartis.net/parkinsons.disease/history.htm; Pearce, 1989). The former, a Dutch physician, wrote in 1680 that tremor can be of two kinds, and suggested, "... *tremors which are produced by attempts at voluntary motion, and those which occur whilst the body is at rest.*" He called the former "*motus tremulous*" and the latter "*tremor coactus*," and this distinction is useful even to this day (http://www.viartis.net/parkinsons.disease/history.htm; Koehler & Keyser, 1997; Pearce, 1989; Stern, 1989). Sauvages was a French physician and a botanist who described *scelotyrbe festinans*, whereby,

> *"patients, whilst wishing to walk in the ordinary mode, are forced to run... I think cannot be more fitly named than hastening or hurrying... the tremulous part leaps, and as it were vibrate, even when supported: whilst every other tremor, he observes, ceases, when the voluntary exertion for moving the limb stops... but returns when we will the limb move;"*
>
> ***Pearce (1989)***

The works of Gerhardt van Swieten in 1749 alluded to an identical gait as well. The festinant gait, however, was described by Hieronymus David Gaubius of Germany (1705–80), nearly 10 years earlier in 1758, and in 1776 Johannes Baptiste Sagar (1732–1813) from France wrote in his treatise,

"*An Ariadne's Thread for Students of the Sick*," "*In Vienna, I saw a man above the age of fifty who was running involuntarily, being also incapable of keeping direction so as to avoid obstacles; in addition he suffered from ptyalism*" and this is a clear description of festination, gait incoordination, and hypersalivation (Cedarbaum & Gancher, 1992; Currier, 1996; Pearce, 1989; Stern, 1989). William Cullen (1710–90) of Scotland mentioned a few features in some patient who might have been suffering from PD (Pearce, 1989).

Very recently, medical historians have unearthed an account, closely resembling that of PD, written by the Hungarian physician, Ferenc Pápai Páriz (1649–1716), where tremor, rigidity, bradykinesia, and postural instability, all the four cardinal features of PD, were adequately described in 1690, though there is no reference to it in Parkinson's original description (Bereczki, 2010; http://www.viartis.net/parkinsons.disease/history.htm). It is said that this is the first complete description of the disease but since it was written in the Hungarian language, it received little attention and has been somewhat ignored. George Cheyne (1671–1743), a Scottish physician, possibly described PD in his book, "*The English Malady*," and wrote,

> *"... a disease wherein the body, or some of its members lose their motion, and sometimes their sensation of feeling. The disease is never acute, often tedious and in old people, almost incurable; and the patient for the most part drags a miserable life... he totters and shakes, and becomes a dismal sight; as if no longer a man, but an animal half dead."*
>
> ***http://www.viartis.net/parkinsons.disease/history.htm***

Interestingly, Caleb Hillier Parry (1755–1824), Parkinson's contemporary and codescriber of Parry-Romberg syndrome, practiced in the rural area of Bath and described a case in 1815. He stated that the "*head and limbs shake, more especially on any muscular exertion*," though later day historians feel that it was a case of essential tremor (Larner, 2014b).

It is on record that Nicolas Poussin (1594–1665), a French painter, suffered from tremulousness in hands which, perhaps, lent his later works, a certain added filigree. His tremor started in 1650 when he was 56 years of age and sophisticated analysis of the tremor in recent times has shown that there was a progressive decline in the speed of his movements. This feature coupled with the age of onset is, one feels, consistent with the diagnosis of PD (Haggard & Rodgers, 2000; Larner, 2014b). Donald Calne, from Vancouver, and his coworkers feel that the incomparable Leonardo da Vinci (1452–1517) might have described a case of PD. It has been unearthed in a manuscript, preserved in Windsor Castle, which reads,

> *"... how nerves sometimes operate by themselves without any command from soul. This is clearly apparent for you will see paralytics and those who are shivering and benumbed by cold move their trembling parts such as their head and hands without permission of the soul, the soul with all its forces cannot prevent them from trembling..."*
>
> ***http://www.viartis.net/parkinsons.disease/history.htm, Larner (2014b), and Calne, Dubini, and Stern (1989)***

Others might have seen such cases and, with their extraordinary percipience and perspicacity, penned vivid accounts of the maladies (Bereczki, 2010; Larner, 2014b). William Shakespeare (1564–1616) gave an account of shaking palsy in Henry VI, and Charles Dickens (1812–70) might have described progressive supranuclear palsy in 1857, 107 years before J.C. Steele, J.C. Richardson, and J. Olszewski described the illness in *Archives of Neurology* in 1964 (Haan, 2013; http://www.viartis.net/parkinsons.disease/history.htm; Larner, 2002a, 2002b, 2014b; Steele, Richardson, & Olszewski, 1964; Van der Brugger & Widdershaven, 2004). It has often been observed that even the Bible contains reference to PD. The Old Testament says in the Gospel of Luke,

> *"When the guardians of the house tremble, and strong men are bent..." in Ecclesiastes and the New Testament describes, "There was a woman who for eighteen years had been crippled by a spirit... bent and completely incapable of standing erect."*
>
> ***http://www.viartis.net/parkinsons.disease/history.htm***

In Greece, the greatest poet Homer of the 8th century BC in his epic, *The Iliad*, portrayed the old Kind Nestor with symptoms suggestive of PD, and Erasistratus of Ceos (304–250 BC), a Greek anatomist, who founded a school of anatomy in Alexandria along with the physician Herophilus (335–280 BC), is reported to have described freezing which he named *paradoxos*, and defined it as a kind of paralysis, where a person suddenly stops while moving and, after some hesitation, continues his gait (http://www.viartis.net/parkinsons.disease/history.htm). Roman history mentions that Aulus Cornelius Celsus (25 BC–50 AD), an encyclopedist, famed for his description of the features of inflammation (*rubor, calor, dolor, tumor*), distinguished fine tremor from the coarse one, the latter, independent of voluntary movement, thus resembling rest tremor of PD (http://www.viartis.net/parkinsons.disease/history.htm). Pedanius Dioscorides, a Roman physician, noticed that the aged people exhibited tremor owing to decline in their power to control the motion of the limbs (http://www.viartis.net/parkinsons.disease/history.htm). In the medieval history the writings of Paul of Aegina (625–690), the Byzantine Greek physician and Ibn Sina (980–1037), the Persian polymath and physician hint at tremor which might indicate PD (http://www.viartis.net/parkinsons.disease/history.htm).

John Aubrey (1626–97), the British writer, compiled a biography of the philosopher Thomas Hobbes (1588–1679) and gave a succinct account of his terminal days in *Brief Lives*, and "*Life of Mr Thomas Hobbes of Malmesbury*." He wrote,

> *"... had the shaking palsy in his hands which began in France before the year 1650, and has grown upon him in degree ever since, so that he has not been able to write very legibly since 1665 or 1666, as I find by some of his letters to me."*
>
> ***http://www.viartis.net/parkinsons.disease/history.htm and Palfreman (2015)***

Giuseppe Longhi (1766–1831), an Italian engraver, remarked that the innkeeper in the painting of Rembrandt van Rijn's (1606–69) "*The Good Samaritan*" stood flexed while greeting the visitor and holding his right hand, as if it had been trembling and Johann Wolfgang von Goethe (1749–1832), the great German writer too, commented likewise in his essay "*Rembrandt The Thinker*" (Cedarbaum & Gancher, 1992). Wilhelm von Humboldt (1767–1835), a German academic reformer, statesman, and writer, described the disease in himself who lived more or less at the same time with James Parkinson and never saw him. He wrote to Goethe, his friend, in 1924, the year of Parkinson's death, that his handwriting was getting worse with time, the letters were becoming smaller, and he had difficulty in turning in bed. Curiously, his handwriting was worse while writing in German than in Latin. He died at the age of 68 of pneumonia and his intellect remained clear (Horowski, Horowski, Vogel, Poewe, & Kielhorn, 1995; Lakke, 1996).

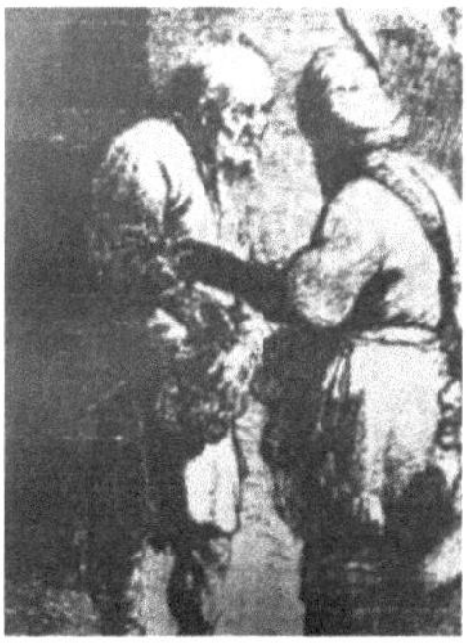

The good Samaritan

Source: Cedarbaum, J. M., & Gancher, S. T. (Eds.) (1992). *Neurologic clinics: Parkinson's disease* (Vol. 10, p. 301). Philadelphia, USA: WB Saunders Company.

It took nearly 40 years before the giants in Salpétrière, Paris, were awakened to the entity of PD. Armánd Trousseau (1801–67) described rigidity, a sign that escaped Parkinson's attention, possibly because of the paucity of cases he could actually examine, in the *15th Lecture on Clinical Medicine* (Pearce, 1989). Jean Martin Charcot (1825–93), in collaboration with his peers, Alfred Vulpian (1826–87), and Leopold Ordenstein (1835–1902) noted some more features in 1862 in addition to what had been described by Parkinson and it has been compiled in Lecture 5 of Charcot's celebrated *Lecons sure les maladies du systême nerveux faites a la Salpétrière* in 1880 (Charcot, 1880). He wrote that tremor was the cardinal symptom:

> *"... limited at first to one member, then little by little becoming generalized ... almost pathognomonic, the patient closes the fingers on the thumb as though in the act of spinning wool ... or crumbling bread... The movements are slow and seem feeble ..."*
>
> ***Pearce (1989)***

Furthermore, he wrote,

> *"... a tendency to propulsion and retropulsion ... the individual is unable to stop ... being apparently forced to follow a flying center of gravity... a peculiar attitude of the body and its members, a fixed look, and immobile features ... Speech was slow, jerky and short, jolted out as it were, like an inexperienced rider on horseback, when the animal is trotting."*
>
> ***Charcot (1880)***

Charcot conferred the eponym, which was till then known as *shaking palsy* or *paralysis agitans*, as Parkinson and William Gowers from Queen Square, London, described it, respectively. It was Charcot who first described rigidity-dependent PD without tremor, and since the patient he examined was not paralyzed, he advocated elimination of the term paralysis agitans, preferring the use of the famed eponym and wrote, "... *paralysis agitans is indisputably a very little known disease.*" Importantly, he separated the entity of pyramidal dysfunction, characterized by weakness and spasticity from extrapyramidal disorders, characterized by bradykinesia and rigidity. He wrote,

> *"According to that author, Parkinson, decreased muscle strength always accompanies the disease, and it is probably true for a good number of cases. But this is far from being the rule. Many patients, including ours today, maintain, at least for a long time, good muscular strength."*
>
> ***Louis (1997)***

And again, he wrote,

> *"More commonly, muscular rigidity only comes on or predominates in the most advanced stage of paralysis agitans. Yet, long before rigidity actually develops, patients have significant difficulty performing ordinary activities; ... a cursory examination demonstrates that their problem refers more to slowness in execution of movements rather than to real weakness... These phenomena have often been interpreted as weakness, but ... until late in the disease these patients are remarkably strong."*
>
> ***Louis (1997)***

Paul Richer (1849–1933), a student of Charcot and an artist, drew sketches of a patient named Marie Anne Gavr in a span of 3 years from 1874 to 1877 and brilliantly illustrated the progress from stooped posture to camptocormia, in order to illustrate the clinical picture (Pearce, 1989), and Lebert Claveleira highlighted bradykinesia as a distinctive symptom, while Sigismond Jaccoud (1830–1913), a Swiss physician, referred to this symptom as akinesia in 1873. Jean René Cruchet (1875–59), a French pathologist, emphasized that bradykinesia should be treated as one of the fundamental signs of PD and Jules Froment (1878–1946), a French neurologist, contributed liberally to the study of rigidity (http://www.viartis.net/parkinsons.disease/history.htm). William Gowers, an expert in shorthand and sketching, drew representative pictures of the stooped and the flexed posture in PD which he reproduced in his famous book, *Manual of the Nervous System*, published in 1888 (Gowers, 1893).

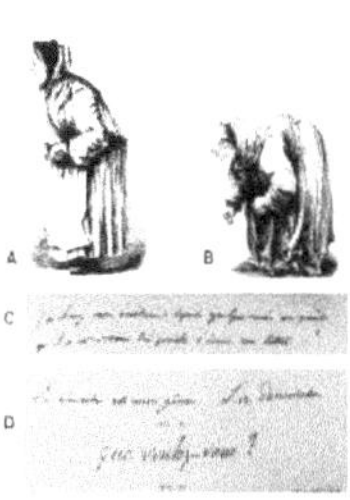

Paul Richter's illustration of Mary Anne Gavr

Source: www.federaljack.com

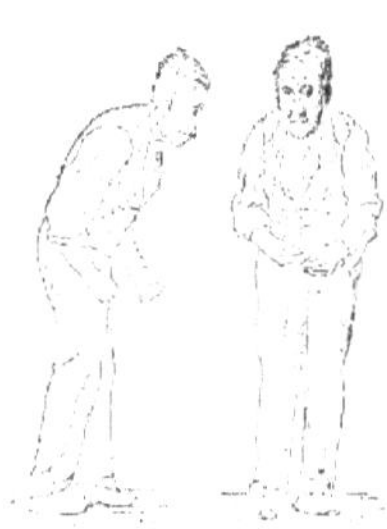

William Gower's sketch of stooped posture

Source: www.viartis.net

In an exhaustive review, entitled, "*The Shaking Palsy, the First Forty-Five Years: A Journey Through the British Literature*," Elan D. Louis brought to light that during that period, only 27 references were found on this disease,

Parkinson's own account included, and most of them reiterated what Parkinson had already observed (Louis, 1997). All of them gave due credit to the original treatise; for example, J. Cooke wrote in his monograph "*A Treatise on Nervous Disease*" that "*A disease has been lately described by Mr. Parkinson, under the title, paralysis agitans, which appears to me highly deserving of our attention*" (Cooke, 1820). There were some articles, which contained added information on the disease. J. Elliotson, a practitioner at St. Thomas' Hospital, London, described one case as "*... and suddenly he brings out his words with extreme rapidity and such is the effort that he cannot stop himself ... It is a phenomenon analogous to the running which occurs on the attempt to walk.*" Obviously, he was referring to festination, which Parkinson described as "*walking on running pace*" in one of his observed cases and the rush of words has been described as tachyphemia (Elliotson, 1830). Marshall Hall described a 28-year-old man as hemiplegic paralysis agitans and wrote,

> *"... is affected by weakness and agitation of the right arm and leg; augmented on any occasion of agitation, and on moving; it is observed as he walks or when he passes his cane from one hand to the other; there is besides, a peculiar lateral rocking of the eyes, a degree of stammering and defective articulation."*
>
> **Hall (1841)**

Parkinson and some other notable physicians described emphatically that the motor system bore the brunt of the disease and the poverty of movements and bradykinesia were the result of weakness and paralysis of muscles, and hence the term paralysis agitans seemed apposite (Louis, 1997). Parkinson wrote that the patients had "*lessened muscular power*" (Parkinson, 1817), while J. Cooke noted "*... this disease begins with some degree of weakness*" (Cooke, 1820). Marshall Hall too felt that "*... the first symptom of this insidious disease is weakness and tremor,*" and Paget described a patient as "*... tendency to lean forwards, and fall on his face*" (Hall, 1841; Paget, 1855). However, T. Watson wrote,

> *"there is no truth in paralysis," and a few years later J.R. Reynolds wrote in 1865, "The term paralysis agitans is essentially bad, as paralysis does not necessarily exist in the condition referred to, and when present, as in some cases, is not primary... The patient can do little with his affected limbs; but it is because of their constant agitation, not because of their paralysis"*
>
> **Watson (1872) and Reynolds (1865)**

In 1865, W.R. Sanders suggested alternate names for the conditions like *paralysis agitans festinia, paralysis agitans senilis, and paralysis agitans Parkinsonii* (Sanders, 1865). T.C. Gowry described one such case and named it *paralysis agitans intermittens.* He described a 26-year-old lady and wrote,

> *"Involuntary tremor of upper and lower extremities, continuing for about five to six minutes, occurring twice or three every hour, and attended with complete loss of power of limbs ... and tongue partially protruded with a corresponding sound, and inability to articulate; orbicular muscles of eyelids, during some of the paroxysms, are similarly affected; paroxysm terminates in a heavy sigh ... During intermission is ready to able to raise hands to head, but this is done slowly, and with great consequent fatigue."*
>
> ***Gowry (1831)***

Elan D. Louis wrote that in all likelihood, Gowry described a case of seizure disorder, where the term paralysis was used for the cessation of activity, and agitans for the clonic component (Louis, 1997) !!

1.2 The 20th Century

The clinical features of parkinsonism took a turn when physicians were startled to see a novel condition following the worldwide outbreak of influenza in 1918 which lasted till 1920. In the wake of this global disaster a new variety of movement disorders were observed by the Rumanian psychiatrist, Constantin von Economo (1876–1931) in 1917. He presented his paper before the Viennese Society of Psychiatry and published his observations in the journal, "*Wiener Klinische Wochenschrift*" the same year and later, in 1929, wrote a monogram, "*Die Encephalitis lethargica, ihre Nachkrankheiten und ihre Behandlung*" (Bhattacharyya, 2011). He classified the clinical features into three categories, somnolent-ophthalmoplegic, hyperkinetic, and amyostatic, of which the last variety bore many of the features of parkinsonism, while the second entity presented with myoclonic twitches and choreiform movements. He wrote,

> *"...a rigidity, without a real palsy and without symptoms arising from the pyramidal tract. This form of encephalitis lethargica is particularly common in the chronic cases, dominating the clinical picture of parkinsonism... To look at these patients one would suppose them to be in a state of profound secondary dementia. Emotions are scarcely noticeable in the face, but they are mentally intact."*
>
> ***Bhattacharyya (2011)***

Incidentally, von Economo's publication was preceded only 2 weeks ago by the description of the same condition by Jean René Cruchet of Bordeaux (1875–1959), who insisted that the honor of describing the condition first should be bestowed on him. However, Van Bogaert (1897–1989) from Belgium was appointed as the adjudicator and he extended his palm to von Economo with the verdict that only he defined the condition as a single entity, which Cruchet did not. However, some historians refer to encephalitis lethargica as "*Cruchet's disease.*"

Wilfred Harris (1869–1960), Frederick Batten (1865–1918), Kinnier Wilson, Edward Farquhar Buzzard (1871–1945), and others reported cases of encephalitis lethargica resembling parkinsonism from England in 1918 (Dimsdale, 1946). In 1946, Helen Dimsdale (1907–77) from the Maida Vale Hospital for Nervous Diseases, London, wrote an exhaustive article in the *Quarterly Journal of Medicine*, after studying 320 patients of parkinsonism collected from records in the 20th century (Dimsdale, 1946). It was observed that in the earlier part of the century, paralysis agitans constituted the predominant form, while postencephalitic parkinsonism was the dominant variety from 1920 to 1930. Thereafter, though the incidence of the postencephalitic variety declined, sporadic cases still occurred. Psychiatric problems, emotional lability, rigidity, oculogyric crisis, and sialorrhea were the principal symptoms observed. In 1924, Kinnier Wilson and William Cobb reported few cases of parkinsonism in association with tabes dorsalis (Dimsdale, 1946).

In 1929, MacDonald Critchley wrote an article in the journal *Brain*, entitled, "*Arteriosclerotic Parkinsonism*" that generated more heat than light. He wrote,

> *"... Hitherto scant attention has been paid to the occurrence of Parkinsonism among the syndromes of cerebro-vascular disease. It is the object of this paper to emphasize the importance of this syndrome as being one of the most frequent objective manifestations of a protean disease. It is not essential to find Parkinsonian syndrome in its entirety in cerebral arteriosclerosis. Incomplete forms are more common ..."*
>
> ***Critchley (1929)***

In later years when the existence of this entity was disputed, he remained firm in his convictions, and with subtle changes in emphasis, he wrote,

> *"In 1929, my paper on arteriosclerotic Parkinsonism ... attracted no little attention and this expression passed smoothly into the currency of neurology. However, since the significance of dopamine began to unfold... some went so far as to express the view that it was an imaginary disorder... I am well aware that there are mythical maladies of the nervous system... but arteriosclerotic Parkinsonism, I strongly submit, does not belong to that category."*
>
> ***Bhattacharyya (2011) and Critchley (1929)***

In order to avert this controversy, a term, *arteriosclerotic pseudoparkinsonism*, has been introduced later in the parlance of neurology. In an eminently readable review in 1995 in the *British Medical Journal*, Niall Quinn of Queen Square, London, wrote that elderly and usually hypertensive patients are often afflicted with a disorder which resembles PD, but certain red flags help to distinguish it from the classical disorder (Quinn, 1995). These patients are generally hypertensive and while walking, the upper half of the body does not seem to follow that of the lower half, as if it is being held back. This has been likened to the upper half of a Dalmatian dog superimposed on the feet of a hippopotamus, and the gait has been named by Quinn as *Dalmatamus gait*. The gait is short and is often known as *marché a petit pas*, or short march, and is often ataxic and broad based, as opposed to the unmistakable shuffling gait of idiopathic PD. Gait ignition failure and start hesitancy may be seen, but the upper part of the body is usually remarkably free from Parkinsonian features, and thus hypophonia, hypomimia, rigidity, bradykinesia, and loss of arm swing are not seen. This condition is, therefore, often known as *Lower Body Parkinsonism*.

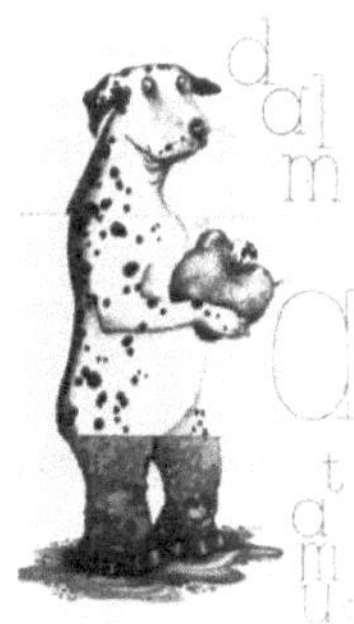

Dalmatamus

Source: www.bmj.com

One of the most important contributions to the motor aspects of PD in the last century is the work of Margaret Hoehn and Melvin Yahr for a period of 15 years from 1949 to 1964 from the Columbia University, and they published their observations in 1967 in a seminal paper in the journal *Neurology* (Hoehn & Yahr, 1967). In a robust study on 56 patients, they classified the degree of disability into five stages from stage I to stage V, starting from unilateral involvement to confinement in chair or bed. In a nutshell, they observed that two-thirds of the patients had their onset of illness between 50 and 69 years of age without any sex predilection, 80% of the patients were severely disabled within 10–14 years of illness, tremor was the most frequent symptom, mortality was three times higher when compared with age and sex matched population, tremor dominant PD had lesser risk of mortality compared to those with rigidity or bradykinesia, there was no improvement in prolongation of life with newer modalities of treatment, and bronchopneumonia and urinary tract infection were the usual modes of termination.

One of the landmarks in the assessment of motor problems in PD in the 20th century has been the "*pull test*" in order to assess postural instability. Hunt et al. wrote that this test was first proposed by Moritz Romberg from Germany in 1853, and thereafter, Charcot attempted at a quantitative measurement by pulling the clothes of the patients and observing their response in 1880. Hoehn and Yahr pushed at the sternum in the 1960s, but Stanley Fahn from Columbia described the test the way it is done today in the 1980s (Hunt & Sethi, 2006).

One of the spectacular advances in the assessment of the motor symptoms in the 20th century has been the development of the Unified Parkinson's Disease Rating Scale (UPDRS). It owes its genesis primarily to Stanley Fahn, from Columbia University and a giant in the field of movement disorders in contemporary world, who felt the need of a unified rating scale after surveying various scales which lacked in uniformity. The issue was broached in a meeting in Bermuda in 1984, and after hours of animated discussion, Fahn videotaped patients, wrote to the members, asked them to score, and came to a compromise and published his views in the proceedings in a subsequent meeting sponsored by the Sandoz Pharmaceuticals at Hawaii in 1987. Finally, after lots of trials and tribulations, the paper was published in 1992 (Fahn, Marsden, Goldstein, & Calne, 1987). The scale was used for the longitudinal assessment of the progress of motor and other problems thereafter, and it embraced within its ambit, six subsets like: (1) evaluation of mentation, behavior, and mood; (2) self-evaluation of the activities of daily living, including speech, swallowing, handwriting, dressing, hygiene, fall, salivation, turning in bed, walking, and cutting food; (3) motor evaluation; (4) complications of therapy; (5) Hoehn and Yahr staging of severity; and (6) Schwab and England Activity of Daily Living scale. In 2003, The Movement Disorder Task Force for Rating Scales for Parkinson's Disease felt the need to prepare a revised and updated version of the scale after scrupulously scrutinizing some of its inadequacies and identifying some flaws like absence of nonmotor symptoms, inadequate instructions for raters, metric limitations, and some ambiguities in the instructions (Movement Disorder Society Task Force on Rating Scales for Parkinson's Disease, 2003), and based on their recommendations, a new scale MDS-UPDRS was devised in 2007 (Goetz et al., 2007). The scales are now named (1) nonmotor experiences of daily living; (2) motor experiences with daily living; (3) motor examination; (4) motor complications and each one is assigned numbers like 0 or normal, 1 or slight, 2 or mild, 3 or moderate, and 4 or severe.

2. INTRODUCTION OF LEVODOPA AND NEW MOTOR FEATURES

Following the hypothesis advanced by Arvid Carlsson (1923–) from Sweden, the Nobel Laureate in 2000, that deficiency of dopamine in the substantia nigra is the root cause of PD (Carlsson, Lindqvist, Magnusson, & Waldeck, 1958), Herbert Ehringer (1932–) and Oleh Hornykiewicz (1926–) from Austria discovered the striatal dopamine loss in the human brain (Goetz, 2011). W. Birkmayer received a steady supply of levodopa synthesized in the laboratory of Hornykiewicz and used the intravenous preparation for the first time in 1961 with good result (Goetz, 2011). The use of oral levodopa was initiated by André Barbeau (1931–86) from Canada (Barbeau, 1969), George Cotzias (1918–77) from the United States (Cotzias, Papavasiliou, & Gellene, 1969), and Melvin Yahr, also from the United States independently in 1969 (Yahr et al., 1969), and in a few years the long-term motor complications were reported by C. David Marsden (1938–98) and David Parks from King's College, Hospital, London (Marsden & Parkes, 1977). It was estimated that around 10% of patients develop motor fluctuations like on–off phenomenon and dyskinesias, with the initiation of levodopa therapy, and in clinic-based studies, it was observed that around 50% of patients suffer after 5 years of treatment (Marsden, 1994; Sweet & McDowell, 1975). However, there is some controversy whether these are the results of long-term therapy with levodopa or part of the disease process itself, and whether lowering the dose of levodopa reduces complications (Barbeau, 1976; Cederbaum, Gandy, & McDowell, 1991; Fahn & Bressman, 1984; Lees & Stern, 1983; Markham & Diamond, 1986; Melamed, 1986; Poewe, Lees, & Stern, 1986; Weiner, 1999). Studies have shown higher incidence of levodopa-induced complications in younger patients, longer duration of therapy, higher dose, and greater severity of the disease (Claveria, Calne, & Allen, 1973; Hardie, Lees, & Stern, 1984; Kostic, Przedborski, Flaster, & Sternic, 1991; Lesser et al., 1979; Miyawaki et al., 1997; Schrag & Quinn, 2000). The risk is lesser with other anti-Parkinsonian agents (Rascol et al., 2000; Rinne, 1989).

2.1 The Conundrum of Atypical Parkinsonism: A Diagnostic Riddle

In a landmark paper, published in *Archives in Neurology* in 1963, entitled, "*Progressive supranuclear palsy. A heterogeneous degeneration involving the brain, basal ganglia and cerebellum with vertical gaze and pseudobulbar palsy, nuchal dystonia and dementia,*" John Steele, J. Clifford Richardson, and Jerzy Olszewski described a classic syndrome after studying eight cases that resemble idiopathic PD in many ways but perhaps differ more (Steele et al., 1964). The name was assigned by J.C. Richardson, a pathologist, while Steele was a clinician, and Olszewski performed the autopsy. However, it is on record that William Campbell Posey and William Spiller described a similar condition in 1904 and 1905, respectively, and these are often cited as the earliest description of the disease (Siderowf, Galetta, Hurtig, & Liu, 1998). Subsequent autopsy by Spiller himself demonstrated a tumor in the right cerebral peduncle and the periaqueductal area (Siderowf et al., 1998). Early fall, vertical gaze palsy, nuchal extension, reptilian stare, growling dysarthria, pseudobulbar palsy, applause sign, and the procerus and omega sign on the forehead are the distinguishing features.

In the year 1900, Joseph Jules Dejerine (1849–1917) and his pupil, André Thomas (1867–1963) from Salpêtrière, Paris, described a few cases of Parkinsonism and cerebellar ataxia which, on autopsy, showed neuronal loss in the ventral pons, inferior olive, and cerebral cortex, and they named the condition, *olivopontocerebellar atrophy* or OPCA (Dejerine & Thomas, 1900). In 1960, Raymond Delacy Adams (1911–2008) from the United States described a condition which he named striatonigral degeneration or SND which had features like onset after 40 years, duration of the disease for less than 10 years, poor response to levodopa, autonomic failure, absence of dementia, apraxia, and supranuclear ophthalmoplegia (Aotsuka & Paulson, 1993). Milton Shy and Glenn Drager from the United States described a condition in *Archives of Neurology* in 1960, where profound autonomic failure in the form of postural hypotension, along with urinary incontinence, impotence, and Parkinsonian features, was the presenting features (Shy & Drager, 1960). Rummaging through all available literature and studying the clinical profile, J.G. Graham and D.R. Oppenheimer from Radcliffe Infirmary, Oxford, lumped the disparate conditions under the ambit of the term, *multiple system atrophy* or MSA for this group of diseases (Graham & Oppenheimer, 1969). In more recent times, MSA is subclassified into MSA A, where autonomic features are predominant; MSA C, where the brunt falls on the cerebellum or its connections; and MSA P, where the Parkinsonism is the dominant presentation. Apart from Parkinsonian features, some of the distinctive signs of the condition are prominent antecollis or dropped head phenomenon, Pisa syndrome, camptocormia, stimulus-sensitive cortical myoclonus, chorea, facial or oromandibular dystonia, or chorea with levodopa therapy, as opposed to axial dystonia in idiopathic PD, focal reflex myoclonus induced by a pinprick laryngeal inspiratory stridor due to paradoxical movement of the vocal chords or Gerhardt's syndrome. The cold hand or the cold feet sign, manifested by dusky and violaceous look of the hands or feet, is a characteristic feature.

One last comment that deserves mentioning is the identification of the gene in a cohort of patients of PD by Polymeropoulos et al., in 1996. Though William Gowers from the United Kingdom first recognized the familial nature of the disease (Gowers, 1893), finding the specific genetic locus for the first time took a long time and these investigators after studying genomic scan in a large number of kindreds of Italian decent found the locus at 4q21–q23 (Polymeropoulos et al., 1996). In a later work, Polymeropoulos alluded to the gene, alpha-synuclein, as a result of missense mutation in the gene. Alpha-synuclein is a presynaptic protein of unknown function. The author conceived that the mutation in PD results in self-aggregation or altered degradation of the protein, which leads to the accumulation of intracytoplasmic inclusion bodies and cell death (Polymeropoulos, 1998).

3. CONCLUDING REMARKS

James Parkinson's description of the disease did not bring him much fame and honor during his lifetime and he left the world unwept and unsung. However, it caught the imagination of future physicians, particularly in England and France, and their pertinacious inquiry into the clinical details of the motor aspects led to the unraveling of many new aspects of the disease. Much glitter and sheen have illumined the body of literature of this disease in the last 200 years, and atypical Parkinsonism has emerged as a distinct clinical entity in the last 50 years or so. It is likely that many more new insights will enrich our knowledge and some of the established and treasured facts of today will be thrown into the shopworn shibboleths of the future. However, everything gainsaid, the initial description by James Parkinson remains the benchmark, the model of acute clinical acumen, and there lies the indisputable and indelible legacy of James Parkinson, the "*Villager's Friend and Physician*" in the early 19th century.

REFERENCES

Aotsuka, A., & Paulson, G. W. (1993). Striatonigral degeneration. In M. B. Stern & W. C. Koller (Eds.), *Parkinsonian syndromes* (pp. 33–42). New York: Marcel Dekker.

Barbeau, A. (1969). L-Dopa therapy in Parkinson's disease. *Canadian Medical Association Journal, 101*, 59–68.

Barbeau, A. (1976). Six years of high-level levodopa therapy in severely akinetic parkinsonian patients. *Archives of Neurology*, *33*, 333–338.
Bereczki, D. (2010). The description of all four cardinal signs of Parkinson's disease in a Hungarian medical text published in 1690. *Parkinsonism & Related Disorders*, *16*, 290–293.
Bhattacharyya, K. B. (2011). *Eminent neuroscientists: Their lives & works* (1st ed.). Kolkata: Academic Publishers.
Calne, D. B., Dubini, A., & Stern, G. (1989). Did Leonardo describe Parkinson's disease? *The New England Journal of Medicine*, *320*, 594.
Carlsson, A., Lindqvist, M., Magnusson, T., & Waldeck, B. (1958). On the presence of 3-hydroxytyramine in brain. *Science*, *127*, 471.
Cedarbaum, J. M., & Gancher, S. T. (Eds.), (1992). *Neurologic clinics: Parkinson's disease*: *Vol. 10* (p. 301). Philadelphia, USA: WB Saunders Company.
Cederbaum, J. M., Gandy, S. E., & McDowell, F. H. (1991). 'Early initiation' of levodopa treatment does not promote the development of motor response fluctuations, dyskinesias, or dementia in Parkinson's disease. *Neurology*, *41*, 622–629.
Charcot, J. M. (1880). *Lecons sure les maladies du système nerveux faites a la Salpétrière*. (p.186). Paris: Bourneville, Delahaye et LeCrosnier.
Claveria, L. E., Calne, D. B., & Allen, J. G. (1973). On-off phenomenon related to high plasma levodopa. *British Medical Journal*, *2*, 641–643.
Cooke, J. (1820). *A treatise on nervous disease*, *Vol. 207*. London: Longman.
Cotzias, G. C., Papavasiliou, P. S., & Gellene, R. (1969). Modifications of parkinsonism: Chronic treatment with L-dopa. *The New England Journal of Medicine*, *280*, 337–345.
Critchley, M. (1929). Arteriosclerotic parkinsonism. *Brain*, *52*, 23–83.
Currier, R. D. (1996). Did John Hunter give James Parkinson an idea? *Archives of Neurology*, *53*, 377–379.
Dejerine, J., & Thomas, A. (1900). L'atrophie olivo-ponto-cérébelleuse. *Nouvre Iconographie Salpetriere*, *330*, 370.
Dimsdale, H. (1946). Changes in the Parkinsonian syndrome in the twentieth century. *The Quarterly Journal of Medicine*, *59*, 155–170.
Elliotson, J. (1830). Clinical lecture on paralysis agitans. *The Lancet*, *8*, 119–123.
Fahn, S., & Bressman, S. B. (1984). Should levodopa therapy for Parkinsonism be started early or late? Evidence against early treatment. *The Canadian Journal of Neurological Sciences*, *11*, 200–205.
Fahn, S., Marsden, C. D., Goldstein, M., & Calne, D. (Eds.), (1987). *Recent developments in Parkinson's disease*: *Vol. II*. Florham Park, NJ: McMillan Health Care Information.
Goetz, C. G. (2011). The history of Parkinson's disease: Early clinical descriptions and neurological therapies. *Cold Spring Harbor Perspectives in Medicine*, *1*, 1–21.
Goetz, C. G., Fahn, S., Martinez-Martin, P., Poewe, W., Sampaio, C., Stebbins, G. T., et al. (2007). Movement disorder society-sponsored revision of the unified Parkinson's disease rating scale (MDS-UPDRS): Process, format, and clinimetric testing plan. *Movement Disorders*, *22*, 41–47.
Gowers, W. R. (1893). *A manual of diseases of the nervous system* (1st ed.). Philadelphia: Blackstone.
Gowry, T. C. (1831). Case of paralysis agitans intermittens. *The Lancet*, *2*, 651.
Graham, J. G., & Oppenheimer, D. R. (1969). Orthostatic hypotension and nicotinic sensitivity in a case of multiple system atrophy. *Journal of Neurology, Neurosurgery & Psychiatry*, *32*, 28–34.
Haan, J. (2013). Protagonists with Parkinson's disease. In J. Bogousslavsky & S. Dieguez (Eds.), *Frontiers of neurology and neuroscience*: *Vol. 31*. *Literary medicine: Brain disease and doctors in novels, theater, and film* (pp. 178–187). Basel: Karger.

Haggard, P., & Rodgers, S. (2000). The movement disorder of Nicolas Poussin. *Movement Disorders, 15*, 328–334.

Hall, M. (1841). *On the diseases and derangements of the nervous system* (pp. 320–321). London: H. Baillière.

Hardie, R. J., Lees, A. J., & Stern, G. M. (1984). *On-off fluctuations in Parkinson's disease. Brain, 107*, 487–506.

Hoehn, M., & Yahr, M. (1967). Parkinsonism: Onset, progression, and mortality. *Neurology, 17*, 427–442.

Horowski, R., Horowski, L., Vogel, S., Poewe, W., & Kielhorn, F. W. (1995). An essay on Wilhelm von Humboldt and the shaking palsy: First comprehensive description of Parkinson's disease by a patient. *Neurology, 45*, 565–568.

Hunt, A. L., & Sethi, K. D. (2006). The pull test: A history. *Movement Disorders, 21*, 894–899.

Jefferson, M. (1973). James Parkinson 1755–1824. *British Medical Journal, 2*, 601–603.

Koehler, P. J., & Keyser, A. (1997). Tremor in Latin texts of Dutch physicians: 16th–18th centuries. *Movement Disorders, 12*, 798–806.

Kostic, V., Przedborski, S., Flaster, E., & Sternic, N. (1991). Early development of levodopa-induced dyskinesias and response fluctuations in young-onset Parkinson's disease. *Neurology, 41*, 202–205.

Lakke, J. P. (1996). Wilhelm von Humboldt and James Parkinson. An appraisal of observation and creativity. *Parkinsonism & Related Disorders, 2*, 225–229.

Larner, A. J. (2002a). Did Charles Dickens describe progressive supranuclear palsy in 1857? *Movement Disorders, 17*, 832–833.

Larner, A. J. (2002b). Charles Dickens qua neurologist. *Advances in Clinical Neuroscience & Rehabilitation, 2*, 22.

Larner, A. J. (2014a). History of neurology: Parkinson's disease before James Parkinson. In *Vol. 13. 24th annual meeting of the European Charcot foundation.* (pp. 24–25).

Larner, A. J. (2014b). Parkinson's disease before James Parkinson. *Advances in Clinical Neuroscience & Rehabilitation, 13*, 24–25.

Lees, A. J. (2007). Unresolved issues relating to the shaking palsy on the celebration of James Parkinson's 250th birthday. *Movement Disorders, 22*(Suppl. 17), S327–S334.

Lees, A. J., & Stern, G. M. (1983). Sustained low-dose levodopa therapy in Parkinson's disease: A 3-year follow-up. *Advances in Neurology, 37*, 9–15.

Lesser, R. P., Fahn, S., Snider, S. R., Cote, L. J., Isgreen, W. P., & Barrett, R. E. (1979). Analysis of the clinical problems in Parkinsonism and the complications of long-term levodopa therapy. *Neurology, 29*, 1253–1260.

Louis, E. D. (1997). The shaking palsy, the first forty-five years: A journey through the British literature. *Movement Disorders, 12*, 1068–1072.

Manyam, B. (1990). Paralysis agitans and levodopa in "Ayurveda": Ancient Indian medical treatise. *Movement Disorders, 5*, 47–48.

Markham, C. H., & Diamond, S. G. (1986). Long-term follow up of early dopa treatment in Parkinson's disease. *Annals of Neurology, 19*, 365–372.

Marsden, C. D. (1994). Problems with long-term levodopa therapy for Parkinson's disease. *Clinical Neuropharmacology, 17*(Suppl. 2), S32–S44.

Marsden, C. D., & Parkes, J. D. (1977). Success and problems of long-term therapy in Parkinson's disease. *The Lancet, 12*, 345–349.

Melamed, E. (1986). Initiation of levodopa therapy in parkinsonian patients should be delayed until advanced stages of the disease. *Archives of Neurology, 43*, 402–405.

Miyawaki, E., Lyons, K., Pahwa, R., Tröster, A. I., Hubble, J., Smith, D., et al. (1997). Motor complications of chronic levodopa therapy. *Clinical Neuropharmacology, 20*, 523–530.

Movement Disorder Society Task Force on Rating Scales for Parkinson's Disease. (2003). The unified Parkinson's disease rating scale (UPDRS): Status and recommendations. *Movement Disorders, 18*, 738–750.

Paget, G. E. (1855). Case of involuntary tendency to fall precipitately forwards: With remarks. *The Medical Times and Gazette, 10*, 178–180.

Palfreman, J. (2015). *Brain storms: The race to unlock the mysteries of Parkinson's disease*. USA: Farrar, Strauss, Giroux LLC.

Parkinson, J. (1817). *An essay on the shaking palsy*. London: Sherwood, Neely & Jones.

Parkinson, J. W. K. (Ed.), (1833). *Parkinson J. Hunterian reminiscences*. London, England: Sherwood, Gilbert & Piper.

Pearce, J. M. S. (1989). Aspects of the history of Parkinson's disease. *Journal of Neurology, Neurosurgery & Psychiatry, 52*(Suppl.), 6–10.

Poewe, W. H., Lees, A. J., & Stern, G. M. (1986). Low-dose L-dopa therapy in Parkinson's disease. *Neurology, 36*, 1528–1536.

Polymeropoulos, M. H. (1998). Autosomal dominant Parkinson's disease and alpha-synuclein. *Annals of Neurology, 44*(Suppl. 1), S63–S64.

Polymeropoulos, M. H., Higgins, J. J., Golbe, L. I., Johnson, W. G., Lorio, G. D., Sanges, G., et al. (1996). Mapping of a gene for Parkinson's disease to chromosome 4q21–q23. *Science, 274*, 1197–1198.

Quinn, N. (1995). Parkinsonism: Recognition and differential diagnosis. *British Medical Journal, 310*, 447–452.

Rana, A. Q. (2016). *Natural therapies for Parkinson's disease*. USA: FriesenPress Inc.

Rascol, O., Brooks, D. J., Korczyn, A. D., De Deyn, P. P., Clarke, C. E., & Lang, A. E. (2000). A five-year study of the incidence of dyskinesia in patients with early Parkinson's disease who were treated with ropinirole or levodopa. *The New England Journal of Medicine, 18*, 1484–1491.

Reynolds, J. R. (1865). *The diagnosis of diseases of the brain, spinal cord, nerves and their appendages*. (pp.163–164). London: John Churchill.

Rinne, U. K. (1989). Early dopamine agonist therapy in Parkinson's disease. *Movement Disorders, 4*, S86–S94.

Sanders, W. R. (1865). Case of an unusual form of nervous disease, dystaxia or pseudo-paralysis agitans, with remarks. *Edinburgh Medical Journal, 10*, 987–997.

Schrag, A., & Quinn, N. (2000). Dyskinesias and motor fluctuation in Parkinson's disease. A community-based study. *Brain, 123*, 2297–2305.

Scott Simon, R. W. (2015). The wrong James Parkinson. *Practical Neurology, 1*, 1136.

Shy, G. M., & Drager, G. A. (1960). A neurological syndrome associated with orthostatic hypotension: A clinic-pathological study. *Archives of Neurology, 2*, 511–527.

Siderowf, A. D., Galetta, S. L., Hurtig, H. I., & Liu, G. T. (1998). Posey and Spiller and progressive supranuclear palsy: An incorrect attribution. *Movement Disorders, 13*, 170–174.

Steele, J. C., Richardson, J. C., & Olszewski, J. (1964). Progressive supranuclear palsy: A heterogeneous degeneration involving brain stem, basal ganglia and cerebellum with vertical gaze and pseudobulbar palsy, nuchal dystonia and dementia. *Archives of Neurology, 10*, 333–359.

Stern, G. (1989). Did Parkinsonism occur before 1817? *Journal of Neurology, Neurosurgery & Psychiatry, 52*(Suppl.), 11–12.

Sweet, R. D., & McDowell, F. H. (1975). Five years' treatment of Parkinson's disease with levodopa. Therapeutic results and survival of 100 patients. *Annals of Internal Medicine, 83*, 456–463.

Thorpe-Gardner, C. (2010). James Parkinson (1755–1824). *Journal of Neurology, 257*, 492–493.

Vaidya, A. B., Rajgopalan, T. S., Mankodi, N. A., et al. (1978). Treatment of Parkinson's disease with the cowhage plant—Mucuna pruriens (Bak). *Neurology India, 36*, 171–176.

Van der Brugger, H., & Widdershaven, G. (2004). Being a Parkinson's patient: Immobile and unpredictably whimsical. Literature and existential analysis. *Medicine, Health Care, and Philosophy*, 7, 289–301.

Watson, T. (1872). In *Lectures on the principles and practice of physic delivered at King's College: Vol. 1* (5th ed., pp. 629–631). London: Henry C Lea.

Weiner, W. J. (1999). The initial treatment of Parkinson's disease should begin with levodopa. *Movement Disorders*, *14*, 716–724.

Yahr, M. D., Duvoisin, R. C., Myma, J., Schear, M., Barrett, R. E., & Hoehn, M. M. (1969). Treatment of parkinsonism with levodopa. *Archives of Neurology*, *21*, 343–354.

CHAPTER TWO

The Motor Syndrome of Parkinson's Disease

Roberto Erro*,†,1, Maria Stamelou‡,§,¶
*Center for Neurodegenerative Diseases (CEMAND), University of Salerno, Fisciano, Italy
†Institute of Neurology, UCL, London, United Kingdom
‡University of Athens Medical School, Hospital Attikon, Athens, Greece
§HYGEIA Hospital, Athens, Greece
¶Philipps University, Marburg, Germany
[1]Corresponding author: e-mail address: erro.roberto@gmail.com

Contents

Abstract

The clinical diagnosis of Parkinson's disease (PD) is centered on a specific motor syndrome that is characterized by the presence of bradykinesia, plus rest tremor, muscle rigidity, or both. Recently, novel criteria for diagnosing PD have been released that rehearse the motor syndrome as the core feature of PD. Beyond these three main symptoms, other motor features might be present in PD including gait difficulties and postural instability. Moreover, patients with PD usually develop motor complications 5–10 years into their disease. These motor complications are the strongest predictor of PD pathology and are in fact used clinically to support the diagnosis.

Ancillary investigations are usually of little utility and to perform only in selected cases, which remarks the importance of the clinical examination for making the diagnosis of PD or suspect other condition that can be masquerading it.

International Review of Neurobiology, Volume 132
ISSN 0074-7742
http://dx.doi.org/10.1016/bs.irn.2017.01.004

1. INTRODUCTION

Parkinson's disease (PD) is a progressive, neurodegenerative movement disorder, which in its most classical manifestation is characterized by motor symptoms (Kalia & Lang, 2015). Although it is now widely accepted that PD pathology is widespread (Braak & Braak, 2000) and therefore gives rise to a number of nonmotor symptoms (Zis, Erro, Walton, Sauerbier, & Chaudhuri, 2015), the clinical diagnosis of PD has been always centered on a specific motor syndrome that features the presence of two or more signs/symptoms among bradykinesia, rest tremor, muscle rigidity, and postural instability. While the definitive diagnosis of PD relies on postmortem confirmation of cell loss in the substantia nigra along with the presence of Lewy body (Kalia & Lang, 2015), the clinical diagnosis is in fact based on the presence of the aforementioned clinical features. Several attempts have been therefore made to define clinical diagnostic criteria, e.g., by the UK Parkinson's Disease Society Brain Bank (Hughes, Daniel, Kilford, & Lees, 1992) or the National Institute of Neurological Disorders and Stroke (Gelb, Oliver, & Gilman, 1999). More recently, novel diagnostic criteria have been proposed by the International PD and Movement Disorder Society (MDS-PD criteria) (Postuma, Berg, Stern, et al., 2015). This proposal rehearses the motor syndrome as the core feature of PD and suggests a two-step process for diagnosing PD. First, parkinsonism is established on the presence of bradykinesia in combination with rest tremor, rigidity, or both. Then, the criteria define through a number of supportive features or red flags whether this parkinsonism is in fact attributable to PD (Table 1) (Postuma et al., 2015). For clinical practice, the implementation of these criteria appears useful, but it has to be kept in mind that even if the diagnosis is made by movement disorder experts, the diagnostic certainty ranges between 75% and 90% when compared with the results of the autopsy (Dickson, Braak, Duda, et al., 2009; Hughes, Daniel, & Lees, 2001). While looking for biomarkers that might increase diagnostic certainty, the initial diagnosis of PD remains a clinical one and is purely based on medical history and clinical examination.

Thus, the first step is to define whether or not a parkinsonian syndrome is present. As mentioned earlier, parkinsonism is defined as bradykinesia, in combination with rest tremor, rigidity, or both. These features have to be

Table 1 Summary of the Motor Features That Are Used for the Diagnosis of PD (or Against It)

Definition of Parkinsonism
Presence of bradykinesia plus either rest tremor or rigidity
Supportive features
Clear and dramatic benefit from L-dopa therapy on motor symptoms
Unequivocal and marked on/off fluctuations that must include wearing-off
L-Dopa-induced dyskinesias
Rest tremor of a limb, documented on clinical examination (in past or on current examination)[a]
Absolute exclusion criteria
Absence of response to L-dopa at high doses
Absence of spread of motor symptoms (that are confined for more than 3 years in the lower limbs)
Red flags
Rapid progression of gait impairment
A complete absence of progression of motor symptoms or signs over 5 or more years
Recurrent (>1/year) falls because of impaired balance within 3 years of onset
Bilateral symmetric parkinsonism (no side predominance is observed on objective examination)

[a]Rest tremor is also included among the supported features since the criterion of dramatic response to L-dopa therapy might be hard to meet in tremor-dominant patients and also because it is less common in alternate conditions.
Modified from Postuma, R. B., Berg, D., Stern, M., et al. (2015). MDS clinical diagnostic criteria for Parkinson's disease. *Movement Disorders, 30*, 1591–601.

clearly demonstrable and should not be attributable to confounding factors. There is evidence in fact that a proportion of elderly have mild parkinsonian signs in the absence of PD (Erro, Schneider, Stamelou, Quinn, & Bhatia, 2016): examiner judgment should be hence used to decide whether examination findings are entirely attributable to confounding features. In this regard, the presence of *true* bradykinesia, as defined later, is most useful to discriminate between parkinsonism and other causes that can produce movement slowness (e.g., weakness, psychomotor slowness, etc.).

2. MOTOR SYMPTOMS OF PD

The initial presentation of PD may vary, with tremor being the most common motor symptom in patients, in whom the diagnosis of PD has been verified postmortem (Hughes, Daniel, Blankson, & Lees, 1993). A recent community-based study in 358 patients identified tremor as the initially leading symptom in approximately half of the patients. Up to 44% showed an akinetic-rigid phenotype, while only 7% presented initially with gait disturbances (Wickremaratchi, Knipe, Sastry, et al., 2011). Classically, the motor symptoms of PD develop unilaterally in keeping with the asymmetric striatonigral denervation detectable in vivo with DaTscan SPECT imaging (Kalia & Lang, 2015). However, it should be noted that a proportion of PD patients might present with a symmetric akinetic-rigid syndrome. Asymmetry in symptoms/sign distribution is generally lost over time and, in fact, it is regarded as a red flag for PD when persistent on the long term (Postuma et al., 2015).

2.1 Bradykinesia

Bradykinesia is defined as the slowness of movement and the progressive reduction of either frequency or amplitude of repetitive movements (Postuma et al., 2015). This renders the presence of the *decrement* component mandatory and makes the definition of bradykinesia different from its etymological meaning. Bradykinesia literally describes only slowness in movements. Moreover, in clinical practice, it is erroneously often used interchangeably with either hypokinesia (small amplitude movements) or akinesia (absence or poverty of expected spontaneous voluntary movement). It has to be made clear that, while a number of patients may have all of these three features, the term *bradykinesia* (and consequently the diagnosis of PD) should be only applied if decrement is present. The MDS-PD criteria further state that limb bradykinesia must be documented to establish a diagnosis of PD, although it can be present also in the face, voice, and axial/gait domains. Beyond specifically testing for bradykinesia in the limbs, signs of hypokinesia and/or akinesia are usually easily recognized as the clinician initially interviews and examines the patient: facial masking with reduced blinking, soft speech, lack of gesturing while talking, and hesitancy when the patient rises from the chair are all clues for suspecting a parkinsonian syndrome. Moreover, micrographia can be observed on writing.

2.2 Tremor

The characteristic parkinsonian rest tremor is a low-frequency (4–6 Hz) tremor that manifests in fully resting limb and dampens with movement initiation. Phenomenologically, parkinsonian rest tremor has been also defined as pill-rolling tremor since the fingers and wrist move in a manner reminiscent of a rhythmic voluntary manipulation of small objects or pills in the hand. Classically, there is no tremor on action or on posture. However, one type of "postural" tremor (that appears to be specific of PD) is characterized by tremor that re-emerges after a variable delay while maintaining posture, hence defined "re-emergent tremor" (Jankovic, Schwartz, & Ondo, 1999). Electrophysiological studies have demonstrated that the re-emergent tremor of PD shares pathophysiological mechanisms with the more typical rest tremor rather than being a true postural tremor (Jankovic et al., 1999).

As the disease progresses, other tremor forms, such as action tremor and postural tremor, may also occur (Jankovic et al., 1999). However, there is a general tendency in the course of the disease for a reduction of tremor intensity that gives way to the bradykinetic symptoms. Worth of note, about 25% of PD patients do not develop tremor during the entire course of the disease (Hughes et al., 1993).

2.3 Rigidity

Rigidity refers to "lead-pipe" resistance, that is, velocity-independent resistance (hence being different from spasticity) to passive movement not solely reflecting failure to relax (hence being distinct from paratonia). Many PD patients complain about unilateral back and/or shoulder pain as a consequence of the asymmetric muscular rigidity, which may result in the consultation of an orthopedic specialist before final referral to a neurologist (Madden & Hall, 2010). On examination, there might be the presence of the "cogwheel phenomenon." While this has been formerly interpreted as a distinctive feature of parkinsonian rigidity, it reflects the combination of rigidity and tremor incidentally felt while examining tone (Deuschl, Bain, & Brin, 1998). Thus, isolated "cogwheeling" without "lead-pipe" rigidity does not fulfill minimum requirements for rigidity (Postuma et al., 2015).

2.4 Gait and Axial Disturbances

Although the definition of a parkinsonian syndrome according to current criteria relies on the presence of the three symptoms mentioned earlier,

PD patients might manifest with additional motor symptoms including gait and axial disturbances (Kalia & Lang, 2015). These might be present in the very early stage of the disease but become usually more prominent at a later stage (Coelho & Ferreira, 2012).

Patients with PD commonly have gait hesitancy with the first step and, if severe, it might give the appearance of gait freezing. In the early stage, however, reduced arm swing, shortened stride, and stooped posture during walking are more common (Coelho & Ferreira, 2012; Kalia & Lang, 2015). The short steps, in which the heel lands less than one foot length ahead of the toes of the other foot, observed in the parkinsonian gait account for the definition of "shuffling gait." During walking, patients might also have anteropulsion, meaning that the center of gravity is ahead of the feet, hence causing forward acceleration, the so-called festination, which is characterized by short but hasty steps attempting to compensate for displaced center of gravity.

The stooped posture of PD patients might worsen over time and results in camptocormia that is currently defined by a bending angle more than 45 degrees (Doherty, van de Warrenburg, Peralta, et al., 2011). Other postural abnormalities such as lateral flexion of the trunk (the so-called Pisa syndrome) can occur, usually at a later stage (Tinazzi, Fasano, Geroin, et al., 2015). As the disease progresses, postural instability affects the majority of PD patients and can lead to falls (Coelho & Ferreira, 2012). It can be appreciated with the pull test. Normal subjects respond to a quick pull backward on their shoulders, simply arching the trunk or making a step backward. PD patients have the tendency to retropulsion or to fall in the examiner's arm. Pronounced postural instability at the initial presentation is an indicator for alternative diagnoses (Stamelou & Hoeglinger, 2013) and therefore has to be carefully set into context with other motor features.

2.5 Motor Complications of PD

The classic motor syndrome of PD is exquisitely responsive to L-dopa treatment in the early stage. Such a dramatic and sustained L-dopa response is considered a supportive feature for PD diagnosis (Postuma et al., 2015). However, as the disease progresses, a number of motor complications arise (Kalia & Lang, 2015). These include the wearing-off phenomenon in which motor symptoms start to return or worsen before the next dose of L-dopa is due, delayed-on in which there is a delay in the onset of benefit of a L-dopa dose, unpredictable off periods, and off-dystonia. The aforementioned features reflect a hypodopaminergic state, whereas patients can also manifest with hyperkinesias, namely L-dopa-induced dyskinesias that can occur either concomitant to the plasmatic L-dopa peak (peak dyskinesias) or when the drug concentration rises or falls (diphasic dyskinesias). It is beyond the aims of this chapter to provide details about the motor complications of PD and their management, but it has to be noted here that these are the strongest indicators of Lewy body pathology (Selikhova, Kempster, Revesz, et al., 2013) and are in fact considered supportive features for the clinical diagnosis of PD (Table 1) (Postuma et al., 2015). Thus, if a treated patient does not develop motor complication 5–10 years into the disease, it is recommended to revise the diagnosis and consider alternative conditions.

3. SUMMARY

The clinical diagnosis of PD is mostly based on its motor syndrome. When the latter has been established, other conditions that can be masquerading PD need to be excluded based on the presence of features atypical for PD or the absence of other features that are instead typical for PD such as motor fluctuations and L-dopa-induced dyskinesias (Table 1). Ancillary investigations including olfactory testing, MRI, sympathetic cardiac SPECT, and DaTscan SPECT imaging are usually of little utility and to perform only in selected cases, which remarks the importance of the clinical examination for making the diagnosis of PD.

REFERENCES

Braak, H., & Braak, E. (2000). Pathoanatomy of Parkinson's disease. *Journal of Neurology, 247*(Suppl. 2), II3–II10.

Coelho, M., & Ferreira, J. J. (2012). Late-stage Parkinson disease. *Nature Reviews. Neurology, 8*, 435–442.

Deuschl, G., Bain, P., & Brin, M. (1998). Consensus statement of the Movement Disorder Society on Tremor. Ad Hoc Scientific Committee. *Movement Disorders, 13*(Suppl. 3), 2–23.

Dickson, D. W., Braak, H., Duda, J. E., et al. (2009). Neuropathological assessment of Parkinson's disease: Refining the diagnostic criteria. *The Lancet Neurology, 8*, 1150–1157.

Doherty, K. M., van de Warrenburg, B. P., Peralta, M. C., et al. (2011). Postural deformities in Parkinson's disease. *The Lancet Neurology, 10*, 538–549.

Erro, R., Schneider, S. A., Stamelou, M., Quinn, N. P., & Bhatia, K. P. (2016). What do patients with scans without evidence of dopaminergic deficit (SWEDD) have? New evidence and continuing controversies. *Journal of Neurology, Neurosurgery, and Psychiatry, 87*, 319–323.

Gelb, D. J., Oliver, E., & Gilman, S. (1999). Diagnostic criteria for Parkinson disease. *Archives of Neurology, 56*, 33–39.

Hughes, A. J., Daniel, S. E., Blankson, S., & Lees, A. J. (1993). A clinicopathologic study of 100 cases of Parkinson's disease. *Archives of Neurology, 50*, 140–148.
Hughes, A. J., Daniel, S. E., Kilford, L., & Lees, A. J. (1992). Accuracy of clinical diagnosis of idiopathic Parkinson's disease: A clinico-pathological study of 100 cases. *Journal of Neurology, Neurosurgery, and Psychiatry, 55*, 181–184.
Hughes, A. J., Daniel, S. E., & Lees, A. J. (2001). Improved accuracy of clinical diagnosis of Lewy body Parkinson's disease. *Neurology, 57*, 1497–1499.
Jankovic, J., Schwartz, K. S., & Ondo, W. (1999). Re-emergent tremor of Parkinson's disease. *Journal of Neurology, Neurosurgery, and Psychiatry, 67*, 646–650.
Kalia, L. V., & Lang, A. E. (2015). Parkinson's disease. *The Lancet, 386*, 896–912.
Madden, M. B., & Hall, D. A. (2010). Shoulder pain in Parkinson's disease: A case-control study. *Movement Disorders, 25*, 1105–1106.
Postuma, R. B., Berg, D., Stern, M., et al. (2015). MDS clinical diagnostic criteria for Parkinson's disease. *Movement Disorders, 30*, 1591–1601.
Selikhova, M., Kempster, P. A., Revesz, T., et al. (2013). Neuropathological findings in benign tremulous parkinsonism. *Movement Disorders, 28*, 145–152.
Stamelou, M., & Hoeglinger, G. U. (2013). Atypical parkinsonism: An update. *Current Opinion in Neurology, 26*, 401–405.
Tinazzi, M., Fasano, A., Geroin, C., et al. (2015). Italian Pisa Syndrome Study Group. Pisa syndrome in Parkinson disease: An observational multicenter Italian study. *Neurology, 85*, 1769–1779.
Wickremaratchi, M. M., Knipe, M. D., Sastry, B. S., et al. (2011). The motor phenotype of Parkinson's disease in relation to age at onset. *Movement Disorders, 26*, 457–463.
Zis, P., Erro, R., Walton, C. C., Sauerbier, A., & Chaudhuri, K. R. (2015). The range and nature of non-motor symptoms in drug-naive Parkinson's disease patients: A state-of-the-art systematic review. *NPJ Parkinson's Disease, 1*, 15013.

CHAPTER THREE

The Nonmotor Features of Parkinson's Disease

Nataliya Titova*, Mubasher A. Qamar†,‡,§, K. Ray Chaudhuri†,‡,§,1

*Federal State Budgetary Educational Institution of Higher Education "N.I. Pirogov Russian National Research Medical University" of the Ministry of Healthcare of the Russian Federation, Moscow, Russia
†National Parkinson Foundation International Centre of Excellence, Kings College and Kings College Hospital, London, United Kingdom
‡Maurice Wohl Clinical Neuroscience Institute, Kings College, London, United Kingdom
§National Institute for Health Research (NIHR) Mental Health Biomedical Research Centre (BRC) and Dementia Unit at South London and Maudsley NHS Foundation Trust, London, United Kingdom
[1]Corresponding author: e-mail address: ray.chaudhuri@nhs.net

Contents

Abstract

Nonmotor symptoms (NMS) of Parkinson's disease (PD) were recognized by the great James Parkinson himself who mentioned symptoms such as sleep dysfunction, delirium, dementia, and dysautonomia, in his seminal 1817 essay, "An Essay on the Shaking Palsy" (Parkinson, 1817). In spite of the key impact of PD NMS on quality of life, there was little holistic research and awareness till the validation and use of comprehensive tools such as the NMS questionnaire, scale, and the revised version of the unified PD rating scale. Research studies using these tools highlighted the key impact of the burden of NMS on quality of life of PD patients and the need for NMS to be routinely assessed in clinic. We now define PD as a motor and nonmotor disorder, and the natural history includes a long prodromal phase of PD dominated by a range of NMS. The prodromal phase is the subject of much research particularly in relation to neuroprotection and identifying

International Review of Neurobiology, Volume 132
ISSN 0074-7742
http://dx.doi.org/10.1016/bs.irn.2017.02.016

subjects at risk. Use of NMS tools has also validated burden grading of NMS with cutoff values, which can be used as outcome measure in clinical trials. Finally, the complex multineurotransmitter dysfunction that is seen in PD has been shown to manifest clinically as nonmotor subtypes. Recognition of such subtypes is likely to lead to the emergence of personalized and precision medicine in PD.

Key Points

- Virtually every patient with PD will have NMS, and these can range from 8 to 12 different symptoms.
- NMS can be caused by the disease process and can be drug induced. Origin of NMS is due to a multineurotransmitter deficit in the brain and periphery, not just dopamine.
- NMS can be measured in clinic by validated tools and clinical examination should include patient declared NMS questionnaire for screening as recommended by the Movement Disorders Society.
- NMS burden can be graded using validated cutoff scores on NMS questionnaire and scales and can be used as outcome measure in clinical trials.
- Nonmotor subtypes of PD are emerging and are being supported by specific biomarkers.
- NMS can be treated by dopaminergic and nondopaminergic strategies.

1. IMPACT OF NONMOTOR SYMPTOMS ON QUALITY OF LIFE IN PARKINSON'S DISEASE

James Parkinson, a London general practitioner, described Parkinson's disease he called Paralysis Agitans 200 years ago (Parkinson, 1817). Parkinson's disease (PD) is the second commonest neurodegenerative disorder in the world with a global prevalence ranging from 200 per 100,000 individuals (Alves, Forsaa, Pedersen, Dreetz Gjerstad, & Larsen, 2008; Berger et al., 2000). Largely it is regarded as a condition related to aging, with 1 in 50 over 80 likely to be affected; however, about 10% of the diagnosis is made in those below 40 years of age (Alves et al., 2008). In the United Kingdom, the estimate is that about 128,000 people are diagnosed with PD (Berger et al., 2000). Worldwide, the number of people diagnosed with PD is expected to double by 2030 most likely related to longer lifespan in the modern era.

The impact of increasing number of people diagnosed with PD will be reflected in the overall societal burden of NMS as virtually every patient with PD has NMS ranging from 8 to 12 different symptoms (Chaudhuri, Healy, & Schapira, 2006; Chaudhuri, Odin, Antonini, & Martinez-Martin, 2011; Jankovic, 2008). Importantly PD is now recognized to be as much a nonmotor disorder as a motor disorder with a complex range of NMS being present in the prodromal stage and in the various stages of the motor disorder of PD (Titova, Padmakumar, Lewis, & Chaudhuri, 2016) (see Chapter "Biomarkers of PD" by Titova, Qamar, and Chaudhuri). Rather than considering a single NMS, it has become apparent that it is the burden of NMS that is a crucial factor for driving quality of life of patients in PD (Todorova, Jenner, & Ray Chaudhuri, 2014). Using a multiple linear regression analysis, Martinez-Martin and colleagues showed that quality of life measures in PD correlated most closely with NMS total score as measured by the nonmotor symptom scale (NMSS) considering motor symptoms as well as complications (Martinez-Martin, Rodriguez-Blazquez, Kurtis, & Chaudhuri, 2011). International validation studies of the NMSS previously have also shown a robust and highly significant association of worsening quality of life scores as total score of the NMSS (reflecting NMS burden (NMSB)) increased (Fig. 1) (Chaudhuri et al., 2007; Martinez-Martin et al., 2009). In the late and palliative stage of PD, the impact of NMS is particularly relevant and contributes to hospitalization and institutionalization with great societal costs (Hagell, Nordling, Reimer, Grabowski, & Persson, 2002; Schrag, Jahanshahi, & Quinn, 2000).

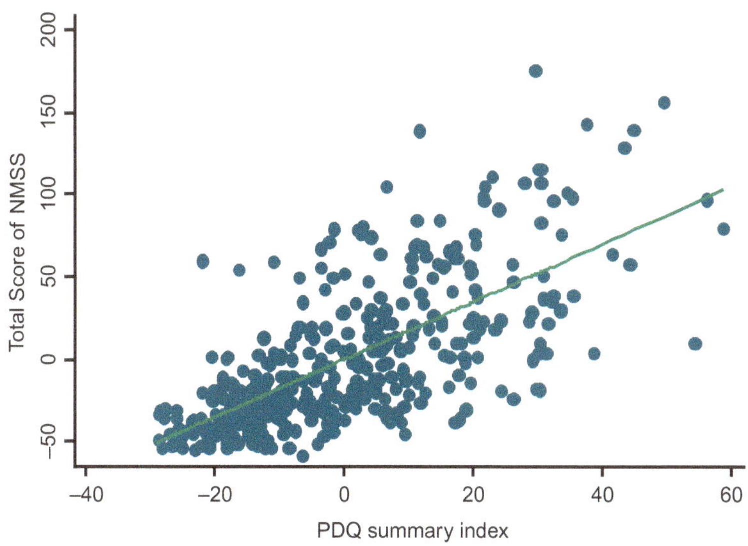

Fig. 1 The highly significant correlation of NMSS total score with worsening quality life scores (PDQ-39). *NMSS*, nonmotor symptom scale; *PDQ*, Parkinson's disease questionnaire. *From Martinez-Martin, P., Rodriguez-Blazquez, C., Abe, K., Bhattacharyya, K. B., Bloem, B. R., Carod-Artal, F. J., et al. (2009). International study on the psychometric attributes of the non-motor symptoms scale in Parkinson disease.* Neurology, *73, 1584–1591.*

A large-scale Italian study, the PRIAMO study, also confirmed that quality of life was significantly worse in those with NMS being present vs those without (Barone et al., 2009).

2. PD IS A NONMOTOR AND MOTOR DISORDER: *ASPECTS OF PATHOPHYSIOLOGY*

A range of pathophysiological mechanisms are likely to set up the neurodegenerative process of PD. From a neurochemical perspective, much of it is based on dysfunctions in the dopamine pathways in the brain and periphery but also other key neurotransmitters such as acetylcholine, noradrenaline, and serotonin among others. Six various pathways of propagation of the pathological process in PD have been proposed and are centered on "bottom-up" initiation as proposed in the seminal works of Braak and colleagues and Jellinger (Braak et al., 2003; Braak, Ghebremedhin, Rub, Bratzke, & Del Tredici, 2004; Jellinger, 2015). The Braak theory has proposed a six-stage pathological process based on Lewy body deposition in the brain. Stage 1 is associated with involvement of the olfactory bulb and the anterior olfactory nucleus in addition to the lower medulla. Stage 2 involves the lower brainstem containing non-dopaminergic nuclei such as the median raphe (serotonin) and locus coeruleus (noradrenaline) among many others. Neurodegeneration is likely to accompany Lewy body deposition and clinically could express late-onset hyposmia as well as rapid eye movement (REM) sleep behavior disorder (RBD). RBD is now recognized as one of the key prodromal clinical biomarkers for the development of dementia as well as synucleinopathy with over 80% risk of phenoconverting at 10 years (Figs. 2 and 3) (Postuma et al., 2015).

The brainstem is thus a key area for the initiation of the neurodegenerative process in PD, and more recently a gut brain axis has been suggested, whereby it is posited that an inflammatory process may spread from the upper gut to the brainstem by the vagus nerve (Klingelhoefer & Reichmann, 2015). The theory has gained clinical support from the reports of people who have had truncal vagotomy having a lesser risk of PD compared to those without (Svensson et al., 2015).

Several reports now suggest Parkinsonian pathology and α-synuclein deposition is seen peripheral organs such as the heart, gut, submandibular glands, and skin, indicating the widespread involvement of the peripheral nervous system in PD. An elegant summary of the spread of α-synuclein deposition and consequent clinical nonmotor effect could be found in a review by Jellinger (2015). The key effects are shown in Table 1.

A key problem toward our understanding of the NMS in PD is the lack of a robust animal model that expresses progressive neurodegeneration with Lewy body formation and NMS. Experimental models to assist in understanding pathogenesis of the range of NMS in PD with potential approaches to treatment of NMS remain an unmet need. Animal models that reflect the neuropathology of PD (central and peripheral), the multineurotransmitter involvement, and progression continue to be problematic. A list of potential animal models that express NMS are shown in Table 2.

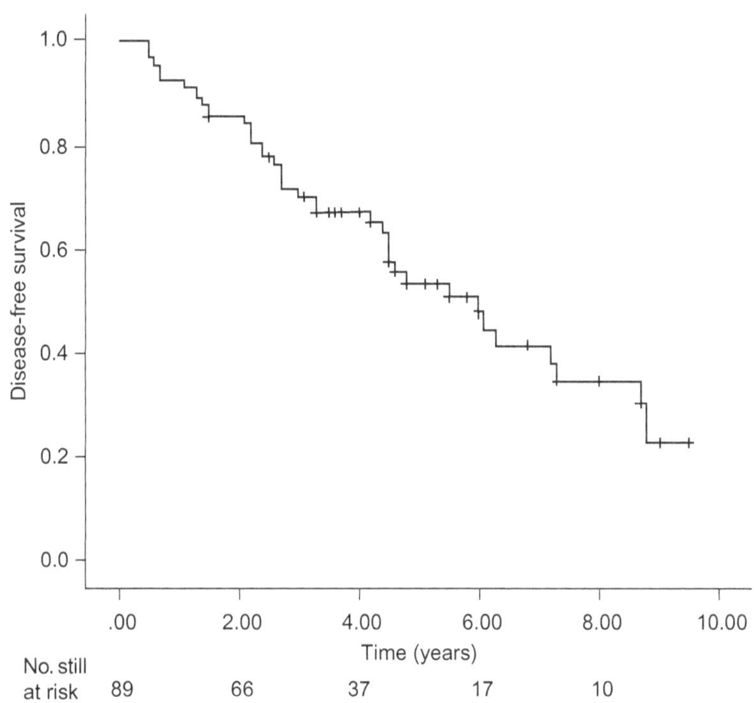

Fig. 2 The risk of development of a neurodegenerative disorder in patients diagnosed with RBD in a Kaplan–Meier plot. *No*, number; *RBD*, rapid eye movement behavior sleep disorder. *From Postuma, R. B., Iranzo, A., Hogl, B., Arnulf, I., Ferini-Strambi, L., Manni, R., et al. (2015). Risk factors for neurodegeneration in idiopathic rapid eye movement sleep behavior disorder: A multicenter study.* Annals of Neurology, *77, 830–839.*

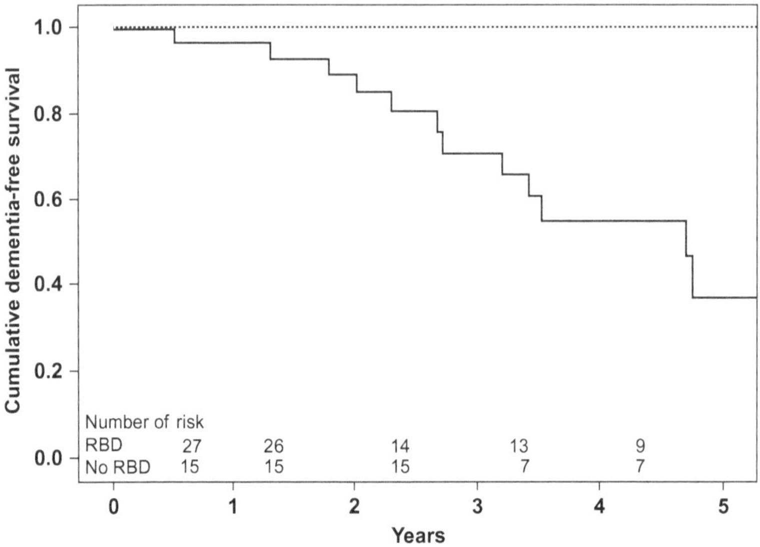

Fig. 3 The risk of development of dementia after RBD. The *dotted line* represents patients with no RBD and the *solid line* represents RBD, Kaplan–Meier plot. *RBD*, rapid eye movement behavior sleep disorder. *From Postuma, R. B., Bertrand, J. A., Montplaisir, J., Desjardins, C., Vendette, M., Rios Romenets, S., et al. (2012). Rapid eye movement sleep behavior disorder and risk of dementia in Parkinson's disease: A prospective study.* Movement Disorders, 27, *720–726.*

Table 1 The Relationship of α-Synuclein Deposition and Braak Stages to Nonmotor Symptoms in Parkinson's Disease

Anatomical Region	α-Synuclein Pathology	Braak Parkinson's Disease Stage	Nonmotor Symptoms
Autonomic nervous system			
Sympathetic ganglia	LN, LB	1–6	Autonomic: Orthostatic hypotension, postural intolerance, cardiac rhythm abnormalities
Gastroesophageal/ enteric plexus	LN, LB	1–6	Constipation, postpranidal hypotension
Pelvic plexus	LN, LB	1–6	Nocturia, impotence, urgency of urination, erectile failure
Cardiac sympathetic nerves	LN, LB	Unknown	Orthostatic hypotention
Adrenal gland	LB	1–6	Fatigue Poor exercise tolerance

Table 1 The Relationship of α-Synuclein Deposition and Braak Stages to Nonmotor Symptoms in Parkinson's Disease—cont'd

Anatomical Region	α-Synuclein Pathology	Braak Parkinson's Disease Stage	Nonmotor Symptoms
Skin			
Epidermal nerves	LN	2–6	Abnormal sensitivity to pain, cutaneous hyperalgesia (allodynia)
Olfactory bulb			
Anterior olfactory nucleus (olfactory brain nuclei)	LN, LB	1	Hyposmia or anosmia
Medulla			
Dorsal motor n. vagus (parasympathetic)	LB, iLB	1	Dysautonomia (gastrointestinal tract, bladder-related symptoms)
Pons			
Locus coeruleus, raphe, lateral tegmental nuclei	LB, LN	2	Depression, anxiety non-REM parasomnias, RBD
Midbrain			
Substantia nigra	LB, LN	3	Extrapyramidal motor
Diencephalon	LB, LN	3, 4	Sleep disorders (insomnia, parasomnias), weight changes
Thalamus			Pain modulation
Hypothalamus			Appetite
Basal forebrain			
Nucleus basalis Meynert	cLB	4	Executive dysfunction, emotional, behavior
Amygdala, hippocampus	cLB		
Neocortex			
Prefrontal cortex	cLB	5	Agnosia, apraxia
Temporal parietal cortex	cLB	6	Dementia Psychosis
Retina	LN	Unknown	Diplopia, reading difficulties

cLB, cortical LB; *iLB*, incidental LB; *LB*, Lewy bodies; *LN*, Lewy neurites; *RBD*, rapid eye movement behavior sleep disorder.

Modified From Jellinger, K. A. (2015). Neuropathobiology of non-motor symptoms in Parkinson disease. *Journal of Neural Transmission, 122*, 1429–1440.

Table 2 Parkinsonian Animal Models That Could Address a Range of Nonmotor Symptoms and Underlying Pathophysiology

Animal Model	Nonmotor Symptoms	References
6-OHDA-lesioned rodents	• Olfaction • Sensory/pain threshold • Sleep/wakefulness • Circadian rhythms • Cognitive function • *(Altered cardiovascular function)* • *(Bladder hyperactivity)* • *(Altered motility of gastrointestinal tract)*	Duty and Jenner (2011); Branchi et al. (2008); Tadaiesky et al. (2008)
α-Synuclein overexpression (ASO = Thy1-αSYN) mice	• Olfaction • Autonomic • Constipation • Sleep *(Circadian dysfunction)* • Cognition	Chesselet et al. (2012); Fleming et al. (2008); Kudo, Loh, Truong, Wu, and Colwell (2011)
MPTP-treated primates	• Bladder hyperreflexia • Constipation • Drooling • Altered cardiovascular function • Sleep disturbance • Cognitive disturbance	Duty and Jenner (2011)
Mice model of intragastric rotenone administration	• α-Synuclein accumulation in dorsal vagal nucleus • Potential for investigating autonomic symptoms such as constipation • Sleep disturbances	Pan-Montojo et al. (2010); Zhang, Zhang, Yeh, Richardson, and Bo (2007)
Göttingen minipigs (Ellegaard Minipigs ApS)	• Cognition • Sleep disturbances	Lind et al. (2007)
GBA-deficiency mouse models	• Memory problems • Cognition problems	Cullen et al. (2011); Sardi et al. (2011)
Transgenic mouse model overexpressing LRRK2 gene mutation	• Gastrointestinal dysfunction • Olfactory dysfunction	Bichler, Lim, Zeng, and Tan (2013)
DJ-1 knockedout	• Cognition disturbances	Pham et al. (2010)

Table 2 Parkinsonian Animal Models That Could Address a Range of Nonmotor Symptoms and Underlying Pathophysiology—cont'd

Animal Model	Nonmotor Symptoms	References
Parkin knockedout	• Anxiety • Cognition	Zhu et al. (2007)
VMAT2-deficient mice	• Olfactory discrimination • Delayed gastric emptying • Sleep disturbances • Anxiety-like behavior • Depression	Taylor et al. (2009)
Cycad-fed rats	• Excessive daytime somnolence • RBD	McDowell et al. (2010)

GBA, glucocerebrosidase; *LRRK2*, leucine-rich repeat kinase 2; *MPTP*, 1-methyl-4-phenyl-1,2,3,6-tetrahydropyridine; *OHDA*, hydroxydopamine; *RBD*, rapid eye movement behavior sleep disorder; *VMAT*, vesicular monoamine transporter.

Adapted from Todorova, A., Jenner, P., & Ray Chaudhuri, K. (2014). Non-motor Parkinson's: Integral to motor Parkinson's, yet often neglected. *Practical Neurology, 14*, 310–322.

3. NONMOTOR SYMPTOMS IN PD: *THE CLINICAL ASPECTS*

Patients consistently rate NMS as most bothersome (Politis et al., 2010) and this is reflected in several studies, which have used the NMS questionnaire (NMSQuest) as a screening tool. Yet unfortunately NMS may remain undeclared as shown in a European study largely because of lack of patient and clinician awareness (Chaudhuri et al., 2010; Todorova et al., 2014).

4. NONMOTOR SYMPTOMS AND GENDER ASSOCIATION

Gender and PD gender differences have already been widely discussed in the context of motor symptoms, whereby men have a higher frequency in PD (Lyons, Hubble, Troster, Pahwa, & Koller, 1998; Scott, Borgman, Engler, Johnels, & Aquilonius, 2000). There has been evidence that an association between nonmotor features of PD and gender too exists. A cross-sectional observational study by Martinez-Martin and colleagues found that in their cohort of 950 patients (62.6% males), there was a higher prevalence and burden of cardiovascular, sleep disturbances, fatigue, mood/apathy, perceptual problems, weight changes, and olfactory dysfunction in women than in men (Martinez-Martin et al., 2012). However, men had a higher prevalence of attention/memory problems, gastrointestinal dysfunction, urinary dysfunction, and sexual dysfunction. In a recent study by Nicoletti and colleagues, they evaluated 585 patients and report women to have a higher frequency of depression and urinary dysfunction than men, while men had more cognitive impairment, sleep disorders, and perceptual problems (Nicoletti et al., 2016). In general, men appear to have more cognitive dysfunction, while women have more neuropsychiatric-related problems in PD. However, a clear gender-related difference for nonmotor features of PD is unclear and further studies are required to explore this further.

5. CLASSIFICATION OF NONMOTOR SYMPTOMS OF PD

NMS occur from nondopaminergic and dopaminergic sources and thus are varied in its range and nature (Chaudhuri, Healy, et al., 2006). It is important however not to lump all NMS together and a classification has been proposed by Todorova and colleagues (2014) (Table 3).

Table 3 A Modern Classification of Nonmotor Symptoms in Parkinson's Disease

Related to the disease process or pathophysiology • Dopaminergic NMS *(depression, pain, anxiety, aspects of sleep dysfunction, NMS of nonmotor fluctuation)* • Nondopaminergic NMS *(dementia. RBD, dysautonomia. Aspects of pain, apathy, fatigue)*
Related to nonmotor fluctuations *(cognitive, autonomic, and sensory subtypes)*
Related to dopaminergic drug therapy • Hallucinations (*benign and malignant*) • Delirium • Impulse control disorders • Dopamine agonist withdrawal syndrome
Possibly genetically determined • Higher risk of dementia in cases or carriers with glucocerebrosidase mutation • Higher risk of depression and sleep disorders in cases with leucine-rich repeat kinase-2 mutation

NMS, nonmotor symptoms; *RBD*, rapid eye movement behavior sleep disorder.

Adapted from Todorova, A., Jenner, P., & Ray Chaudhuri, K. (2014). Non-motor Parkinson's: Integral to motor Parkinson's, yet often neglected. *Practical Neurology, 14*, 310–322.

6. NONMOTOR SYMPTOMS MEASUREMENT IN CLINICS

Holistic and widely validated NMS tools such as the NMSS (Chaudhuri et al., 2007) and NMSQuest (Chaudhuri, Martinez-Martin, et al., 2006) are available and are recommended by the Movement Disorders Society (MDS). NMSQuest is a self-reporting tool completed by patients and thus instrumental as a flagging tool, and data from over 2500 patients in worldwide studies suggest that irrespective of the motor stage of PD a typical PD patient will suffer from 8 to 12 different NMS (Todorova et al., 2014).

Holistic measurements of NMS have been enhanced by validation of the grading of NMSB by the NMSQuest and the NMSS as well as the MDS Unified PD rating scale (UPDRS) (Fig. 4) (Chaudhuri et al., 2013, 2015; Martinez-Martin et al., 2015).

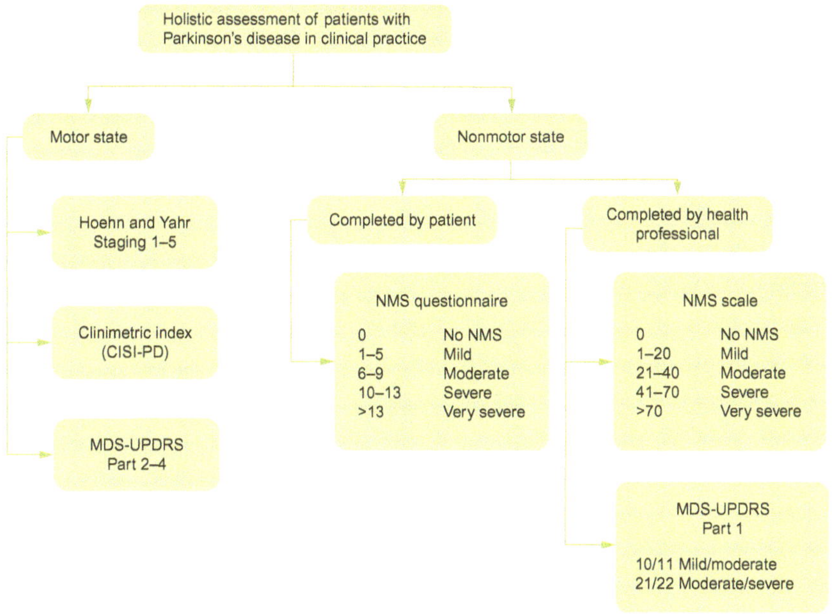

Fig. 4 A holistic clinical strategy using validated tools to obtain a patients' "nonmotor status." All cutoff's quoted are validated from clinical studies. *CISI*, clinical impression of severity index; *MDS*, Movement Disorders Society; *NMS*, nonmotor symptoms; *PD*, Parkinson's disease; *UPDRS*, unified Parkinson's disease rating scale. *From Sauerbier, A., Qamar, M. A., Rajah, T., & Chaudhuri, K. R. (2016). New concepts in the pathogenesis and presentation of Parkinson's disease.* Clinical Medicine (London, England), 16, *365–370.*

To ensure that the NMS status of PD patients is assessed parallel to their motor symptoms, recent guidelines have recommended that NMS assessment tools (NMSS and NMSQuest) be used in combination with motor assessment tools such as the Hoehn and Yahr (HY) staging. This holistic approach to managing a patient will provide a rapid real-time clinical picture of a patient, which ultimately allows physicians to make better decisions in managing patient's symptoms and expectations. While NMSQuest is patient completed and thus easy to use in the clinic, NMSS can be used when more detailed NMS data capture is required such as in a research setting (Fig. 4). A key recommendation would be to combine HY staging with NMSQuest grading for patients, preformed at least once a year. A suggested paradigm for use in clinic is shown in Fig. 4. Additional tools such as the nonmotor section of MDS UPDRS or a short validated clinimetric index such as Clinical Impression Of Severity Index PD (CISI-PD) can also be used.

7. NONMOTOR FLUCTUATIONS

Nonmotor fluctuations (NMF) almost always accompany motor fluctuations and have been classified as autonomic, sensory, and cognitive symptoms. Storch and colleagues have described NMS that are present exclusively during "off" periods, while others present at "on" worsening during motor "off" period (Storch et al., 2013). NMF could also manifest in the early morning known as the "early morning off" state where awakening is associated with a range of NMS (Rizos et al., 2014) (Fig. 5).

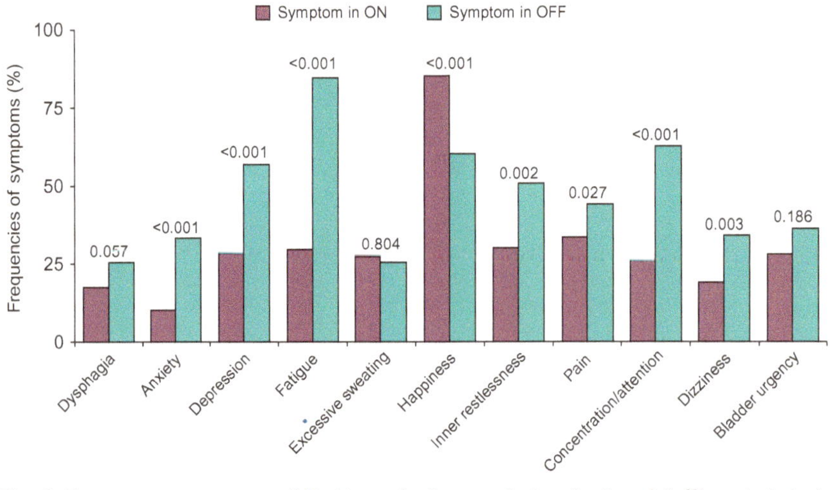

Fig. 5 Nonmotor symptoms of Parkinson's disease during "on" and "off" period. As in the NoMoFlu study from Storch and colleagues. *From Storch, A., Schneider, C. B., Wolz, M., Sturwald, Y., Nebe, A., Odin, P., et al. (2013). Nonmotor fluctuations in Parkinson disease: Severity and correlation with motor complications.* Neurology, 80, *800–809.*

8. BIOMARKERS

Detailed discussion of various clinical, genetics, biochemical, and imaging biomarkers for NMS of PD is beyond the scope of this chapter and is dealt with elsewhere in this book. Dopaminergic transporter (DaT) scan is commonly used in clinical practice and is a useful marker for the motor disorder of PD. Recent evidence suggests that DaT scan may be useful for addressing some NMS in PD and has been extensively discussed in a recent review by Qamar et al. (2017) who report there to be 12 NMS with DaT evidence supportive for some dopaminergic basis to the pathophysiology. Excessive daytime somnolence (Pavese et al., 2012), RBD (Eisensehr et al., 2003), restless leg syndrome (RLS) (Moccia et al., 2016), anxiety (Weintraub et al., 2005), attention deficit (Rinne et al., 2000), urinary dysfunction (Sakakibara et al., 2001), olfactory dysfunction (Bohnen et al., 2007), and weight changes (Lee et al., 2016) are some key NMS identified in this review.

9. TREATMENT OF NONMOTOR SYMPTOMS

Management of NMS in PD presents one of the key challenges in clinical practice. The evidence-based medicine task force of the MDS (Seppi et al., 2011) as well as a recent review of the topic by Schrag and colleagues has been published and highlights key unmet needs (Schrag, Sauerbier, & Chaudhuri, 2015). The role of various nonpharmacological therapies such as exercise, cognitive behavioral therapy, and transcranial magnetic stimulation is also being explored particularly for depression, anxiety, and cognitive problems. However, for many NMS, such as fatigue, sexual dysfunction, apathy, and urinary dysfunction, there is insufficient evidence of treatment (Table 4).

Table 4 A Snapshot View of Varying Treatment Strategies for a Range of Nonmotor Symptoms

Nonmotor Symptoms	Commonly Used Strategies
Memory and cognition	
Cognition, dementia	• Rivastigmine transdermal or oral (recommended by the Movement Disorders Society) (oral or transdermal patch) • Donepezil • Memantine • Other acetylcholinesterase inhibitor

Continued

Table 4 A Snapshot View of Varying Treatment Strategies for a Range of Nonmotor Symptoms—cont'd

Nonmotor Symptoms	Commonly Used Strategies
Neuropsychiatry	
Depression and anxiety	• Antidepressants ○ Tricyclic antidepressant (recommended by Movement Disorders Society) ○ Nortriptyline ○ Desipramine • SSRIs (selective serotonin reuptake inhibitors) ○ Citalopram • SNRIs (selective noradrenalin reuptake inhibitors) ○ Venlafaxine XR, Mirtazapine • Pramipexole
Psychosis (hallucination and delusion)	• Quetiapine (often used first line, based on clinical experience, despite of unconvincing trial data) • Clozapine (atypical antipsychotic that need regular control of blood level) • Exclusion of concomitant systemic infection or illness, which may precipitate psychosis Pimavanserin (serotonin 2A receptor inverse agonist) (recently approved in the United States)
Sleep disturbances	
Excessive daytime sleepiness	• Sleep hygiene • Modafinil • Caffeine intake (unproven) • Sodium oxybate—taken at night, only under specialist supervision (potential for abuse) • Bright light therapy (in specialized centers, investigational)
Insomnia	• Sleep hygiene • Short-acting benzodiazepines ○ Nonbenzodiazepine hypnotics Zopiclone • Tricyclic antidepressants ○ Amitriptyline ○ Melatonin (investigational)
REM sleep behavior disorder	• Sleep in a safe environment while in bed (remove all sharp and breakable objects) • Clonazepam (usually considered first line) • Melatonin

Table 4 A Snapshot View of Varying Treatment Strategies for a Range of Nonmotor Symptoms—cont'd

Nonmotor Symptoms	**Commonly Used Strategies**
Fatigue	• Methylphenidate (recommended by American Academy of Neurology, although considerable side effect profile) • Modafinil (weak evidence)
Autonomic dysfunction	
Dribbling of saliva	• Oral atropine drops (2–3 times/day) • Swallow timer and upright positioning of head • Glycopyrrolate for short-term treatment (recommended by the Movement Disorders Society) • Ipratropium bromide spray (Atrovent) (1–2 doses per day sublingually)
Orthostatic hypotension	• Volume replenishment, drinks of water, rehydration • Avoid prolonged bed rest • Avoid alcohol, diuretics, antihypertensives • Waist-high support stockings • Sodium chloride supplementation of meal • Pharmacotherapy ○ Fludrocortisone ○ Indometacin ○ Ephedrine ○ Midodrine (with specialist supervision) ○ Domperidone in addition to fludrocortisone • L-Threo-3,4-dihydroxyphenylserine for refractory orthostatic ○ Hypotension
Constipation	• Fiber-rich diet • Avoid dehydration • Macrogol (Movicol in the United Kingdom) (recommended by the American Academy of Neurology and the Movement Disorders Society) • Lactulose (Duphalac) • Senna (Senokot) • Avoid constipating opiates for pain • Lubiprostone (Amitiza)
Bladder dysfunction (nocturia)	• Avoid nighttime diuretics • Desmopressin spray for troublesome nocturia (beware of nocturnal hypertension)

Continued

Table 4 A Snapshot View of Varying Treatment Strategies for a Range of Nonmotor Symptoms—cont'd

Nonmotor Symptoms	Commonly Used Strategies
Bladder dysfunction (urgency, frequency)	• Anticholinergic agents (use with caution in patients with hallucinations and cognitive decline) ○ Oxybutynin ○ Tolterodine XL
Erectile dysfunction	• Phosphodiesterase-5 inhibitors (use with caution in patients with postural hypotension) • Sildenafil (recommended by the American Academy of Neurology) • Psychological assessment
Miscellaneous	
Pain	• Analgesics and dopaminergic drugs for nonmotor fluctuation-related pain such as off related dystonic pain • Baclofen (muscular pain aggravated by rigidity, anecdotal evidence) • Opiates (Tramadol) • Central pain: ○ Oxycodone with naloxone

REM, rapid eye movement.

Adapted from Sauerbier, A., & Chaudhuri, K. R. (2014). Non-motor symptoms: The core of multi-morbid Parkinson's disease. *British Journal of Hospital Medicine (London, England), 75*, 18–24; Todorova, A., Jenner, P., & Ray Chaudhuri, K. (2014). Non-motor Parkinson's: Integral to motor Parkinson's, yet often neglected. *Practical Neurology, 14*, 310–322; Trotti, L. M., & Bliwise, D. L. (2014). Treatment of the sleep disorders associated with Parkinson's disease. *Neurotherapeutics, 11*, 68–77; Schrag, A., Sauerbier, A., & Chaudhuri, K. R. (2015). New clinical trials for nonmotor manifestations of Parkinson's disease. *Movement Disorders*, 30, 1490–1504.

10. NONMOTOR SUBTYPING OF PARKINSON'S

This is a new concept and is based on several cluster analyses studies in untreated and early PD patients showing discrete clusters of patients often expressing specific NMS (Erro et al., 2013; Pont-Sunyer et al., 2015). Clinical characterization of these clusters has suggested seven specific NMS-dominant phenotypes: Park cognition, Park apathy, Park depression/anxiety, Park sleep, Park pain, Park fatigue, and Park autonomic (Sauerbier, Jenner, Todorova, & Chaudhuri, 2016; Sauerbier, Qamar, Rajah, & Chaudhuri, 2016; Zis et al., 2015). Further cohort studies are required to define the specific clinical characteristics of these subtypes as well as biomarkers and natural history.

11. MULTIDISCIPLINARY CARE AND NONMOTOR SYMPTOMS OF PD

Multidisciplinary care team (MDT) support is integral to the modern management of PD and involves combined input from speech and language, physiotherapists, and occupational therapists with interface Liaison carried out by the PD specialist nurses (Carne et al., 2005; van der Marck et al., 2009, 2013). In addition, with longer life span, palliative care is also an essential aspect of PD care. Physical exercise benefits motor and several nonmotor aspects of PD (Tajiri et al., 2010), while NMSQuest use should trigger specific MDT-led pathways such as therapy with speech and language specialists to help social communication as well as address problems of dribbling of saliva, which can lead to swallowing dysfunction.

MDT also addresses comorbidity-related issues in PD such as bone health, associated diabetes, and other conditions. As mentioned previously, the PD nurse specialist is pivotal to a holistic care model of PD and particularly when advanced therapies are contemplated. MDT in the context of PD is discussed in more detail elsewhere by Qamar and colleagues.

Table 5 Nonmotor Symptoms That May Be Made Worse on Using Dopaminergic-Based Treatment for Parkinson's Disease

Nonmotor Features	Complication
Autonomic	Parkinson hyperpyrexia syndrome Neuroleptic malignant syndrome Serotonin syndrome Malignant parkinsonism Symptomatic orthostatic hypotension
Neuropsychiatric	Hallucinations Delusions Delirium Dopamine dysregulation syndrome Punding Impulse control disorders Dopamine agonist withdrawal syndrome (DAWS)
Sleep related	Excessive daytime somnolence Sudden onset of sleep
Gastrointestinal	Nausea Diarrhea (often related to intake of COMT inhibitors)

COMT, catechol-*O*-methyl transferase.

12. DRUG-INDUCED NONMOTOR SYMPTOMS OF PD

These are important to recognize and range from benign hallucinations to frank psychosis, delirium, impulse control disorders, as well as the dopamine agonist withdrawal syndrome (Table 5). Detailed discussion of these problems is beyond the scope of this review, but recognition is key to management.

13. CONCLUSIONS

PD is a mixture of motor and a nonmotor disorder right from the onset of the condition. Indeed, the prodromal PD is largely nonmotor. Key advances include the development of validated tools for holistic measure of NMS, the grading of NMS burden in addition to a focus on multimodal biomarkers to define nonmotor subtypes of PD. The latter concept is likely to lead to better management of NMS in PD, still a key unmet need.

REFERENCES

Alves, G., Forsaa, E. B., Pedersen, K. F., Dreetz Gjerstad, M., & Larsen, J. P. (2008). Epidemiology of Parkinson's disease. *Journal of Neurology*, *255*(Suppl. 5), 18–32.

Barone, P., Antonini, A., Colosimo, C., Marconi, R., Morgante, L., Avarello, T. P., et al. (2009). The PRIAMO study: A multicenter assessment of nonmotor symptoms and their impact on quality of life in Parkinson's disease. *Movement Disorders*, *24*, 1641–1649.

Berger, K., Breteler, M. M., Helmer, C., Inzitari, D., Fratiglioni, L., Trenkwalder, C., et al. (2000). Prognosis with Parkinson's disease in Europe: A collaborative study of population-based cohorts. Neurologic diseases in the elderly research group. *Neurology*, *54*, S24–S27.

Bichler, Z., Lim, H. C., Zeng, L., & Tan, E. K. (2013). Non-motor and motor features in LRRK2 transgenic mice. *PLoS One*, *8*, e70249.

Bohnen, N. I., Gedela, S., Kuwabara, H., Constantine, G. M., Mathis, C. A., Studenski, S. A., et al. (2007). Selective hyposmia and nigrostriatal dopaminergic denervation in Parkinson's disease. *Journal of Neurology*, *254*, 84–90.

Braak, H., Del Tredici, K., Rub, U., De Vos, R. A., Jansen Steur, E. N., & Braak, E. (2003). Staging of brain pathology related to sporadic Parkinson's disease. *Neurobiology of Aging*, *24*, 197–211.

Braak, H., Ghebremedhin, E., Rub, U., Bratzke, H., & Del Tredici, K. (2004). Stages in the development of Parkinson's disease-related pathology. *Cell and Tissue Research*, *318*, 121–134.

Branchi, I., D'Andrea, I., Armida, M., Cassano, T., Pezzola, A., Potenza, R. L., et al. (2008). Nonmotor symptoms in Parkinson's disease: Investigating early-phase onset of behavioral dysfunction in the 6-hydroxydopamine-lesioned rat model. *Journal of Neuroscience Research*, *86*, 2050–2061.

Carne, W., Cifu, D., Marcinko, P., Pickett, T., Baron, M., Qutubbudin, A., et al. (2005). Efficacy of a multidisciplinary treatment program on one-year outcomes of individuals with Parkinson's disease. *NeuroRehabilitation*, *20*, 161–167.

Chaudhuri, K. R., Healy, D. G., & Schapira, A. H. V. (2006). Non-motor symptoms of Parkinson's disease: Diagnosis and management. *Lancet Neurology, 5*, 235–245.
Chaudhuri, K. R., Martinez-Martin, P., Brown, R. G., Sethi, K., Stocchi, F., Odin, P., et al. (2007). The metric properties of a novel non-motor symptoms scale for Parkinson's disease: Results from an international pilot study. *Movement Disorders, 22*, 1901–1911.
Chaudhuri, K. R., Martinez-Martin, P., Schapira, A. H., Stocchi, F., Sethi, K., Odin, P., et al. (2006). International multicenter pilot study of the first comprehensive self-completed nonmotor symptoms questionnaire for Parkinson's disease: The NMSQuest study. *Movement Disorders, 21*, 916–923.
Chaudhuri, K. R., Odin, P., Antonini, A., & Martinez-Martin, P. (2011). Parkinson's disease: The non-motor issues. *Parkinsonism & Related Disorders, 17*, 717–723.
Chaudhuri, K. R., Prieto-Jurcynska, C., Naidu, Y., Mitra, T., Frades-Payo, B., Tluk, S., et al. (2010). The nondeclaration of nonmotor symptoms of Parkinson's disease to health care professionals: An international study using the nonmotor symptoms questionnaire. *Movement Disorders, 25*, 704–709.
Chaudhuri, K. R., Rojo, J. M., Schapira, A. H. V., Brooks, D. J., Stocchi, F., Odin, P., et al. (2013). A proposal for a comprehensive grading of Parkinson's disease severity combining motor and non-motor assessments: Meeting an unmet need. *PLoS One, 8*, e57221.
Chaudhuri, K. R., Sauerbier, A., Rojo, J. M., Sethi, K., Schapira, A. H. V., Brown, R. G., et al. (2015). The burden of non-motor symptoms in Parkinson's disease using a self-completed non-motor questionnaire: A simple grading system. *Parkinsonism & Related Disorders, 21*, 287–291.
Chesselet, M. F., Richter, F., Zhu, C., Magen, I., Watson, M. B., & Subramaniam, S. R. (2012). A progressive mouse model of Parkinson's disease: The Thy1-aSyn ("Line 61") mice. *Neurotherapeutics, 9*, 297–314.
Cullen, V., Sardi, S. P., Ng, J., Xu, Y. H., Sun, Y., Tomlinson, J. J., et al. (2011). Acid beta-glucosidase mutants linked to Gaucher disease, Parkinson disease, and Lewy body dementia alter alpha-synuclein processing. *Annals of Neurology, 69*, 940–953.
Duty, S., & Jenner, P. (2011). Animal models of Parkinson's disease: A source of novel treatments and clues to the cause of the disease. *British Journal of Pharmacology, 164*, 1357–1391.
Eisensehr, I., Linke, R., Tatsch, K., Kharraz, B., Gildehaus, J. F., Wetter, C. T., et al. (2003). Increased muscle activity during rapid eye movement sleep correlates with decrease of striatal presynaptic dopamine transporters. IPT and IBZM SPECT imaging in subclinical and clinically manifest idiopathic REM sleep behavior disorder, Parkinson's disease, and controls. *Sleep, 26*, 507–512.
Erro, R., Vitale, C., Amboni, M., Picillo, M., Moccia, M., Longo, K., et al. (2013). The heterogeneity of early Parkinson's disease: A cluster analysis on newly diagnosed untreated patients. *PLoS One, 8*, e70244.
Fleming, S. M., Tetreault, N. A., Mulligan, C. K., Hutson, C. B., Masliah, E., & Chesselet, M. F. (2008). Olfactory deficits in mice overexpressing human wildtype alpha-synuclein. *The European Journal of Neuroscience, 28*, 247–256.
Hagell, P., Nordling, S., Reimer, J., Grabowski, M., & Persson, U. (2002). Resource use and costs in a Swedish cohort of patients with Parkinson's disease. *Movement Disorders, 17*, 1213–1220.
Jankovic, J. (2008). Parkinson's disease: Clinical features and diagnosis. *Journal of Neurology, Neurosurgery, and Psychiatry, 79*, 368–376.
Jellinger, K. A. (2015). Neuropathobiology of non-motor symptoms in Parkinson disease. *Journal of Neural Transmission, 122*, 1429–1440.
Klingelhoefer, L., & Reichmann, H. (2015). Pathogenesis of Parkinson disease—The gut-brain axis and environmental factors. *Nature Reviews. Neurology, 11*, 625–636.

Kudo, T., Loh, D. H., Truong, D., Wu, Y., & Colwell, C. S. (2011). Circadian dysfunction in a mouse model of Parkinson's disease. *Experimental Neurology*, *232*, 66–75.

Lee, J. J., Oh, J. S., Ham, J. H., Lee, D. H., Lee, I., Sohn, Y. H., et al. (2016). Association of body mass index and the depletion of nigrostriatal dopamine in Parkinson's disease. *Neurobiology of Aging*, *38*, 197–204.

Lind, N. M., Moustgaard, A., Jelsing, J., Vajta, G., Cumming, P., & Hansen, A. K. (2007). The use of pigs in neuroscience: Modeling brain disorders. *Neuroscience and Biobehavioral Reviews*, *31*, 728–751.

Lyons, K. E., Hubble, J. P., Troster, A. I., Pahwa, R., & Koller, W. C. (1998). Gender differences in Parkinson's disease. *Clinical Neuropharmacology*, *21*, 118–121.

Martinez-Martin, P., Chaudhuri, K. R., Rojo-Abuin, J. M., Rodriguez-Blazquez, C., Alvarez-Sanchez, M., Arakaki, T., et al. (2015). Assessing the non-motor symptoms of Parkinson's disease: MDS-UPDRS and NMS scale. *European Journal of Neurology*, *22*, 37–43.

Martinez-Martin, P., Falup Pecurariu, C., Odin, P., Van Hilten, J. J., Antonini, A., Rojo-Abuin, J. M., et al. (2012). Gender-related differences in the burden of non-motor symptoms in Parkinson's disease. *Journal of Neurology*, *259*, 1639–1647.

Martinez-Martin, P., Rodriguez-Blazquez, C., Abe, K., Bhattacharyya, K. B., Bloem, B. R., Carod-Artal, F. J., et al. (2009). International study on the psychometric attributes of the non-motor symptoms scale in Parkinson disease. *Neurology*, *73*, 1584–1591.

Martinez-Martin, P., Rodriguez-Blazquez, C., Kurtis, M. M., & Chaudhuri, K. R. (2011). The impact of non-motor symptoms on health-related quality of life of patients with Parkinson's disease. *Movement Disorders*, *26*, 399–406.

McDowell, K. A., Hadjimarkou, M. M., Viechweg, S., Rose, A. E., Clark, S. M., Yarowsky, P. J., et al. (2010). Sleep alterations in an environmental neurotoxin-induced model of parkinsonism. *Experimental Neurology*, *226*, 84–89.

Moccia, M., Erro, R., Picillo, M., Santangelo, G., Spina, E., Allocca, R., et al. (2016). A four-year longitudinal study on restless legs syndrome in Parkinson disease. *Sleep*, *39*, 405–412.

Nicoletti, A., Vasta, R., Mostile, G., Nicoletti, G., Arabia, G., Iliceto, G., et al. (2016). Gender effect on non-motor symptoms in Parkinson's disease: Are men more at risk? *Parkinsonism & Related Disorders*, *35*, 69–74.

Pan-Montojo, F., Anichtchik, O., Dening, Y., Knels, L., Pursche, S., Jung, R., et al. (2010). Progression of Parkinson's disease pathology is reproduced by intragastric administration of rotenone in mice. *PLoS One*, *5*, e8762.

Parkinson, J. (1817). An essay on the shaking palsy. *London Medical and Physical Journal*, 38.

Pavese, N., Metta, V., Simpson, B. S., Marphy, T. A., Ramlackhansingh, A., Chaudhuri, K. R., et al. (2012). Sleep regulatory centres dysfunction in Parkinson's disease patients with excessive daytime sleepiness. An in vivo PET study. *Parkinsonism & Related Disorders*, *18*, S24–S25.

Pham, T. T., Giesert, F., Rothig, A., Floss, T., Kallnik, M., Weindl, K., et al. (2010). DJ-1-deficient mice show less TH-positive neurons in the ventral tegmental area and exhibit non-motoric behavioural impairments. *Genes, Brain, and Behavior*, *9*, 305–317.

Politis, M., Wu, K., Molloy, S., Bain, P. G., Chaudhuri, K. R., & Piccini, P. (2010). Parkinson's disease symptoms: The patient's perspective. *Movement Disorders*, *25*, 1646–1651.

Pont-Sunyer, C., Hotter, A., Gaig, C., Seppi, K., Compta, Y., Katzenschlager, R., et al. (2015). The onset of nonmotor symptoms in Parkinson's disease (the ONSET PD study). *Movement Disorders*, *30*, 229–237.

Postuma, R. B., Iranzo, A., Hogl, B., Arnulf, I., Ferini-Strambi, L., Manni, R., et al. (2015). Risk factors for neurodegeneration in idiopathic rapid eye movement sleep behavior disorder: A multicenter study. *Annals of Neurology*, *77*, 830–839.

Qamar, M. A., Sauerbier, A., Politis, M., Carr, H., Loehrer, P., & Chaudhuri, K. R. (2017). Presynaptic dopaminergic terminal imaging and non-motor symptoms assessment of Parkinson's disease: Evidence for dopaminergic basis? *npj Parkinson's Disease*, *3*, 5. http://dx.doi.org/10.1038/s41531-016-0006-9.

Rinne, J. O., Portin, R., Ruottinen, H., Nurmi, E., Bergman, J., Haaparanta, M., et al. (2000). Cognitive impairment and the brain dopaminergic system in Parkinson disease: [18F]fluorodopa positron emission tomographic study. *Archives of Neurology*, *57*, 470–475.

Rizos, A., Martinez-Martin, P., Odin, P., Antonini, A., Kessel, B., Kozul, T. K., et al. (2014). Characterizing motor and non-motor aspects of early-morning off periods in Parkinson's disease: An international multicenter study. *Parkinsonism & Related Disorders*, *20*, 1231–1235.

Sakakibara, R., Shinotoh, H., Uchiyama, T., Yoshiyama, M., Hattori, T., & Yamanishi, T. (2001). SPECT imaging of the dopamine transporter with [(123)I]-beta-CIT reveals marked decline of nigrostriatal dopaminergic function in Parkinson's disease with urinary dysfunction. *Journal of the Neurological Sciences*, *187*, 55–59.

Sardi, S. P., Clarke, J., Kinnecom, C., Tamsett, T. J., Li, L., Stanek, L. M., et al. (2011). CNS expression of glucocerebrosidase corrects alpha-synuclein pathology and memory in a mouse model of Gaucher-related synucleinopathy. *Proceedings of the National Academy of Sciences of the United States of America*, *108*, 12101–12106.

Sauerbier, A., Jenner, P., Todorova, A., & Chaudhuri, K. R. (2016). Non motor subtypes and Parkinson's disease. *Parkinsonism & Related Disorders*, *22*(Suppl. 1), S41–S46.

Sauerbier, A., Qamar, M. A., Rajah, T., & Chaudhuri, K. R. (2016). New concepts in the pathogenesis and presentation of Parkinson's disease. *Clinical Medicine (London, England)*, *16*, 365–370.

Schrag, A., Jahanshahi, M., & Quinn, N. (2000). What contributes to quality of life in patients with Parkinson's disease? *Journal of Neurology, Neurosurgery, and Psychiatry*, *69*, 308–312.

Schrag, A., Sauerbier, A., & Chaudhuri, K. R. (2015). New clinical trials for nonmotor manifestations of Parkinson's disease. *Movement Disorders*, *30*, 1490–1504.

Scott, B., Borgman, A., Engler, H., Johnels, B., & Aquilonius, S. M. (2000). Gender differences in Parkinson's disease symptom profile. *Acta Neurologica Scandinavica*, *102*, 37–43.

Seppi, K., Weintraub, D., Coelho, M., Perez-Lloret, S., Fox, S. H., Katzenschlager, R., et al. (2011). The movement disorder society evidence-based medicine review update: Treatments for the non-motor symptoms of Parkinson's disease. *Movement Disorders*, *26*(Suppl. 3), S42–S80.

Storch, A., Schneider, C. B., Wolz, M., Sturwald, Y., Nebe, A., Odin, P., et al. (2013). Nonmotor fluctuations in Parkinson disease: Severity and correlation with motor complications. *Neurology*, *80*, 800–809.

Svensson, E., Horvath-Puho, E., Thomsen, R. W., Djurhuus, J. C., Pedersen, L., Borghammer, P., et al. (2015). Vagotomy and subsequent risk of Parkinson's disease. *Annals of Neurology*, *78*, 522–529.

Tadaiesky, M. T., Dombrowski, P. A., Figueiredo, C. P., Cargnin-Ferreira, E., Da Cunha, C., & Takahashi, R. N. (2008). Emotional, cognitive and neurochemical alterations in a premotor stage model of Parkinson's disease. *Neuroscience*, *156*, 830–840.

Tajiri, N., Yasuhara, T., Shingo, T., Kondo, A., Yuan, W., Kadota, T., et al. (2010). Exercise exerts neuroprotective effects on Parkinson's disease model of rats. *Brain Research*, *1310*, 200–207.

Taylor, T. N., Caudle, W. M., Shepherd, K. R., Noorian, A., Jackson, C. R., Iuvone, P. M., et al. (2009). Nonmotor symptoms of Parkinson's disease revealed in an animal model with reduced monoamine storage capacity. *The Journal of Neuroscience*, *29*, 8103–8113.

Titova, N., Padmakumar, C., Lewis, S. J. G., & Chaudhuri, K. R. (2016). Parkinson's: A syndrome rather than a disease? *Journal of Neural Transmission*. http://dx.doi.org/10.1007/s00702-016-1667-6.

Todorova, A., Jenner, P., & Ray Chaudhuri, K. (2014). Non-motor Parkinson's: Integral to motor Parkinson's, yet often neglected. *Practical Neurology*, *14*, 310–322.

van der Marck, M. A., Kalf, J. G., Sturkenboom, I. H., Nijkrake, M. J., Munneke, M., & Bloem, B. R. (2009). Multidisciplinary care for patients with Parkinson's disease. *Parkinsonism & Related Disorders*, *15*(Suppl. 3), S219–S223.

van der Marck, M. A., Munneke, M., Mulleners, W., Hoogerwaard, E. M., Borm, G. F., Overeem, S., et al. (2013). Integrated multidisciplinary care in Parkinson's disease: A non-randomised, controlled trial (IMPACT). *Lancet Neurology*, *12*, 947–956.

Weintraub, D., Newberg, A. B., Cary, M. S., Siderowf, A. D., Moberg, P. J., Kleiner-Fisman, G., et al. (2005). Striatal dopamine transporter imaging correlates with anxiety and depression symptoms in Parkinson's disease. *Journal of Nuclear Medicine*, *46*, 227–232.

Zhang, Y., Zhang, X., Yeh, J., Richardson, P., & Bo, X. (2007). Engineered expression of polysialic acid enhances Purkinje cell axonal regeneration in L1/GAP-43 double transgenic mice. *The European Journal of Neuroscience*, *25*, 351–361.

Zhu, X. R., Maskri, L., Herold, C., Bader, V., Stichel, C. C., Gunturkun, O., et al. (2007). Non-motor behavioural impairments in parkin-deficient mice. *The European Journal of Neuroscience*, *26*, 1902–1911.

Zis, P., Martinez-Martin, P., Sauerbier, A., Rizos, A., Sharma, J. C., Worth, P. F., et al. (2015). Non-motor symptoms burden in treated and untreated early Parkinson's disease patients: Argument for non-motor subtypes. *European Journal of Neurology*, *22*, 1145–1150.

CHAPTER FOUR

The New Diagnostic Criteria for Parkinson's Disease[☆]

Ronald B. Postuma*,[1], Daniela Berg[†]
*L7-305 Montreal General Hospital, Montreal, Canada
[†]Christian-Albrechts-University of Kiel, Kiel, Germany
[1]Corresponding author: e-mail address: ron.postuma@mcgill.ca

Contents

Abstract

This chapter summarizes the advances in diagnosis of Parkinson's disease (PD) that were encapsulated in new International Parkinson Disease and Movement Disorders Society diagnostic criteria for PD. Numerous changes in our understanding of PD have occurred, including our understanding of the nonmotor profile of disease, the recognition of PD as a synucleinopathy, identification of genetic causes, novel hypotheses about spread of disease, etc. These have been reflected in a new definition of PD, which includes a clinicogenetic subtype of PD, removes dementia with Lewy Bodies as an exclusion criterion against PD, and recognizes multiple stages of early disease. The Clinical Diagnostic Criteria for PD reflect these changes and offer a new standardized diagnostic method for use in clinical research and even clinical practice. The criteria for prodromal PD use a method not seen in previous diagnostic criteria; they rely upon published studies of PD predictors to calculate the probability that any individual will develop PD. The field of PD

[☆]This chapter will begin with a brief introduction regarding the diagnosis of PD and existing criteria. We will then summarize the new diagnostic criteria for PD for its clinical and the research criteria for its prodromal stage.

International Review of Neurobiology, Volume 132
ISSN 0074-7742
http://dx.doi.org/10.1016/bs.irn.2017.01.008

is constantly advancing, and our methods of diagnosis need to advance with it; one hopes for a future filled with constant revisions and updates in our diagnostic methodology.

1. PARKINSON'S DISEASE DIAGNOSIS: HOW ACCURATE ARE WE?

There have been several studies assessing the accuracy of clinical diagnosis in Parkinson's disease (PD). The most comprehensive use pathologic validation, which generally require synuclein deposition.

Overall, positive predictive value of diagnosis by neurologists ranges from 65% to 90% at first diagnosis and 75%–99% at final diagnosis (Hughes, Ben-Shlomo, Daniel, & Lees, 1992; Hughes, Daniel, Ben-Shlomo, & Lees, 2002; Hughes, Daniel, Kilford, & Lees, 1992; Jellinger, Logroscino, Rizzo, et al., 2016; Tolosa, Wenning, & Poewe, 2006; Ward & Gibb, 1990). A recent meta-analysis found overall accuracy of 81% compared to pathologic gold standard (Rizzo et al., 2016). Recent studies may find slightly better results, with some exceptions (Adler, Beach, Hentz, et al., 2014; Rizzo et al., 2016), and specialist services generally perform better than nonspecialists (Tolosa et al., 2006). Other than level of expertise, disease duration is clearly important for accuracy. One recent study suggested that only 58% of diagnoses of probable PD coming to autopsy in the first 5 years were correct (compared to 88% of those with duration >5 years) (Adler et al., 2014). However, there are important caveats, including small sample size (i.e., 15 patients), advanced age in which confounds and nonspecific degeneration are common (average = 81 years at symptom onset), potential bias resulting from the fact that these patients who died in their first 5 years of illness had a malignant course (like one would see in atypical parkinsonisms), and inconsistency with the known prevalence of PD (PD accounts for 70%–80% of true parkinsonism in autopsy series).

The commonest discrete neurodegenerative pathological alternative diagnoses are progressive supranuclear palsy (PSP), multiple system atrophy (MSA), and secondary parkinsonisms such as "vascular parkinsonism," and intriguingly, frequent diagnoses of absent or nonspecific neurodegeneration (which may include nonparkinsonian conditions like essential tremor or medication-induced parkinsonism, but also true clinicogenetic PD—see later). Moreover, many series consider other Lewy body conditions (e.g., DLB) to be a false-negative diagnosis. This is no longer a diagnostic exclusion for PD (see later) (Berg, Postuma, Bloem, et al., 2014). Finally, pathology series may skew toward recruiting more atypical (i.e., difficult to diagnose) patients. All of these factors imply that accuracy may be somewhat higher than most studies estimate, particularly once new definitions of PD are taken into account.

2. PRIOR DIAGNOSTIC CRITERIA

Several diagnostic criteria for PD have been developed in the past (Calne, Snow, & Lee, 1992; Gelb, Oliver, & Gilman, 1999; Gibb & Lees, 1988; Litvan, Bhatia, Burn, et al., 2003). By far the commonest used are the UK brain bank criteria (Gibb & Lees, 1988). These criteria were designed to be used for assigning diagnosis in a pathologic series (i.e., they were not designed to be used by the broad PD community, but have been adapted by the community). They start with criteria for diagnosis of parkinsonism (bradykinesia, plus at least one of tremor, rigidity, or postural instability). A list of 16 exclusionary features is included, all of which rule out the diagnosis absolutely. A list of 8 supportive features is then listed (i.e., features that argue for parkinsonism). Probable PD can be defined by the absence of exclusionary features. A combination of 3 supportive and 0 exclusionary features makes a diagnosis of clinically definite PD.

In pathologic studies, the positive predictive value of UK brain bank is high (at least at death), in one study, 99% of patients who met clinically definite criteria had pathologic confirmation (Hughes, Daniel, et al., 1992). The reliability of *early* diagnosis with UK brain bank criteria has not been well studied; one would predict that since many exclusionary features take time to emerge, the reliability would be lower. For sensitivity, one study, approximately 90% of patients with PD at death met UK brain bank criteria. Of note, in this study the expert clinician's diagnosis was more sensitive than the criteria, without any loss of specificity (Hughes et al., 2002).

3. RATIONALE FOR NEW CRITERIA

Given the good performance of the UK brain bank criteria, why are new criteria needed? The obvious answer is that they are over 25 years old, and the field has moved immensely since then. Since the creation of these criteria, we now have identified synuclein as the hallmark of the disease, have recognized the vast nonmotor profile (including nonmotor markers that help diagnosis considerably), and have identified clear genetic forms of PD. Essentially this means that criteria are frequently invoked, but rarely followed accurately (for example, manuscripts may state that UK brain bank criteria were followed; however, patients exposed to atypical neuroleptics or those with familial PD are often nevertheless included).

In recognition of this, the MDS decided to create new diagnostic criteria for PD. These first criteria were created with the full understanding that science constantly advances. It is presumed (and hoped) that as our knowledge advances, these criteria will become outdated, and so will require constant revision.

4. UNDERLYING ASSUMPTIONS OF MDS CRITERIA: DEFINITION OF PD

As part of generating the new diagnostic criteria, the task force examined whether the core definition of PD itself needed to be changed. An introductory definition paper was published in 2014, outlining this process (Berg et al., 2014). The primary conclusions were:

1. It was recognized that the clinicopathologic diagnosis of PD (i.e., substantia nigra neuronal loss, accompanied by synuclein deposition) remains the predominant phenotype of PD. However, it is unclear if synuclein deposition is truly required, as there are exceptions. For example, patients with LRRK-2 mutations commonly have no synuclein on autopsy, despite having a clinical course indistinguishable from sporadic PD. Patients with parkin mutations almost never have synuclein deposition, despite having a progressive levodopa-responsive parkinsonism. To account for these exceptions, a category of "clinicogenetic PD" was created, as a PD subtype; this is defined as a genetic parkinsonism with neuronal degeneration of substantia nigra in which patients meet clinical diagnostic criteria for PD (as do most symptomatic gene carriers), but synuclein deposition may be absent. Depending on study context, this subtype may be included or excluded. The complex issue of genetic movement disorders and its nomenclature has recently been addressed by an MDS task force (Marras, Lang, van de Warrenburg, et al., 2016).
2. Early disease stages were defined. Early PD was divided into preclinical, prodromal, and clinical disease (see Section 9). Preclinical disease refers to a state in which neurodegeneration has started, but no symptoms or signs are evident (i.e., a biomarker diagnosis like a CSF, blood, or imaging marker, which is not yet generally possible). Clinical PD was defined as the presence of neurodegenerative parkinsonism (i.e., bradykinesia

plus one of rest tremor or rigidity). In between is prodromal PD; that is, symptoms or signs of neurodegeneration are present but are not at threshold for clinical PD. It was recognized that nonmotor features were crucial to the diagnosis of PD in these early stages and that criteria should be created for both prodromal and clinical stages.

3. It was recognized that there were clinical and pathologic subtypes of PD. However, the current means to define them was considered not sufficiently strong to create a formal subtype classification. This includes current classifiers; the task force considered that evidence is still insufficient to consider tremor-dominant vs akinetic–rigid disease, since prognosis and clinical features overlap strongly, and since patients often move from one subtype to the other.
4. Dementia with Lewy bodies should no longer be considered an exclusion criterion for PD. It was recognized that dementia is a common nonmotor symptom of PD that can occur at any stage. Many nonmotor manifestations (e.g., REM sleep behavior disorder, constipation, etc.) occur either before or after parkinsonism onset. Yet, these features never exclude PD if they are the first predominant symptom. By the same logic, dementia should be treated this way. Dementia with Lewy bodies certainly exists and should remain as a valid diagnosis (arguably PD patients with dementia might also be referred to as having DLB). However, the conditions are no longer mutually exclusive: patients with both PD and DLB can validly carry both diagnoses (just as RBD and PD, for example, are valid diagnoses that can be applied to one patient).

5. CLINICAL DIAGNOSTIC CRITERIA: OVERALL DESIGN

In generating the criteria, a clinical expert diagnosis was set as benchmark. It was recognized that although biomarkers are improving, they have not replaced the expert clinical diagnosis. The goal of the criteria was thus to mimic the diagnostic process of an expert clinician, codifying and standardizing this process. This implied the inclusion of both negative and positive features, differential weighting of features according to diagnostic strength, and allowance for clinical interpretation of individual criteria. In addition, time components were built into the criteria, so that features that were atypical in early disease were not inappropriately applied to late disease, and vice versa. Finally, because biomarkers are becoming increasingly used, and will expand in the future, the criteria now include diagnostic tests. These consist of one supportive criteria category (which currently includes olfaction and

MIBG scintigraphy), and an exclusion criterion for normal dopaminergic imaging.

What follows is a summary of the individual features of the criteria, along with a rationale for their use. For selected criteria, we have also outlined areas of discussion and interpretation.

5.1 Supportive Criteria

The main rationale for this set of criteria is to include those markers that increase likelihood of Parkinsonism, but which are frequently absent in true PD (and therefore cannot simply be delineated as "red flags" in reverse). Few previous diagnostic criteria incorporated these positive diagnostic features (the UK brain bank being a notable exception). There are four supportive criteria.

5.1.1 Clear and Dramatic Response to Dopamine Therapy

Levodopa response is the hallmark of PD, and arguably the most important key to diagnosis. However, defining what this means is by no means simple. Subtle benefits of dopaminergic treatment are common in other parkinsonian conditions like PSP and MSA. So, to meet this supportive criterion, there must be a dramatic response. The central definition of a dramatic response was a return to normal or near-normal function with treatment. Note that absence of any dopamine response is an absolute exclusion criterion (see later). Anything between these two states is not to be used in criteria.

There can be situations in which assessment is difficult. Patients may not recognize benefit even when clearly evident to bystanders; if the clinician feels that a reliable witness endorses dramatic benefit, the criteria can be applied. Also, in the case of very mild disease, benefits may not be obvious. Or, if treatment is started gradually, particularly with less potent agents, patients may not experience a dramatic effect, or may never return to near-normal function if they are undertreated. Moreover, some symptoms such as rest tremor and postural instability are often unpredictably responsive to medications. Therefore, we added additional situations that could represent an unequivocal response. These included marked responses to dose changes (i.e., generally 30% of UPDRS Part III scores), or clear and typical levodopa fluctuations (meaning starting with predictable end-of-dose off periods).

5.1.2 Levodopa-Induced Dyskinesia

There is no question that dyskinesia argue in favor of PD and are very unusual in atypical parkinsonism. It should be noted, this is not absolute, as patients particularly with MSA can experience dyskinesia. Facial dyskinesia/dystonia is especially common in MSA, and isolated facial dyskinesia should not be used as a supportive criterion.

5.1.3 Rest Tremor of a Limb

Although rest tremor is a core feature of parkinsonism, it also is useful in differential diagnosis. Clearly, the presence of an unequivocal rest tremor is less common in atypical parkinsonisms. The criteria specified occurrence in the limb because rest tremor in the face is harder to assess (i.e., it is difficult to define a resting state, making essential tremor a potential confound). Another reason to include tremor is that it is occasionally resistant to dopaminergic treatment, meaning that definition of a dramatic response to therapy is potentially confounded in tremor-dominant patients.

5.1.4 Diagnostic Testing

This is a feature that is new to criteria and is a sign of advances in the field of PD diagnosis. Hopefully, this section can be expanded upon considerably in the future. For inclusion in the criteria, the task force erred on the side of caution. Inclusion of a diagnostic test as a supportive feature requires at least three studies documenting that the test was 80% specific in the differential diagnosis of PD (i.e., not just distinguishing PD patients from controls) in studies that included at least 30 non-PD patients. A meta-analysis including smaller studies could substitute for one of these three studies.

On review of the literature, we found two diagnostic biomarkers that met this criterion. These included olfactory loss (which should be defined as unequivocal hyposmia, after adjustment for age) and abnormal cardiac MIBG scintigraphy.

It is hoped that this list would expand over time. Also, if multiple reliable tests are developed (and are independent of one another) future iterations of criteria could allow diagnostic testing to constitute more than one supportive criterion. Moreover, some normal diagnostic tests could be used as red flags or absolute exclusions, if they are sufficiently sensitive. For example, many studies of olfaction find sensitivity estimates that exceed 80%, especially with longer disease duration. It is certainly possible that normal olfaction after 5 years disease duration might be eventually be added as a red flag.

6. NEGATIVE CRITERIA

These are meant to outline the most important features that can reliably flag alternative syndromes. The main focus was on features of atypical parkinsonisms. However, we also included features that may indicate that the initial diagnosis of neurodegenerative parkinsonism was incorrect.

Atypical features vary considerably in their diagnostic importance; some essentially rule out the diagnosis of PD, whereas others make it somewhat less likely but are still seen in true PD. The full range of diagnostic importance cannot be easily captured in criteria designed for general use. However, we did divide negative features into absolute exclusions (rare in true PD, therefore incompatible with a diagnosis of probable PD) and red flags (relatively uncommon in true PD, but still occasionally seen). Red flags can still be compatible with a diagnosis of PD if at least an equal number of supporting features are present. The addition of a relatively weighted red flags category is new to diagnostic criteria. As opposed to simple checklists of negative features, they are a way to more accurately weight diagnostic information of intermediate specificity.

Just to note; in early drafts, some had difficulty understanding the time components. One does not need to wait until a time-restricted absolute exclusion is applied (if so, PD could not be diagnosed until at least 10 years duration!). So, if for example, severe orthostatic hypotension in the first 10 years is a red flag. If there is no severe orthostatic hypotension after 5 years of disease, one does not apply this red flag (i.e., not need to wait until 10 years to see if it emerges). If a patient has severe orthostatic hypotension at year 2, apply the red flag (i.e., no need to wait to ensure it is still present at 10 years). Finally, if severe orthostatic hypotension syndrome emerges only after 10 years of disease, do not apply the red flag.

We encourage some clinical judgment in application of negative criteria, just, as an expert would use all information available to weigh symptoms and signs. If there is an alternate *clear* explanation for an abnormality, then the clinician can choose to not apply it. Examples would be progressive gait impairment due to severe orthopedic abnormalities, urinary incontinence due to previous prostate cancer surgery, etc.

Finally, implicit in this criteria is that the evaluating clinician should have sufficient expertise to define the features. In general, the criteria should only be applied by physicians with special training in the recognition of subtle atypical signs (i.e., usually a neurologist would be required).

7. ABSOLUTE EXCLUSIONS

These rule out a diagnosis of probable PD, regardless of any supportive features. There are nine absolute exclusions:

1. Unequivocal cerebellar abnormalities on examination. These include cerebellar gait, limb ataxia, or cerebellar oculomotor abnormalities (e.g., sustained gaze-evoked nystagmus, macro square wave jerks, hypermetric saccades).

   This exclusion primarily will identify patients with MSA and spinocerebellar ataxia type 3. In general, it would be unusual for patients with neurodegenerative parkinsonism to have any clear cerebellar abnormalities.
2. Downward vertical supranuclear gaze palsy or selective slowing of downward vertical saccades.

   This is the hallmark feature of PSP, but can also be seen in other disorders like Niemann Pick Type C or Whipple's disease. Note that isolated loss of optokinetic response with otherwise normal saccades is of uncertain specificity, and probably would not constitute an absolute exclusion criterion.
3. Diagnosis of the probable behavioral variant of frontotemporal dementia or primary progressive aphasia, defined according to consensus criteria (Rascovsky, Hodges, Knopman, et al., 2011) within the first 5 years of disease.

   This particular criterion reflects the definition change of PD. Since DLB is no longer an exclusion criteria for PD, dementia per se is no longer considered an exclusion criterion. However, some forms of dementia can be signs of alternative disease. The most classic is frontotemporal dementia, which can be related to tau deposition, TDP-43 deposition, etc. Because dementia syndromes can be more difficult to delineate in advanced disease, we considered only early frontotemporal dementia as an absolute exclusion.

   This current exclusion criterion is relatively conservative; the consensus criteria are quite specific (and therefore may be insensitive). Mitigating this, most patients with dementia related to alternate pathology will have other negative features; for example, TDP-43-associated dementia syndromes might also have pyramidal tract signs, resulting in exclusion. Regardless, it is possible that future additions might include a broader definition for nonsynuclein-mediated dementia syndromes, perhaps as a red flag.

4. Parkinsonian features restricted to the lower limbs for more than 3 years.

   The pattern of "parkinsonism in the legs" can be seen in "vascular parkinsonism," normal pressure hydrocephalus, and other conditions particularly involving frontal lobe gait control. Typically, these patients have relatively normal facial expression and relatively preserved hand function. This pattern has not been found in pathologically confirmed PD.

5. Treatment with a dopamine receptor blocker or a dopamine-depleting agent in a dose and time-course consistent with drug-induced parkinsonism.

   Exclusion criteria targeted at drug-induced parkinsonism are part of many previous criteria. However since the development of atypical neuroleptics, adaptation is needed. The wording here explicitly asks the clinician to use clinical judgment. In the case of completely atypical neuroleptics such as clozapine, these criteria would presumably never be applied. However, certain "atypical" neuroleptics still have dopamine-blocking capability (e.g., risperidone, olanzpine), and so may be applied if the situation warrants. Also, clinicians frequently see patients with apparent drug-induced parkinsonism that improves when the agent is stopped, only to see the patient again several years later with true PD. This unmasking of latent PD can still be diagnosed as PD if the clinician feels the neuroleptic exposure no longer explains the parkinsonism.

6. Absence of observable response to high-dose levodopa despite at least moderate severity of disease.

   This is the converse of an excellent dopamine response. Again, this criteria required careful writing and careful interpretation to prevent it from being incorrectly invoked. Here, we stipulated that the medication must be levodopa, since it is the most reliably effective of PD medications. Moreover, the dose must be sufficient to ensure no response could have been seen (defined as at least 600 mg per day). In addition, the disease has to be severe enough to improve; which means there must be at least moderate rigidity or bradykinesia, corresponding to a UPDRS score of 3 of 1 of these items in the limbs (tremor was not included in this definition because it responds variably to therapy in true PD). Clinical judgment is required to ensure that the history is reliable; be particularly vigilant when there is no caregiver or second witness, or very gradual dose increases could have made benefit invisible. In the case of an unclear history, withdrawal of medications (± a second restart) can be used; a benchmark of absent response would be a difference of three points or less on the UPDRS Part III.

7. Unequivocal cortical sensory loss (i.e., graphesthesia, stereognosis with intact primary sensory modalities), clear limb ideomotor apraxia, or progressive aphasia.

   These are the hallmarks of the corticobasal syndrome, which is predominantly associated with either 4-repeat tauopathies (PSP, CBD), TDP-43 deposition, or Alzheimer pathology. Caution is needed to ensure that apraxia is not confused with primary sensory abnormalities, severe motor disability due to true parkinsonism, or inability to understand instructions due to cognitive impairment or language barrier.

8. Normal functional neuroimaging of the presynaptic dopaminergic system.

   This is another novel criterion, reflecting the utility of diagnostic testing in diagnosis of PD. A couple of essential points in interpreting this criterion should be understood. This criterion refers to a normal scan—that is, one clearly in the normal range. If the scan results are uncertain (i.e., borderline low levels), the criterion should not be applied (note that the scan could also be repeated some months later in the case of uncertain results). Second, the task force wished to emphasize that inclusion of the criterion was in no way to be interpreted as a requirement (or even an encouragement) to perform dopaminergic functional testing for diagnosis. In the practice of many task force members, such scans are ordered only in a small minority of patients. The utility of adding dopaminergic scans to clinical diagnosis remains unproven. Of note, abnormal scans are not helpful in the differential diagnosis of parkinsonism (the scan only helps diagnose the presence of neurodegenerative parkinsonism).

   Note that previous studies have strongly suggested that the large majority of SWEDD patients did not have PD (Erro, Schneider, Stamelou, Quinn, & Bhatia, 2015); however, recent studies, particularly from the PPMI are documenting that some SWEDD patients have substantial nonmotor features. Studies of the diagnostic reliability of dopaminergic imaging have also suggested specificities below the threshold for an absolute exclusion; however, these studies would include borderline patients, which are excluded here. Regardless, depending upon results of future research, future iterations could include borderline results as red flags, or even downgrade normal scans from absolute exclusions to red flags.

9. Documentation of an alternative condition known to produce parkinsonism and plausibly connected to the patient's symptoms, or the expert evaluating physician, based on the full diagnostic assessment, believes that an alternative syndrome is more likely than PD.

   This criterion essentially allows a clinician to override a diagnosis of probable PD. It was included mainly as a back-up, in the case that some diagnostic information or clinical findings not included in the criteria makes a diagnosis of PD unlikely. Obviously, this would require considerable clinical judgment and expertise before applying this exclusion criterion, again reinforcing why experts are needed to apply the criteria. Finally, as a reminder, DLB is not considered an alternative diagnosis in the definition of PD. Therefore, a patient carrying a diagnosis of DLB can still be diagnosed with PD, and this exclusion criterion should not be applied.

8. RED FLAGS

These features rule out PD if they are multiple (i.e., more than 2), or if the number of red flags exceeds the number of supportive criteria.

1. Rapid progression of gait impairment requiring regular use of wheelchair within 5 years of onset.

   Severe gait impairment is a hallmark feature of many of the atypical parkinsonisms, especially PSP and MSA. "Regular use" implies that the patient requires a wheelchair frequently (i.e., shopping, medical appointments, etc.), but does not require that a patient be completely confined to the wheelchair. This feature can be seen in PD, particularly in older persons with the postural-instability-gait-predominant subtype, so did not warrant an absolute exclusion.

2. A complete absence of progression of motor symptoms or signs over 5 or more years unless stability is related to treatment.

   This red flag was meant to highlight those who may have been initially diagnosed with parkinsonism, but who have no underlying neurodegeneration. This could involve cases of dopamine-responsive dystonia, essential tremor with rest overflow, dystonic tremor, etc. Some true PD patients are relatively slow progressors, so a minimum duration of 5 years was added to ensure these were not flagged as non-PD. In addition, there must be some in-person documentation of the lack of progression (since some patients may not notice progression, or may inaccurately perceive symptom onset).

3. Early bulbar dysfunction, defined as one of severe dysphonia, dysarthria (speech unintelligible most of the time), or severe dysphagia (requiring soft food, nasogastral tube, or gastrostomy feeding) within the first 5 years of disease.

   Although PD patients often experience swallowing dysfunction and dysphonia, these are usually relatively mild in early stages of disease. Such severe bulbar dysfunction is classic of PSP as well as MSA. It is important to emphasize that the red flag is only triggered if the dysfunction is very severe in early stages of disease.

4. Inspiratory respiratory dysfunction defined as either diurnal or nocturnal inspiratory stridor or frequent inspiratory sighs.

   Inspiratory stridor is a classic sign of MSA. It usually predominates at nighttime, but can also be heard during wakefulness. It is related to disco-ordination of laryngeal relaxation, such that the vocal cords close during inspiration. The task force felt that clear inspiratory stridor is best considered an absolute exclusion feature, as it is almost never seen in PD. However, since documentation of this feature requires a reliable witness (and a caregiver observed the feature during nighttime when they themselves may not be fully alert), we were concerned that sounds other than true stridor may be inaccurately called stridor. Therefore, this was downgraded to a red flag.

5. Severe autonomic failure in the first 5 years of disease. This can include:
   - Orthostatic hypotension: orthostatic decrease of blood pressure within 3 min of standing by at least 30 mm Hg systolic or 15 mm Hg diastolic, in the absence of dehydration, medication, or other diseases that could plausibly explain autonomic dysfunction.
   - Severe urinary incontinence or urinary retention (excluding long-standing low-volume stress incontinence in women), which is not simply functional incontinence (i.e., inability to get to the bathroom in a reasonable time). In men, urinary retention must not be caused by prostate disease, and this must be associated with erectile dysfunction.

     Severe autonomic dysfunction is a defining feature of MSA. In some previous criteria, even moderate autonomic denervation served as an exclusion criterion, and orthostatic hypotension is the core of MSA criteria (Gilman, Lost, Low, et al., 2008). However, recent research has found that orthostatic hypotension is quite common in PD, occurring in approximately 30% (Velseboer, de Haan, Wieling, Goldstein, & de Bie, 2011). Therefore, this criteria were worded carefully to make sure that only severe and early orthostatic hypotension was identified, ensuring no clear alternate explanation for the finding was present, and delineating it a red flag rather than an absolute exclusion.

The urinary section was worded carefully to avoid confounds already assessed in other red flags; for example, functional incontinence resulting from reduced mobility would already be captured in the wheelchair red flag. In men with MSA, urinary incontinence of this severity is almost always accompanied by severe erectile dysfunction (erectile dysfunction usually occurs first). Therefore, to prevent misdiagnosis of prostate disease, etc., we inserted the erectile dysfunction requirement. Unlike stress incontinence, in which small amounts of urine leak from cough or straining, the urinary incontinence in PD is generally urge incontinence. Note that urinary retention is usually not related to PD, but is a common feature of MSA.

6. Recurrent (>1/year) falls because of impaired balance within 3 years of onset.

   This is another feature in which the time course is of essence. Falls occur in most patients with PD at some point in their illness; however, the presence of early falls is one of the most commonly defined signs of an alternative diagnosis. Note that this criterion requires clinical judgment to determine that impaired balance was critical to generating the fall. So, falls on ice in winter, or while playing tennis, or because someone is knocked down do not constitute red flag, if the clinician feels that someone with preserved balance would have fallen down in the same circumstance. Syncope should also not be counted, to prevent double-counting of orthostatic hypotension.

7. The presence of disproportionate anterocollis (dystonic in nature) or contractures of hand or feet within the first 10 years.

   The "dropped head" sign is a classic feature of MSA; it can be seen occasionally in advanced PD, but generally not within the first 10 years. Note that this is distinct from the stooped posture that is a classic feature of PD (which is generally more truncal). Contractures are often seen in MSA as well, as well as other very severe atypical parkinsonisms, but are uncommon in PD.

8. Absence of any of the common nonmotor features of disease despite 5 years disease duration. These include:

- Sleep dysfunction: sleep-maintenance insomnia, excessive daytime somnolence, symptoms of rapid eye movement sleep behavior disorder.
- Autonomic dysfunction: constipation, daytime urinary urgency (i.e., not simply nocturia), symptomatic orthostasis.
- Hyposmia.
- Psychiatric dysfunction: depression, anxiety, or hallucinations.

  This red flag is novel to any criteria and reflects our advances in the understanding of nonmotor PD. Occasionally, one sees a patient with PD who has complete absence of nonmotor symptoms, but it is unusual for this state to persist beyond a few years. The nonmotor features listed here have prevalence well over 40% in most studies, and hyposmia is seen in most patients with PD. Collectively, 10% or less of PD patients will not have a single one of these at 5 years disease duration. Like the "nonprogression" red flag, this will predominantly target those misdiagnosed with neurodegenerative parkinsonism (essential tremor, dystonic tremor, etc).

9. Otherwise unexplained pyramidal tract signs, defined as pyramidal weakness or clear pathologic hyperreflexia (excluding mild reflex asymmetry in the more affected limb, and isolated extensor plantar response).

   Pyramidal dysfunction is a classic feature of MSA and also can be seen in "vascular parkinsonism." Note the exceptions to this red flag are important. It is common to see a mild increase in deep tendon reflexes on the affected side, perhaps suggesting an effect of motor activation. In severe parkinsonism, one can often see a "striatal toe," which is an isolated upgoing first toe that can occur independent of plantar stimulation; this should not be included. Finally, many elderly patients may have increased reflexes due to cervical stenosis, or unrelated strokes; these should not be included.

10. Bilateral symmetric parkinsonism throughout the disease course. The patient or caregiver reports bilateral symptom onset with no side predominance, and no side predominance is observed on objective examination.

    This red flag reflects the (as yet unexplained) phenomenon of unilaterality in PD. The majority of PD patients will either have onset of symptoms on one side, or a side predominance on objective examination. Caution is suggested here in the case of very well-treated parkinsonism, in which signs are minimal; it is important to check the medical record to ensure that the pretreatment examination was truly symmetric. On the other hand, it is possible that in very advanced disease, signs are "at floor" and so appear symmetric. In this case, one would query patients and caregivers for reports of asymmetry. As with all features, if the examiner is uncertain, the red flag should not be applied. For example, if no reliable history is available, the red flag does not apply.

A summary of the criteria, from the original publication are presented in Table 1 (Postuma, Berg, Stern, et al., 2015).

9. THE MDS PRODROMAL CRITERIA

The prodromal criteria have a different purpose, which is to identify patients who are in the neurodegenerative state, which may eventually lead to clinical PD. Thus, they have signs or symptoms of Parkinson's disease, but these are not yet advanced enough to define full clinical PD. Currently, identification of prodromal PD is of uncertain clinical benefit, since neuroprotective therapy is not available. So, for now these are intended as research criteria only, for example, to identify candidates for neuroprotective trials against early PD stages or as candidates for cohort studies designed to better understand the course of the prediagnostic phase.

These criteria became possible because of impressive advances in the understanding of how to predict clinical PD. There are now many markers that have been proven to identify prodromal stages in prospective cohort studies. Much of these markers are nonmotor, and derive from the fact that the substantia nigra may be involved relatively late in the disease process, after olfactory, peripheral autonomic, and lower brainstem areas are affected (Braak & Del, 2008). However, most prodromal features of PD are relatively nonspecific; that is, patients may have an abnormal marker for reasons that have nothing to do with neurodegenerative synucleinopathy. Therefore, it is impossible to be certain that any patient with any combination of markers has prodromal PD.

In defining the state of prodromal PD, the task force considered that probable prodromal PD would be defined as an 80% likelihood of neurodegenerative Lewy body disease being present (although different probability thresholds might be defined by researchers depending on the specific nature of the research study). The difficulty is how to define this, given that many possible combinations of prodromal markers could be present or absent in any given patient.

Table 1 MDS Clinical Diagnostic Criteria for PD—Executive Summary/Completion Form

The first essential criterion is parkinsonism, which is defined as bradykinesia, in combination with at least one of rest tremor or rigidity. Examination of all cardinal manifestations should be carried out as described in the MDS-Unified Parkinson Disease Rating Scale (Goetz, Tilley, Shaftman, et al., 2008). Once parkinsonism has been diagnosed:

Diagnosis of Clinically Established PD requires:

(1) absence of absolute exclusion criteria,
(2) at least two supportive criteria, and
(3) no red flags

Diagnosis of Clinically Probable PD requires:

(1) absence of absolute exclusion criteria
(2) presence of red flags counterbalanced by supportive criteria
  - If one red flag is present there must also be at least one supportive criterion.
  - If two red flags, at least two supportive criteria are needed.
  - No more than two red flags are allowed for this category.

Supportive criteria (Check box if criteria met)

☐ 1. Clear and dramatic beneficial response to dopaminergic therapy. During initial treatment, patient returned to normal or near-normal level of function. In the absence of clear documentation of initial response a dramatic response can be classified as:
  (a) Marked improvement with dose increases or marked worsening with dose decreases. Mild changes do not qualify. Document this either objectively (>30% in UPDRS III with change in treatment) or subjectively (clearly documented history of marked changes from a reliable patient or caregiver).
  (b) Unequivocal and marked on/off fluctuations, which must have at some point included predictable end-of-dose wearing off.

☐ 2. Presence of levodopa-induced dyskinesia.

☐ 3. Rest tremor of a limb, documented on clinical examination (in past, or on current exam)

☐ 4. The presence of either olfactory loss or cardiac sympathetic denervation on MIBG scintigraphy

Absolute exclusion criteria: The presence of any of these features rules out PD:

☐ 1. Unequivocal cerebellar abnormalities, such as cerebellar gait, limb ataxia, or cerebellar oculomotor abnormalities (e.g., sustained gaze-evoked nystagmus, macro square wave jerks, hypermetric saccades).

☐ 2. Downward vertical supranuclear gaze palsy or selective slowing of downward vertical saccades.

Continued

Table 1 MDS Clinical Diagnostic Criteria for PD—Executive Summary/Completion Form—cont'd

☐ 3. Diagnosis of probable behavioral variant frontotemporal dementia or primary progressive aphasia, defined according to consensus criteria (Rascovsky et al., 2011) within the first 5 years of disease.
☐ 4. Parkinsonian features restricted to the lower limbs for more than 3 years.
☐ 5. Treatment with a dopamine receptor blocker or a dopamine-depleting agent in a dose and time-course consistent with drug-induced parkinsonism.
☐ 6. Absence of observable response to high-dose levodopa despite at least moderate severity of disease.
☐ 7. Unequivocal cortical sensory loss (i.e., graphesthesia, stereognosis with intact primary sensory modalities), clear limb ideomotor apraxia, or progressive aphasia.
☐ 8. Normal functional neuroimaging of the presynaptic dopaminergic system.
☐ 9. Documentation of an alternative condition known to produce parkinsonism and plausibly connected to the patient's symptoms, or, the expert evaluating physician, based upon the full diagnostic assessment feels that an alternative syndrome is *more likely* than PD.
Red flags
☐ 1. Rapid progression of gait impairment requiring regular use of wheelchair within 5 years of onset.
☐ 2. A complete absence of progression of motor symptoms or signs over 5 or more years unless stability is related to treatment.
☐ 3. Early bulbar dysfunction: *severe* dysphonia/dysarthria (speech unintelligible most of the time) and/or severe dysphagia (requiring soft food, NG tube, or gastrostomy feeding) within first 5 years.
☐ 4. Inspiratory respiratory dysfunction: either diurnal or nocturnal inspiratory stridor and/or frequent inspiratory sighs.
☐ 5. Severe autonomic failure in the first 5 years of disease. This can include: (a) Orthostatic hypotension (Gilman et al., 2008)—orthostatic decrease of blood pressure within 3 min of standing by at least 30 mm Hg systolic or 15 mm Hg diastolic, in the absence of dehydration, medication, or other diseases that could plausibly explain autonomic dysfunction, or (b) Severe urinary retention or urinary incontinence in the first 5 years of disease (excluding long-standing or small amount stress incontinence in women), that is not simply functional incontinence. In men, urinary retention must not be due to prostate disease, and must be associated with erectile dysfunction.

Table 1 MDS Clinical Diagnostic Criteria for PD—Executive Summary/Completion Form—cont'd

☐	6. Recurrent (>1/year) falls due to impaired balance within 3 years of onset.
☐	7. Disproportionate anterocollis (dystonic) and/or contractures of hand or feet within the first 10 years.
☐	8. Absence of any of the common nonmotor features of disease despite 5 years disease duration. These include sleep dysfunction (sleep-maintenance insomnia, excessive daytime somnolence, symptoms of REM sleep behavior disorder), autonomic dysfunction (constipation, daytime urinary urgency, symptomatic orthostasis), hyposmia, or psychiatric dysfunction (depression, anxiety, or hallucinations).
☐	9. Otherwise unexplained pyramidal tract signs, defined as pyramidal weakness and/or clear pathologic hyperreflexia (excluding mild reflex asymmetry and isolated extensor plantar response).
☐	10. Bilateral symmetric parkinsonism. The patient or caregiver reports bilateral symptom onset with no side predominance, *and* no side predominance is observed on objective examination.

Criteria Application:

1. Does the patient have parkinsonism, as defined by the MDS criteria?	Yes ☐ No ☐
If no, *neither* probable PD nor clinically established PD can be diagnosed. *If yes*:	
2. Are any absolute exclusion criteria present?	Yes ☐ No ☐
If "yes," *neither* probable PD nor clinically established PD can be diagnosed. *If no*:	
3. Number of red flags present	____
4. Number of supportive criteria present	____
5. Are there at least two supportive criteria *and* no red flags?	Yes ☐ No ☐
If yes, patient meets criteira for *clinically established PD*. *If no*:	
6. Are there more than two red flags?	Yes ☐ No ☐
If "yes," probable PD *cannot* be diagnosed. *If no*:	
7. Is the number of red flags equal to, or less than, the number of supportive criteria?	Yes ☐ No ☐
If yes, patient meets criteria for *probable PD*	

Since each prodromal marker would be included based on prospective studies that documented its diagnostic utility, the task force elected to use the information embedded in these studies to calculate probability. Each study would have estimates of predictive power, including sensitivity and specificity of each marker (although for some studies, this would have to be estimated based upon other information). Assuming these markers are independent (which appears to be largely true for most categories of markers based upon estimates in the general population and in populations with idiopathic RBD), markers can be combined to estimate probability.

The means to combine diagnostic information together is termed the Bayesian naive classifier. In this classifier, one starts with a pretest probability; in this case, the chance of prodromal PD without any other information. We calculated this as an age-dependent variable, using published estimates of PD prevalence, PD incidence, lifetime PD risk, and prospective cohort studies and assuming an average prodromal PD duration of 10 years. Because of low baseline probability, and the uncertainty in interpreting markers at young ages, we applied this only to those 50 years and older. We estimate baseline probability of prodromal PD in Table 3.

The next step is to add diagnostic information. Sensitivities and specificities of each diagnostic marker are converted into likelihood ratios (LR). A LR+ is a positive diagnostic test which increases likelihood of PD; LR+ is calculated as sensitivity/1—specificity. A LR− is a negative test that decreases likelihood; LR− is calculated as 1—sensitivity/specificity. The advantage of LR is that unlike relative risk, they can be multiplied by each other. Based upon published papers, the LR for each marker was calculated. We assessed both risk markers and prodromal markers; however, the disease cannot be diagnosed based upon risk alone. Prodromal markers with a total LR+ of at least four must also be present in order to diagnose PD. Although the criteria are valid regardless of the amount of diagnostic information available, it is important to try and collect all available information (e.g., sex should always be added to the model, and easily assessed factors such as smoking/constipation should be known in most patients). Moreover, it is recognized that cutoffs for abnormal values can vary between contexts and test procedures; in general, results of any testing must be clearly normal or abnormal compared to controls, before LR for any test is applied.

The prodromal markers are summarized in Table 2. This has been updated as of 2016, to reflect several new studies that were not included in the original criteria (Gibbons & Freeman, 2015; Postuma et al., 2016).

Table 2 Prodromal Markers of PD

	LR +	LR −
Risk markers		
Male sex	1.2 (male)	0.8 (female)
Regular pesticide exposure	1.5	n/a
Occupational solvent exposure	1.5	n/a
Nonuse of caffeine	1.35	0.88
Smoking		
Current smoker	n/a	0.45
Never smoker	1.25	n/a
Former smoker	n/a	0.8
Sibling had PD with age onset <50	7.5	n/a
Any other first degree relative with PD	2.5	n/a
Known gene mutation	Berg et al. (2015)	n/a
Substantia nigra hyperechogenicity	4.7	0.45
Prodromal markers		
Polysomnogram-proven RBD or Positive RBD screen questionnaire with >80% specificity or Probable RBD diagnosed on expert interview (specialist in sleep medicine)	130 2.3 50	0.62 0.76 0.62
Dopaminergic PET/SPECT clearly abnormal (e.g., <65% normal, 2 SD below mean)	40	0.65
Possible subthreshold parkinsonism (UPDRS >3 excluding action tremor) or Abnormal quantitative motor testing	10 3.5	0.7 0.60
Olfactory loss	4.0	0.43
Constipation	2.2	0.80
Excessive daytime somnolence	2.2	0.88
Symptomatic hypotension	5.2	0.80
Severe erectile dysfunction	2	0.90
Urinary dysfunction	1.9	0.90
Depression (± anxiety)	1.8	0.85

Table 3 Likelihood Ratio Thresholds for Diagnosis of Prodromal PD

Age	Prior Probability (%)	LR for Probable Prodromal PD
50–54	0.4	1000
55–59	0.75	515
60–64	1.25	300
65–69	2.0	180
70–74	2.5	155
75–79	3.5	110
>80	4.0	95

Please see the original criteria for the references used in generating LR (Berg, Postuma, Adler, et al., 2015).

Each test is considered independently and added to the overall diagnostic picture. This is done by multiplying all LR by each other, to generate a total LR for that patient. If no information for a prodromal marker is present, or if results of testing are borderline or uncertain, it is not added to the equation (i.e., LR for that variable is 1). The total LR for the patient is then compared with the LR needed to obtain a diagnosis of probable prodromal PD (Table 3). If above the threshold, probable prodromal PD can be calculated. If desired, the exact probability can also be calculated; the mathematics is relatively simple, and many Bayesian calculators are available online (e.g., http://araw.mede.uic.edu/cgi-bin/testcalc.pl).

Here is an illustrative example.

A 58-year-old man is being evaluated for possible prodromal PD. He reports no occupational pesticide exposure, does not drink coffee, and was a former smoker. He has idiopathic RBD, olfactory loss, constipation, preserved erectile function, no depression or anxiety, and no daytime somnolence. Quantitative motor testing was in the borderline/low-normal range (there was no expert examination available), so results were uncertain. One would then calculate as follows:

Step 1 Establish the prior from the table = 0.75%.

Step 2 Calculate total LR = 1.2 (male) × 1.0 (pesticide) × 1.35 (coffee) × 0.8 (former smoker) × 130 (RBD) × 4.0 (olfaction) × 2.2 (constipation) × 0.90 (normal erection) × 0.85 (no depression or anxiety) × 0.88 (no somnolence) × 1.0 (borderline motor testing – result omitted) = 998.

Step 3 Check against the threshold—This exceeds the threshold for his age (515), so he meets criteria for probable prodromal PD.

As a final caution, although it is quite simple and tempting to apply the LR to any individual who fears PD, at this stage, this approach is only meant be applied for research. It is the first time a statistical approach has been used to define the presence of a neurological disease. Further studies are needed to validate the criteria and especially to improve precision of probability estimates. Moreover, as long as there is no way to intervene in the prodromal stage of neurodegenerative diseases, the benefit of a prodromal diagnosis is very unclear. Nevertheless, this approach is a first step toward development and testing of disease-modifying therapies for the earliest phases of PD.

10. CONCLUSIONS

The field of PD is rapidly advancing, and so is our definition of PD. The current conception of PD has now been reflected in new diagnostic criteria. The goal of the clinical criteria is to help advance research and clinical care, by improving diagnostic accuracy in clinical settings where expertise in PD may be less, and standardizing diagnosis for clinical trials. The goal of the prodromal criteria is to open up a new area of PD treatment at the earliest stages of disease, where it may be most effective.

It should never be forgotten that the field of PD is rapidly advancing and much will change. Clinical criteria will change as we develop new diagnostic procedures. Prodromal criteria will change even more as we discover new markers and refine estimates of sensitivity and specificity. Nevertheless, the structures of criteria represent a scaffold for future advances and are a step along the journey to a fuller understanding of PD.

REFERENCES

Adler, C. H., Beach, T. G., Hentz, J. G., et al. (2014). Low clinical diagnostic accuracy of early vs advanced Parkinson disease: Clinicopathologic study. *Neurology*, *83*(5), 406–412.

Berg, D., Postuma, R. B., Adler, C. H., et al. (2015). MDS research criteria for prodromal Parkinson's disease. *Movement Disorders*, *30*(12), 1600–1611.

Berg, D., Postuma, R. B., Bloem, B., et al. (2014). Time to redefine PD? Introductory statement of the MDS Task Force on the definition of Parkinson's disease. *Movement Disorders*, *29*(4), 454–462.

Braak, H., & Del, T. K. (2008). Invited article: Nervous system pathology in sporadic Parkinson disease. *Neurology*, *70*(20), 1916–1925.

Calne, D. B., Snow, B. J., & Lee, C. (1992). Criteria for diagnosing Parkinson's disease. *Annals of Neurology*, *32*(Suppl.), S125–S127.

Erro, R., Schneider, S. A., Stamelou, M., Quinn, N. P., & Bhatia, K. P. (2015). What do patients with scans without evidence of dopaminergic deficit (SWEDD) have? New evidence and continuing controversies. *Journal of Neurology, Neurosurgery, and Psychiatry, 87*, 319–323.

Gelb, D. J., Oliver, E., & Gilman, S. (1999). Diagnostic criteria for Parkinson disease. *Archives of Neurology, 56*(1), 33–39.

Gibb, W. R., & Lees, A. J. (1988). The relevance of the Lewy body to the pathogenesis of idiopathic Parkinson's disease. *Journal of Neurology, Neurosurgery, and Psychiatry, 51*(6), 745–752.

Gibbons, C. H., & Freeman, R. (2015). Clinical implications of delayed orthostatic hypotension: A 10-year follow-up study. *Neurology, 85*(16), 1362–1367.

Gilman, S., Lost, D., Low, P. A., et al. (2008). Second consensus statement on the diagnosis of multiple system atrophy. *Neurology, 71*(9), 670–676.

Goetz, C. G., Tilley, B. C., Shaftman, S. R., et al. (2008). Movement Disorder Society-sponsored revision of the Unified Parkinson's Disease Rating Scale (MDS-UPDRS): Scale presentation and clinimetric testing results. *Movement Disorders, 23*(15), 2129–2170.

Hughes, A. J., Ben-Shlomo, Y., Daniel, S. E., & Lees, A. J. (1992). What features improve the accuracy of clinical diagnosis in Parkinson's disease: A clinicopathologic study. *Neurology, 42*(6), 1142–1146.

Hughes, A. J., Daniel, S. E., Ben-Shlomo, Y., & Lees, A. J. (2002). The accuracy of diagnosis of parkinsonian syndromes in a specialist movement disorder service. *Brain, 125*(Pt. 4), 861–870.

Hughes, A. J., Daniel, S. E., Kilford, L., & Lees, A. J. (1992). Accuracy of clinical diagnosis of idiopathic Parkinson's disease: A clinico-pathological study of 100 cases. *Journal of Neurology, Neurosurgery, and Psychiatry, 55*(3), 181–184.

Jellinger, K. A., Logroscino, G., Rizzo, G., et al. (2016). Accuracy of clinical diagnosis of Parkinson disease: A systematic review and meta-analysis. *Neurology, 87*(2), 237–238.

Litvan, I., Bhatia, K. P., Burn, D. J., et al. (2003). Movement disorders society scientific issues committee report: SIC Task Force appraisal of clinical diagnostic criteria for Parkinsonian disorders. *Movement Disorders, 18*(5), 467–486.

Marras, C., Lang, A., van de Warrenburg, B. P., et al. (2016). Nomenclature of genetic movement disorders: Recommendations of the international Parkinson and movement disorder society task force. *Movement Disorders, 31*(4), 436–457.

Postuma, R. B., Berg, D., Stern, M., et al. (2015). MDS clinical diagnostic criteria for Parkinson's disease. *Movement Disorders, 30*(12), 1591–1600.

Postuma, R. B., Pelletier, A., Berg, D., Gagnon, J.-F., Escudier, F., & Montplaisir, J. (2016). Screening for prodromal Parkinson's disease in the general community: A sleep-based approach. *Sleep Medicine, 21*, 101–105.

Rascovsky, K., Hodges, J. R., Knopman, D., et al. (2011). Sensitivity of revised diagnostic criteria for the behavioural variant of frontotemporal dementia. *Brain, 134*(Pt. 9), 2456–2477.

Rizzo, G., Copetti, M., Arcuti, S., Martino, D., Fontana, A., & Logroscino, G. (2016). Accuracy of clinical diagnosis of Parkinson disease: A systematic review and meta-analysis. *Neurology, 86*(6), 566–576.

Tolosa, E., Wenning, G., & Poewe, W. (2006). The diagnosis of Parkinson's disease. *Lancet Neurology, 5*(1), 75–86.

Velseboer, D. C., de Haan, R. J., Wieling, W., Goldstein, D. S., & de Bie, R. M. (2011). Prevalence of orthostatic hypotension in Parkinson's disease: A systematic review and meta-analysis. *Parkinsonism & Related Disorders, 17*(10), 724–729.

Ward, C. D., & Gibb, W. R. (1990). Research diagnostic criteria for Parkinson's disease. *Advances in Neurology, 53*, 245–249.

CHAPTER FIVE

Advances in the Clinical Differential Diagnosis of Parkinson's Disease

Sebastian R. Schreglmann*, Kailash P. Bhatia*, Maria Stamelou[†,‡,§,1]
*Institute of Neurology, UCL, London, United Kingdom
†University of Athens Medical School, Hospital Attikon, Athens, Greece
‡HYGEIA Hospital, Athens, Greece
§Philipps University, Marburg, Germany
[1]Corresponding author: e-mail address: mariastamelou@gmail.com

Contents

Abstract

The differential diagnosis of Parkinson's disease has widened considerably in recent years. This chapter aims to summarize the current knowledge on the clinical differential diagnoses of sporadic Parkinson's disease. As the number of monogenic familial Parkinson's disease variants and risk factors is growing, so is the number of appreciated etiologies of atypical parkinsonian and other pallidopyramidal syndromes. This work aims at summarizing the current knowledge on both motor and nonmotor neurological signs and symptoms that aid the clinical diagnosis of Parkinson's disease and its differential diagnoses.

International Review of Neurobiology, Volume 132
ISSN 0074-7742
http://dx.doi.org/10.1016/bs.irn.2017.01.007

ABBREVIATIONS

AD Alzheimer's disease
CBD corticobasal degeneration
CBS corticobasal syndrome
DLB dementia with Lewy bodies
DRPLA dentate-rubro-pallidoluysian atrophy
ET essential tremor
FBS frontal behavioral-spatial syndrome
GBA glucocerebrosidase
HD Huntington's disease
NAV nonfluent, agrammatic variant of primary progressive aphasia
MSA multiple system atrophy
NBIA neurodegeneration with brain iron accumulation
NMS nonmotor symptoms
PD Parkinson's disease
PDD Parkinson's disease dementia
PPTg pedunculopontine tegmental nuclei
POLG polymerase gamma
PIGD postural instability gait disorder
PSP progressive supranuclear palsy
RBD REM-sleep behavior disorder
SWEDDs scans without evidence of dopaminergic deficit

1. INTRODUCTION

Parkinson's disease (PD) is the second most common neurodegenerative disease in the developed world. In neurological practice its recognition and treatment form a major part of daily routine work for clinicians around the globe. Recent years were marked especially by the increasing recognition of genetic factors playing a role as susceptibility risk factors as well as monogenic causes of parkinsonian conditions (Bras, Guerreiro, & Hardy, 2015), and it is now generally acknowledged that around 10% of cases of PD are of familial origin (de Lau & Breteler, 2006), with the remaining 90% bulk of cases being sporadic. Without doubt, the additional knowledge of the genetics of this disease has shaped our understanding of PD as a disease process and has shed light on a number of processes involved in its pathophysiology (Singleton & Hardy, 2016). At the same time, the scope of differential diagnoses has widened and poses a particular challenge, as their identification mainly relies on clinical characteristics. With the ever-growing number of phenotypical descriptions of parkinsonian syndromes with and without associated genetic ramifications, a sound phenotypical classification based predominantly on symptoms and clinical findings remains key to the establishment of the correct diagnosis. A meta-analysis of the clinicopathological studies for the diagnosis of PD of the past 25 years revealed that the diagnostic accuracy for PD is still suboptimal and reaches 74% in an nonexpert and around 84% in a specialist setting, with other tremor disorders, atypical parkinsonian conditions, and secondary parkinsonism being the most frequent misdiagnoses (Rizzo et al., 2016).

As PD is increasingly conceptualized as several different diseases within a phenotypic spectrum (Berg et al., 2014), clinical skills will remain quintessential to identify subgroups with potentially different cause and—possibly in the future—treatment. Similarly, in the absence of a universally available PD biomarker and the growing recognition of parkinsonian conditions beyond PD and the classical atypical parkinsonian disorders, clinicians continue to depend on their clinical assessment, using all information accessible. This increasing knowledge has led to new clinical criteria for PD and for prodromal PD (Postuma et al., 2015). This chapter aims at helping in the clinical differential diagnosis of PD from other parkinsonian conditions.

2. PHENOTYPIC VARIABILITY AND CLINICAL HETEROGENEITY OF PARKINSON'S DISEASE

2.1 Age at Onset

Since the very first clinical description of PD by its namesake 200 years ago (Parkinson, 2002), a connection between PD prevalence and advancing age has been established. While sporadic PD is only rarely diagnosed before the age of 50 (Van Den Eeden et al., 2003), its annual incidence in both sexes has been reported to increase with advancing age from 3.1 per 100,000 for the age of 40–49 years to 17.4 per 100,000 (50–59 years), 52.5 per 100,000 (60–69 years), and 93.1 per 100,000 (70–79 years) in a large, community-based cohort (Bower, Maraganore, McDonnell, & Rocca, 1999, 2000). In terms of absolute incidence rate this might still be an underestimation, as door-to-door prevalence studies showed consistently 39%–53% higher incidences than record-based studies (Benito-León et al., 2004; de Lau et al., 2004). Similarly, worldwide PD prevalence increases with advancing age, as corroborated in a methodologically sound meta-analysis on all published door-to-door or population-based random sampling assessments of the condition: 41 per 100,000 (40–49 years), 107 per 100,000 (50–59 years),

428 per 100,000 (60–69 years), 1078 per 100,000 (70–79 years), and 1903 per 100,000 above 80 years of age (Pringsheim, Jette, Frolkis, & Steeves, 2014).

Conscious of the association with age, in clinical practice patients presenting with earlier onset of suggestive clinical features have been labeled as "early/young-onset" referring to <45 years of age and "juvenile onset" (<20 years), highlighting the importance of age at onset for differential diagnostic thinking (Muthane et al., 1994; Schrag & Schott, 2006; Wickremaratchi, Ben-Shlomo, & Morris, 2009). Advanced age at onset in PD has also been implicated with a poorer rate of levodopa response (Wickremaratchi et al., 2009) and a potentially different pattern of dopaminergic terminal loss throughout putamen and caudate nucleus (Liu et al., 2015). Furthermore, the higher occurrence of alternative proteinopathies and vascular events in the aging brain is documented in community-based pathological studies (Kovacs et al., 2013) and has been proposed as one of the causes for potentially more complex PD diagnosis with advanced age, as mixed brain pathology increases (Rizzo et al., 2016).

2.2 Motor Phenotypes

Phenotypic classification of sporadic PD is so far based predominantly on motor phenotype. To this end, tremor-dominant, indeterminate and postural instability gait disorder (PIGD)/akinetic-rigid subtypes are differentiated (Stebbins et al., 2013). However, postural instability generally occurs later in the evolution, and therefore, it is no longer considered an essential diagnostic feature (Postuma et al., 2015). Confirmation of the validity of this classification system has come from imaging studies that proved different activation patterns in functional MRI (Prodoehl et al., 2013) as well as cortical gray matter volume (Rosenberg-Katz et al., 2013) between tremor-dominant and PIGD PD patients. Data also suggest that motor phenotypes at the time of diagnosis may be associated with different rates of progression, with the akinetic-rigid phenotype displaying faster progression and more cognitive symptoms (Baumann, Held, Valko, Wienecke, & Waldvogel, 2014) than the tremor-dominant type (Tremblay, Achim, Macoir, & Monetta, 2013). Differentiation of PD subtypes has been achieved using empirical approaches based on clinical observations and data-driven approaches without an a priori hypothesis—the latter, however, has so far not been used to guide subsequent etiological or even treatment studies. Alternative subtyping approaches have considerably progressed in recent years with regard to genotype, while characterization based on biomarkers is awaited still.

The current data on the validity of subtyping based on motor symptoms alone, however, most likely do not allow definitive conclusions, as with disease progression the predominant motor phenotype can change (Vu, Nutt, & Holford, 2012) and there are controversies in the literature in this regard, as it has been suggested that this clinical heterogeneity of different phenotypes may rather represent different stages of the disease as opposed to distinct biological subtypes (Nutt, 2016).

In clinical reality, motor phenotypes are part of a spectrum. The degree to which motor symptoms are levodopa-responsive can be different between individual patients and the reasons for this difference between subtypes are poorly understood, but seems to be a function of age, with advanced age at onset being associated with poorer response rates (Wickremaratchi et al., 2009). Over time, motor symptoms invariably progress and may include levodopa-nonresponsive motor symptoms such as speech and swallowing problems. Furthermore, cognitive and behavioral symptoms add to the multisystemic presentation of the disease. Data from a meta-analysis suggest that patients with nontremor predominant motor symptoms and depression have more and more severe cognitive symptoms (Tremblay et al., 2013).

2.3 Response to Dopaminergic Medication

One of the hallmark features of PD is the sustained and marked response of motor symptoms to dopaminergic medication, as stated in several versions of published diagnostic criteria (Calne, Snow, & Lee, 1992; Gelb, Oliver, & Gilman, 1999; Gibb & Lees, 1989; Litvan et al., 2003). There have, however, been reports about PD patients nonresponsive to levodopa, which warrant closer attention: From 95 pathologically proven PD cases the initial levodopa response to an adequate trial of "usually 1000 mg/day in divided doses over several months" was recorded to be "nil" to "moderate" in 23% of cases (Hughes, Daniel, Ben-Shlomo, & Lees, 2002). In a similar study, 23% of 100 pathologically confirmed PD and 58% of 38 pathologically confirmed multiple system atrophy (MSA) patients had an initially poor levodopa response (Wenning et al., 2000). In general, bradykinesia is the motor sign considered to be most consistently responsive to levodopa.

Over decades, levodopa-responsiveness has been used as a feature to differentiate PD from atypical parkinsonian conditions, but it is important to note that there is a substantial fraction of MSA, but also progressive supranuclear palsy (PSP) patients that experience some symptomatic relief from levodopa. One study reported up to 70% of clinically confirmed MSA patients with an at least transient benefit from levodopa (Albanese et al., 1995). This percentage has been more consistently reported to be around 30%–40% of MSA patients and in particular among its MSA-P phenotype—characteristically, the response is modest and nonsustained and levodopa-induced dyskinesia seems to affect more facial than limb muscles (Constantinescu, Richard, & Kurlan, 2007).

Similarly, 32% of 103 pathologically proven cases of PSP had a modest or good response to levodopa, while none had an excellent response. As suggested by the authors, and consistent with the current PSP classification, these patients' clinical features were suggestive of PSP-P and less likely of the classical Richardson's syndrome phenotype (Williams et al., 2005). Smaller studies found similar rates of levodopa-responsiveness between 26% and 38% of PSP patients (Collins, Ahlskog, Parisi, & Maraganore, 1995; Kompoliti, Goetz, Litvan, Jellinger, & Verny, 1998; Lang, 2005; Litvan et al., 1996). Unlike in MSA and PD, there have been reports of motor symptom worsening with PSP (Constantinescu et al., 2007). There is only a handful of reports of levodopa response in autopsy-proven corticobasal degeneration (CBD)/corticobasal syndrome (CBS) (Frucht, Fahn, Chin, Dhawan, & Eidelberg, 2000; Kompoliti, Goetz, Boeve, et al., 1998; Wenning et al., 1998).

The familial monogenic forms of PD due to *GBA*, *VPS35*, parkin, *PINK1*, and *DJ-1* show drastic and sustained positive response to levodopa but also display levodopa-induced dyskinesia very early on in their course (see Table 1). Most of the recessive PD mutations including *PLA2G6*, *ATP13A2*, and *FBX07* have a clear levodopa response early on in their course with early levodopa-induced dyskinesia but a more variable response in due course (Ferreira & Massano, 2017; Schneider et al., 2013; Schneider et al., 2010). Among *LRRK2* PD patients levodopa response can be variable, while the great majority of them are responsive (Wider, Dickson, & Wszolek, 2010). Cases of *DNAJC6*-positive PD show either no response to levodopa if onset is juvenile, or good response if onset is in late adulthood (Köroğlu, Baysal, Cetinkaya, Karasoy, & Tolun, 2013; Olgiati et al., 2016). The few cases of parkinsonism caused by *SYNJ1* mutations showed marked

Table 1 Monogenic Familial PD

Gene Symbol (Disease Name)	Gene Name	Mean Age at Onset	Characteristic Clinical Features	*Postmortem* Pathology	Pathophysiology
Autosomal dominant					
SNCA p.A30P p.H50Q p.E46K	Alpha-synuclein p. A30P, p.H50Q, p. E46K mutations	6th–7th decade	Depending on genotype	Widespread alpha-synuclein-positive Lewy neurites and Lewy bodies, also tau inclusions, brain stem, and cortical cell loss	Synaptic/ mitochondrial function, autophagy
SNCA p.A53E p.A53T	Alpha-synuclein p. A53E, p.A53T mutations	3rd–6th decade	PD + cognitive involvement	Similar to other SNCA mutations, A53T can show TDP43 inclusions	—
SNCA p.G51D	Alpha-synuclein p.G51D	2nd–4th decade	Aggressive PD + spasticity, cognitive involvement + seizures	Alpha-synuclein-positive Lewy neurites and Lewy bodies without tau	—
SNCA multiplications	Alpha-synuclein	Depending on gene number	Similar to PD, but more cognitive involvement with increasing gene copy number	Widespread alpha-synuclein-positive Lewy neurites and Lewy bodies with tau inclusions	—
LRRK2	Leucine-rich repeat kinase 2	Mostly 6th decade, variable	Majority indistinguishable from sporadic PD, single CBS, PSP cases described	Majority neuronal degeneration with Lewy bodies, minority without Lewy bodies, individual cases with PSP, MSA, and FTD pathology	Synaptic function, inflammation, autophagy
VPS35 pD620N	Vacuolar protein sorting 35 homolog	53 years	Similar to sporadic PD with slow progression	n.k.	Autophagy, endocytosis

Continued

Table 1 Monogenic Familial PD—cont'd

Gene Symbol (Disease Name)	Gene Name	Mean Age at Onset	Characteristic Clinical Features	*Postmortem* Pathology	Pathophysiology
Autosomal recessive					
GBA p.N370S	Glucocerebrosidase	4th decade	Similar to sporadic PD + hepatosplenomegaly, anemia, thrombocytopenia	Alpha-synuclein pathology in brainstem, hippocampus, and cortex	Inflammation, autophagy, metabolic
Parkin	Parkin RBR E3 ubiquitin protein ligase	~35 years	Similar to sporadic PD, but frequent (foot) dystonia, slower disease progression, and early levodopa-induced dyskinesia	Severe substantia nigra cell loss, often without Lewy body pathology, occasional cortical and brainstem neurofibrillary tangles	Mitochondrial/ synaptic function, ubiquitination
PINK1	PTEN-induced putative kinase 1	~35 years	Slowly progressive, levodopa-responsive PD, often prominent dystonia	Substantia nigra cell loss, brainstem Lewy body pathology	Mitophagy
DJ-1	Daisuke-Junko 1 gene	~35 years	Similar to sporadic PD with slow disease progression, frequent focal dystonia	n.k.	Inflammation, mitochondrial function

PLA2G6	Phospholipase A2, group VI	2nd–3rd decade	Subacute onset dystonia parkinsonism, pyramidal signs, eye movement abnormalities, cognitive decline, initially levodopa-responsive	Prominent basal ganglia and cortical alpha-synuclein ± tau, axonal spheroids	Mitochondrial function
FBX07	F-box protein 7	Childhood onset equinovarus, parkinsonism in 2nd–3rd decade	Equinovarus deformity, lower limb spasticity, pyramidal signs + parkinsonism	Degeneration of pallidum, substantia nigra, and pyramidal tract without inclusions	Ubiquitination, mitochondrial function
ATP13A2 (Kufor-Rakeb)	ATPase type 13A2	12–16 years	Rapid progressive parkinsonism + pyramidal signs, cognitive decline, (incomplete) supranuclear gaze palsy, usually levodopa-responsive	One study showed neuronal ceroid lipofuscinosis pathology (Guerreiro et al., 2015)	Mitochondrial function, autophagy

Continued

Table 1 Monogenic Familial PD—cont'd

Gene Symbol (Disease Name)	Gene Name	Mean Age at Onset	Characteristic Clinical Features	*Postmortem* Pathology	Pathophysiology
DNAJC6	DnaJ (Hsp40) homolog, subfamily C, member 6	Some families <11 years, others 3rd–5th decade	Dependent on age at onset: juvenile onset: rapid progression, levodopa-nonresponsive, dominant dystonia, pyramidal features, seizures, and mental retardation; late adulthood onset: slow progression, levodopa-responsive	n.k.	Synaptic vesicle function, endocytosis
SYNJ1	Synaptojanin 11	22–28 years	Rapidly progressive bradykinesia, fatigue, leg rigidity, cognitive decline and dysarthria, supranuclear gaze palsy, levodopa-induced severe oromandibular and limb dystonia	n.k.	Synaptic vesicle function, endocytosis

VPS13C	Vacuolar protein sorting 13C	25–46 years	Rapid and severe progression with early cognitive decline, dysarthria, dysautonomia	Diffuse alpha-synuclein throughout + brainstem, hippocampus, and motor cortex tau-positive neurofibrillary tangles	PINK1/Parkin-dependent mitophagy
X-linked					
RAB39B	RAB39B, member RAS oncogene family	Childhood onset intellectual disability; parkinsonism <45 years	Variable degree of intellectual disability and parkinsonism	Widespread classic alpha-synuclein, iron accumulation, tau immunoreactivity, axonal spheroids	Alpha-synuclein homeostasis, synapse formation/ maintenance
X-linked dystonia parkinsonism (Lubag)	Xq13.1	4th–5th decade	Starts with focal dystonia progressing into generalized dystonia, action/rest tremor, only minority show parkinsonism	n.k.	n.k.

Continued

Table 1 Monogenic Familial PD—cont'd

Gene Symbol (Disease Name)	Gene Name	Mean Age at Onset	Characteristic Clinical Features	*Postmortem* Pathology	Pathophysiology
High-risk variants (odds ratio 5–8)					
GBA	Glucocerebrosidase	1–6 years younger than sporadic PD	Similar to sporadic PD but higher incidence of cognitive impairment, anxiety, depression; more rapid disease progression	Alpha-synuclein pathology in brainstem, hippocampus, and cortex	Inflammation, autophagy, metabolic
Additionally established genetic associations with prominent parkinsonism					
GCH-1 (dopa-responsive dystonia)	GTP-cyclohydroxylase 1	~46 years	Similar to sporadic PD	n.k.	Dopamine synthesis
22q11.2 deletion	*22q11.2*	~37 years	Childhood cognitive impairment, psychotic features, early drug-related dyskinesia, with or without orofacial dysmorphia	n.k.	n.k.

n.k., not known.

worsening of oromandibular and limb dystonia as well as orthostatic hypotension (Quadri et al., 2013), while the three patients with *VPS13C*-related parkinsonism had some degree of functional improvement with levodopa (Lesage et al., 2016).

Dopaminergic medication only rarely results in relevant relief of symptoms in neurodegeneration with brain iron accumulation (NBIA), even if parkinsonism is the prominent clinical feature (see Table 2). It often causes levodopa-induced dyskinesia and neuropsychiatric side effects, particularly in the case of dopamine agonists (Hogarth, 2015). Kufor-Rakeb (*ATP13A2*) is an exception, as it has been described to be levodopa-responsive, but similarly with early motor fluctuations and dyskinesia (Hogarth, 2015). *ATP1A3* (rapid-onset dystonia parkinsonism) displays very poor response to dopaminergic medication—benzodiazepines provide some symptomatic relief (Heinzen et al., 2014). Similarly, infantile-onset parkinsonism due to dopamine transporter deficiency (Kurian et al., 2009; Lohr, Masoud, Salahpour, & Miller, 2017), early-onset dystonia parkinsonism (Charlesworth, Bhatia, & Wood, 2013), Perry syndrome (Wider & Wszolek, 2008), and Lubag (Rosales, 2010) (some symptomatic benefit by zolpidem in the latter) show no levodopa response.

2.4 Nonmotor Phenotypes

Recent years have seen the increasing recognition of nonmotor symptoms (NMS) not only in sporadic (Adler, 2005) but also in monogenic forms of PD. It is now accepted that a considerable disease burden in PD is caused by NMS (Gallagher, Lees, & Schrag, 2010). A cluster-driven analysis of untreated de novo PD patients showed around 27% initially presented with an NMS-dominant phenotype (Erro et al., 2013). A differentiation of six different NMS-dominant PD phenotypes in the early and untreated phase has been proposed, which differentiates predominant autonomic, cognitive, apathetic, depression/anxiety, sleep, pain, and fatigue involvement, but awaits corroboration (Sauerbier, Jenner, Todorova, & Chaudhuri, 2016) (see Fig. 1). More importantly, even the identification of this easily accessible additional clinical information has led to profound considerations with regard to the definition of the condition—a process which ultimately influenced the current diagnostic criteria (Berg et al., 2014). Several lines of evidence indicate that a diagnosis of PD based on motor symptoms

Table 2 Neurodegeneration With Brain Iron Accumulation (NBIA)

Disease Name/Gene Symbol	Gene Name (Inheritance)	Mean Age at Onset	Characteristic Clinical Features	Postmortem Pathology	Classical Findings
Pantothenate-kinase-associated neurodegeneration (PKAN)	PANK2 (AR)	<6 years (classic, rapid progressive)	Lower limb dystonia, opisthotonus, mild cognitive impairment pyramidal tract signs, pigmentary retinopathy, progressive	Perivascular globus pallidus iron accumulation, neuroaxonal spheroids, alpha-synuclein negative	Eye of the tiger sign on T2-weighed MRI; +/− acanthocytes
	—	Adolescence (atypical, slowly progressive)	Change in speech pattern, eating dystonia, progressive tics, neuropsychiatric symptoms, mixed degree of dystonia, parkinsonism, spasticity	—	—
Phospholipase A2-associated neurodegeneration (PLAN)	PLA2G6 (AR)	6 months to 3 years (INAD)	Slowing and cessation of development, regression in all domains, pronounced cerebellar features, death before 10 years	Dystrophic axonal spheroids in peripheral and central nervous tissue	Cerebellar atrophy, thinning of corpus callosum and optic chiasma; iron deposition often only on SWI-weighed MRI
	—	Adolescence (adult form)	Dystonia parkinsonism, cognitive and psychiatric features	Prominent basal ganglia and cortical alpha-synuclein ± tau	Globus pallidus iron accumulation

Mitochondrial membrane protein-associated neurodegeneration (MPAN)	C19orf12 (AR)	0–10 years	Spastic gait, optic atrophy, cognitive impairment, distal dystonia	Prominent generalized alpha-synuclein in basal ganglia and neocortex (protein load 40 × more than sporadic PD), globus pallidus iron	Imaging: T2-weighed hypointense signal (iron deposition) in globus pallidus and substantia nigra
		Early adulthood	Parkinsonism, cognitive and behavioral changes	—	—
Beta-propeller protein-associated neurodegeneration (BPAN; previously called "static encephalopathy with neurodegeneration in childhood," SENDA)	WDR45 (X-linked dominant)	Biphasic course with childhood onset and decline in adolescence	Global developmental delay, pyramidal signs, disordered sleep in childhood; parkinsonism, dystonia, dementia in adolescence	Axonal spheroids, tau-positive neurofibrillary tangles	Imaging: T2-weighed hypointensities in globus pallidus, cerebral peduncles, and particularly substantia nigra; T1-weighed hyperintense "halo" in substantia nigra
Fatty acid hydroxylase-associated neurodegeneration (FAHN)	FA2H (AR)	0–10 years	Progressive spasticity, dystonia, cerebellar dysfunction, dysarthria, dysphagia, cognitive decline, optic atrophy	n.k.	Imaging: T2-weighed hypointensity in globus pallidus, white matter lesions, thinning of corpus callosum, atrophy of cerebellum, pons, medulla, and cord

Continued

Table 2 Neurodegeneration With Brain Iron Accumulation (NBIA)—cont'd

Disease Name/Gene Symbol	Gene Name (Inheritance)	Mean Age at Onset	Characteristic Clinical Features	Postmortem Pathology	Classical Findings
Coenzyme A synthase protein-associated neurodegeneration (CoPAN)	COASY (AR)	0–10 years	Gait difficulties, cognitive impairment, dysarthria, spasticity, axonal neuropathy, parkinsonism	n.k.	n.k.
Kufor-Rakeb	ATP13A2 (AR)	11–22 years	Slowly progressive, fatigue, gait difficulties, parkinsonism, facial-faucial finger mini-myoclonus, supranuclear gaze palsy, visual hallucinations	n.k.	Generalized brain atrophy, hypointensities in lentiform nucleus
Woodhouse–Sakati syndrome	DCAF17 (AR)	10–20 years	Progressive alopecia, hypogonadism, choreoathetosis, dystonia, dysarthria, dysphagia, diabetes mellitus, sensorineural deafness	n.k.	Basal ganglia hypointensities, extensive white matter hypertintensities on T2-weighed MRI

Neuroferritinopathy	FTL (AR)	Mid-life	Asymmetric chorea, predominant orofacial dystonia, parkinsonism, cognitive decline, low serum ferritin	n.k.	T2-weighed hypointensities in putamen, caudate, thalamus, globus pallidus, substantia nigra, and red nucleus
Aceruloplasminemia	CP (AR)	Adulthood	Microcytic anemia, diabetes, retinal disease, facial dystonia, chorea, tremor, parkinsonism, ataxia, cognitive decline Low or absent serum ceruloplasmin, elevated ferritin, low iron, low serum copper but normal urinary copper	n.k.	Basal ganglia T2-weighed hypointensities

n.k., not known.

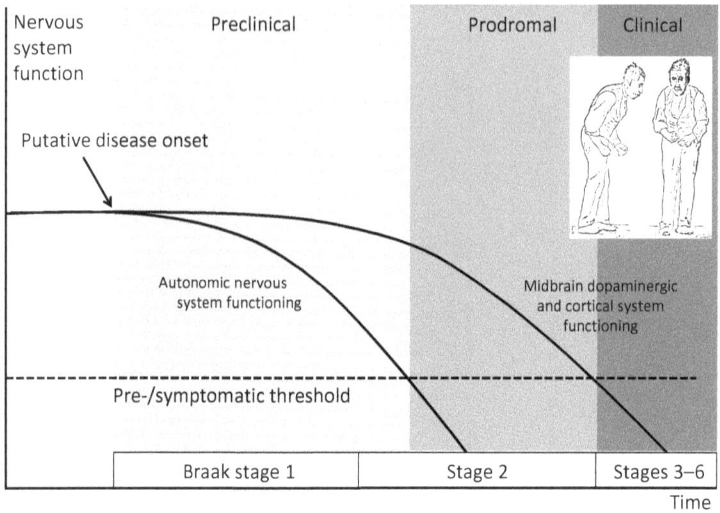

Fig. 1 Current conceptualization of Parkinson's disease. Recognition of a preclinical, a premotor, and a motor stage of disease.

alone falls short to capture important aspects of this multisystem disorder: (a) the fact that clinically defining motor symptoms only occur after around 60% of substantia nigra neurons have already disappeared, (b) Braak's observation of a continuous spread of alpha-synuclein pathology which does not begin in the substantia nigra but in the peripheral autonomic nervous system, dorsal motor nucleus of the vagal nerve, and olfactory bulb (Braak, Ghebremedhin, Rüb, Bratzke, & Del Tredici, 2004; Del Tredici & Braak, 2016), (c) which concurs with the clinical observation that NMS often predate PD motor symptoms (Mollenhauer et al., 2013; Sauerbier et al., 2016).

This has led to the conceptualization of a premotor or prodromal phase of PD, encompassing clinical nonmotor as well as motor symptoms that not yet fulfill PD diagnostic criteria (Mahlknecht, Seppi, & Poewe, 2015; Siderowf & Stern, 2008). The current evidence supports a particular usefulness of the following prodromal symptoms (sensitivity/specificity to detect future PD), possibly in the order of predictive value: REM-sleep behavior disorder (RBD) (low to moderate/high), hyposmia (high/low), constipation (moderate/low), depression, and anxiety (low/low) (Mahlknecht et al., 2015). The combination of several markers has been shown to even increase the area under the receiver operating characteristic curve (AUC) for PD prediction in the prodromal stages (Mollenhauer et al., 2013). The future challenge to identify subjects in the preclinical disease stage, however, will have to rely on disease biomarkers from tissue samples, which are still to be established.

Cognitive symptoms typically associated with PD are executive dysfunction in planning, inhibition, working memory, and learning, which has been known for some time (Taylor, Saint-Cyr, & Lang, 1986). A multicenter study with over 1300 PD patients reported a 25.8% prevalence of mild cognitive impairment, defined as a deviation of more than 1.5 standard deviations of their age- and education-corrected *z* score in one or more domains (Aarsland et al., 2010), rendering cognitive symptoms among a frequent nonmotor manifestation of the disease.

Dementia with Lewy bodies (DLB) and Parkinson's disease dementia (PDD) are characterized by the combination of PD with pronounced cognitive symptoms, which predominantly affect executive function, visuospatial function, verbal fluency, and visual hallucinations, while memory remains relatively unaffected. The pathological hallmark features are alpha-synuclein accumulation in neocortical and brain stem neuronal somata (Lewy bodies) and processes (Lewy neurites). According to a recent meta-analysis, the DLB prevalence in the population above the age of 65 is 36 per 100,000, accounting for 4.2% of all dementia cases in the general population (Vann Jones & O'Brien, 2013). The incidence has been reported as 3.5 per 100,000 person-years for DLB and 2.5 per 100,000 person-years for PDD (Savica, Boeve, & Logroscino, 2016). As the chronological sequence of cognitive vs motor symptom development follows a continuous spectrum, the arbitrary rule of whether cognitive impairment preceded motor symptoms by 1 year is generally accepted to differentiate DLB from PDD (Levin, Kurz, Arzberger, Giese, & Höglinger, 2016), but has recently been challenged to accommodate for the increasingly recognized similarity between PD, DLB, and PDD (Postuma et al., 2016). Accordingly, the recently published new clinical criteria for PD diagnosis (Berg et al., 2015, 2014) do not include dementia any longer as an exclusion criterion. DLB has been invariably described in the literature as an atypical parkinsonian condition, as a PD "phenotype" or as one end of the spectrum of "Lewy body diseases." Indeed, DLB, PDD, and PD share common pathological and clinical features, and rather represent a spectrum reflecting the distribution of Lewy body pathology, which is now acknowledged and taken into account in the recently proposed PD clinical criteria (Postuma et al., 2015).

The exact attribution of cognitive symptoms in the context of PD has so far been following arbitrary rules and therefore will potentially change in the future (Postuma et al., 2016).

2.5 Genetic Parkinson's Disease

Around 10% of PD cases are familial and their clinical characteristics can aid their identification. The knowledge about different underlying molecular mechanisms contributes to the appreciation that PD is most likely not a single disease but a multitude of entities with shared clinical characteristics (Ferreira & Massano, 2017). As the recognition of a molecular mechanism is easier once an underlying genetic deficit has been identified, this population of patients has generated particular interest in the most recent past. Diagnosing these PD subtypes not only will aid finding presymptomatic carriers but also select subjects for therapeutic interventions aiming at a particular molecular mechanism in the near future.

Ethnic background, age at onset, clinical features, and family history are important clues to suspect genetic forms of PD. For example, *SNCA* mutation carriers are more commonly of Greek or Italian ethnic background, have a variable disease onset, and usually a more aggressive course with cognitive and autonomic dysfunction earlier than expected in sporadic PD (Papadimitriou et al., 2016). In contrast, mutations in the leucine-rich repeat kinase 2 (*LRRK2*), which have been confirmed to be the most frequent autosomal-dominant genetic cause of PD in the Caucasian population, are more common in North-Africa and Ashkenazi Jewish ancestry, and usually manifest with a clinical picture indistinguishable of classic sporadic, levodopa-responsive PD (Wider et al., 2010). The most common genetic risk factor that has also been considered as a dominant form of PD with reduced penetrance is heterozygous *GBA* mutations (odds ratio 5.8) (Sidransky et al., 2009) with a strong preponderance among populations of Ashkenazi Jewish descent. Clinically, a slightly younger age at onset and higher incidence of cognitive impairment, as well as psychiatric symptoms (depression and anxiety) and a steeper rate of progression have been shown (Brockmann & Berg, 2014). *VPS31* seems to be rare (Sharma et al., 2012), whereas *VPS13C* has been recently added (Lesage et al., 2016).

Mutations in recessive genes mainly comprise parkin, *PINK1*, and *DJ1*, presenting mostly with early-onset levodopa-responsive parkinsonism with variable other features. Because of their presentation, the following autosomal-recessive PD mutations have been described as pallidopyramidal disease: in addition to parkinsonian features, patients exhibit various degrees of pyramidal involvement with hyperreflexia, spasticity, and equinovarus deformities, in particular in cases of *ATP13A2*, parkin, *PINK1*, *DJ-1*, *PLA2G6*, and *FBX07* mutations (Deng, Liang, & Jankovic, 2013). The term pallidopyramidal syndrome similarly links these conditions to some of the NBIAs (Kara, Hardy, & Houlden, 2013).

3. DIFFERENTIAL DIAGNOSIS OF PARKINSON'S DISEASE

Clinicopathological studies have repeatedly been used over the years to validate the clinical diagnosis in the field of PD. It is a sobering fact that a recent meta-analysis of 13 studies with pathology confirmation indicated that the diagnostic accuracy of PD has remained the same for the last 25 years (Rizzo et al., 2016). The UK Brain Bank diagnostic clinical criteria were more sensitive (90.8% vs 81.3%), but less specific (34%) compared to the expert clinical diagnosis (83.5%)—other tremor disorders, atypical parkinsonian conditions, and secondary parkinsonism were found to be the most frequent misdiagnoses (Rizzo et al., 2016).

3.1 Tremor Syndromes

Tremor is one of the most obvious clinical features in PD, but tremor also can cause considerable confusion as to its etiological origin—tremor disorders are most commonly misdiagnosed as PD.

Classic essential tremor (ET) with young-onset, bilateral symmetric, postural or action tremor of the arm, a positive alcohol response, and a positive family history are rarely confused with PD. But cases with a slightly asymmetric picture, some rest component and later age at onset can be confusing. In this regard the importance to establish bradykinesia through documentation of decrement/fatigability—a continuous reduction in amplitude and/or speed of a repetitive movement—is imperative for the clinician. Furthermore, reemerging tremor—i.e., the lapse of some time after the establishment of a new arm/hand posture until a tremor becomes apparent—is another feature, described to distinctly differentiate postural tremor in PD from the classically immediately apparent postural tremor in ET.

The group of patients initially described with asymmetric rest tremor and normal DaTSCANs (Scans Without evidence of Dopaminergic Deficit, SWEDDs) can mimic parkinsonian rest tremor and have been reported to account for up to 15% of patients clinically diagnosed as PD (Schwingenschuh et al., 2010). Most likely, SWEDDs are an umbrella term for different etiologies: among the majority of SWEDD cases that present with dominant asymmetrical tremor, dystonia and dystonic tremor is one of the most frequent diagnosis found, supported by the fact that some of these patients have been shown to have electrophysiological features of dystonia (Schwingenschuh et al., 2010), the description of single cases of *TOR1A* (Cáceres-Redondo, Carrillo, Palomar, & Mir, 2012; Stamelou, Edwards, & Bhatia, 2013), *ANO3* (Stamelou et al., 2014), or *SGCE* mutation carriers (Cilia et al., 2014) presenting as SWEDDs, and the clinical description of subtle dystonic features in numerous SWEDD cases (Erro, Schneider, Stamelou, Quinn, & Bhatia, 2016). Other cases have been subsequently diagnosed as ET, fragile X premutation carriers, or tardive syndromes (Erro et al., 2016). The minority of SWEDD patients that do not show a predominant tremor component have been subsequently diagnosed as having secondary parkinsonism, including normal pressure hydrocephalus and vascular parkinsonism (Erro et al., 2016). A small proportion of SWEDD cases, however, have been described to show a conversion to nigrostriatal deficit on DaTSCAN follow-up, which is suggestive of a slow progression toward PD in at least a subset of SWEDD patients over time. Conversion rates have been described from 3% after follow-up of 2.4 years (Marshall, Patterson, Hadley, Grosset, & Grosset, 2006), 13% after around 3 years (Menéndez-González, Tavares, Zeidan, Salas-Pacheco, & Arias-Carrión, 2014), and 12.5% after a mean of 7.5 years (Batla et al., 2014).

Clinically, the presence of true bradykinesia with decrement/fatiguing, a good response to dopaminergic medication, the presence of a reemerging tremor, and classical PD nonmotor features (Schwingenschuh et al., 2010) are suggestive of PD, while motor fluctuations and levodopa-induced dyskinesia have been described as the only reliable clinical features to predict PD pathology in tremulous patients (Selikhova, Kempster, Revesz, Holton, & Lees, 2013).

3.2 Atypical Parkinsonism

In early disease stages the establishment of a diagnosis can be particularly difficult in atypical parkinsonism, i.e., MSA, PSP, and CBS. One of the main problems with the differential diagnosis of these conditions is the fact that characteristic clinical features may only become obvious in later stages of the disease. Again age of onset and ethnic background are of help for the differential diagnosis. For example, in Japan, the prevalence of MSA-C seems to be higher than MSA-P, which deviates from the general worldwide distribution (Fanciulli & Wenning, 2015). A new subgroup of PSP-C of patients with postmortem-confirmed PSP pathology and clinically predominant cerebellar involvement has also been described in Japan (Kanazawa et al., 2009; Koga et al., 2015). For a tabular summary, see Table 3.

3.2.1 Multiple System Atrophy

MSA, which had been reported as Shy–Drager syndrome, olivopontocerebellar atrophy, and striatonigral degeneration before its seminal description in 1969, is a sporadic neurodegenerative disorder with the clinical hallmark features of progressive autonomic, parkinsonian, cerebellar, and pyramidal features of variable intensity—parkinsonian (MSA-P) and cerebellar (MSA-C) subtypes are defined by the predominant symptom at onset and early stages of the disease (Wenning, Colosimo, Geser, & Poewe, 2004). The prevalence in the general population has been reported at around 3.4–4.9 per 100,000 and the mean incidence at 0.7 per 100,000 person-years (Fanciulli & Wenning, 2015). According to consensus criteria, the definitive diagnosis of MSA requires postmortem evidence of widespread glial alpha-synuclein accumulation with pontine and cerebellar atrophy or striatonigral degeneration. Current diagnostic criteria define MSA as a sporadic, adult-onset, progressive disorder with poorly levodopa-responsive parkinsonism or cerebellar syndrome with autonomic failure—depending on the number and severity of autonomic symptoms and supportive imaging features, the difference between probable and possible MSA (Gilman et al., 2008).

Sleep changes in sporadic PD have been studied extensively and are described above. Sleep, however, can be also useful in the differential diagnosis of atypical parkinsonism. Atypical parkinsonian disorders appear to share excessive daytime sleepiness as a frequent feature but without further power to differentiate between them (Abbott & Videnovic, 2014). RBD on the other hand is a much more frequent finding in alpha-synucleinopathies,

Table 3 Sporadic Atypical Parkinsonian Disorders

Disease Name	Mean Age at Onset	Characteristic Clinical Features	*Postmortem* Pathology	Brain Magnetic Resonance Imaging (MRI)
Multiple system atrophy-parkinsonism (MSA-P; 60% of MSA cases worldwide, 30% in Japan)	53 years	Parkinsonism > cerebellar (gait or limb ataxia, ataxic dysarthria, cerebellar oculomotor signs), autonomic (orthostatic hypotension, urinary incontinence, erectile dysfunction), pyramidal features, nocturnal stridor, REM-sleep behavior disorder	Oligodendroglial cytoplasmic alpha-synuclein inclusions	Pontine "hot cross bun" sign, atrophy of middle cerebellar peduncle, putamen, pons, cerebellum
Multiple system atrophy-cerebellar (MSA-C; 30% of MSA cases worldwide, 60% in Japan)	53 years	Cerebellar > parkinsonism, autonomic, pyramidal features, nocturnal stridor, REM-sleep behavior disorder	Oligodendroglial cytoplasmic alpha-synuclein inclusions	Hyperintense "putaminal rim" (MSA-P), atrophy of middle cerebellar peduncle, putamen, pons
Progressive supranuclear palsy (PSP)	63 years	Combination of supranuclear gaze palsy, gait abnormalities with falls within first 3 years	4-repeat tau aggregates in astrocytes (tufts), oligodendrocytes (coiled bodies), and neurons (neurofibrillary tangles)	Midbrain atrophy—mickey mouse/penguin sign

PSP phenotypes				
PSP-Richardson's syndrome (PSP-RS; 40% of all PSP cases)	65.9 years	Symmetric, axial, akinetic-rigid, levodopa-resistant parkinsonism, early postural instability, and vertical supranuclear gaze palsy	PSP pathology predominantly in globus pallidus, substantia nigra, subthalamic nucleus, red nucleus, pontine tegmentum, oculomotor nucleus, dentate nucleus	Midbrain atrophy—mickey mouse/penguin sign
PSP-parkinsonism (PSP-P; 20% of all PSP cases)	64 years	Initially levodopa-responsive, asymmetric, limb-predominant parkinsonism, and late-onset postural instability, falls, and supranuclear gaze palsy	Less severe tau pathology in midbrain (substantia nigra and ventral tegmentum)	—
Pure akinesia with gait freezing (PAGF; <5% of all PSP cases)	6th decade	Gait freezing without rigidity and late-onset supranuclear gaze palsy	Severe atrophy and neuronal loss in globus pallidus, substantia nigra, and subthalamic nucleus only	—
PSP-behavioral variant frontotemporal dementia phenotype (bvFTD; 15% of all PSP cases)	6th decade	Apathy, social disinhibition, loss of empathy and impaired executive functions, parkinsonism within 3–7 years of onset, late supranuclear gaze palsy	n.k.	—

Continued

Table 3 Sporadic Atypical Parkinsonian Disorders—cont'd

Disease Name	Mean Age at Onset	Characteristic Clinical Features	*Postmortem* Pathology	Brain Magnetic Resonance Imaging (MRI)
PSP-progressive nonfluent Aphasia phenotype (PNFA; 5% of PSP cases)	6th decade	Nonfluent speech production and agrammatism	Additional severe temporal cortex and superior frontal gyrus cortical tau pathology	—
PSP-corticobasal syndrome phenotype (PSP-CBS; <5% of cases)	65.9 years	Combination of cortical and extrapyramidal symptoms, aphasia, ataxia, asymmetric	Additional severe mid-frontal and inferior parietal cortical tau pathology	—
PSP-cerebellar phenotype (PSP-C; rare)	69 years	Prominent gait and limb ataxia up to 7 years before onset of parkinsonian features, sometimes before onset of supranuclear gaze palsy	Additional tau-positive inclusion bodies in Purkinje cells	—
PSP-primary lateral sclerosis phenotype (PSP-PLS)	71 years	Mixture of prominent parkinsonian and pyramidal signs	Additional PSP pathology in precentral gyrus and pyramidal tract	—
PSP-pallido-nigro-luysian atrophy phenotype (PSP-PNLA; rare)	57.1 years	Similar presentation to PSP-RS but earlier gait abnormalities, handwriting difficulties and freezing, falls late feature	Severe degeneration and axonal dystrophy in pallido-nigro-luysial distribution	—

Corticobasal degeneration (CBD)	63.7 years	Variable; at least one cortical (apraxia, loss of cortical sensitivity, alien limb) and one extrapyramidal (akinesia, rigidity, myoclonus, dystonia) symptom	Astrocytic, oligodendrocytic, and neuronal 4-repeat tau protein aggregation in basal ganglia and neocortex	—
CBD phenotypes				
Corticobasal syndrome (CBS)		Markedly asymmetric combination of symptoms of cortical (apraxia, astereognosis, myoclonus, alien limb) and basal ganglia dysfunction (rigidity, akinesia, dystonia, myoclonus), levodopa-unresponsive	Astrocytic, oligodendrocytic, and neuronal 4-repeat tau protein aggregation in basal ganglia and neocortex	—
CBD-frontal behavioral-spatial syndrome (fBS; ca 10% of all CBD cases)	?	Executive dysfunction, behavioral/personality changes, visuospatial deficits	CBD pathology more in the frontal cortex	—

Continued

Table 3 Sporadic Atypical Parkinsonian Disorders—cont'd

Disease Name	Mean Age at Onset	Characteristic Clinical Features	*Postmortem* Pathology	Brain Magnetic Resonance Imaging (MRI)
CBD-Richardson's syndrome (RS; ca 40% of all CBD cases)	?	Symmetric axial, akinetic-rigid, levodopa-resistant parkinsonism with early-onset postural instability and vertical supranuclear gaze palsy	CBD pathology prominent in the brainstem	—
CBD-progressive nonfluent aphasia (PNFA; <5% of all CBD cases)	?	Additional nonfluent speech production with agrammatism	CBD pathology	—

n.k., not known.

such as PD, DLB, and MSA (64%) than nonalpha-synucleinopathies such as Alzheimer's disease (AD), CBD, FTD, or PSP (3%)—this results in a positive predictive value for the presence of alpha-synucleinopathy between 91% (based on clinical features) and 100% (based on histopathology) (Boeve, Silber, Ferman, Lucas, & Parisi, 2001). It has its neuropathological origin mainly in the loss of brainstem cholinergic neurons in the pedunculopontine tegmental nuclei (PPTg). PSP has been associated repeatedly with sleep architecture changes such as decreased total sleep time and decreased sleep efficiency, while very little is known about sleep changes in CBD (Abbott & Videnovic, 2014). Thus in a patient with parkinsonism the presence of RBD would strongly point to PD or MSA, whereas the absence of RBD is not helpful to differentiate PD from atypical parkinsonian syndromes.

Nocturnal stridor, a potentially fatal but treatable symptom due to laryngeal dysfunction, is highly specific of MSA and is more frequent (42%) than obstructive sleep apnea (37%) in MSA (Vetrugno et al., 2004). A loss in the physiological nocturnal dip in blood pressure is an additional suggestive nocturnal feature of MSA (Abbott & Videnovic, 2014; Fanciulli & Wenning, 2015; Wenning et al., 2004). In the absence of cerebellar or parkinsonian features in a patient with progressive autonomic involvement, the differential diagnosis of pure autonomic failure (PAF), an alpha-synucleinopathy, only affecting the autonomic nervous system, is likely (Chung & Kim, 2015).

Nonsupportive features for MSA diagnosis are in particular age at onset >75 years, hallucinations not induced by drugs, "pill-rolling" rest tremor, a clinically significant neuropathy, and family history of ataxia, parkinsonism, and dementia. Depending on the predominant clinical presentation, i.e., parkinsonism or cerebellar syndrome, features that could suggest the presence of the following differentials should be actively sought in order to consolidate the diagnosis. In the context of a cerebellar syndrome, this includes a suggestive family history of cognitive impairment reminiscent of fragile-X-associated tremor ataxia syndrome, neuropathy and foot deformities as in Friedreich's ataxia, or neuropathy and family history as in SCA1, 2, 3, 6, and 17, which can similarly also present with parkinsonian features (Fanciulli & Wenning, 2015; Kim, Stamelou, & Jeon, 2016; Stamelou, Quinn, & Bhatia, 2013). Idiopathic late-onset idiopathic cerebellar ataxia (ILOCA) is a difficult differential of MSA-C, as it similarly presents in mid-life (age at onset >20 years) with a slowly progressive cerebellar ataxia, in the absence of a family history and exclusion of known acquired and hereditary ataxia forms but can include some autonomic features. A recent comparison of the natural course of autopsy-confirmed MSA-C vs ILOCA suggested that age at onset (41.1 years for ILOCA), presence of corticospinal tract signs, bradykinesia, constipation, pathological laughter, and atrophy of brainstem and of the cerebellar peduncle distinguished the two entities significantly. Interestingly, the presence of oculomotor abnormalities, urinary autonomic symptoms/erectile dysfunction, and RBD was found to distinguish the two early on (Lin, Hermann, & Schmahmann, 2016).

The differentiation of MSA-P and PD is difficult and predominantly based on the evaluation of autonomic involvement. Electrophysiologically, reduced elicitation rates and prolonged latencies of the bulbocavernosus reflex have been described to differentiate between MSA and PD in early stages (Cai et al., 2016). Also, cardiovascular autonomic tests including head-up tilt test and Valsalva maneuver have been described to discriminate the two entities with 91% sensitivity and 92% specificity in single centers (Baschieri et al., 2015).

(123)-I-myocardial meta-iodobenzylguanidine (MIBG) scintigraphy has been described to reliably differentiate MSA from PD—the pooled sensitivity and specificity for this differentiation have been found to be 90.2% and 81.9%, respectively, in a recent review (Chung & Kim, 2015). Results from a Japanese study suggest that olfactory testing is superior in differentiating MSA-C and MSA-P from PD, while MIBG scintigraphy was able to detect differences between MSA-C, but not MSA-P and PD (Kikuchi et al., 2011). However, prospective neuropathologically confirmed studies are largely missing.

3.2.2 Progressive Supranuclear Palsy

PSP has been established as a disease entity in 1964 and was described as a characteristic combination of progressive parkinsonism with early falls, supranuclear vertical gaze palsy, pseudobulbar dysfunction, axial rigidity, and mild cognitive impairment (Steele, Richardson, & Olszewski, 1964), now called Richardson's syndrome (PSP-R). The prevalence is estimated to be 5–6 per 100,000. The classic neuropathological changes of PSP are tau aggregates in astrocytes (tufts), oligodendrocytes (coiled bodies), and neurons (neurofibrillary tangles), which are distinct from other tauopathies. PSP is a sporadic condition in the vast majority of cases; however, a number of familial PSP cases have been reported from different groups: while mutations in the *MAPT* gene have been found in both sporadic and familial PSP cases, patients with a PSP phenotype have rarely been found in kindreds with *LRRK2* gene mutations and otherwise classical PD presentations (Im, Kim, & Kim, 2015).

Since 2005 further phenotypes have been described (Williams et al., 2005; Williams & Lees, 2009): Apart from PSP-R, which represents the classic PSP phenotype PSP-parkinsonism, characterized by a slower disease progression, more asymmetric presentation and initial levodopa-responsiveness, pure akinesia with gait freezing (PAGF), progressive non-fluent aphasia (PNFA), PSP-CBS and further phenotypes have been described (Respondek et al., 2014). Since 1996 clinical diagnostic criteria according to the National Institute of Neurological Disorders and Stroke (NINDS)-PSPS have been widely used and the combined use of postural instability and supranuclear gaze palsy is appreciated as very specific but not sensitive to differentiate PSP from sporadic PD (Lopez, Bayulkem, & Hallett, 2016; Williams & Lees, 2009). PSP pathology with phenotypes overlapping with primary lateral sclerosis via prominent corticospinal tract involvement (PSP-PLS) (Josephs et al., 2006), and pallido-nigro-luysian atrophy (PSP-PNLA) presenting with a somewhat slower progression of symptoms but earlier gait involvement (Ahmed, Josephs, Gonzalez, DelleDonne, & Dickson, 2008) have been described (Lopez et al., 2016). Although initially an exclusion criterion for PSP diagnosis, patients with postmortem-confirmed PSP pathology but clinically predominant cerebellar involvement have been described, forming the novel subgroup PSP-C, initially reported and confirmed from Japan (Kanazawa et al., 2009; Koga et al., 2015). A consensus has recently been reached for new clinical diagnostic criteria for PSP, but remains to be published (Stamelou & Bhatia, 2016).

The latency to correct diagnosis has been reported to be 4.9 years for PSP, while PSP-P (10 years) and PSP-CBS (7 years) had the longest latency, suggesting that the diagnostic verification of these subtypes proved most challenging (Respondek et al., 2014). In general, recently published diagnostic criteria for PD (Postuma et al., 2015) have included "red flags" to account for potentially useful clinical features that might help differentiate between PD and PSP: postural instability is no longer considered a criterion for the definition of parkinsonism but a "red flag" for an atypical condition if present within the first 3 years, as it has been shown that while highly specific, early falls within the first year only occur in a minority of PSP patients. The heterogeneity of PSP subtypes and their different evolution during disease progression complicates early diagnostic identification further (Respondek et al., 2014). While the latencies to develop dysarthria have been reported around 24 months for MSA and PSP, CBD (40 months) and PD (84 months) are much longer—this allows for differentiation between PD and atypical parkinsonian conditions, but is not useful for differentiation between the latter (Grijalvo-Perez & Litvan, 2014).

3.2.3 Corticobasal Degeneration

CBD, first described as "cortico-dentato-nigral degeneration with neuronal achromasia" in 1967 (Rebeiz, Kolodny, & Richardson, 1967), is a pathological entity characterized by astrocytic, oligodendrocytic, and neuronal four-repeat (4R) tau accumulation in the basal ganglia and cortex. CBD is a sporadic disorder, while some familial cases due to *MAPT* (Bugiani et al., 1999; Spillantini et al., 2000) and progranulin (*PGRN*) gene mutations have been described (Masellis et al., 2006; Spina et al., 2007). There are no population-based epidemiological data regarding CBS or CBD available, while the incidence for CBS has been reported around 0.02 per 100,000 patient-years in a report from Russia (Winter et al., 2010) and the prevalence around 9 per 100,000 in a study from Japan (Osaki, Morita, Kuwahara, Miyano, & Doi, 2011).

CBS describes the typical clinical presentation (Grijalvo-Perez & Litvan, 2014). This includes an asymmetric presentation with early onset and often severe limb rigidity in 57% of cases, and unilateral ideomotor apraxia (45%) or other cortical signs such as alien limb phenomena and cortical sensory loss. Mixed action-/postural- and resting tremor, often clearly deviating from typical PD rest tremor, has been reported to be present in around 39% of patients. Dystonia starting in an upper limb is one of the typical early motor features in CBS, commonly occurring within 2 years of onset. Stimulus-sensitive, cortical myoclonus is often described as classical, whereas clinic-pathological series ascribe its prevalence at around 27% only. A similar fraction of patients displays eye movement abnormalities at disease onset, especially increase latency of horizontal saccades ipsilateral to the apraxic limb with preserved velocity (Grijalvo-Perez & Litvan, 2014).

However, CBD pathology has been described in patients with further phenotypes, e.g., frontal behavioral-spatial syndrome (FBS), Richardson's syndrome (RS), and progressive nonfluent aphasia (PNFA) (Armstrong et al., 2013). Conversely, CBS has repeatedly been described to be associated with AD, FTLD-TDP43, and mixed Lewy body/AD pathology (Alexander et al., 2014; Armstrong et al., 2013). In an attempt to increase the sensitivity of diagnosis of CBD taking into account all these phenotypes, new clinical criteria have been proposed (Armstrong et al., 2013). However, first evidence from pathology-confirmed cases indicates that the new consensus criteria for CBD have not led to an improvement in diagnostic specificity (Alexander et al., 2014). The large phenotypic variability among CBD cases and the large pathology variability underlying CBS such as FTLD-TDP43 and AD have been identified as most problematic (Stamelou & Bhatia, 2016).

3.3 Secondary Parkinsonism

Drug-induced parkinsonism has been suggested to occur in around 15% of patients on long-term neuroleptic treatment. In addition to a suggestive history (all neuroleptics apart from clozapine are potential culprits), normal DaTSCAN imaging and olfactory testing can differentiate this entity from PD, although neuroleptic exposure has been reported to unmask presymptomatic PD. Similarly, drugs derived from this class of medication, such as cinnarizine, can similarly cause parkinsonism (Wenning, Litvan, & Tolosa, 2011).

Vascular parkinsonism is supposed to account conservatively for about 3%–4% of cases of parkinsonism and is clinically characterized by lower body parkinsonism with early urinary incontinence and cognitive decline with often impaired postural reflexes and pyramidal signs in the lower limbs. Tremor is usually absent and DaTSCANs usually normal, unless lesions affect the striatum (Korczyn, 2015). The literature on levodopa response is conflicting (Zijlmans, Katzenschlager, Daniel, & Lees, 2004), although most authors deny any meaningful effect on lower body parkinsonism (Korczyn, 2015). Recently, the validity of the umbrella term vascular parkinsonism, which likely includes different subtypes, has been challenged (Vizcarra, Lang, Sethi, & Espay, 2015).

In addition to the mentioned, most important and frequent differential diagnoses there is a continuously increasing list of heredodegenerative disorders that result in parkinsonism (see Table 4). Differentiation is often difficult in early disease stages, whereas the phenotype becomes clearer with time. Metabolic, toxic, and structural causes of parkinsonism should always be excluded (see Table 5).

4. OTHER RARER DIFFERENTIAL DIAGNOSES

Fragile-X tremor ataxia syndrome affects around 40% of male premutation carriers (55–200 CGG repeat expansion in *FMR1* gene)

Table 4 Other Heredodegenerative Causes of Parkinsonism

Syndrome (Gene)	Onset	Clinical Features	Pathology	Suggestive Features
Fragile-X tremor ataxia syndrome (*FMR1* CGG 55–200 repeat expansions)	60 years (men), unknown in women	Action > intention > rest tremor, cerebellar gait and eye movement abnormalities, parkinsonism, neuropathy	Spherical, eosinophilic, ubiquitin-positive neuronal and astrocytic inclusions throughout the brain, Purkinje cell loss	Ovarian failure, family history of cognitive impairment, MCP sign on T2-weighed MRI
Perry syndrome (*DCTN1*)	46 years	Rapid-progressive, levodopa-nonresponsive parkinsonism, apathy, depression, weight loss, nocturnal central apnea	Massive cell loss in substantia nigra, locus coeruleus, dorsal raphe nucleus, caudate, pallidum, putamen, and pre-Bötzinger complex (medullar respiratory pacemaker) with few or no Lewy bodies	—
X-linked dystonia parkinsonism (DYT3, Lubag)	39–40 years	Male:female 100:1; starting predominantly as progressive, generalizing dystonia, over time more parkinsonian features, after 15 years predominantly akinetic-rigid, often tremor, myoclonus, chorea, and myorhythmia	Atrophy in striatum, caudate nucleus, changing pattern of involvement of striosome and matrix over time	Depression, high suicide rate; MRI: hyperintense putaminal ring (dystonic and parkinsonian phase), atrophy in caudate and putamen in parkinsonian phase

Dopa-responsive dystonia (*GCH1*, DYT5a)	4.5 years	Slowly progressive lower limb onset dystonia, generalizing, late-onset parkinsonism	Reduction in nigral melanin and dopamine content without cell loss or degeneration	Diurnal fluctuations, excellent and sustained effect of low doses of levodopa on motor features
Rapid-onset dystonia parkinsonism (*ATP1A3*, DYT12)	75% <25 years	Abrupt onset of dystonia parkinsonism, cranial–caudal severity gradient, triggered by acute illness or event	Possible channelopathy located at cortical interneurons	—
Autosomal-recessive, early-onset dystonia parkinsonism (*PRKRA*, DYT16)	Childhood	Variable parkinsonism + dystonia, generalization	n.k.	—
Dopamine transporter deficiency syndrome (*SLC6A3*)	Infancy	Complex disorder with progressive parkinsonism dystonia	n.k.	—
Huntington's disease (CAG repeat expansion in *HTT*)	1st decade 2nd decade	Westphal variant: developmental delay, cognitive dysfunction, behavioral difficulties, followed by parkinsonism	Predominant striatal medium spiny neuron pathology	—
Huntington's disease-like type 3 (chr. 4p15.3)	3–4 years	Parkinsonism, dystonia, chorea, pyramidal signs	n.k.	—

Continued

Table 4 Other Heredodegenerative Causes of Parkinsonism—cont'd

Syndrome (Gene)	Onset	Clinical Features	Pathology	Suggestive Features
Chorea-acanthocytosis (*VPS13A*)	2nd–3rd decade	Chorea, "feeding" dystonia with tongue protrusion, tics, subcortical dementia, eye movement abnormalities, self-mutilation, parkinsonism in minority	n.k.	Acanthocytes on blood film, elevated creatine kinase, hepatomegaly
MacLeod (*XK*)	25–60 years	Chorea, facial dyskinesia, tongue biting, dysphagia, dystonia, or parkinsonism	n.k.	Acanthocytes on blood film, elevated creatine kinase; cardiac: atrial fibrillations, dilatative cardiomyopathy
SCA 3, 6, 8, 13, 17	Variable, 3rd–5th decade	Adult onset gait and limb ataxia, slowed saccades, lower limb spasticity $\pm$ parkinsonism	Variable	—
Dentato-rubro-pallido-luysian atrophy (CAG repeat expansion in *ATN1*)	20–30 years	Chorea, ataxia, myoclonus	n.k.	—

Hereditary spastic paraparesis type 11 (*KIAA1840*, SPG11)	Early infancy–adulthood	Progressive lower limb weakness and spasticity + ataxia, early-onset levodopa-responsive parkinsonism in singular patients	n.k.	Thin corpus callosum on MRI
Hereditary spastic paraparesis type 11 (*ZFYVE26*, SPG15)	1st–2nd decade	Progressive lower limb weakness and spasticity + intellectual disability, dysarthria, parkinsonism, axonal neuropathy	n.k.	Thin corpus callosum on MRI
Frontotemporal dementia with parkinsonism (*MAPT*, FTDP-17)	Variable	Behavior/personality change, cognitive dysfunction, atypical parkinsonism	Cortical and subcortical neuronal and glial hyperphosphorylated tau inclusions	—
Creutzfeldt–Jakob disease	Sporadic/familial/infectious	Subacute, rapidly progressive, cognitive decline, cerebellar symptoms, visual changes ± parkinsonism, alien limb, supranuclear gaze palsy, dystonia, myoclonus	Generalized atrophy, cell loss, vacuolation	CSF protein 14-3-3, EEG: periodic sharp waves, cortical ribboning on DWI-MRI

Continued

Table 4 Other Heredodegenerative Causes of Parkinsonism—cont'd

Syndrome (Gene)	Onset	Clinical Features	Pathology	Suggestive Features
Gerstmann–Sträussler–Scheinker (*PRNP*)	4th–6th decade	Slightly slower progressive course with subacute progressive ataxia or parkinsonism	Generalized atrophy, cell loss, vacuolation	CSF protein 14-3-3, EEG: periodic sharp waves, limbic DWI-hyperintensities
Parkinsonism-dementia-ALS-complex of Guam	52 years	Parkinsonism, upper motor neuron signs, dementia, apathy, supranuclear gaze palsy	Substantia nigra degeneration, severe tau neurofibrillary tangles, inconsistent beta-amyloid pathology	—
Fahr's disease	3rd–5th decade	Parkinsonism, chorea, tremor, cognitive, neuropsychiatric symptoms	Basal ganglia calcifications	—

n.k., not known.

Table 5 Metabolic, Toxic, and Structural Causes of Parkinsonism

Metabolic
Wilson's disease, acquired hepatolenticular degeneration, maple syrup urine disease, neuronal ceroid lipofuscinosis, mitochondrial (e.g., POLG), Niemann–Pick type C, GM1 gangliosidosis, phenylketonuria, cerebrotendinous xanthomatosis, hemiparkinsonism–hemiatrophy syndrome
Structural
Vascular parkinsonism, posttraumatic, postencephalitic, postanoxic
Toxic
MPTP, ephedrine, manganese, cyanide, carbon monoxide
Drug induced
Typical antipsychotics (haloperidol, chlorpromazine), atypical antipsychotics (risperidone, olanzapine), metoclopramide, valproate, tetrabenazine, reserpine, antihistamines (flunarizine, cinnarizine), lithium

of fragile-X (>200 CGG repeat expansions), the most frequent heritable cause of mental retardation (1:3600 live births), and 8% of females >40 years of age. It is often misdiagnosed as one of the atypical parkinsonian disorders because of its age at onset above 55 years with prominent action > intention > rest tremor, cerebellar gait ataxia, and frequently parkinsonism. Additional neuropathy, family history of a tremor disorder, cognitive impairment, or ovarian failure are additional suggestive features (Leehey & Hagerman, 2012).

When chorea is an additional clinical feature, Huntington's disease (HD) (in particular juvenile) and HD-like syndromes, neuroacanthocytosis and McLeod syndrome, but also dentate-rubro-pallidoluysian atrophy (DRPLA) and neuroferritinopathy should be kept in mind. Acanthocytes, hepatomegaly, and parkinsonism raise the suspicion of neuroacanthocytosis or McLeod syndrome (Schneider, Walker, & Bhatia, 2007), while cardiac involvement points to the latter (Jung, Danek, & Walker, 2011). In case of predominant dystonic features, the list of potential differentials considerably widens and further differential thinking should be based on age at onset; in the context of a positive family history for PD, autosomal-recessive hereditary causes should be investigated for; and in case of suggestive MRI findings on susceptibility- or T2 star-weighed sequences, NBIAs should be assessed (see Table 3). Neuropathy plus alopecia, parkinsonism, and basal ganglia iron accumulation on MR imaging point at Woodhouse–Sakati syndrome (Al-Semari & Bohlega, 2007; Woodhouse & Sakati, 1983). Additional microcytic anemia together with elevated ferritin, low serum, and urine copper with normal urinary copper in the context of basal ganglia iron deposition is suggestive of aceruloplasminemia (Schneider et al., 2013). Rarer forms of dystonia parkinsonism include dopa-responsive dystonias, rapid-onset parkinsonism, dopamine transporter deficiency syndrome, Lubag, and early-onset dystonia parkinsonism (see Table 4).

Orofacial dysmorphic features in the context of childhood onset cognitive impairment and early-onset PD can be indicative of a 22q deletion syndrome (Mok et al., 2016). External ophthalmoplegia in combination with parkinsonism and neuropathy is suggestive of mitochondrial disease, such as in *POLG* mutations (Dolhun, Presant, & Hedera, 2013; Hudson et al., 2007; Invernizzi et al., 2008; Sato et al., 2011). Additional nocturnal central apnea/hypoventilation, especially in the context of parkinsonism with prominent depression and apathy, is indicative of autosomal-dominant Perry syndrome (Wider & Wszolek, 2008). Hepatosplenomegaly, anemia, and thrombocytopenia in a PD patient should prompt the differential of *GBA* mutation-related PD, as these are frequent features especially in carriers of the p.N370S *GBA* mutation (Brockmann & Berg, 2014).

Ethnic background may be again an important clue in some of these rare disorders, e.g., neuroferritinopathy shows geographical clustering in Cumbria in northern Britain (Hogarth, 2015), neuroacanthocytosis seems to be more frequent in Japan and the French-Canadian population (Jung et al., 2011), DRPLA is particularly prevalent in Japan but very rare elsewhere (Schneider et al., 2007). The Philippine island of Panay has been identified as the origin of X-linked dystonia parkinsonism (Evidente et al., 2002; Rosales, 2010) and the Mariana island Guam is home to the only population that harbors parkinsonism-dementia-ALS-complex of Guam (Lee, 2011). Kufor-Rakeb (*ATP13A2* mutations) has been originally described in a Jordanian family, but cases with origin from Chile, Brazil, Japan, and Pakistan have been confirmed since (Schneider et al., 2010). Most of cases of Woodhouse–Sakati syndrome (Al-Semari & Bohlega, 2007; Hogarth, 2015; Woodhouse & Sakati, 1983) and the only family with HD-like 3 have so far been described from Saudi-Arabia (Schneider et al., 2007).

5. SUMMARY

Still today the diagnosis of PD largely relies on the correct interpretation of findings from history and clinical examination that aim at the correct phenotypical characterization of individual cases. Recent years have proven that the correct identification of sporadic PD, its familial variants, and especially the atypical parkinsonian disorders can still pose a considerable challenge for clinicians. Albeit increasing the possibilities of genetic analysis that have so tremendously enlarged and enriched the differential diagnosis of PD, the need for a precise phenotypical description remains and will by no mean render clinical skills redundant. Quite the opposite—as appreciable from the often overlapping clinical presentation—the need for a careful phenomenological classification of an individual patient has become more important than ever to guide the necessary steps in finding the correct diagnosis and ultimately the correct treatment.

REFERENCES

Aarsland, D., Bronnick, K., Williams-Gray, C., Weintraub, D., Marder, K., Kulisevsky, J., et al. (2010). Mild cognitive impairment in Parkinson disease: A multicenter pooled analysis. *Neurology*, *75*(12), 1062–1069. http://doi.org/10.1212/WNL.0b013e3181f39d0e.

Abbott, S. M., & Videnovic, A. (2014). Sleep disorders in atypical parkinsonism. *Movement Disorders Clinical Practice*, *1*(2), 89–96. http://doi.org/10.1002/mdc3.12025.

Adler, C. H. (2005). Nonmotor complications in Parkinson's disease. *Movement Disorders*, *20*(Suppl. 11), S23–S29. http://doi.org/10.1002/mds.20460.

Ahmed, Z., Josephs, K. A., Gonzalez, J., DelleDonne, A., & Dickson, D. W. (2008). Clinical and neuropathologic features of progressive supranuclear palsy with severe pallido-nigro-luysial degeneration and axonal dystrophy. *Brain*, *131*(Pt. 2), 460–472. http://doi.org/10.1093/brain/awm301.

Albanese, A., Bentivoglio, A. R., Fenici, R., Melillo, G., Colosimo, C., & Tonali, P. (1995). Multiple system atrophy presenting as parkinsonism: Clinical features and diagnostic criteria. *Journal of Neurology, Neurosurgery & Psychiatry*, *59*(2), 144–151.

Alexander, S. K., Rittman, T., Xuereb, J. H., Bak, T. H., Hodges, J. R., & Rowe, J. B. (2014). Validation of the new consensus criteria for the diagnosis of corticobasal degeneration. *Journal of Neurology, Neurosurgery, and Psychiatry*, *85*(8), 925–929. http://doi.org/10.1136/jnnp-2013-307035.

Al-Semari, A., & Bohlega, S. (2007). Autosomal-recessive syndrome with alopecia, hypogonadism, progressive extra-pyramidal disorder, white matter disease, sensory neural deafness, diabetes mellitus, and low IGF1. *American Journal of Medical Genetics. Part A*, *143A*(2), 149–160. http://doi.org/10.1002/ajmg.a.31497.

Armstrong, M. J., Litvan, I., Lang, A. E., Bak, T. H., Bhatia, K. P., Borroni, B., et al. (2013). Criteria for the diagnosis of corticobasal degeneration. *Neurology*, *80*(5), 496–503. http://doi.org/10.1212/WNL.0b013e31827f0fd1.

Baschieri, F., Calandra-Buonaura, G., Doria, A., Mastrolilli, F., Palareti, A., Barletta, G., et al. (2015). Cardiovascular autonomic testing performed with a new integrated instrumental approach is useful in differentiating MSA-P from PD at an early stage. *Parkinsonism & Related Disorders*, *21*(5), 477–482. http://doi.org/10.1016/j.parkreldis.2015.02.011.

Batla, A., Erro, R., Stamelou, M., Schneider, S. A., Schwingenschuh, P., Ganos, C., et al. (2014). Patients with scans without evidence of dopaminergic deficit: A long-term follow-up study. *Movement Disorders*, *29*(14), 1820–1825. http://doi.org/10.1002/mds.26018.

Baumann, C. R., Held, U., Valko, P. O., Wienecke, M., & Waldvogel, D. (2014). Body side and predominant motor features at the onset of Parkinson's disease are linked to motor and nonmotor progression. *Movement Disorders*, *29*(2), 207–213. http://doi.org/10.1002/mds.25650.

Benito-León, J., Bermejo-Pareja, F., Morales-González, J. M., Porta-Etessam, J., Trincado, R., Vega, S., et al. (2004). Incidence of Parkinson disease and parkinsonism in three elderly populations of central Spain. *Neurology*, *62*(5), 734–741.

Berg, D., Postuma, R. B., Adler, C. H., Bloem, B. R., Chan, P., Dubois, B., et al. (2015). MDS research criteria for prodromal Parkinson's disease. *Movement Disorders*, *30*(12), 1600–1611. http://doi.org/10.1002/mds.26431.

Berg, D., Postuma, R. B., Bloem, B., Chan, P., Dubois, B., Gasser, T., et al. (2014). Time to redefine PD? Introductory statement of the MDS task force on the definition of Parkinson's disease. *Movement Disorders*, *29*(4), 454–462. http://doi.org/10.1002/mds.25844.

Boeve, B. F., Silber, M. H., Ferman, T. J., Lucas, J. A., & Parisi, J. E. (2001). Association of REM sleep behavior disorder and neurodegenerative disease may reflect an underlying synucleinopathy. *Movement Disorders*, *16*(4), 622–630.

Bower, J. H., Maraganore, D. M., McDonnell, S. K., & Rocca, W. A. (1999). Incidence and distribution of parkinsonism in Olmsted County, Minnesota, 1976-1990. *Neurology*, *52*(6), 1214–1220.

Bower, J. H., Maraganore, D. M., McDonnell, S. K., & Rocca, W. A. (2000). Influence of strict, intermediate, and broad diagnostic criteria on the age- and sex-specific incidence of Parkinson's disease. *Movement Disorders*, *15*(5), 819–825. http://dx.doi.org/10.1002/1531-8257(200009)15:5<819::AID-MDS1009>3.0.CO;2-P.

Braak, H., Ghebremedhin, E., Rüb, U., Bratzke, H., & Del Tredici, K. (2004). Stages in the development of Parkinson's disease-related pathology. *Cell and Tissue Research*, *318*(1), 121–134. http://doi.org/10.1007/s00441-004-0956-9.

Bras, J., Guerreiro, R., & Hardy, J. (2015). SnapShot: Genetics of Parkinson's disease. *Cell*, *160*(3), 570–570.e1. http://doi.org/10.1016/j.cell.2015.01.019.

Brockmann, K., & Berg, D. (2014). The significance of GBA for Parkinson's disease. *Journal of Inherited Metabolic Disease*, *37*(4), 643–648. http://doi.org/10.1007/s10545-014-9714-7.

Bugiani, O., Murrell, J. R., Giaccone, G., Hasegawa, M., Ghigo, G., Tabaton, M., et al. (1999). Frontotemporal dementia and corticobasal degeneration in a family with a P301S mutation in tau. *Journal of Neuropathology and Experimental Neurology*, *58*(6), 667–677.

Cáceres-Redondo, M. T., Carrillo, F., Palomar, F. J., & Mir, P. (2012). DYT-1 gene dystonic tremor presenting as a "scan without evidence of dopaminergic deficit". *Movement Disorders*, *27*(11), 1469. http://doi.org/10.1002/mds.25171.

Cai, Z.-Y., Niu, X.-T., Pan, J., Ni, P.-Q., Wang, X., & Shao, B. (2016). The value of the bulbocavernosus reflex and pudendal nerve somatosensory evoked potentials in distinguishing between multiple system atrophy and Parkinson's disease at an early stage. *Acta Neurologica Scandinavica*. http://doi.org/10.1111/ane.12710. (Epub ahead of print).

Calne, D. B., Snow, B. J., & Lee, C. (1992). Criteria for diagnosing Parkinson's disease. *Annals of Neurology*, *32*(Suppl.), S125–S127.

Charlesworth, G., Bhatia, K. P., & Wood, N. W. (2013). The genetics of dystonia: New twists in an old tale. *Brain, 136*(Pt. 7), 2017–2037. http://doi.org/10.1093/brain/awt138.

Chung, E. J., & Kim, S. J. (2015). (123)I-metaiodobenzylguanidine myocardial scintigraphy in Lewy body-related disorders: A literature review. *Journal of Movement Disorders, 8*(2), 55–66. http://doi.org/10.14802/jmd.15015.

Cilia, R., Reale, C., Castagna, A., Nasca, A., Muzi-Falconi, M., Barzaghi, C., et al. (2014). Novel DYT11 gene mutation in patients without dopaminergic deficit (SWEDD) screened for dystonia. *Neurology, 83*(13), 1155–1162. http://doi.org/10.1212/WNL.0000000000000821.

Collins, S. J., Ahlskog, J. E., Parisi, J. E., & Maraganore, D. M. (1995). Progressive supranuclear palsy: Neuropathologically based diagnostic clinical criteria. *Journal of Neurology, Neurosurgery & Psychiatry, 58*(2), 167–173.

Constantinescu, R., Richard, I., & Kurlan, R. (2007). Levodopa responsiveness in disorders with parkinsonism: A review of the literature. *Movement Disorders, 22*(15), 2141–2148. http://doi.org/10.1002/mds.21578.

de Lau, L. M. L., & Breteler, M. M. B. (2006). Epidemiology of Parkinson's disease. *Lancet Neurology, 5*(6), 525–535. http://doi.org/10.1016/S1474-4422(06)70471-9.

de Lau, L. M. L., Giesbergen, P. C. L. M., de Rijk, M. C., Hofman, A., Koudstaal, P. J., & Breteler, M. M. B. (2004). Incidence of parkinsonism and Parkinson disease in a general population: The Rotterdam Study. *Neurology, 63*(7), 1240–1244.

Del Tredici, K., & Braak, H. (2016). Review: Sporadic Parkinson's disease: Development and distribution of α-synuclein pathology. *Neuropathology and Applied Neurobiology, 42*(1), 33–50. http://doi.org/10.1111/nan.12298.

Deng, H., Liang, H., & Jankovic, J. (2013). F-box only protein 7 gene in parkinsonian-pyramidal disease. *JAMA Neurology, 70*(1), 20–24. http://doi.org/10.1001/jamaneurol.2013.572.

Dolhun, R., Presant, E. M., & Hedera, P. (2013). Novel polymerase gamma (POLG1) gene mutation in the linker domain associated with parkinsonism. *BMC Neurology, 13*(1), 92. http://doi.org/10.1186/1471-2377-13-92.

Erro, R., Schneider, S. A., Stamelou, M., Quinn, N. P., & Bhatia, K. P. (2016). What do patients with scans without evidence of dopaminergic deficit (SWEDD) have? New evidence and continuing controversies. *Journal of Neurology, Neurosurgery & Psychiatry, 87*(3), 319–323. http://doi.org/10.1136/jnnp-2014-310256.

Erro, R., Vitale, C., Amboni, M., Picillo, M., Moccia, M., Longo, K., et al. (2013). The heterogeneity of early Parkinson's disease: A cluster analysis on newly diagnosed untreated patients. *PLoS One, 8*(8), e70244. http://doi.org/10.1371/journal.pone.0070244.

Evidente, V. G. H., Advincula, J., Esteban, R., Pasco, P., Alfon, J. A., Natividad, F. F., et al. (2002). Phenomenology of "Lubag" or X-linked dystonia-parkinsonism. *Movement Disorders, 17*(6), 1271–1277. http://doi.org/10.1002/mds.10271.

Fanciulli, A., & Wenning, G. K. (2015). Multiple-system atrophy. *The New England Journal of Medicine, 372*(3), 249–263. http://doi.org/10.1056/NEJMra1311488.

Ferreira, M., & Massano, J. (2017). An updated review of Parkinson's disease genetics and clinicopathological correlations. *Acta Neurologica Scandinavica, 135*(3), 273–284. http://doi.org/10.1111/ane.12616.

Frucht, S., Fahn, S., Chin, S., Dhawan, V., & Eidelberg, D. (2000). Levodopa-induced dyskinesias in autopsy-proven cortical-basal ganglionic degeneration. *Movement Disorders, 15*(2), 340–343.

Gallagher, D. A., Lees, A. J., & Schrag, A. (2010). What are the most important nonmotor symptoms in patients with Parkinson's disease and are we missing them? *Movement Disorders, 25*(15), 2493–2500. http://doi.org/10.1002/mds.23394.

Gelb, D. J., Oliver, E., & Gilman, S. (1999). Diagnostic criteria for Parkinson disease. *Archives of Neurology*, *56*(1), 33–39.

Gibb, W. R., & Lees, A. J. (1989). The significance of the Lewy body in the diagnosis of idiopathic Parkinson's disease. *Neuropathology and Applied Neurobiology*, *15*(1), 27–44.

Gilman, S., Wenning, G. K., Low, P. A., Brooks, D. J., Mathias, C. J., Trojanowski, J. Q., et al. (2008). Second consensus statement on the diagnosis of multiple system atrophy. *Neurology*, *71*(9), 670–676. http://doi.org/10.1212/01.wnl.0000324625.00404.15.

Grijalvo-Perez, A., & Litvan, I. (2014). Corticobasal degeneration. *Seminars in Neurology*, *34*(02), 160–173. http://doi.org/10.1055/s-0034-1381734.

Guerreiro, R., Brás, J., & Hardy, J. (2015 Feb 12). SnapShot: Genetics of ALS and FTD. *Cell*, *160*(4), 798.e1. http://dx.doi.org/10.1016/j.cell.2015.01.052.

Heinzen, E. L., Arzimanoglou, A., Brashear, A., Clapcote, S. J., Gurrieri, F., Goldstein, D. B., et al. (2014). Distinct neurological disorders with ATP1A3 mutations. *The Lancet Neurology*, *13*(5), 503–514. http://doi.org/10.1016/S1474-4422(14)70011-0.

Hogarth, P. (2015). Neurodegeneration with brain iron accumulation: Diagnosis and management. *Journal of Movement Disorders*, *8*(1), 1–13. http://doi.org/10.14802/jmd.14034.

Hudson, G., Schaefer, A. M., Taylor, R. W., Tiangyou, W., Gibson, A., Venables, G., et al. (2007). Mutation of the linker region of the polymerase gamma-1 (POLG1) gene associated with progressive external ophthalmoplegia and Parkinsonism. *Archives of Neurology*, *64*(4), 553–557. http://doi.org/10.1001/archneur.64.4.553.

Hughes, A. J., Daniel, S. E., Ben-Shlomo, Y., & Lees, A. J. (2002). The accuracy of diagnosis of parkinsonian syndromes in a specialist movement disorder service. *Brain*, *125*(Pt. 4), 861–870.

Im, S. Y., Kim, Y. E., & Kim, Y. J. (2015). Genetics of progressive supranuclear palsy. *Journal of Movement Disorders*, *8*(3), 122–129. http://doi.org/10.14802/jmd.15033.

Invernizzi, F., Varanese, S., Thomas, A., Carrara, F., Onofrj, M., & Zeviani, M. (2008). Two novel POLG1 mutations in a patient with progressive external ophthalmoplegia, levodopa-responsive pseudo-orthostatic tremor and parkinsonism. *Neuromuscular Disorders: NMD*, *18*(6), 460–464. http://doi.org/10.1016/j.nmd.2008.04.005.

Josephs, K. A., Katsuse, O., Beccano-Kelly, D. A., Lin, W.-L., Uitti, R. J., Fujino, Y., et al. (2006). Atypical progressive supranuclear palsy with corticospinal tract degeneration. *Journal of Neuropathology and Experimental Neurology*, *65*(4), 396–405. http://doi.org/10.1097/01.jnen.0000218446.38158.61.

Jung, H. H., Danek, A., & Walker, R. H. (2011). Neuroacanthocytosis syndromes. *Orphanet Journal of Rare Diseases*, *6*(1), 68. http://doi.org/10.1186/1750-1172-6-68.

Kanazawa, M., Shimohata, T., Toyoshima, Y., Tada, M., Kakita, A., Morita, T., et al. (2009). Cerebellar involvement in progressive supranuclear palsy: A clinicopathological study. *Movement Disorders*, *24*(9), 1312–1318. http://doi.org/10.1002/mds.22583.

Kara, E., Hardy, J., & Houlden, H. (2013). The pallidopyramidal syndromes. *Current Opinion in Neurology*, *26*(4), 381–394. http://doi.org/10.1097/WCO.0b013e3283632e83.

Kikuchi, A., Baba, T., Hasegawa, T., Sugeno, N., Konno, M., & Takeda, A. (2011). Differentiating Parkinson's disease from multiple system atrophy by [123I] meta-iodobenzylguanidine myocardial scintigraphy and olfactory test. *Parkinsonism and Related Disorders*, *17*(9), 698–700. http://doi.org/10.1016/j.parkreldis.2011.07.011.

Kim, H.-J., Stamelou, M., & Jeon, B. (2016). Multiple system atrophy-mimicking conditions: Diagnostic challenges. *Parkinsonism and Related Disorders*, *22*(Suppl. 1), S12–S15. http://doi.org/10.1016/j.parkreldis.2015.09.003.

Koga, S., Aoki, N., Uitti, R. J., van Gerpen, J. A., Cheshire, W. P., Josephs, K. A., et al. (2015). When DLB, PD, and PSP masquerade as MSA: An autopsy study of 134 patients. *Neurology*, *85*(5), 404–412. http://doi.org/10.1212/WNL.0000000000001807.

Kompoliti, K., Goetz, C. G., Boeve, B. F., Maraganore, D. M., Ahlskog, J. E., Marsden, C. D., et al. (1998a). Clinical presentation and pharmacological therapy in corticobasal degeneration. *Archives of Neurology*, *55*(7), 957–961.

Kompoliti, K., Goetz, C. G., Litvan, I., Jellinger, K., & Verny, M. (1998b). Pharmacological therapy in progressive supranuclear palsy. *Archives of Neurology*, *55*(8), 1099–1102.

Korczyn, A. D. (2015). Vascular parkinsonism—Characteristics, pathogenesis and treatment. *Nature Reviews. Neurology*, *11*(6), 319–326. http://doi.org/10.1038/nrneurol.2015.61.

Köroğlu, Ç., Baysal, L., Cetinkaya, M., Karasoy, H., & Tolun, A. (2013). DNAJC6 is responsible for juvenile parkinsonism with phenotypic variability. *Parkinsonism and Related Disorders*, *19*(3), 320–324. http://doi.org/10.1016/j.parkreldis.2012.11.006.

Kovacs, G. G., Milenkovic, I., Wöhrer, A., Höftberger, R., Gelpi, E., Haberler, C., et al. (2013). Non-Alzheimer neurodegenerative pathologies and their combinations are more frequent than commonly believed in the elderly brain: A community-based autopsy series. *Acta Neuropathologica*, *126*(3), 365–384. http://doi.org/10.1007/s00401-013-1157-y.

Kurian, M. A., Zhen, J., Cheng, S.-Y., Li, Y., Mordekar, S. R., Jardine, P., et al. (2009). Homozygous loss-of-function mutations in the gene encoding the dopamine transporter are associated with infantile parkinsonism-dystonia. *The Journal of Clinical Investigation*, *119*(6), 1595–1603. http://doi.org/10.1172/JCI39060.

Lang, A. E. (2005). Treatment of progressive supranuclear palsy and corticobasal degeneration. *Movement Disorders*, *20*(Suppl. 1), S83–S91. http://doi.org/10.1002/mds.20545.

Lee, S. E. (2011). Guam dementia syndrome revisited in 2011. *Current Opinion in Neurology*, *24*(6), 517–524. http://doi.org/10.1097/WCO.0b013e32834cd50a.

Leehey, M. A., & Hagerman, P. J. (2012). Fragile X-associated tremor/ataxia syndrome. *Handbook of Clinical Neurology*, *103*, 373–386. http://doi.org/10.1016/B978-0-444-51892-7.00023-1.

Lesage, S., Drouet, V., Majounie, E., Deramecourt, V., Jacoupy, M., Nicolas, A., et al. (2016). Loss of VPS13C function in autosomal-recessive parkinsonism causes mitochondrial dysfunction and increases PINK1/parkin-dependent mitophagy. *American Journal of Human Genetics*, *98*(3), 500–513. http://doi.org/10.1016/j.ajhg.2016.01.014.

Levin, J., Kurz, A., Arzberger, T., Giese, A., & Höglinger, G. U. (2016). The differential diagnosis and treatment of atypical parkinsonism. *Deutsches Arzteblatt International*, *113*(5), 61–69. http://doi.org/10.3238/arztebl.2016.0061.

Lin, D. J., Hermann, K. L., & Schmahmann, J. D. (2016). The diagnosis and natural history of multiple system atrophy, cerebellar type. *The Cerebellum*, *15*, 663–679. http://doi.org/10.1007/s12311-015-0728-y.

Litvan, I., Bhatia, K. P., Burn, D. J., Goetz, C. G., Lang, A. E., McKeith, I., et al. (2003). Movement Disorders Society Scientific Issues Committee report: SIC Task Force appraisal of clinical diagnostic criteria for Parkinsonian disorders. *Movement Disorders: Official Journal of the Movement Disorder Society*, *18*, 467–486. http://doi.org/10.1002/mds.10459.

Litvan, I., Mangone, C. A., McKee, A., Verny, M., Parsa, A., Jellinger, K., et al. (1996). Natural history of progressive supranuclear palsy (Steele-Richardson-Olszewski syndrome) and clinical predictors of survival: A clinicopathological study. *Journal of Neurology, Neurosurgery & Psychiatry*, *60*(6), 615–620.

Liu, S.-Y., Wu, J.-J., Zhao, J., Huang, S.-F., Wang, Y.-X., Ge, J.-J., et al. (2015). Onset-related subtypes of Parkinson's disease differ in the patterns of striatal dopaminergic dysfunction: A positron emission tomography study. *Parkinsonism and Related Disorders*, *21*(12), 1448–1453. http://doi.org/10.1016/j.parkreldis.2015.10.017.

Lohr, K. M., Masoud, S. T., Salahpour, A., & Miller, G. W. (2017). Membrane transporters as mediators of synaptic dopamine dynamics: Implications for disease. *The European Journal of Neuroscience*, *45*(1), 20–33. http://doi.org/10.1111/ejn.13357.

Lopez, G., Bayulkem, K., & Hallett, M. (2016). Progressive supranuclear palsy (PSP): Richardson syndrome and other PSP variants. *Acta Neurologica Scandinavica*, *134*(4), 242–249. http://doi.org/10.1111/ane.12546.

Mahlknecht, P., Seppi, K., & Poewe, W. (2015). The concept of prodromal Parkinson's disease. *Journal of Parkinson's Disease*, *5*(4), 681–697. http://doi.org/10.3233/JPD-150685.
Marshall, V. L., Patterson, J., Hadley, D. M., Grosset, K. A., & Grosset, D. G. (2006). Two-year follow-up in 150 consecutive cases with normal dopamine transporter imaging. *Nuclear Medicine Communications*, *27*(12), 933–937. http://doi.org/10.1097/01.mnm.0000243374.11260.5b.
Masellis, M., Momeni, P., Meschino, W., Heffner, R., Elder, J., Sato, C., et al. (2006). Novel splicing mutation in the progranulin gene causing familial corticobasal syndrome. *Brain*, *129*(Pt. 11), 3115–3123. http://doi.org/10.1093/brain/awl276.
Menéndez-González, M., Tavares, F., Zeidan, N., Salas-Pacheco, J. M., & Arias-Carrión, O. (2014). Diagnoses behind patients with hard-to-classify tremor and normal DaT-SPECT: A clinical follow up study. *Frontiers in Aging Neuroscience*, *6*, 56. http://doi.org/10.3389/fnagi.2014.00056.
Mok, K. Y., Sheerin, U., Simón-Sánchez, J., Salaka, A., Chester, L., Escott-Price, V., et al. (2016). Deletions at 22q11.2 in idiopathic Parkinson's disease: A combined analysis of genome-wide association data. *The Lancet Neurology*, *15*(6), 585–596. http://doi.org/10.1016/S1474-4422(16)00071-5.
Mollenhauer, B., Trautmann, E., Sixel-Doring, F., Wicke, T., Ebentheuer, J., Schaumburg, M., et al. (2013). Nonmotor and diagnostic findings in subjects with de novo Parkinson disease of the DeNoPa cohort. *Neurology*, *81*(14), 1226–1234. http://doi.org/10.1212/WNL.0b013e3182a6cbd5.
Muthane, U. B., Swamy, H. S., Satishchandra, P., Subhash, M. N., Rao, S., & Subbakrishna, D. (1994). Early onset Parkinson's disease: Are juvenile- and young-onset different? *Movement Disorders*, *9*(5), 539–544. http://doi.org/10.1002/mds.870090506.
Nutt, J. G. (2016). Motor subtype in Parkinson's disease: Different disorders or different stages of disease? *Movement Disorders*, *31*(7), 957–961. http://doi.org/10.1002/mds.26657.
Olgiati, S., Quadri, M., Fang, M., Rood, J. P. M. A., Saute, J. A., Chien, H. F., et al. (2016). DNAJC6 mutations associated with early-onset Parkinson's disease. *Annals of Neurology*, *79*(2), 244–256. http://doi.org/10.1002/ana.24553.
Osaki, Y., Morita, Y., Kuwahara, T., Miyano, I., & Doi, Y. (2011). Prevalence of Parkinson's disease and atypical parkinsonian syndromes in a rural Japanese district. *Acta Neurologica Scandinavica*, *124*(3), 182–187. http://doi.org/10.1111/j.1600-0404.2010.01442.x.
Papadimitriou, D., Antonelou, R., Miligkos, M., Maniati, M., Papagiannakis, N., Bostantjopoulou, S., et al. (2016). Motor and nonmotor features of carriers of the p. A53T alpha-synuclein mutation: A longitudinal study. *Movement Disorders*, *31*(8), 1226–1230. http://doi.org/10.1002/mds.26615.
Parkinson, J. (2002). An essay on the shaking palsy. 1817. *The Journal of Neuropsychiatry and Clinical Neurosciences*, *14*(2), 223–236. Discussion 222. http://doi.org/10.1176/jnp.14.2.223.
Postuma, R. B., Berg, D., Stern, M., Poewe, W., Olanow, C. W., Oertel, W., et al. (2015). MDS clinical diagnostic criteria for Parkinson's disease. *Movement Disorders*, *30*(12), 1591–1601. http://doi.org/10.1002/mds.26424.
Postuma, R. B., Berg, D., Stern, M., Poewe, W., Olanow, C. W., Oertel, W., et al. (2016). Abolishing the 1-year rule: How much evidence will be enough? *Movement Disorders*, *31*(11), 1623–1627. http://doi.org/10.1002/mds.26796.
Pringsheim, T., Jette, N., Frolkis, A., & Steeves, T. D. L. (2014). The prevalence of Parkinson's disease: A systematic review and meta-analysis. *Movement Disorders*, *29*(13), 1583–1590. http://doi.org/10.1002/mds.25945.
Prodoehl, J., Planetta, P. J., Kurani, A. S., Comella, C. L., Corcos, D. M., & Vaillancourt, D. E. (2013). Differences in brain activation between tremor- and

nontremor-dominant Parkinson disease. *JAMA Neurology*, *70*(1), 100–106. http://doi.org/10.1001/jamaneurol.2013.582.

Quadri, M., Fang, M., Picillo, M., Olgiati, S., Breedveld, G. J., Graafland, J., et al. (2013). Mutation in the SYNJ1 gene associated with autosomal recessive, early-onset parkinsonism. *Human Mutation*, *34*(9), 1208–1215. http://doi.org/10.1002/humu.22373.

Rebeiz, J. J., Kolodny, E. H., & Richardson, E. P. (1967). Corticodentatonigral degeneration with neuronal achromasia: A progressive disorder of late adult life. *Transactions of the American Neurological Association*, *92*, 23–26.

Respondek, G., Stamelou, M., Kurz, C., Ferguson, L. W., Rajput, A., Chiu, W. Z., et al. (2014). The phenotypic spectrum of progressive supranuclear palsy: A retrospective multicenter study of 100 definite cases. *Movement Disorders*, *29*(14), 1758–1766. http://doi.org/10.1002/mds.26054.

Rizzo, G., Copetti, M., Arcuti, S., Martino, D., Fontana, A., & Logroscino, G. (2016). Accuracy of clinical diagnosis of Parkinson disease: A systematic review and meta-analysis. *Neurology*, *86*(6), 566–576. http://doi.org/10.1212/WNL.0000000000002350.

Rosales, R. L. (2010). X-linked dystonia parkinsonism: Clinical phenotype, genetics and therapeutics. *Journal of Movement Disorders*, *3*(2), 32–38. http://doi.org/10.14802/jmd.10009.

Rosenberg-Katz, K., Herman, T., Jacob, Y., Giladi, N., Hendler, T., & Hausdorff, J. M. (2013). Gray matter atrophy distinguishes between Parkinson disease motor subtypes. *Neurology*, *80*(16), 1476–1484. http://doi.org/10.1212/WNL.0b013e31828cfaa4.

Sato, K., Yabe, I., Yaguchi, H., Nakano, F., Kunieda, Y., Saitoh, S., et al. (2011). Genetic analysis of two Japanese families with progressive external ophthalmoplegia and parkinsonism. *Journal of Neurology*, *258*(7), 1327–1332. http://doi.org/10.1007/s00415-011-5936-x.

Sauerbier, A., Jenner, P., Todorova, A., & Chaudhuri, K. R. (2016). Non motor subtypes and Parkinson's disease. *Parkinsonism & Related Disorders*, *22*(Suppl. 1), S41–S46. http://doi.org/10.1016/j.parkreldis.2015.09.027.

Savica, R., Boeve, B. F., & Logroscino, G. (2016). Epidemiology of alpha-synucleinopathies: From Parkinson disease to dementia with Lewy bodies. *Handbook of Clinical Neurology*, *138*, 153–158. http://doi.org/10.1016/B978-0-12-802973-2.00009-4.

Schneider, S. A., Dusek, P., Hardy, J., Westenberger, A., Jankovic, J., & Bhatia, K. P. (2013). Genetics and pathophysiology of neurodegeneration with brain iron accumulation (NBIA). *Current Neuropharmacology*, *11*(1), 59–79. http://doi.org/10.2174/157015913804999469.

Schneider, S. A., Paisan-Ruiz, C., Quinn, N. P., Lees, A. J., Houlden, H., Hardy, J., et al. (2010). ATP13A2 mutations (PARK9) cause neurodegeneration with brain iron accumulation. *Movement Disorders*, *25*(8), 979–984. http://doi.org/10.1002/mds.22947.

Schneider, S. A., Walker, R. H., & Bhatia, K. P. (2007). The Huntington's disease-like syndromes: What to consider in patients with a negative Huntington's disease gene test. *Nature Clinical Practice Neurology*, *3*(9), 517–525. http://doi.org/10.1038/ncpneuro0606.

Schrag, A., & Schott, J. M. (2006). Epidemiological, clinical, and genetic characteristics of early-onset parkinsonism. *The Lancet Neurology*, *5*(4), 355–363. http://doi.org/10.1016/S1474-4422(06)70411-2.

Schwingenschuh, P., Ruge, D., Edwards, M. J., Terranova, C., Katschnig, P., Carrillo, F., et al. (2010). Distinguishing SWEDDs patients with asymmetric resting tremor from Parkinson's disease: A clinical and electrophysiological study. *Movement Disorders*, *25*(5), 560–569. http://doi.org/10.1002/mds.23019.

Selikhova, M., Kempster, P. A., Revesz, T., Holton, J. L., & Lees, A. J. (2013). Neuropathological findings in benign tremulous parkinsonism. *Movement Disorders*, *28*(2), 145–152. http://doi.org/10.1002/mds.25220.

Sharma, M., Ioannidis, J. P. A., Aasly, J. O., Annesi, G., Brice, A., Bertram, L., et al. (2012). A multi-centre clinico-genetic analysis of the VPS35 gene in Parkinson disease indicates reduced penetrance for disease-associated variants. *Journal of Medical Genetics*, *49*(11), 721–726. http://doi.org/10.1136/jmedgenet-2012-101155.

Siderowf, A., & Stern, M. B. (2008). Premotor Parkinson's disease: Clinical features, detection, and prospects for treatment. *Annals of Neurology*, *64*(Suppl. 2), S139–S147. http://doi.org/10.1002/ana.21462.

Sidransky, E., Nalls, M. A., Aasly, J. O., Aharon-Peretz, J., Annesi, G., Barbosa, E. R., et al. (2009). Multicenter analysis of glucocerebrosidase mutations in Parkinson's disease. *The New England Journal of Medicine*, *361*(17), 1651–1661. http://doi.org/10.1056/NEJMoa0901281.

Singleton, A., & Hardy, J. (2016). The evolution of genetics: Alzheimer's and Parkinson's diseases. *Neuron*, *90*(6), 1154–1163. http://doi.org/10.1016/j.neuron.2016.05.040.

Spillantini, M. G., Yoshida, H., Rizzini, C., Lantos, P. L., Khan, N., Rossor, M. N., et al. (2000). A novel tau mutation (N296N) in familial dementia with swollen achromatic neurons and corticobasal inclusion bodies. *Annals of Neurology*, *48*(6), 939–943.

Spina, S., Murrell, J. R., Huey, E. D., Wassermann, E. M., Pietrini, P., Grafman, J., et al. (2007). Corticobasal syndrome associated with the A9D Progranulin mutation. *Journal of Neuropathology and Experimental Neurology*, *66*(10), 892–900. http://doi.org/10.1097/nen.0b013e3181567873.

Stamelou, M., & Bhatia, K. P. (2016). Atypical parkinsonism—New advances. *Current Opinion in Neurology*, *29*(4), 480–485. http://doi.org/10.1097/WCO.0000000000000355.

Stamelou, M., Charlesworth, G., Cordivari, C., Schneider, S. A., Kägi, G., Sheerin, U.-M., et al. (2014). The phenotypic spectrum of DYT24 due to ANO3 mutations. *Movement Disorders*, *29*(7), 928–934. http://doi.org/10.1002/mds.25802.

Stamelou, M., Edwards, M. J., & Bhatia, K. P. (2013a). Late onset rest-tremor in DYT1 dystonia. *Parkinsonism & Related Disorders*, *19*(1), 136–137. http://doi.org/10.1016/j.parkreldis.2012.05.026.

Stamelou, M., Quinn, N. P., & Bhatia, K. P. (2013b). "Atypical" atypical parkinsonism: New genetic conditions presenting with features of progressive supranuclear palsy, corticobasal degeneration, or multiple system atrophy—A diagnostic guide. *Movement Disorders*, *28*(9), 1184–1199. http://doi.org/10.1002/mds.25509.

Stebbins, G. T., Goetz, C. G., Burn, D. J., Jankovic, J., Khoo, T. K., & Tilley, B. C. (2013). How to identify tremor dominant and postural instability/gait difficulty groups with the movement disorder society unified Parkinson's disease rating scale: Comparison with the unified Parkinson's disease rating scale. *Movement Disorders*, *28*(5), 668–670. http://doi.org/10.1002/mds.25383.

Steele, J. C., Richardson, J. C., & Olszewski, J. (1964). Progressive supranuclear palsy. A heterogeneous degeneration involving the brain stem, basal ganglia and cerebellum with vertical gaze and pseudobulbar palsy, nuchal dystonia and dementia. *Archives of Neurology*, *10*, 333–359.

Taylor, A. E., Saint-Cyr, J. A., & Lang, A. E. (1986). Frontal lobe dysfunction in Parkinson's disease. The cortical focus of neostriatal outflow. *Brain*, *109*(Pt. 5), 845–883.

Tremblay, C., Achim, A. M., Macoir, J., & Monetta, L. (2013). The heterogeneity of cognitive symptoms in Parkinson's disease: A meta-analysis. *Journal of Neurology, Neurosurgery, and Psychiatry*, *84*(11), 1265–1272. http://doi.org/10.1136/jnnp-2013-305021.

Van Den Eeden, S. K., Tanner, C. M., Bernstein, A. L., Fross, R. D., Leimpeter, A., Bloch, D. A., et al. (2003). Incidence of Parkinson's disease: Variation by age, gender, and race/ethnicity. *American Journal of Epidemiology*, *157*(11), 1015–1022.

Vann Jones, S. A., & O'Brien, J. T. (2013). The prevalence and incidence of dementia with Lewy bodies: A systematic review of population and clinical studies. *Psychological Medicine*, *44*(04), 673–683. http://doi.org/10.1017/S0033291713000494.

Vetrugno, R., Provini, F., Cortelli, P., Plazzi, G., Lotti, E. M., Pierangeli, G., et al. (2004). Sleep disorders in multiple system atrophy: A correlative video-polysomnographic study. *Sleep Medicine*, *5*(1), 21–30.

Vizcarra, J. A., Lang, A. E., Sethi, K. D., & Espay, A. J. (2015). Vascular parkinsonism: Deconstructing a syndrome. *Movement Disorders*, *30*(7), 886–894. http://doi.org/10.1002/mds.26263.

Vu, T. C., Nutt, J. G., & Holford, N. H. G. (2012). Progression of motor and nonmotor features of Parkinson's disease and their response to treatment. *British Journal of Clinical Pharmacology*, *74*(2), 267–283. http://doi.org/10.1111/j.1365-2125.2012.04192.x.

Wenning, G. K., Ben-Shlomo, Y., Hughes, A., Daniel, S. E., Lees, A., & Quinn, N. P. (2000). What clinical features are most useful to distinguish definite multiple system atrophy from Parkinson's disease? *Journal of Neurology, Neurosurgery & Psychiatry*, *68*(4), 434–440. http://doi.org/10.1136/jnnp.68.4.434.

Wenning, G. K., Colosimo, C., Geser, F., & Poewe, W. (2004). Multiple system atrophy. *The Lancet Neurology*, *3*(2), 93–103.

Wenning, G. K., Litvan, I., Jankovic, J., Granata, R., Mangone, C. A., McKee, A., et al. (1998). Natural history and survival of 14 patients with corticobasal degeneration confirmed at postmortem examination. *Journal of Neurology, Neurosurgery & Psychiatry*, *64*(2), 184–189.

Wenning, G. K., Litvan, I., & Tolosa, E. (2011). Milestones in atypical and secondary parkinsonisms. *Movement Disorders*, *26*(6), 1083–1095. http://doi.org/10.1002/mds.23713.

Wickremaratchi, M. M., Ben-Shlomo, Y., & Morris, H. R. (2009). The effect of onset age on the clinical features of Parkinson's disease. *European Journal of Neurology*, *16*(4), 450–456. http://doi.org/10.1111/j.1468-1331.2008.02514.x.

Wider, C., Dickson, D. W., & Wszolek, Z. K. (2010). Leucine-rich repeat kinase 2 gene-associated disease: Redefining genotype-phenotype correlation. *Neuro-Degenerative Diseases*, 7(1–3), 175–179. http://doi.org/10.1159/000289232.

Wider, C., & Wszolek, Z. K. (2008). Rapidly progressive familial parkinsonism with central hypoventilation, depression and weight loss (Perry syndrome)—A literature review. *Parkinsonism & Related Disorders*, *14*(1), 1–7. http://doi.org/10.1016/j.parkreldis.2007.07.014.

Williams, D. R., de Silva, R., Paviour, D. C., Pittman, A., Watt, H. C., Kilford, L., et al. (2005). Characteristics of two distinct clinical phenotypes in pathologically proven progressive supranuclear palsy: Richardson's syndrome and PSP-parkinsonism. *Brain*, *128*(Pt. 6), 1247–1258. http://doi.org/10.1093/brain/awh488.

Williams, D. R., & Lees, A. J. (2009). Progressive supranuclear palsy: Clinicopathological concepts and diagnostic challenges. *The Lancet Neurology*, *8*(3), 270–279. http://doi.org/10.1016/S1474-4422(09)70042-0.

Winter, Y., Bezdolnyy, Y., Katunina, E., Avakjan, G., Reese, J. P., Klotsche, J., et al. (2010). Incidence of Parkinson's disease and atypical parkinsonism: Russian population-based study. *Movement Disorders*, *25*(3), 349–356. http://doi.org/10.1002/mds.22966.

Woodhouse, N. J., & Sakati, N. A. (1983). A syndrome of hypogonadism, alopecia, diabetes mellitus, mental retardation, deafness, and ECG abnormalities. *Journal of Medical Genetics*, *20*(3), 216–219.

Zijlmans, J., Katzenschlager, R., Daniel, S. E., & Lees, A. J. (2004). The L-dopa response in vascular parkinsonism. *Journal of Neurology, Neurosurgery, and Psychiatry*, *75*(4), 545–547. http://doi.org/10.1136/jnnp.2003.018309.

CHAPTER SIX

Clinical Assessments in Parkinson's Disease: Scales and Monitoring

Roongroj Bhidayasiri[*,†,1], **Pablo Martinez-Martin**[‡]
[*]Chulalongkorn Center of Excellence for Parkinson's Disease & Related Disorders, Faculty of Medicine, Chulalongkorn University and King Chulalongkorn Memorial Hospital, Thai Red Cross Society, Bangkok, Thailand
[†]Juntendo University, Tokyo, Japan
[‡]National Center of Epidemiology and CIBERNED, Carlos III Institute of Health, Madrid, Spain
[1]Corresponding author: e-mail address: rbh@chulapd.org

Contents

Abstract

Measurement of disease state is essential in both clinical practice and research in order to assess the severity and progression of a patient's disease status, effect of treatment, and alterations in other relevant factors. Parkinson's disease (PD) is a complex disorder expressed through many motor and nonmotor manifestations, which cause disabilities that can vary both gradually over time or come on suddenly. In addition, there is a wide interpatient variability making the appraisal of the many facets of this disease difficult.

International Review of Neurobiology, Volume 132
ISSN 0074-7742
http://dx.doi.org/10.1016/bs.irn.2017.01.001

Two kinds of measure are used for the evaluation of PD. The first is subjective, inferential, based on rater-based interview and examination or patient self-assessment, and consist of rating scales and questionnaires. These evaluations provide estimations of conceptual, nonobservable factors (e.g., symptoms), usually scored on an ordinal scale. The second type of measure is objective, factual, based on technology-based devices capturing physical characteristics of the pathological phenomena (e.g., sensors to measure the frequency and amplitude of tremor). These instrumental evaluations furnish appraisals with real numbers on an interval scale for which a unit exists. In both categories of measures, a broad variety of tools exist. This chapter aims to present an up-to-date summary of the most relevant characteristics of the most widely used scales, questionnaires, and technological resources currently applied to the assessment of PD. The review concludes that, in our opinion: (1) no assessment methods can substitute the clinical judgment and (2) subjective and objective measures in PD complement each other, each method having strengths and weaknesses.

1. INTRODUCTION

Quantification of patients' health status and severity of disease state is a vital tool in the monitoring of changes in a disease's course, or treatment effects, over time. Measurements are relevant for diagnosis (e.g., blood glucose level for diabetes); determining the state of the condition (e.g., severity of cognitive impairment), functional performance (e.g., arterial oxygen saturation of hemoglobin), or ability to perform activities (e.g., disability level); tracking disease evolution (e.g., the size of a tumor) or the effect of a treatment (e.g., change in severity of pain with an analgesic); and advancing a prognosis (e.g., biomarkers for long-term prognosis after myocardial infarction), as well as assisting data recording and interprofessional communication about a patient's condition.

2. MEASUREMENT: CONCEPTS AND NEED

Measurement is an essential requisite for any scientific study and for the implementation of the scientific method, a research process based on the formulation of a hypothesis, collection and analysis of empirical evidence, and interpretation of the results in order to support or refute a theory. Measurement has been defined as "the assignment of numerals to aspects of objects or events according to rules" (Stevens, 1959). For health, and following the Stevens' quotation, measurement could be expressed as "the assignment of corresponding quantitative levels to a health indicator according to rules," where the indicator reflects a condition's aspects or events.

Information captured by qualitative means (e.g., a question about the current health state: how is your pain today?) may be useful for pragmatic management and planning, but quantification is necessary for precise monitoring and research.

There are two kinds of objects to be measured: those with material existence and those with conceptual existence. For the first group, an object exists in a measurable unit and it is possible to obtain a physical measure of that object that can then be compared (e.g., a distance in kilometers using a "meter" as unit). Many aspects of human health can be measured either by means of biological assays or performance measures, or objective procedures using units and providing results in real numbers on an interval scale. In an interval scale, all divisions in the scale are equal (e.g., milligrams), and the difference between points on the scale is also identical throughout the scale (e.g., 3 m will be the same distance from 0 to 3 m as from 26 to 29 m). Objects belonging to the second, conceptual, group are not directly observable and do not have any measurable unit. These abstract concepts (constructs) can only be measured subjectively and indirectly, through variables related to them can be operationalized and quantified in some way. Values for these variables are on an ordinal scale (e.g., first, second, third, and fourth). This requires the assignment of a rank order, but differences between contiguous values are unknown and may be not equivalent (e.g., difference between no pain and mild pain compared to difference between moderate and severe pain).

These general principles are also applicable to patient evaluations in general, and have, for decades, been applied to assess Parkinson's disease (PD) patients (Lang & Fahn, 1989; LaRocca, n.d; Marsden & Schachter, 1981; Teravainen & Calne, 1980). A combination of both objective and subjective approaches was expressly recommended for evaluation of PD, by Barbeau et al. (1981).

3. PD AS AN OBJECT FOR MEASUREMENT

PD is a disorder characterized by a multitude of manifestations categorized as motor and nonmotor symptoms (NMS). The disease progresses over time, with symptoms not only increasing in severity but also in number experienced thus causing increasing disability and severe complications.

Importantly, the combined effect of these features deteriorates the patients' quality of life and creates an increasing burden on their caregivers and on the consumption of social resources. Close monitoring of these many changing facets is vital for improving disease knowledge and, therefore, treatment of PD patients.

Some aspects of the disorder can be measured by means of physical, objective measures (e.g., computerized analysis of movement, oscillography, timed tests). The main advantages of this type of approach are reliability and objectivity as the results are expressed in physical units, but frequently they require sophisticated and expensive equipment and standardized test conditions. In addition, they only offer data which are restricted to a specific body region (e.g., tremor in hands) at the specific time the test was performed.

Due to these limitations, most of the evaluations used for clinical daily practice and research studies are based on subjective judgments. These appraisals provide valuations in which the assignment of values is based on estimations from the professional observer, the patient him/herself, or the caregiver. They are relatively rapid and simple to apply, do not require sophisticated instruments, and furnish global data on current state and wide time frames (e.g., the last 2 weeks). These evaluation tools are designed as rating scales or questionnaires and they have been employed by practitioners to evaluate signs, symptoms, complications, disability, health-related quality of life, and other constructs (satisfaction with treatment, satisfaction with life, living with a chronic disease, etc.).

3.1 Subjective Measures for PD: Rating Scales and Questionnaires

The need to measure the main features of PD was evident more than 50 years ago. It was evident that it was essential to quantify patients' symptoms, signs, and disability caused by the disease, in order to monitor the course of the disease and the effect of therapeutic interventions. The early rating scales that were designed and used from 1960 up to the second half of the 1980s decade, almost exclusively focused on the motor aspects of the disease (Alba, Trainor, Ritter, & Dacso, 1968; Canter, De La Torre, & Mier, 1961; Cotzias, Papavasiliou, Fehling, Kaufman, & Mena, 1970; Hoehn & Yahr, 1967; Klawans & Garvin, 1969; Larsen, Calne, & Calne, 1984; Lieberman et al., 1980; McDowell et al., 1970; Petrinovich & Hardyck, 1964; Schwab, 1960; Schwab & England, 1969; Walker et al., 1972; Webster, 1968). However, generally these scales were not formally validated after their elaboration and, in addition, were frequently and arbitrarily modified from one study to other by the developers themselves or other users, a fact that prevented objective comparisons.

In 1987 two new scales were developed with the intention of making a common assessment tool that could be used by most studies. One of these scales, Unified Parkinson's Disease Rating Scale (UPDRS) offered a comprehensive evaluation of four relevant dimensions in PD: mentation, behavior, and mood; activities of daily living; motor examination; and complications (Fahn & Elton, 1987). The other scale, Intermediate Scale for Assessment of Parkinson's Disease (ISAPD) was developed to offer a short scale that could be included as a shared tool in clinical trials and practice together with other scales (Martinez-Martin, 1987). Formal validations of both scales were published several years later (Martinez-Martin et al., 1994, 1995). The UPDRS became the reference scale for over 20 years, but was substituted by a revised scale, the Movement Disorder Society-Unified Parkinson's Disease Rating Scale (MDS-UPDRS), which was published in 2008 (Goetz et al., 2007; Goetz, Tilley, et al., 2008; Movement Disorder Society Task Force on Rating Scales for Parkinson's Disease, 2003).

Several other scales have appeared over the past 20 years, looking for more sound, simple, or comprehensive evaluations which focus on motor and nonmotor disturbances (Chaudhuri et al., 2007; Friedberg, Zoldan, Weizman, & Melamed, 1998; Goetz et al., 1994; Marinus et al., 2004; Marinus, Visser, Verwey, et al., 2003; Martinez-Martin et al., 1997; Pagonabarraga et al., 2008; Rabey et al., 1997; Visser et al., 2007). In addition, health-related quality-of-life evaluation tools and other patient-reported outcomes have been developed (Ambrosio et al., 2016; Brown, Dittner, Findley, & Wessely, 2005; Calne et al., 1996; Chaudhuri et al., 2006, 2002; de Boer, Wijker, Speelman, & de Haes, 1996; Giladi et al., 2000; Jenkinson, Fitzpatrick, Peto, Greenhall, & Hyman, 1997; Katzenschlager et al., 2007; Leentjens et al., 2014; Marinus, Visser, van Hilten, Lammers, & Stiggelbout, 2003; Peto, Jenkinson, Fitzpatrick, & Greenhall, 1995; Reddy et al., 2014; Stacy et al., 2005; Visser, Marinus, Stiggelbout, & Van Hilten, 2004).

In this chapter, given the high number of scales used in the assessment of PD patients, only the most relevant specific PD instruments will be considered. For each one, reference of the original publication, description, a judgment on its clinimetric properties, and additional information is provided.

3.2 Global Evaluations

3.2.1 Hoehn and Yahr Staging Scale (HY)

This rater-based scale places the patient in one of five stages of disease between 1 (unilateral involvement, usually with minimal or no functional impairment) and 5 (confined to bed or wheelchair unless aided) (Hoehn & Yahr, 1967). Each stage is briefly defined in terms of motor impairment severity and disability/dependence. A seven-level modification was added to complement the UPDRS, including stages 1.5 and 2.5, but the clinimetric attributes of this modified version have not been explored. Therefore, the MDS recommends the use of the original version (Goetz et al., 2004).

Due to its simplicity and ability to determine the motor and functional group to which the patient can be assigned, the HY is universally used to classify patients throughout the phases of disease progression. Despite the fact that it has been scarcely tested in regard to its metric attributes, it is considered reliable and valid (Goetz et al., 2004).

The HY ranks are not lineal in progression and their amplitude between ranks is variable and does not assess NMS. However, it remains the reference classification for PD progression, is included in the MDS-UPDRS, and could be complemented with a NMS classification (Goetz, Tilley, et al., 2008; Ray Chaudhuri et al., 2013). Recently, a "Wii"-based assessment has been proposed for scoring the HY (Kocer & Oktay, 2016). HY is in the public domain and can be freely used.

3.2.2 Clinical Impression of Severity Index

The Clinical Impression of Severity Index (CISI-PD) is a global, rater-based assessment composed of four items: motor signs, disability, motor complications, and cognitive status (Martinez-Martin, Forjaz, Cubo, Frades, & de Pedro Cuesta, 2006; Martinez-Martin, Rodriguez-Blazquez, Forjaz, & de Pedro, 2009). Each item scores from 0 (not at all) to 6 (very severe) and a total CISI-PD score (0–24) is obtained from the sum of the items scores. This score represents PD severity as perceived by the clinician at the time of assessment and is designed to be applied after carrying out an interview and examination, as the last evaluation. In these circumstances, CISI-PD scoring takes less than a minute and explains over 90% of the Clinical Global Impression-Severity variance (Martinez-Martin et al., 2006). It possesses very satisfactory clinimetric properties and a unifactorial structure (Martinez-Martin et al., 2006; Martinez-Martin, Rodriguez-Blazquez,

Forjaz, et al., 2009). Recently, the CISI-PD demonstrated the most satisfactory performance in comparison with other global evaluations and the highest association with measures of PD impairment, disability, and quality of life (Martinez-Martin, Rojo-Abuin, et al., 2016).

The main advantages of this measure are its simplicity and excellent clinimetric attributes, providing a profile (the scores of the four components) and a total score. However, its interrater reliability and responsiveness have not been formally tested and, up to now, has only been used by the developers. The CISI-PD is in public domain and can be used freely.

3.3 Comprehensive Scales

3.3.1 Unified Parkinson's Disease Rating Scale

The UPDRS has been the most used PD scale and the reference measure for regulatory agencies since its development; however, it is being progressively displaced by its revised version, the MDS-UPDRS (Fahn & Elton, 1987; Goetz, Tilley, et al., 2008). It consists of 42 items in four subscales: Section I: Mentation, behavior, and mood (4 items); Section II: Activities of daily living (13 items; it may be scored in "on" and "off" states); Section III: Motor examination (14 items that provide 27 scores, as several signs are separately evaluated in both sides and different body parts); Section IV: Complications of therapy (11 items including 4 for dyskinesias, 4 for fluctuations, and 3 for other complications). The scoring range for each item of the Sections I at III is from 0 (normal) to 4 (severe). The scoring of those items in Section IV is irregular, with some items scoring 0 (absence) or 1 (he/she witnesses) and others, referred to duration or intensity, from 0 to 4. The total score of the subscales is Section I: 16 points; Section II: 52; Section III: 108; and Section IV: 23. Therefore, the UPDRS total score ranges between 0 and 199 points. Sections I and II are scored by interview; Section III is scored through a structured neurological examination; and the scores for Section IV are based on interview and observation. The UPDRS is complemented with the Hoehn and Yahr staging, and the Schwab and England scale (SES) (Hoehn & Yahr, 1967; Schwab & England, 1969). The UPDRS shows floor effect in Sections I and IV, but most of its clinimetric properties have been found acceptable or satisfactory (Forjaz & Martinez-Martin, 2006; Martinez-Martin & Forjaz, 2006; Movement Disorder Society Task Force on Rating Scales for Parkinson's Disease, 2003). However, it assesses very few nonmotor items, lacks of instructions for standardized application, includes in Section II items that would be allocated in Section III, and has cultural bias in Section II. These weaknesses promoted the revision of the scale by a MDS Task Force (Movement Disorder Society Task Force on Rating Scales for Parkinson's Disease, 2003). The UPDRS is in the public domain, available in many languages.

3.3.2 Movement Disorders Society Sponsored Revision of the Unified Parkinson's Disease Rating Scale

The MDS-UPDRS is a new version of the UPDRS, more complete, homogeneous, and with better clinimetric properties than its predecessor (Goetz, Tilley, et al., 2008). At present, the scale is available in 15 languages, besides the original in English (http://www.movementdisorders.org/MDS/Education/Rating-Scales/Rating-Scales-By-Disorder.htm), a figure that is continuously increasing. The MDS-UPDRS consists of four parts: Part I: Nonmotor Aspects of Experiences of Daily Living; Part II: Motor Aspects of Experiences of Daily Living; Part III: Motor Examination; and Part IV: Motor complications.

Part I contains 13 items (6 rater-based, evaluated through interview, and 7 through a self-completed patient questionnaire). Part II also consists of 13 items (assessed via a self-completed patient questionnaire). Part III includes 18 items (with 33 scores from separate assessments of body parts, both on right and left sides). Part IV is composed of 6 items (2 for dyskinesias, 4 for fluctuations). In this scale, all items score from 0 (normal) to 4 (severe) have instructions for standardized application and explanations adjusted to each rank of responses. The correlation with the corresponding scales of the UPDRS and the most relevant MDS-UPDRS clinimetric attributes have been explored and found to be satisfactory (Goetz, Tilley, et al., 2008; Martinez-Martin et al., 2013). Several studies have also been carried out on the validity of Part I appended to other scales for assessment of NMS, and methods for conversion of the MDS-UPDRS scores to SCOPA-motor, UPDRS, Nonmotor Symptoms Scale (NMSS) scores and vice versa have been proposed (Gallagher, Goetz, Stebbins, Lees, & Schrag, 2012; Goetz, Stebbins, & Tilley, 2012; Hentz et al., 2015; Martinez-Martin et al., 2015; Verbaan et al., 2011; Weintraut et al., 2016). Interestingly, MDS-UPDRS scores seem to somewhat predicted the time to initiate symptomatic therapy in PD, and relatively high scores have been obtained in the general population, mainly for elderly, women, and patients with specific comorbidities (Keezer, Wolfson, & Postuma, 2016; Simuni et al., 2016). Its length is the main disadvantage for use in daily practice.

The MDS-UPDRS is a benchmark for PD assessment, its application is standardized, possesses satisfactory clinimetric attributes and a certified training program (http://mds.movementdisorders.org/updrs/) (Goetz et al., 2010). It is owned by the International Parkinson and Movement Disorder Society, IPMDS), and permission for use is needed (https://mds.movementdisorders.org/publications/rating_scales/request_form.php).

3.4 Scales for Motor and Functional Assessment

3.4.1 Scales for Outcomes in Parkinson's Disease-Motor (SCOPA-Motor)

This scale is composed of 21 items included in three domains: (A) Motor evaluation, with the scores of eight items attained through clinical examination and for two additional items by historical information; (B) Activities of daily living, composed of seven rater-based items following interview; and (C) Motor complications, including two items for dyskinesias and two for fluctuations, evaluated by interview and observation (Marinus et al., 2004). The scoring range for all items is 0 (normal, absent) to 3 (severe, intense). Summative scores are obtained for the domains and the complete scale (the range of the total score is 0–75, as four items are assessed in both sides).

The SCOPA-Motor (originally, SPES/SCOPA) was based on the UPDRS, but developed as a shorter and clinimetrically more sound instrument than that scale. As a consequence, the SCOPA-Motor has satisfactory clinimetric properties, including a close concurrent validity with the corresponding components of the UPDRS (Marinus et al., 2004; Martinez-Martin et al., 2005). However, its responsiveness has been hardly explored (Hudson, Seeman, & Seeman, 2014). A formula for conversion of SCOPA-Motor to MDS-UPDRS scores or vice versa has been proposed (Verbaan et al., 2011). The scale is available in several languages (www.scopa-propark.eu), but has been scarcely used by researchers other than the developers.

3.4.2 Schwab & England Activities of Daily Living Scale

The SES is an interview-based scale, although it may be completed by the patient or even the caregiver (Schwab & England, 1969). It assesses the degree of functional independence of patients on a range of 11 response options (from 100%, completely independent, to 0%, vegetative functions are not functioning, bedridden). Despite the use of a percentage format and difference of 10% applied to successive levels, the scoring system is not an interval scale but an ordinal one (in fact, the "%" could be entirely dispensed with). It is available in many languages, has been widely used due to its simplicity of application and interpretation, and was added as a complementary evaluation to the UPDRS. Due to these reasons and despite the fact the SES is not specific for PD, it was included in this review.

The SES lacks instructions for users (McRae, Diem, Vo, O'Brien, & Seeberger, 2000), and its psychometric properties have been scarcely explored in a systematic manner (Forjaz & Martinez-Martin, 2006; Martinez-Martin & Forjaz, 2006; McRae et al., 2000). However, there are data suggesting satisfactory responsiveness, and the SES meets the criteria of "Recommended" by the IPMDS Task Force (Schrag, Spottke, Quinn, & Dodel, 2009; Shulman et al., 2016).

3.4.3 Self-Assessment Parkinson's Disease Disabilities Scale

The Self-Assessment Parkinson's Disease Disabilities Scale (SPDDS) is a patient-based questionnaire composed of 24 items evaluating the patients' ability to perform activities of daily living (Brown, MacCarthy, Gotham, Der, & Marsden, 1988). Response options for each item are from 1 "able to do alone without difficulty" to 5 "unable to do at all." Summative total scores run from 25 to 125. Scale reliability, construct validity, and responsiveness were found to be satisfactory (Biemans, Dekker, & van der Woude, 2001; Gazibara et al., 2013; Stallibrass, Sissons, & Chalmers, 2002). The SPDDS has been "recommended" by the IPMDS Task Force (Shulman et al., 2016).

3.4.4 Postural Instability and Gait Difficulty Score

The Postural Instability and Gait Difficulty Score (PIGD) initially represented the mean of five items of the UPDRS: falling, freezing, walking (three items from Part II-Activities of daily living), gait, and postural instability (from the Part III-Motor examination), but is also used as a summative score ranging from 0 (normal) to 20 (maximal difficulty) (Jankovic et al., 1990). It is frequently used for characterizing the PIGD subtype of PD and tested clinimetric properties have been found to be acceptable. A PIGD index may be also obtained from the MDS-UPDRS derived from the items rating walking/balance and freezing (from the Part II-Motor Aspects of Experiences of Daily Living), plus the scores of the items rating gait, freezing of gait (FOG), and postural stability (Part III-Motor examination) (Stebbins et al., 2013). The performance of both indexes, from UPDRS and MDS-UPDRS, to identify the PIGD subtype is satisfactory and quite close each other (Stebbins et al., 2013). However, as several clinimetric properties of the MDS-UPDRS-derived scores still remain untested, this PIGD score could not reach the "recommended" level of the IPMDS whereas the UPDRS-derived score achieved this grade (Bloem et al., 2016).

3.4.5 Freezing of Gait Questionnaire

The freezing of gait questionnaire (FOGQ) is a 6-item scale for FOG evaluation (Giladi et al., 2000). Scores are obtained through interview, with each item scoring from 0 (normal, none, etc.) to 4 (unable to walk, always, etc.) and the total score ranging from 0 to 24. It showed unidimensionality, satisfactory internal consistency and reproducibility, weak or moderate correlation with UPDRS subscales, and a high correlation with the Hoehn and Yahr staging (Giladi et al., 2000, 2009). Adequate responsiveness and criterion validity have also been described (Frazzitta, Pezzoli, Bertotti, & Maestri, 2013; Giladi et al., 2009; Tomlinson et al., 2013). A new FOGQ has been developed and partially validated (Nieuwboer et al., 2009). However, a recent study has challenged the usefulness of these questionnaires (Shine et al., 2012). The FOGQ is "recommended" by the IPMDS (Bloem et al., 2016).

3.5 Comprehensive NMS Assessments

3.5.1 Nonmotor Symptoms Questionnaire

The nonmotor symptoms questionnaire (NMSQuest) is a patient-based questionnaire designed to screen a range of NMS relevant for PD. It is composed of 30 items grouped in nine domains: digestive (7 items); urinary (2 items); apathy/attention/memory (3 items); hallucinations/delusions (2 items); depression/anxiety (2 items); sexual function (2 items); cardiovascular (2 items); sleep disorders (5 items); and miscellaneous (pain, weight change, swelling, seating, diplopia) (5 items) (Chaudhuri et al., 2006). Response options to the questions refer to the experience of the symptoms in the last month and are binary (yes/no). A total score can be obtained from the sum of the "yes" responses, representing the number of NMS experienced by the patient, and may be used as an immediate index of NMS burden, and can reflect the effect of therapeutic interventions (Chaudhuri et al., 2006, 2015; Dafsari et al., 2016; Martinez-Martin et al., 2007). It has not been tested with diagnostic criteria, but has showed a close association with the NMS Scale, and satisfactory known-groups validity (Chaudhuri et al., 2007, 2006; Martinez-Martin et al., 2007). Due to its design and content, the NMSQuest can be used in disorders other than PD (Günther et al., 2016). The NMSQuest has been translated to a diversity of languages and is owned by the IPMDS thus requires their permission for use (https://mds.movementdisorders.org/publications/rating_scales/request_form.php).

3.5.2 Nonmotor Symptoms Scale

The NMSS is a rater-based scale, scored through interview with the patient/caregiver, for evaluation of the NMS burden over the last month (Chaudhuri et al., 2007). The NMSS includes 30 items in nine domains: cardiovascular (2 items); sleep/fatigue (4 items); mood/apathy (6 items); perceptual problems/hallucinations (3 items); attention/memory (3 items); gastrointestinal (3 items); urinary (3 items); sexual function (2 items); and miscellaneous (4 items). Each item score is obtained from multiplication of frequency (1, rarely, to 4, very frequent) by intensity (0, none, to 3, severe). Summative scores are obtained for the respective domains and the complete scale (theoretical range: 0–360). Validation studies have demonstrated the NMSS has acceptable or satisfactory clinimetric attributes as a whole, including satisfactory responsiveness (Antonini et al., 2015; Bohlega et al., 2015; Carod-Artal & Martinez-Martin, 2013; Chaudhuri et al., 2007; Dafsari et al., 2016; Koh et al., 2012; Martinez-Martin et al., 2015; Martinez-Martin, Rodriguez-Blazquez, Abe, et al., 2009; Martinez-Martin, Rodriguez-Blazquez, Kurtis, Chaudhuri, & NMSS Validation Group, 2011; Ou et al., 2016; Sellami et al., 2016). It has been used to quantify nonmotor fluctuations and to determine the effect of referral to expert care on the NMS burden (Prakash et al., 2015; Storch et al., 2015).

The NMSS is available and validated in many languages. At the time of writing, a validation study of a revised version sponsored by the IPMDS is about to begin. The NMSS is owned by the IPMDS and requires their permission for use (https://mds.movementdisorders.org/publications/rating_scales/request_form.php).

3.6 Scales for Motor Complications

3.6.1 Unified Dyskinesia Rating Scale

The Unified Dyskinesia Rating Scale (UDysRS) is a PD-specific scale with four sections: Part I: Historical On dyskinesia rating (11 items: 1 rater-based, 10 patient-based; 0–44 points); Part II: Historical Off-dystonia rating (4 items: 1 rater-based, 3 patient-based; 0–16 points); Part III: Objective evaluation of impairment by dyskinesia (severity, body regions distribution, and type (choreic or dystonic dyskinesia) during four observed activities; 0–28 points); and Part IV: Objective evaluation of disability by dyskinesia, based in the four activities performed in the Part III (communication, drinking, dressing, and ambulation) (Goetz, Nutt, & Stebbins, 2008). In the original study, acceptable reliability parameters were found (Goetz, Nutt, et al., 2008). It is completed in around 15 min and its historical time frame covers the past week. In the review by the MDS Task Force, the UDysRS was qualified as "suggested" because some clinimetric properties remained untested and the scale had not been used by researchers other than the developers (Colosimo et al., 2010). Since that review, however, new information has appeared about the appropriate stability of the scale, and its sensitivity to change, confirming the high quality of this comprehensive dyskinesia scale (Goetz et al., 2013, 2011). The UDysRS is currently only available in three languages other than English, but has a certificate education program (http://udysrs.movementdisorders.org/Welcome?ReturnUrl=%2f), and is owned by the IPMDS, thereby requiring their permission for use (https://mds.movementdisorders.org/publications/rating_scales/request_form.php) (Goetz, Nutt, Stebbins, & Chmura, 2009).

3.6.2 The Wearing-Off Questionnaires

The first version of the Wearing-Off Questionnaires (WOQ) was a 32-item tool designed to identify patients with wearing-off phenomenon (Stacy et al., 2005). Although this "WOQ-32" showed usefulness in screening, its length was considered excessive and the authors selected 19 items with similar outcome (WOQ-19). This 19-item version was also named QUICK (Martinez-Martin, Tolosa, Hernandez, & Badia, 2008). In addition, even shorter versions have been used with 18, 10, or 9 items (Martinez-Martin & Hernandez, 2012; Santens & de Noordhout, 2006; Stacy et al., 2008). As a whole, all of these versions have shown adequate properties for wearing-off detection.

In all these questionnaires, there is a list of symptoms in which the patient has to mark those he/she is experiencing. In a second list, the patient marks if the previously indicated symptoms improve after the next dose of medication. One positive response is indicative of potential existence of motor and nonmotor wearing-off and the use of these questionnaires can improve the clinical detection in a routine visit. Two positive responses have been proposed for balancing sensitivity and specificity (Martinez-Martin & Hernandez, 2012; Martinez-Martin et al., 2008). Both, the 19- and 9-item versions are recommended by the MDS for screening of wearing-off in PD (Antonini et al., 2011). WOQ-9, WOQ-19 (QUICK), and WOQ-32 are copyrighted by Duke University Medical Center (https://eprovide.mapi-trust.org/instruments/wearing-off-questionnaire).

3.7 Other Scales and Questionnaires

In addition to the measures reviewed, there is a huge amount of generic and specific scales and questionnaires that have been applied to evaluate very different aspects of PD. Their characteristics and quality are very variable and, therefore, careful selection of the scales to be applied in a study is needed. To this purpose, the systematic reviews, like those carried out by the IPMDS and the MDS Task Force provide an invaluable resource. The scales recommended by the IPMDS may be found in: https://mds.movementdisorders.org/publications/rating_scales/. The reviews carried out by the MDS Task Force and Committee on Rating Scales Development appear in: http://www.movementdisorders.org/MDS/About/Committees–Other-Groups/MDS-Committees/Committee-on-Rating-Scales-Development.htm.

4. OBJECTIVE MEASURES FOR PD: THE RATIONALES

4.1 The Rationales

Recently, there has been a growing interest in developing objective assessment of the symptoms in PD, and its health-related outcomes, using new technology-based tools, worn or operated by patients either in a healthcare or domestic environment. These technology-based devices can be classified as wearable, nonwearable, and hybrid devices (Godinho et al., 2016). As the aim of our review is on the clinical applications of these devices, we will focus on the potential application in daily clinical use of wearables, defined as electronic technology or computers designed to be worn on the body, or embedded into watches, bracelets, clothing, and hybrid systems, referred to the blend of technologies combining wearable and nonwearable devices. The term "wearable" in this chapter may be referred to differently as "inertial sensor," or "body-fixed sensor" depending on how it was described in the original chapter. The detailed technological aspects of these devices will not be covered in this chapter. Although some of these technologies are not new, the recent uptake of these technologies is likely a result of the advances and availability of high-speed internet connections, the development of smaller and more compact devices, which are now portable and importantly affordable, and the rising of computer literacy in the general population.

The use of technology-based devices shares similar goals to subjective measures, including scales and questionnaires, in terms of eliciting outcomes that are useful in determining the presence or severity of symptoms in order to improve clinical management of PD. Objective assessment of certain features (e.g., tremor and bradykinesia) may assist physicians in making the correct diagnosis. Additional benefits of objective measurement include its capabilities in providing unbiased measurements, detecting subtle changes, simplifying patient participation, data management, and enabling monitoring in unobtrusive free-living environments (e.g., nighttime and home-based monitoring) (Maetzler, Domingos, Srulijes, Ferreira, & Bloem, 2013; Stamford, Schmidt, & Friedl, 2015). Testing environments during clinic visits can be stressful for patients; thus, altering the symptomatology of patients (Hemmerle, Herman, & Seroogy, 2012). One recent study demonstrated significant differences of motor performance measures in PD subjects between in-home and in-clinic assessments with a tendency toward better motor performance during in-clinic assessments (Toosizadeh et al., 2015). The application of ambulatory monitoring is particularly useful in PD patients when their symptoms fluctuate, limiting the ability for patients and caregivers to adequately recall the symptoms. The use of current clinical instruments for extended monitoring, such as a PD home diary, is associated with fatigue, recalled bias and may not be suitable in certain PD populations, for example, patients with cognitive impairment (Papapetropoulos, 2012; Stone, Shiffman, Schwartz, Broderick, & Hufford, 2002). In addition, certain times of the day (e.g., nighttime) can be particularly challenging for clinical monitoring with scales or questionnaires (Bhidayasiri, Sringean, & Thanawattano, 2016; Maetzler et al., 2013). It is important to realize that subjective and objective measures in PD complement each other as each method has unique strengths and weaknesses. Table 1 provides a comparison of advantages and disadvantages of subjective vs objective assessments in PD. Importantly, a number of studies have demonstrated significant correlations between objective evaluations (e.g., gait velocity) and subjective measures (e.g., HY stage) and this is the area that many researchers are exploring (Toosizadeh et al., 2015). It is, therefore, the judgment of treating physicians to determine what kind of measurement is appropriate in individual patient in a particular clinical situation.

For the purpose of this review, we will describe the uses of objective assessment in PD, divided into the objective measures of cardinal features of PD, nonmotor and associated features, and ambulatory monitoring.

4.2 Objective Measures of Cardinal Features in PD

Although the cardinal features of PD, including rest tremor, bradykinesia, rigidity, and postural instability, are very well recognized by physicians

Table 1 Advantages and Disadvantages of Questionnaires and Scales vs Objective Assessment Tools in Parkinson's Disease

Types	Advantages	Disadvantages
Questionnaires and scales	• Suitable methods for screening a large number of patients in a short period of time • Validated instruments for clinical routines and clinical trials • Several scales are widely accepted and implemented in large clinical trials • Ability to capture subjective symptoms • No risk for physical injury during the test	• Subjective nature • Potential for interrater variability • Difficult if continuous monitoring is indicated • Ratings may fluctuate when performed on the same patient • Certain disease-specific features may affect rater's outcomes • Every components of questionnaire needs to be used together rather than independently
Technology-based assessment	• Provide quantifiable data • Ability for continuous monitoring • Different technology platforms	• Potential high cost for investigations • Increased risks from medical devices • Most devices are not as yet applicable for daily clinical use • Diagnostic accurately for each device has not been performed in large prospective clinical trials • Different setups and criteria have not been standardized

who are regularly involved in the care of PD patients, recent evidence has documented the heterogeneity of these symptoms, leading to a number of classifications defining subtypes of PD, not limited to traditional tremor-predominant and akinetic-rigid subtypes (Marras & Lang, 2013). For example, there are now several forms of tremor in PD associated with the considerable variability of clinical expression (Bhidayasiri, 2005; Deuschl, Bain, & Brin, 1998). Moreover, different clinical presentations of tremors can also be observed in other parkinsonian syndromes, not limited to PD. Bradykinesia is a good example where progressive decrement in amplitude, hesitations, or arrests during ongoing movement assessment may not be easily appreciated by clinical examiners (Fahn & Elton, 1987). These limitations pose significant challenges to the subjective assessments made by clinical examination alone with or without scales and questionnaires. While no instruments can supersede thorough clinical examination, these limitations can be at least partially overcome with the use of objective assessments. Table 2 outlines commonly used questionnaires, scales, and objective tools in the assessment of cardinal features of PD.

4.2.1 Parkinsonian Tremor

Tremor in PD is traditionally evaluated by the UPDRS, or, more recently, by the MDS-UPDRS (Fahn & Elton, 1987; Goetz, Tilley, et al., 2008). The Clinical Tremor Rating Scale (TRS), developed by Fahn, Tolosa, and Marin, is a scale dedicated to the evaluation of tremor, but its clinimetric properties have not been validated in patients with parkinsonian tremor (Fahn, Tolosa, & Marin, 1988). Tremor can be clinically assessed by means of spiral drawings and evaluation of hand writing specimens, frequently exhibiting the features of micrographia in PD, or be quantified as continuous variables in terms of the frequency and magnitude of the oscillatory cycles. In order to capture parkinsonian tremor quantitatively, a device needs to be able to measure both translational and rotational movements with six degree of freedom; thus, requiring at least six one-dimensional transducers.

Objective assessment of parkinsonian tremor has been reported with various transducer-based methods, including accelerometry, gyroscopy, electromyography, electromagnetic tracking, actigraphy, and digitizing tablets (Haubenberger et al., 2016). Among these devices, an inertial sensor, which refers to a pair of triaxial accelerometers and gyroscopes housing in the same unit (an inertial measurement unit, IMU), is the most frequently employed device used in the objective evaluation of tremor due to its ability to measure both linear and angular accelerations in three dimensional (3D) space, commonly involved in parkinsonian tremor (Bhidayasiri, Petchrutchatachart, et al., 2014; Wong, Wong, & Lo, 2007). In addition, as a result of advancing circuit technology, these sensors are becoming smaller in size and better in performance (Fig. 1). The applications for tremor analysis have also been developed in a number of smartphones and smart watches, which nowadays are equipped with accelerometers (Daneault, Carignan, Codere, Sadikot, & Duval, 2012; LeMoyne & Mastroianni, 2015; Wile, Ranawaya, & Kiss, 2014). The functions of the inertial sensor have been explored for different clinical purposes in PD, including assisting in disease diagnosis based on

Table 2 Questionnaires, Scales and Objective Methods for the Evaluation of Cardinal Features of Parkinson's Disease

		Objective Assessment	
Feature	**Questionnaire/Clinical Scales**	**Types of Device**	**Outcome Measures**
Tremor	Clinical score • UPDRS III (tremor subscore) • MDS-UPDRS III • Fahn–Tolosa–Marin tremor rating scale (TRS)	*Wearable inertial sensors* • Low-cost, 3-dimension, office-based inertial sensors (ChulaPD tremor device)	Quantitative tremor parameters from gyroscope including root mean square (RMS) angular rate (degrees/second), RMS angle (degrees), peak frequency (Hz), peak magnitude (degrees/second), and Q (dispersion of frequency). Quantitative tremor parameters from accelerometer including RMS rate (meter/second), RMS velocity (meter/second), peak magnitude (meter/second), peak frequency (Hz), and Q (dispersion of frequency)
		• Kinesia™ system	The objective motor scores for PD symptoms were calculated by clinically validated algorithms and range from 0 (no symptoms) to 4 (severe symptoms)
		• PERFORM system: composed of the wearable multisensor monitor unit (WMSMU) and the local base unit (LBU)	The signals coming from the WMSMU are processed by the Daily Monitoring Processor (DMP) which is composed of the following modules: Tremor (Posture and Resting) Recognizer, LID Recognizer, FOG Recognizers, Bradykinesia Recognizer, and Activity Recognizer
		• Bosch BMA150 triaxial, digital acceleration sensors	Smartphone mobile medical application for monitoring acceleration in all axes
		Nonwearable inertial sensors • Motus movement monitor (two solid-state gyroscopes)	Peak amplitude, RMS of angular velocity, tremor frequency, tremor dispersion score, power spectrum graph

Bradykinesia	Clinical scales • UPDRS III (bradykinesia subscore) • MDS-UPDRS III	*Wearable inertial sensors*	
		• Parkinson's KinetiGraph™ system (PKG)	Graphs of patient's movements with algorithm to determine the severity of dradykinesia and dyskinesia
		• Microsoft Kinect sensors (Kinect Xbox)	The use of the MS Kinect system for movement-data acquisition via selected digital signal- and image-processing methods
		• PERFORM system: composed of the wearable multisensor monitor unit (WMSMU) and the local base unit (LBU)	The signals are processed by the Daily Monitoring Processor (DMP) which is composed of the following modules: Tremor (Posture and Resting) Recognizer, LID Recognizer, FOG Recognizer, Bradykinesia Recognizer, and Activity Recognizer
		Nonwearable inertial sensors • The Motus motion movement monitor includes two solid-state gyroscopes	Peak amplitude, RMS of angular velocity, tremor frequency, tremor dispersion score, power spectrum graph
		• 3D Motion Analysis: Ultrasonic motion measurement system (Zebris Medical GmbH)	Mean segment length, peaks of velocity and acceleration, number of motion changes, segment frequency
		• Vicon motion analysis system: infrared camera	Velocity and acceleration time
Rigidity	Clinical scales • UPDRS III (rigidity subscore) • MDS-UPDRS • Hoehn and Yahr score	*Nonwearable dynamometers*	
		• Biodex isokenetic dynamometer	Maximum torque, Angular position, Torque–velocity relationship, muscle endurance, Reciprocal muscle group ratio

Continued

Table 2 Questionnaires, Scales and Objective Methods for the Evaluation of Cardinal Features of Parkinson's Disease—cont'd

Feature	Questionnaire/Clinical Scales	Objective Assessment	
		Types of Device	**Outcome Measures**
Postural instability, gait difficulty, and balance	Questionnaires • ABC-16 scale Clinical scales • Pull test • Hoehn and Yahr score • UPDRS III (PIGD subscore) • MDS-UPDRS III • Berg Balance scale • Tinetti Balance Scale • Balance Evaluation Systems test (BESTest) • Mini-BESTest • FOG score • Gait and Balance Scale • Dynamic Gait Index (DGI) • 6-min walk tests (6-MWT) • 10-m walk test (10-MWT) • Timed Up and Go • Functional Reach test	*Wearable inertial sensors* • Physilog® 4: gait analysis system combined triaxial accelerometer, triaxial gyroscope, triaxial magnetometer, and barometer	Temporospatial variables, clearance analysis, and turning analysis
		• InvenSense IDG-300 & Freescale Semiconductor MMA7260QT: triaxial accelerometer	Acceleration
		• Axivity AX3: triaxial accelerometer	Acceleration
		• Mobility Lab system: Combined triaxial accelerometer, triaxial gyroscope, and triaxial magnetometer	Cadence, Foot Clearance, Gait Cycle, Duration, Gait Speed, Double Support, Terminal Double Support, Lateral Step, Variability, Circumduction, Dorsiflexion, Plantarflexion, Stance, Step Duration, Stride, Length, Swing, Toe Out Angle, Stride Length Variability
		• DynaPort MoveTest: triaxial accelerometer	Gait pattern analysis with four basis for advanced parameter calculations, including step time asymmetry, bilateral coordination, and stride time fluctuations
		• Mobility Lab system: combined triaxial accelerometer, triaxial gyroscope, and triaxial magnetometer	Cadence, Foot Clearance, Gait Cycle, Duration, Gait Speed, Double Support, Terminal Double Support, Lateral Step, Variability, Circumduction, Dorsiflexion, Plantarflexion, Stance, Step Duration, Stride, Length, Swing, Toe Out Angle, Stride Length Variability

	Nonwearable gait system	
	• GAITRite system	Temporospatial gait variables (gait velocity, Cadence, Stride length, Cycle time, Single support time, Double support time, Swing time, Stance phase time)
	• Zebris Rehalwalk system	Temporospatial variables (gait velocity, Cadence, Stride length, Cycle time, Single support time, Double support time, Swing time, Stance phase time)
	Nonwearable balance analysis system	
	• Balance Master system (NeuroCom, USA)	Sensory integration balance test, Limits of stability test, Rhythmic weight shift test, Weight bearing squat test, Unilateral stance test
	• Biodex dynamic posturography	Postural instability test, Limits of stability test, Single leg stability test, Fall risk test, Sensory integration of balance test
	• Nintendo Wii® balance board	Center of pressure (COP), COP path length

ABC-16, the activities-specific balance confidence scale—16 items; *FOG*, freezing of gait; *LID*, levodopa-induced dyskinesia; *PD*, Parkinson's disease; *RMS*, root mean square; *UPDRS*, The Unified Parkinson's disease Rating Scale.

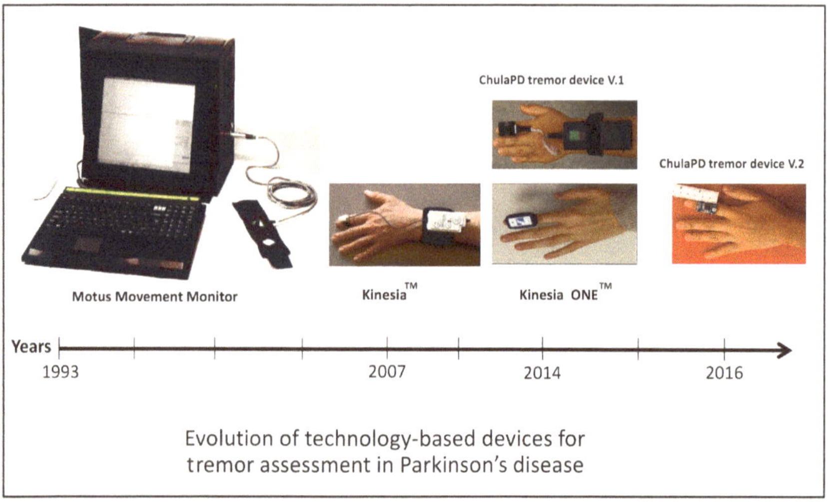

Fig. 1 A set of photographs demonstrating the evolution of technology-based devices for tremor assessment in Parkinson's disease. Note that the unit size becomes much smaller and more portable. The unit examples are Motus Movement Monitor (www.motusbioengineering.com), Kinesia and Kinesia ONE (www.glneurotech.com/kinesia), and ChulaPD tremor devices both version 1 and 2 (Bhidayasiri, Petchrutchatachart, et al., 2014).

tremor parameters, characterization of various forms of parkinsonian tremor (amplitude, frequency, occurrence), measurement of treatment effects in PD, and continuous ambulatory assessment of tremor (Bhidayasiri, Petchrutchatachart, et al., 2014; Elble & McNames, 2016; Haubenberger et al., 2016; Hoff, Wagemans, & van Hilten, 2001; Maetzler et al., 2013; Ossig et al., 2016; Sanchez-Ferro et al., 2016). However, reported outcomes vary greatly among investigators, consisting of spectral peak amplitude, peak frequency, log peak power, area under the peak, and area under the spectrum. Among these variables, tremor amplitudes were found to correlate with clinical ratings and frequency to decrease with time (Elble et al., 2006; Hellwig et al., 2009).

The application of inertial sensors in the diagnosis of parkinsonian tremor has been explored in a number of studies with different platforms and algorithms (Bhidayasiri, Petchrutchatachart, et al., 2014; Hossen et al., 2013; Jang et al., 2013; Martinez Manzanera, Elting, van der Hoeven, & Maurits, 2016; Thanawattano, Pongthornseri, Anan, Dumnin, & Bhidayasiri, 2015; Wharrad & Jefferson, 2000; Wile et al., 2014). Certain waveform characteristics of resting tremor have been identified to differentiate between parkinsonian and drug-induced tremor (Jang et al., 2013).

At least two analytic techniques have been proposed with the diagnostic accuracy of more than 90% in the discrimination between PD and essential tremor (ET), another common tremor disorder frequently mimicking PD (Hossen et al., 2013; Thanawattano et al., 2015). Despite early convincing results, the diagnostic accuracy of the above-mentioned systems has not been established in large-scale clinical trials leading to the implementation in clinical practice for diagnostic purposes. Therefore, its use in routine clinical practice for the diagnosis of parkinsonian tremor cannot be recommended at this stage. However, these devices may find their role in assisting physicians in the evaluation of challenging cases when symptom presentations are not that typical of parkinsonian tremor or in patients with other comorbidities making the interpretation from clinical examination alone difficult.

Inertial sensors may have a place in the evaluation of therapeutic effects in PD with a capability to demonstrate quantitative data for tremor reduction. The feasibility of intraoperative symptom monitoring with inertial sensors for tremor and bradykinesia has been tested in PD patients during deep brain stimulation (DBS) demonstrating its ability to provide quantifiable data of tremor and bradykinesia improvement during macrostimulation (Papapetropoulos, Jagid, Sengun, Singer, & Gallo, 2008). Similar approaches have been used to determine the efficacy of botulinum toxin injection for upper limb parkinsonian tremor (Rahimi, Samotus, Lee, & Jog, 2015). Recently, their role in DBS therapy has expanded to assist physicians in surgical candidate selection, evaluating surgical outcomes during and after surgery, and in optimizing DBS settings (Lieber, Taylor, Appelboom, McKhann, & Connolly, 2015).

With the advances of Microelectro-Mechanical Systems (MEMS), signal processing for continuous monitoring of PD symptoms is now possible. Due to the variability of tremor presentations between clinic and daily life as well as possible fluctuations with treatment, monitoring systems that enable continuous registration of tremor can provide the information on duration and severity of tremor for an extended period of observation including outdoor evaluations or serve as a tool for therapeutic interventions in clinical trials (Hoff et al., 2001; Thielgen, Foerster, Fuchs, Hornig, & Fahrenberg, 2004). At-home testing device (AHTD) is an example of a system which can evaluate a series of motor tasks (tremor, bradykinesia, speech, movement reaction time, and complex motor control) at a regular interval with a promising application for at-home assessment (Goetz, Stebbins, et al., 2009). In an evaluation study, involving early PD patients, the capability to detect change in tremor with AHTD was demonstrated as a significant predictor of change in UPDRS (Goetz, Stebbins, et al., 2009). Although starting with tremor monitoring, the concept of continuous monitoring of PD symptoms has moved rapidly to incorporate many features of motor and NMS in the analysis with good correlations established with various clinical rating scales, which will be discussed later.

4.2.2 Bradykinesia

Bradykinesia, referred to the slowness of initiation of voluntary movement with progressive reduction in speed and amplitude of repetitive actions, and represents a core feature of parkinsonism and a required feature for the diagnosis of parkinsonian syndrome according to the UK Parkinson's Disease Society Brain Bank clinical diagnostic criteria (Bhidayasiri & Reichmann, 2013; Gibb & Lees, 1988). In PD, the presence of bradykinesia has a significant impact on patient's disability and activity of daily living as demonstrated by worsening the HY stage and SE scale (Stebbins & Goetz, 1998). Clinically, bradykinesia can be elicited by standard clinical examination in the UPDRS, and its recent update MDS-UPDRS, in which 3 out of 6 distinct factors of the former, and 4 out of 7 of the latter scales, pertain to bradykinesia (Fahn & Elton, 1987; Goetz, Tilley, et al., 2008). To help quantify bradykinesia more objectively, a variety of different technology-based tools have been developed providing objective scores with continuous variables. These technologies that have been evaluated for bradykinesia and correlated with the UPDRS and MDS-UPDRS as the gold standard, including gyroscopes (e.g., Motus motion analysis system), coordination ability test system (CATS), brain test, quantitative digitography, precision real-time image-based motion analysis, and the AHTD (Pal & Goetz, 2013).

The identification of bradykinesia plays a crucial role in the differential diagnosis of parkinsonism. While bradykinesia refers to a decrement in speed and amplitude during repetitive performance, such as finger tapping, this phenomenon can be difficult to appreciate during clinical examination, resulting in a misinterpretation between bradykinesia and hypokinesia with a latter defined as small amplitude movements without decremented responses. Two recent studies utilizing infrared-emitting diodes and inertial sensors attached to the digits were able to distinguish hypokinesia without decrement in patients with progressive supranuclear palsy (PSP) from the finger tap pattern in PD and multiple system atrophy (Djuric-Jovicic et al., 2016; Ling, Massey, Lees, Brown, & Day, 2012). Similarly, micrographia with a lack of decrement in script size was also more common in patients with PSP than PD (Ling et al., 2012). Bradykinesia can be measured by determining the number of keystrokes per 60s, reported as a Kinesia score (Homann et al., 2000). Gauging the speed and amplitude component of bradykinesia in relation to motor impairment and disability has also been evaluated with an electromagnetic tracking device. While amplitude was disproportionally more affected than speed in the "off" state, levodopa normalized speed to a greater extent than amplitude, suggesting that these two phenomena may not share the same pathophysiological mechanism (Espay et al., 2009). Graded impairments in amplitude tended to correlate with the UPDRS and S&E scales (Espay et al., 2009).

As bradykinesia, particularly distal bradykinesia, has been shown to respond well to dopaminergic medications and DBS, treatment effect on bradykinesia is one of the key outcomes of such treatments. Investigators are, therefore, obviously keen to develop a protocol involving technology-based tools that can reliably determine a significant effect following therapeutic trials. Some examples include quantitative digitography as a method to assess bradykinesia during repetitive alternating finger-tapping task and a gyroscope to evaluate bradykinesia during repetitive wrist pronation–supination during DBS (Koop, Andrzejewski, Hill, Heit, & Bronte-Stewart, 2006; Taylor Tavares et al., 2005). The efficacy of both systems to capture the improvements from both dopaminergic medications and DBS was demonstrated, with a significant correlation with the UPDRS. Moreover, these techniques may be more sensitive in detecting a subtle, but significant, difference of treatment effects compared to the standard UPDRS (Taylor Tavares et al., 2005).

A move toward home testing for bradykinesia was conducted with a computer-based AHTD, which evaluated a series of motor tasks, including bradykinesia at a regular interval over a 6-month period. Although the feasibility of this system has been demonstrated in terms of high patient compliance and satisfaction, measures of AHTD on bradykinesia did not detect changes earlier or more robustly than clinical scales casting doubt on its use as a valid tool for assessment of bradykinesia (Goetz, Stebbins, et al., 2009).

4.2.3 Gait Dysfunction and Postural Instability

Postural instability is an important cardinal feature of PD as it signifies the disability of at least stage 3 by HY and is considered an index of disease progression (Evans et al., 2011; Hoehn & Yahr, 1967). Although postural instability differs from gait dysfunction in terms of pathophysiology and treatment response, both features are tightly connected, and share overlapped clinical symptomatology as well as consequences (e.g., falls). Therefore, gait dysfunction and postural instability are frequently lumped together when referred to in the literature.

As symptoms of gait and balance in PD can be both episodic (e.g., FOG, hesitation, difficult turning) and continuous (e.g., slow gait) associated with variability in performance, clinical examination at a point of time (e.g., Pull test) is often inadequate in elucidating the full spectrum of problems in individual patients. FOG is a good example of this episodic phenomenon, characterized by brief, episodic absence or marked reduction of forward progression of the feet despite the intention to walk (Giladi & Nieuwboer, 2008). The phenomenon of FOG usually manifests during initiation (start hesitation), turning, at the end of a walking journey (destination hesitation), or as shuffling episodes when patients approaches restricted areas, or while performing dual tasks (Nutt et al., 2011). Although the gold standard for assessing the presence and severity of FOG is based on the clinical examination of the number of episodes via video clips, this method represents a challenge for the evaluation of FOG in daily clinical practice (Snijders et al., 2010). As a result, wearable sensors, frequently worn in the lower body segment, have emerged as a novel tool to quantitatively assess FOG during real life with more reliability than clinical measures alone (Moore, MacDougall, & Ondo, 2008; Morris et al., 2012). A number of devices been developed to adopt this approach with expanded applications to provide new metrics, algorithms, and optimal configurations for autonomous identification of FOG (Bachlin et al., 2010; Morris et al., 2012). Moreover, different setups with different periods of recording are now available for research applications (the seven-sensor approach), clinical use (the single-shank sensor), or daily use with a smartphone-based architecture (Capecci, Pepa, Verdini, & Ceravolo, 2016; Ginis et al., 2016; Moore et al., 2013; Weiss, Herman, Giladi, & Hausdorff, 2015).

Early objective assessments of gait and balance in PD are usually performed using large equipment (e.g., 3D-camera-based systems, instrumented walkways) that require heavy installation and a large space to conduct the experiments. For nonresearch purposes, the trend is to utilize much simple devices (e.g., smartphones, tablets) to determine gait and postural parameters that are comparable to sophisticated systems (Ozinga, Machado, Miller Koop, Rosenfeldt, & Alberts, 2015). The details of these studies are not under the scope of this review. Although the findings from the laboratory-based studies have shed several new insights to a better understanding of gait and balance problems in PD, most outcome measures are highly technical based on spatiotemporal parameters that are difficult for physicians in clinical practice to interpret, and importantly, do not always reflect patient's performance in daily situations, such as the in-home environment. Moreover, established gait characteristics (e.g., stance time, swing time) have not been quantified in free-living environments in PD patients. Recently, there is a growing attempt to derive these parameters into more ADL-related outcomes, such as a number of falls that are more closely related to quality of life and morbidity of PD patients. Indeed, number of falls has been included as a primary outcome in recent studies with pharmacologic agents and physical interventions (Ashburn et al., 2007; Chung, Lobb, Nutt, & Horak, 2010). Due to the nature of falls as a sporadic, and episodic events, recalls of fall situations alone based on the diary are often inaccurate. To this end, several studies have investigated the utility of a body-fixed sensor as a "fall detector," providing continuous monitoring in outdoor environments. Certain parameters have been identified from these studies to be associated with significant fall risk, including the presence of missteps, and higher step-to-step variability in both vertical and mediolateral axes (Iluz et al., 2014; Weiss et al., 2013; Weiss, Herman, Giladi, & Hausdorff, 2014). Another initiative, the Parkinson@Home Study protocol, equips PD patients with a set of sensors (smartwatch, smartphone, and fall detector) to estimate a number of falls in relation physical activity over a 3-month period with results to be expected in a near future (Silva de Lima et al., 2016).

4.3 Objective Measures for Nonmotor and Associated Features of PD

Evidence supports the existence of NMS in all stages of PD, from prodromal onto advanced disease stages . From retrospective and longitudinal studies, decreased sense of smell, depression, night-time sleep disturbances, and gastrointestinal complaints are recognized as part of a premotor phase of PD, manifesting years before the classic motor symptoms. NMS (pain, urinary dysfunction, anxiety/depression) have been identified as a presenting complaint in 21% of pathologically proven cases of PD (O'Sullivan et al., 2008). As the disease progresses, the predominant NMS change to neuropsychiatric symptoms (e.g., apathy, psychosis), dementia, fatigue, and dysautonomia, which may be induced or exacerbated by dopaminergic medications. Certain NMS exist in all stages of PD (e.g., sleep disorders). At least one of the above NMS symptoms was reported in a majority of PD patients with this figure reaching 100% of patients with motor fluctuations (Barone et al., 2009; Bhidayasiri, Mekawichai, et al., 2014; Martinez-Martin et al., 2007). While many NMS complaints are subjective (e.g., insomnia, fatigue), many investigators are exploring the possibility of objectively measuring NMS either directly, or indirectly via related outcomes. In this section, we provide an overview of the growing trend to seek objective assessment of common NMS and associated symptoms including some of which may be inclusive of both motor and NMS (e.g., sleep disorders) (Table 3).

4.3.1 Sleep Disorders

Sleep disturbances are very common in PD patients with a reported prevalence of 60%–100% depending on study population (Bhidayasiri, Mekawichai, et al., 2014; Lees, Blackburn, & Campbell, 1988). The manifestations of nocturnal disturbances in PD are myriad, not only restricted to sleep disruption, but also involve motor, neuropsychiatric, and urinary symptoms (Barone, Amboni, Vitale, & Bonavita, 2004). Unfortunately, the recognition of sleep problems in PD is low, importantly due to the inability of patients or caregivers to articulate their night-time problems during consultations (Bhidayasiri, Sringean, & Thanawattano, 2016). Moreover, direct observation of most night-time symptoms by treating physicians is almost impossible in clinical practice with an except in the in-patient situation, or sleep laboratory for those who undergo polysomnographic (PSG) study. However, these settings are not routinely applicable to most PD patients whose care is usually based on an out-patient basis.

In recent years, there has been a growing recognition of night-time symptoms in PD leading to the development of many assessing instruments, for example, Parkinson's Disease Sleep Scale (PDSS) and its modified version (PDSS-2) (Chaudhuri & Martinez-Martin, 2004; Trenkwalder et al., 2011). This progress also extends to the exploration of the use of sensors to determine night-time activity in patients with PD. While early reports with wrist activity monitors suggested an elevated nocturnal activity in PD patients, a number of more recent studies utilizing multisite wearable inertial sensors have been able to delineate the differences between decreased axial and increased limb movements during the night, objectively demonstrating the presence of nocturnal hypokinesia among PD patients (Bhidayasiri, Sringean, Taechalertpaisarn, & Thanawattano, 2016; Louter et al., 2015; Sringean, Taechalertpaisarn, Thanawattano, & Bhidayasiri, 2016a; van Hilten et al., 1994). Moreover, the severity of nocturnal hypokinesia has been found to correlate with clinical rating scales (e.g.,

Table 3 Questionnaires, Scales, and Objective Methods for the Evaluation of Nonmotor and Associated Features of Parkinson's Disease

		Objective Assessment	
Feature	**Questionnaire/Clinical Score**	**Types of Device**	**Outcome Measures**
Sleep disorders	• The Parkinson's disease sleep scale (PDSS) • The Pittsburgh sleep quality index (PSQI) • Epworth Sleepiness Scale (ESS) • Inappropriate Sleep Composite Score (ISCS) • Stanford Sleepiness Scale (SSS) • Nocturnal Akinesia Dystonia and Cramp Score (NADCS)	*Wearable inertial sensors* • ChulaPD-NIGHT Recorder	Leg and arm movements, getting out of bed, Rolling over or turning in bed (number, degree, velocity, duration, acceleration)
		• Dynaport McRoberts	Turning, Axial movement measures (frequency, size, duration, speed)
		• Wrist Actigraph (e.g., Actiwatch, Camntech, Actiwatch AW-64)	Sleep latency, sleep time, sleep efficiency, wake after sleep onset, movement and fragmentation index, nocturnal activity, nocturnal motility time duration of Sleep
Dysautonomia	Recommended Global scale • The Scales for Outcomes in PD-Autonomic (SCOPA-AUT) • Nonmotor Symptoms Questionnaire for PD (NMSQuest) • Nonmotor Symptom Scale (NSS)	The SUEMPATHY device (Suess Medizin-Technik, Germany), Noninvasive blood pressure monitoring CBM3000 device (Nihon Colin Co, Komaki, Japan	– Baroreflex sensitivity (BRS) – Spectral parameters of the heart rate or RR interval and of systolic blood pressure

Continued

Table 3 Questionnaires, Scales, and Objective Methods for the Evaluation of Nonmotor and Associated Features of Parkinson's Disease—cont'd

		Objective Assessment	
Feature	**Questionnaire/Clinical Score**	**Types of Device**	**Outcome Measures**
	Constipation scale • Rome III constipation module	N/A	N/A
	Sialorrhea scale • Drooling Severity and Frequency Scale (DSFS) • Drooling Rating Scale • Sialorrhea Clinical Scale for PD (SCS-PD)	N/A	N/A
	Dysphagia scale • The Swallowing Disturbance Questionnaire (SDQ) • Dysphagia-Specific Quality of Life (SWAL-QOL)	N/A	N/A
Fatigue	For screening • FSS (R), FACIT-F (R), PFS (R), MFI (S), FAI (S)	Physical fatigability Cognitive fatigability	N/A
	For severity rating • FSS (R), MFI (R), FAI (s), FACIT-F (S), PFS (S), D-FIS (S)	N/A	N/A

PD, Parkinson's disease; *UPDRS*, Unified Parkinson's disease Rating Scale.

UPDRS-axial score) (Sringean et al., 2016a). The application of inertial sensors during the night also provides information on the predominance of the supine sleep position in PD, found to be associated with certain comorbidities (e.g., OSA, bed sores), and the severity of nocturnal hypokinesia in the latter part of the night (Sommerauer et al., 2015; Sringean, Taechalertpaisarn, Thanawattano, & Bhidayasiri, 2016b). This information, which is not possible to gather through scales and questionnaires, assists physicians in the identification of those at-risk of sleep-related complications and treatment planning (Bhidayasiri, Sringean, & Thanawattano, 2016).

In an effort to provide an alternative option to PSG, Home Sleep Testing was performed in PD patients who could not undertake PSG for various medical reasons to determine its sensitivity and specificity in an unattended environment (Collop et al., 2007). While it is a good tool to indicate the presence of OSA in PD patients where the complication is suspected, the failure rate was relatively high, particularly in those with mild OSA, but with significant motor disabilities (Gros et al., 2015). Therefore, the suitability of the portable monitoring to exclude OSA in PD patients is still questionable.

4.3.2 Autonomic Dysfunction

Common autonomic dysfunctions in PD include gastrointestinal dysmotility, orthostatic hypotension, urinary incontinence, and among others, impaired heart rate variability, sweating, sialorrhea, and sexual dysfunction (Seppi et al., 2011). A common method for assessment of these complications usually derives from a combination of clinical interviews, and direct measurement with additional questionnaires when available (e.g., Orthostatic Hypotension Symptom Assessment, Arizona Sexual Experience Scale) (Jitkritsadakul, Jagota, & Bhidayasiri, 2015; Merola et al., 2016). However, the evaluation of these symptoms can be particularly challenging as they are subjective, nonspecific, and usually occur in PD patients with multiple comorbidities. Most autonomic function tests (e.g., Head-up tilt test, Valsalva maneuver) tend to evaluate the existence of a symptom at a particular point of time, but their role in objective monitoring has not been established (Rocchi et al., 2015). Attempts have been made to apply wearable sensors in the continuous assessment of heart rate variability yielding the significant finding of a reduced low-frequency/high-frequency ratio in PD patients (Niwa, Kuriyama, Nakagawa, & Imanishi, 2011).

4.3.3 Fatigue

Fatigue in PD refers to self-reported significantly diminished energy levels or increased perceptions of effort that are disproportionate to attempted activities (Kluger et al., 2016). It affects approximately half of PD patients and represents an early sign of diminished quality of life (Martinez-Martin et al., 2011). While fatigue in PD is traditionally assessed by scales focusing on subjective complaints in individual patients, new objective measures have been developed to determine fatigue based on their physical performance on force generation protocols ("physical" fatigability), and cognitive performance on engaging attentional networks ("cognitive" fatigability) (Martino et al., 2016). Early results suggest a link between PD-related fatigue and attention-demanding motor tasks, which may be applied to future therapeutic models of fatigue in PD.

4.3.4 Cognitive Function

Although direct assessment of cognitive function is not possible, cognitive function could be determined indirectly from movements collected from wearable sensors. While not tested in PD patients, poor gait performances have been identified with dual tasking among individuals with mild cognitive impairment (Montero-Odasso et al., 2014). This potential link could be explored as an indirect objective measure for early cognitive decline in PD patients.

4.4 Ambulatory Monitoring in PD: Clinical Implications

With the advances of circuit technology, wearable sensors have been developed to quantitatively capture movement patterns during clinic visit and daily lives of PD patients. This capability has now been extended to ambulatory monitoring of various parkinsonian symptoms for various clinical purposes. This approach has addressed an important unmet need in PD by providing continuous objective assessment that is related to the fluctuating symptoms of an individual patient (Politis et al., 2010). It is not usually possible to obtain this kind of information by clinical interview or standard examination alone, but the requirement for continuous symptom assessment has become increasingly important as part of a 24-h therapeutic concept in PD in which both day- and night-time symptoms should be carefully evaluated and treated when clinically indicated (Chaudhuri, Pal, Bridgman, & Trenkwalder, 2001). In this section, we will review potential applications of ambulatory assessment in PD for the evaluation of motor and nonmotor fluctuations, activity components, and home monitoring for day and night activities.

4.4.1 Ambulatory Assessment of Motor and Nonmotor Fluctuations

Symptom fluctuations are a disabling adverse effect of long-term dopaminergic medications with an estimated prevalence of 50% in PD patients after a mean exposure of 5 years with levodopa treatment (Ahlskog & Muenter, 2001). The manifestations of symptom fluctuations are not limited to the motor component, comprising of dyskinesia, and "off" period, but also include of a range of NMS frequently reported by patients including anxiety, depression, fatigue, restlessness, pain, concentration, and dizziness (Bhidayasiri & Truong, 2008; Storch et al., 2013). Traditionally, the assessment of functional status in patients with fluctuations is performed by completion of a home diary that evaluates the presence of "off," "on without dyskinesia," "on with nontroublesome dyskinesia," "on with troublesome dyskinesia," and "asleep" at half-hour time periods (Hauser et al., 2000). This assessment comes with certain limitations, including interrater variability, limited scope of continuous monitoring to only motor symptoms, and dependence on the compliance and correct understanding of both patients and caregivers (Stone et al., 2002). Moreover, the rating from patients is subjective, heavily relying on the perception of the individual patient whose impression can be different from day-to-day due to many factors (e.g., emotional changes) and is not referenced to normative values of age-matched controls.

The concept of ambulatory assessment on motor fluctuations was first applied to the detection of dyskinesias using wearable sensors when an accuracy of over 90% was demonstrated for the identification of different types of dyskinesias and correlations with clinical rating scales (Keijsers, Horstink, & Gielen, 2003a; Manson et al., 2000). The accelerometer pattern has also been identified to have the capability to distinguish dyskinesias from physiological sway and voluntary movements (Keijsers, Horstink, & Gielen, 2003b; Lopane et al., 2015). The algorithm was later expanded to comprehensively evaluate the presence of both bradykinesia and dyskinesia, giving severity scores over a 10-day monitoring period (Griffiths et al., 2012). The established correlation was also demonstrated between these objective severity scores of both bradykinesia and dyskinesia and clinical rating scales (e.g., UPDRS) (Griffiths et al., 2012). Moreover, the temporal relationship between continuous recording and the timing of medications provided the platform for assessing the effectiveness of a therapeutic invention in an individual patient. The different motor outcomes reported have been combined into a set of motor scores, including ambulatory tremor and fluctuation scores, demonstrating its validity with clinical rating scales (Braybrook et al., 2016; Horne, McGregor, & Bergquist, 2015). In addition to the motor parameters, the use of ambulatory continuous monitoring has been explored in other aspects of PD, including night-time monitoring for axial movements, daytime sleepiness, and impulsive compulsive behaviors (Bhidayasiri, Sringean, Taechalertpaisarn, et al., 2016; Evans et al., 2014; Klingelhoefer et al., 2016; Kotschet et al., 2014; Louter et al., 2015; Sringean et al., 2016a).It is likely that more objective outcomes will be identified with possible applications in future clinical trials.

4.4.2 Ambulatory Activity Assessment

Reduced physical activity and sedentary lifestyle were recently identified in over 90% of PD patients who reported their physical activity to be below the recommended level as proposed by the American College of Sports Medicine and the American Heart Association (Dontje et al., 2013). This figure is particularly concerning as reduced physical activity can potentially lead to several health and social problems in PD patients. While clinical information on physical activity alone is often inaccurate, the application of body-fixed sensors has been utilized to evaluate ambulatory activity in PD patients related to total energy expenditure per day, average daily walking duration, walking/activity bouts, daily steps, and daily living transitions (Bernad-Elazari et al., 2016; Cavanaugh et al., 2012, 2015; Dontje et al., 2013; Klenk et al., 2016; Lord et al., 2013). The findings from these studies were consistent in that ambulatory activity in PD patients was significantly less than healthy controls or recommended activity levels and a significant decline was demonstrated at annual assessments, and when levodopa equivalent dosage was also increased. When comparisons were made with patients with other neurodegenerative disorders, the number of longer walking bouts and walking bout length were least in patients with PSP, followed by PD and degenerative ataxias at the same severity (Klenk et al., 2016).

Although these results need to be confirmed in prospective longitudinal studies, they do concur with our clinical impression that PD patients are less active than healthy age-matched individuals. Several investigators have already moved toward promoting physical activity with different interventions and utilize body-fixed sensors as the activity monitor (Speelman, van Nimwegen, Bloem, & Munneke, 2014; van der Kolk et al., 2014).

4.4.3 Home Monitoring

The capability to providing ambulatory assessment of various PD symptoms and related activities in a continuous fashion has prompted several investigators to explore the feasibility of home monitoring using different sensor setups (Table 4). Looking toward the development of an automatic

Table 4 Questionnaires, Scales and Objective Methods for Ambulatory Monitoring of Parkinson's Disease

		Objective Assessment	
Features	**Questionnaires/Scales**	**Types of Device**	**Outcome Measures**
Fluctuation	• PD diary • The MDS-UPDRS scale • The Unified Dyskinesia Rating Scale • The Fluctuation Score	*Wearable inertial sensors*	
		• Parkinson's KinetiGraph System (PKG)	Tremor (Posture and Resting), LID, FOG, Bradykinesia and Activity Recognizer
		• Kinesia™ system	Clinically validated algorithm to determine the severity of symptoms, ranging from 0 (no symptom) to 4 (severe symptom)
		• PERFORM system: consisting of the wearable multisensor monitor unit (WMSMU) and the local base unit (LBU)	Tremor (Posture and Resting) Recognizer, LID Recognizer, FOG Recognizers, Bradykinesia Recognizer and Activity Recognizer
Activity measurement	• Activity logs and diaries • 7- Days Recall Questionnaire • Physical Activities Questionnaire	*Wearable inertial sensors*	
		• TriTrac RT3, • Stepwatch3 Step Activity Monitor (SAM)	Measure movement across three orthogonal planes: vertical (x), anteroposterior (y), and mediolateral (z), mean acceleration, Activity counts Total number of steps, maximum output for steps, number of minutes with >100 steps, number and duration of walking bouts, peak activity index, % of day spent inactive

Continued

Table 4 Questionnaires, Scales and Objective Methods for Ambulatory Monitoring of Parkinson's Disease—cont'd

Features	Questionnaires/Scales	Objective Assessment	
		Types of Device	**Outcome Measures**
Home-based monitoring	N/A	*Wearable inertial sensors*	
		• Dynaport McRoberts • Senior Mobility Monitor (SMM) • Body sensor AGYRO • Axivity AX3	Number of walking bouts, walking duration, total number of steps, median number of steps per bout, bout duration, cadence, step and stride regularity, frequency domain measures (harmonic ratio, amplitude, slope, and width of dominant frequency), step duration, step symmetry, acceleration range, etc.
		Others devices	
		• Smart Home sensor system and Wall-mounted cameras	Clinical Assessment using Activity Behavior (CAAB) approach
		• Smart beds	N/A
		• Smartphone and self-monitoring application	N/A
		• At-home monitoring device	N/A

FOG, freezing of gait; *LID*, levodopa-induced dyskinesia; *PD*, Parkinson's disease; *UPDRS*, Unified Parkinson's disease Rating Scale.

symptom detection system using artificial neural networks, one recent study compared the data derived from bilateral wrist-worn accelerometers against patient-completed symptom diaries and clinical ratings for the identification of motor symptoms in PD (Fisher, Hammerla, Ploetz, et al., 2016). While specificity for dyskinesia was high in the clinical setting, sensitivity for on/off detection was suboptimal. In addition, a number of studies are being conducted to determine the feasibility of sensors (smartphone, smartwatch, fall detector) in the estimation of physical activity, tremor, sleep quality, and falls in PD patients in their own home environment (Ferreira et al., 2015; Silva de Lima et al., 2016). Another separate system, PERFORM, is currently being validated for continuous remote monitoring and assessment of motor symptoms related to on/off phenomenon and dyskinesias with the aim of providing remote clinician evaluation of a patient's motor status and drug/food intake (Tzallas et al., 2014).

Although the accuracy of the all the above-mentioned systems is, as yet, neither acceptable nor applicable for clinical use, we are starting to see an increasing trend toward moving Parkinson care and assessment into the home environment as and when the technology advances to reached the level of clinical acceptability (Dorsey et al., 2016). Several benefits can be foreseen if Parkinson care can be partially performed in patient's own home, including a reduction of caregiver's burden, more patient-centred individualized care, and a likelihood of budget saving in healthcare cost for authorities.

5. CONCLUSION

Patients with PD experience a vast array of both motor and NMS, superimposed with effects of aging, comorbidities, and polypharmacy. Traditional evaluation of this complex symptomatology is based on periodic clinic interviews with reports of symptoms during the office visit resulting in many gaps in captured information. In clinical situations, subjective information obtained from patients can give physicians a limited and biased view; thus, creating ambiguity around when they need to make therapeutic decision for their patients. A move to quantify individual or sets of symptoms has been initiated with the introduction of home-based diaries, and clinical scales, which have been validated for assessing motor states, NMS, activities of daily living, and quality of life. While these methods have been utilized in a large proportion of clinical studies with the ability to demonstrate long-term changes, the findings come with certain limitations related to recall bias, rater reliability, subjective reporting, accuracy, and insensitivity to subtle changes. Nevertheless, the advantages of these evaluation tools cannot be overlooked as they do not consume large amount of resources and have been thoroughly validated for applications in routine clinical practice and clinical trials, making them ideal for the screening of large numbers of patients in a relatively short period of time (Table 1). However, we, as physicians who encounter the needs of PD patients on a daily basis, have to be aware and ready to adopt what recent technologies have to offer to improve the diagnosis and care of PD patients. The capability of technology-based devices to generate valuable objective data from second-to-second continuous monitoring of multidomain symptoms of PD should be further explored in prospective longitudinal large-scale studies that can also address certain limitations of these devices, for example, compatibility and user's engagement (Espay et al., 2016; Stamford et al., 2015). While results from cross-sectional and short-term studies are already available, some prospective large-scale studies are being conducted or planned and we expect the results to be available in the near future (Silva de Lima et al., 2016). Early findings from the applications of these technologies have been described in this review, showing that cardinal features of PD, certain NMS, gait, mobility, fall risk, daily living transitions, and physical activities can all be tracked, delivering added value to assessments compared with conventional testing. Moreover, from the patient's perspective, long-term monitoring with wearable sensors has been found to be acceptable by PD patients without a negative effect on their health-related quality of life (Fisher, Hammerla, Rochester, Andras, & Walker, 2016; van Uem et al., 2016). The field of technology-based devices is growing rapidly and it is likely that not all studies in this area have been mentioned in this review. However, it is our intention to provide an overview of clinical assessment in PD with scales and monitoring that is up-to-date and relevant to clinical practice to physicians who regularly involve in taking care of PD patients.

It is the belief of the authors that no assessment methods can replace the clinical acumen of an individual physician, consisting of detailed history taking, and thorough examination, surpassed by observing skills. It is a physician's judgement to determine which method, scales or monitoring devices or a combination of both, is most appropriate to individual patient for a particular clinical question that needs to be assessed. No publication can provide a specific answer to each of an individual patient's needs, but clinical experiences together with up-to-date knowledge which this chapter aims to provide, and most importantly, the commitment of an individual physician to do the best for his/her patients remains the best tool for the job, unrivaled by any assessment method either now or in the future.

ACKNOWLEDGMENTS

R.B. is supported by the grant from the National Research Council of Thailand (GRB_APS_05_59_30_04), Chula Research Scholar of the Ratchadapiseksomphot Endowment Fund (GCRS_58_05_30_02), and Chulalongkorn Academic Advancement Fund into its 2nd Century Project of Chulalongkorn University, Bangkok, Thailand.

Conflict of interest: The authors have no conflict of interest.

REFERENCES

Ahlskog, J. E., & Muenter, M. D. (2001). Frequency of levodopa-related dyskinesias and motor fluctuations as estimated from the cumulative literature. *Movement Disorders*, *16*(3), 448–458.

Alba, A., Trainor, F. S., Ritter, W., & Dacso, M. M. (1968). A clinical disability rating for Parkinson patients. *Journal of Chronic Diseases*, *21*(7), 507–522.

Ambrosio, L., Portillo, M. C., Rodriguez-Blazquez, C., Martinez-Castrillo, J. C., Rodriguez-Violante, M., Serrano-Duenas, M., … Martinez-Martin, P. (2016). Satisfaction with life scale (SLS-6): First validation study in Parkinson's disease population. *Parkinsonism and Related Disorders*, *25*, 52–57.

Antonini, A., Martinez-Martin, P., Chaudhuri, R. K., Merello, M., Hauser, R., Katzenschlager, R., … Goetz-Christopher, G. (2011). Wearing-off scales in Parkinson's disease: Critique and recommendations. *Movement Disorders*, *26*(12), 2169–2175.

Antonini, A., Yegin, A., Preda, C., Bergmann, L., Poewe, W., & GLORIA study investigators & coordinators. (2015). Global long-term study on motor and non-motor symptoms and safety of levodopa-carbidopa intestinal gel in routine care of advanced Parkinson's disease patients; 12-month interim outcomes. *Parkinsonism & Related Disorders*, *21*(3), 231–235. http://dx.doi.org/10.1016/j.parkreldis.2014.12.012.

Ashburn, A., Fazakarley, L., Ballinger, C., Pickering, R., McLellan, L. D., & Fitton, C. (2007). A randomised controlled trial of a home based exercise programme to reduce the risk of falling among people with Parkinson's disease. *Journal of Neurology, Neurosurgery, and Psychiatry*, *78*(7), 678–684. http://dx.doi.org/10.1136/jnnp.2006.099333.

Bachlin, M., Plotnik, M., Roggen, D., Maidan, I., Hausdorff, J. M., Giladi, N., & Troster, G. (2010). Wearable assistant for Parkinson's disease patients with the freezing of gait symptom. *IEEE Transactions on Information Technology in Biomedicine*, *14*(2), 436–446. http://dx.doi.org/10.1109/TITB.2009.2036165.

Barbeau, A., Duvoisin, R. C., Gerstenbrand, F., Lakke, J. P., Marsden, C. D., & Stern, G. (1981). Classification of extrapyramidal disorders. Proposal for an international classification and glossary of terms. *Journal of the Neurological Sciences*, *51*(2), 311–327.

Barone, P., Amboni, M., Vitale, C., & Bonavita, V. (2004). Treatment of nocturnal disturbances and excessive daytime sleepiness in Parkinson's disease. *Neurology*, *63*(8 Suppl. 3), S35–S38.

Barone, P., Antonini, A., Colosimo, C., Marconi, R., Morgante, L., Avarello, T. P., … Dotto, P. D. (2009). The PRIAMO study: A multicenter assessment of nonmotor symptoms and their impact on quality of life in Parkinson's disease. *Movement Disorders*, *24*(11), 1641–1649. http://dx.doi.org/10.1002/mds.22643.

Bernad-Elazari, H., Herman, T., Mirelman, A., Gazit, E., Giladi, N., & Hausdorff, J. M. (2016). Objective characterization of daily living transitions in patients with Parkinson's disease using a single body-fixed sensor. *Journal of Neurology*, *263*(8), 1544–1551. http://dx.doi.org/10.1007/s00415-016-8164-6.

Bhidayasiri, R. (2005). Differential diagnosis of common tremor syndromes. *Postgraduate Medical Journal*, *81*(962), 756–762. http://dx.doi.org/10.1136/pgmj.2005.032979.

Bhidayasiri, R., Mekawichai, P., Jitkritsadakul, O., Panyakaew, P., Kaewwilai, L., Boonrod, N., … Setthawatcharawanich, S. (2014). Nocturnal journey of body and mind in Parkinson's disease: The manifestations, risk factors and their relationship to daytime symptoms. Evidence from the NIGHT-PD study. *Journal of Neural Transmission*, *121*(Suppl. 1), 59–68. http://dx.doi.org/10.1007/s00702-014-1199-x.

Bhidayasiri, R., Petchrutchatachart, S., Pongthornseri, R., Anan, C., Dumnin, S., & Thanawattano, C. (2014). Low-cost, 3-dimension, office-based inertial sensors for automated tremor assessment: Technical development and experimental verification. *Journal of Parkinson's Disease*, *4*(2), 273–282. http://dx.doi.org/10.3233/JPD-130311.

Bhidayasiri, R., & Reichmann, H. (2013). Different diagnostic criteria for Parkinson disease: What are the pitfalls? *Journal of Neural Transmission*, *120*(4), 619–625. http://dx.doi.org/10.1007/s00702-013-1007-z.

Bhidayasiri, R., Sringean, J., Taechalertpaisarn, P., & Thanawattano, C. (2016a). Capturing nighttime symptoms in Parkinson disease: Technical development and experimental verification of inertial sensors for nocturnal hypokinesia. *Journal of Rehabilitation Research and Development*, *53*(4), 487–498. http://dx.doi.org/10.1682/JRRD.2015.04.0062.

Bhidayasiri, R., Sringean, J., & Thanawattano, C. (2016b). Sensor-based evaluation and treatment of nocturnal hypokinesia in Parkinson's disease: An evidence-based review. *Parkinsonism & Related Disorders*, *22*(Suppl. 1), S127–S133. http://dx.doi.org/10.1016/j.parkreldis.2015.09.049.

Bhidayasiri, R., & Truong, D. D. (2008). Motor complications in Parkinson disease: Clinical manifestations and management. *Journal of the Neurological Sciences*, *266*(1–2), 204–215. http://dx.doi.org/10.1016/j.jns.2007.08.028. [pii] S0022-510X(07)00573-4.

Biemans, M. A., Dekker, J., & van der Woude, L. H. (2001). The internal consistency and validity of the Self-assessment Parkinson's Disease Disability Scale. *Clinical Rehabilitation*, *15*, 221–228.

Bloem, B. R., Marinus, J., Almeida, Q., Dibble, L., Nieuwboer, A., Post, B., … Movement Disorders Society Rating Scales Committee. (2016). Measurement instruments to assess posture, gait, and balance in Parkinson's disease: Critique and recommendations. *Movement Disorders*, *31*(9), 1342–1355. http://dx.doi.org/10.1002/mds.26572.

Bohlega, S., Abou Al-Shaar, H., Alkhairallah, T., Al-Ajlan, F., Hasan, N., & Alkahtani, K. (2015). Levodopa-carbidopa intestinal gel infusion therapy in advanced Parkinson's disease: Single middle eastern center experience. *European Neurology*, *74*(5–6), 227–236. http://dx.doi.org/10.1159/000442151.

Braybrook, M., O'Connor, S., Churchward, P., Perera, T., Farzanehfar, P., & Horne, M. (2016). An ambulatory tremor score for Parkinson's disease. *Journal of Parkinson's Disease*, *6*(4), 723–731. http://dx.doi.org/10.3233/JPD-160898.

Brown, R. G., Dittner, A., Findley, L., & Wessely, S. C. (2005). The Parkinson fatigue scale. *Parkinsonism & Related Disorders*, *11*(1), 49–55. http://dx.doi.org/10.1016/j.parkreldis.2004.07.007.

Brown, R. G., MacCarthy, B., Gotham, A. M., Der, G. J., & Marsden, C. D. (1988). Depression and disability in Parkinson's disease: A follow-up of 132 cases. *Psychological Medicine*, *18*(1), 49–55.

Calne, S., Schulzer, M., Mak, E., Guyette, C., Rohs, G., Hatchard, S., … Pegler, S. (1996). Validating a quality of life rating scale for idiopathic parkinsonism: Parkinson's Impact Scale (PIMS). *Parkinsonism & Related Disorders*, *2*(2), 55–61.

Canter, G. J., De La Torre, R., & Mier, M. (1961). A method for evaluating disability in patients with Parkinson's disease. *The Journal of Nervous and Mental Disease*, *133*, 143–147.

Capecci, M., Pepa, L., Verdini, F., & Ceravolo, M. G. (2016). A smartphone-based architecture to detect and quantify freezing of gait in Parkinson's disease. *Gait & Posture, 50*, 28–33. http://dx.doi.org/10.1016/j.gaitpost.2016.08.018.

Carod-Artal, F. J., & Martinez-Martin, P. (2013). Independent validation of the non motor symptoms scale for Parkinson's disease in Brazilian patients. *Parkinsonism & Related Disorders, 19*(1), 115–119. http://dx.doi.org/10.1016/j.parkreldis.2012.08.008.

Cavanaugh, J. T., Ellis, T. D., Earhart, G. M., Ford, M. P., Foreman, K. B., & Dibble, L. E. (2012). Capturing ambulatory activity decline in Parkinson's disease. *Journal of Neurologic Physical Therapy, 36*(2), 51–57. http://dx.doi.org/10.1097/NPT.0b013e318254ba7a.

Cavanaugh, J. T., Ellis, T. D., Earhart, G. M., Ford, M. P., Foreman, K. B., & Dibble, L. E. (2015). Toward understanding ambulatory activity decline in Parkinson disease. *Physical Therapy, 95*(8), 1142–1150. http://dx.doi.org/10.2522/ptj.20140498.

Chaudhuri, K. R., & Martinez-Martin, P. (2004). Clinical assessment of nocturnal disability in Parkinson's disease: The Parkinson's disease sleep scale. *Neurology, 63*(8 Suppl. 3), S17–S20.

Chaudhuri, K. R., Martinez-Martin, P., Brown, R. G., Sethi, K., Stocchi, F., Odin, P., … Schapira, A. H. (2007). The metric properties of a novel non-motor symptoms scale for Parkinson's disease: Results from an international pilot study. *Movement Disorders, 22*(13), 1901–1911. http://dx.doi.org/10.1002/mds.21596.

Chaudhuri, K. R., Martinez-Martin, P., Schapira, A. H., Stocchi, F., Sethi, K., Odin, P., … Olanow, C. W. (2006). International multicenter pilot study of the first comprehensive self-completed nonmotor symptoms questionnaire for Parkinson's disease: The NMSQuest study. *Movement Disorders, 21*(7), 916–923. http://dx.doi.org/10.1002/mds.20844.

Chaudhuri, K. R., Pal, S., Bridgman, K., & Trenkwalder, C. (2001). Achieving 24-hour control of Parkinson's disease symptoms: Use of objective measures to improve nocturnal disability. *European Neurology, 46*(Suppl. 1), 3–10.

Chaudhuri, K. R., Pal, S., DiMarco, A., Whately-Smith, C., Bridgman, K., Mathew, R., … Trenkwalder, C. (2002). The Parkinson's disease sleep scale: A new instrument for assessing sleep and nocturnal disability in Parkinson's disease. *Journal of Neurology, Neurosurgery, and Psychiatry, 73*(6), 629–635.

Chaudhuri, K. R., Sauerbier, A., Rojo, J. M., Sethi, K., Schapira, A. H., Brown, R. G., … Martinez-Martin, P. (2015). The burden of non-motor symptoms in Parkinson's disease using a self-completed non-motor questionnaire: A simple grading system. *Parkinsonism & Related Disorders, 21*(3), 287–291. http://dx.doi.org/10.1016/j.parkreldis.2014.12.031.

Chung, K. A., Lobb, B. M., Nutt, J. G., & Horak, F. B. (2010). Effects of a central cholinesterase inhibitor on reducing falls in Parkinson disease. *Neurology, 75*(14), 1263–1269. http://dx.doi.org/10.1212/WNL.0b013e3181f6128c.

Collop, N. A., Anderson, W. M., Boehlecke, B., Claman, D., Goldberg, R., Gottlieb, D. J., … Portable Monitoring Task Force of the American Academy of Sleep Medicine. (2007). Clinical guidelines for the use of unattended portable monitors in the diagnosis of obstructive sleep apnea in adult patients. Portable Monitoring Task Force of the American Academy of Sleep Medicine. *Journal of Clinical Sleep Medicine, 3*(7), 737–747.

Colosimo, C., Martinez-Martin, P., Fabbrini, G., Hauser, R. A., Merello, M., Miyasaki, J., … Goetz, C. G. (2010). Task force report on scales to assess dyskinesia in Parkinson's disease: Critique and recommendations. *Movement Disorders, 25*(9), 1131–1142. http://dx.doi.org/10.1002/mds.23072.

Cotzias, G. C., Papavasiliou, P. S., Fehling, C., Kaufman, B., & Mena, I. (1970). Similarities between neurologic effects of L-dipa and of apomorphine. *The New England Journal of Medicine, 282*(1), 31–33. http://dx.doi.org/10.1056/nejm197001012820107.

Dafsari, H. S., Reddy, P., Herchenbach, C., Wawro, S., Petry-Schmelzer, J. N., Visser-Vandewalle, V., … Timmermann, L. (2016). Beneficial effects of bilateral subthalamic stimulation on non-motor symptoms in Parkinson's disease. *Brain Stimulation, 9*(1), 78–85. http://dx.doi.org/10.1016/j.brs.2015.08.005.

Daneault, J. F., Carignan, B., Codere, C. E., Sadikot, A. F., & Duval, C. (2012). Using a smart phone as a standalone platform for detection and monitoring of pathological tremors. *Frontiers in Human Neuroscience, 6*, 357. http://dx.doi.org/10.3389/fnhum.2012.00357.

de Boer, A. G., Wijker, W., Speelman, J. D., & de Haes, J. C. (1996). Quality of life in patients with Parkinson's disease: Development of a questionnaire. *Journal of Neurology, Neurosurgery, and Psychiatry, 61*(1), 70–74.

Deuschl, G., Bain, P., & Brin, M. (1998). Consensus statement of the Movement Disorder Society on Tremor. Ad Hoc Scientific Committee. *Movement Disorders, 13*(Suppl. 3), 2–23.

Djuric-Jovicic, M., Petrovic, I., Jecmenica-Lukic, M., Radovanovic, S., Dragasevic-Miskovic, N., Belic, M., … Kostic, V. S. (2016). Finger tapping analysis in patients with Parkinson's disease and atypical Parkinsonism. *Journal of Clinical Neuroscience, 30*, 49–55. http://dx.doi.org/10.1016/j.jocn.2015.10.053.

Dontje, M. L., de Greef, M. H., Speelman, A. D., van Nimwegen, M., Krijnen, W. P., Stolk, R. P., … van der Schans, C. P. (2013). Quantifying daily physical activity and determinants in sedentary patients with Parkinson's disease. *Parkinsonism & Related Disorders, 19*(10), 878–882. http://dx.doi.org/10.1016/j.parkreldis.2013.05.014.

Dorsey, E. R., Vlaanderen, F. P., Engelen, L. J., Kieburtz, K., Zhu, W., Biglan, K. M., … Bloem, B. R. (2016). Moving Parkinson care to the home. *Movement Disorders, 31*(9), 1258–1262. http://dx.doi.org/10.1002/mds.26744.

Elble, R. J., & McNames, J. (2016). Using portable transducers to measure tremor severity. *Tremor and Other Hyperkinetic Movements (New York, N.Y.), 6*, 375. http://dx.doi.org/10.7916/D8DR2VCC.

Elble, R. J., Pullman, S. L., Matsumoto, J. Y., Raethjen, J., Deuschl, G., Tintner, R., & Tremor Research, G. (2006). Tremor amplitude is logarithmically related to 4- and 5-point tremor rating scales. *Brain, 129*(Pt. 10), 2660–2666. http://dx.doi.org/10.1093/brain/awl190.

Espay, A. J., Beaton, D. E., Morgante, F., Gunraj, C. A., Lang, A. E., & Chen, R. (2009). Impairments of speed and amplitude of movement in Parkinson's disease: A pilot study. *Movement Disorders, 24*(7), 1001–1008. http://dx.doi.org/10.1002/mds.22480.

Espay, A. J., Bonato, P., Nahab, F. B., Maetzler, W., Dean, J. M., Klucken, J., … Movement Disorders Society Task Force on Technology. (2016). Technology in Parkinson's disease: Challenges and opportunities. *Movement Disorders, 31*(9), 1272–1282. http://dx.doi.org/10.1002/mds.26642.

Evans, A. H., Kettlewell, J., McGregor, S., Kotschet, K., Griffiths, R. I., & Horne, M. (2014). A conditioned response as a measure of impulsive-compulsive behaviours in Parkinson's disease. *PLoS One, 9*(2). e89319. http://dx.doi.org/10.1371/journal.pone.0089319.

Evans, J. R., Mason, S. L., Williams-Gray, C. H., Foltynie, T., Brayne, C., Robbins, T. W., & Barker, R. A. (2011). The natural history of treated Parkinson's disease in an incident, community based cohort. *Journal of Neurology, Neurosurgery, and Psychiatry, 82*(10), 1112–1118. http://dx.doi.org/10.1136/jnnp.2011.240366.

Fahn, S., & Elton, R. L. (1987). Unified Parkinson's disease rating scale. In S. Fahn, C. D. Marsden, D. B. Calne, & M. Goldstein (Eds.), *Recent developments in Parkinson's disease, 2* (pp. 153–164). NJ: Florham Park.

Fahn, S., Tolosa, E., & Marin, C. (1988). Clinical rating scale for tremor. In J. Jankovic & E. Tolosa (Eds.), *Parkinson's disease and movement disorders* (pp. 271–280). Baltimore, Munich: Urban & Schwarzenberg.

Ferreira, J. J., Santos, A. T., Domingos, J., Matthews, H., Isaacs, T., Duffen, J., … Maetzler, W. (2015). Clinical parameters and tools for home-based assessment of

Parkinson's disease: Results from a Delphi study. *Journal of Parkinson's Disease*, *5*(2), 281–290. http://dx.doi.org/10.3233/JPD-140493.
Fisher, J. M., Hammerla, N. Y., Ploetz, T., Andras, P., Rochester, L., & Walker, R. W. (2016a). Unsupervised home monitoring of Parkinson's disease motor symptoms using body-worn accelerometers. *Parkinsonism & Related Disorders*, *33*, 44–50. http://dx.doi.org/10.1016/j.parkreldis.2016.09.009.
Fisher, J. M., Hammerla, N. Y., Rochester, L., Andras, P., & Walker, R. W. (2016b). Body-worn sensors in Parkinson's disease: Evaluating their acceptability to patients. *Telemedicine and E-Health*, *22*(1), 63–69. http://dx.doi.org/10.1089/tmj.2015.0026.
Forjaz, M. J., & Martinez-Martin, P. (2006). Metric attributes of the unified Parkinson's disease rating scale 3.0 battery: Part II, construct and content validity. *Movement Disorders*, *21*(11), 1892–1898. http://dx.doi.org/10.1002/mds.21071.
Frazzitta, G., Pezzoli, G., Bertotti, G., & Maestri, R. (2013). Asymmetry and freezing of gait in parkinsonian patients. *Journal of Neurology*, *260*(1), 71–76. http://dx.doi.org/10.1007/s00415-012-6585-4.
Friedberg, G., Zoldan, J., Weizman, A., & Melamed, E. (1998). Parkinson psychosis rating scale: A practical instrument for grading psychosis in Parkinson's disease. *Clinical Neuropharmacology*, *21*(5), 280–284.
Gallagher, D. A., Goetz, C. G., Stebbins, G., Lees, A. J., & Schrag, A. (2012). Validation of the MDS-UPDRS Part I for nonmotor symptoms in Parkinson's disease. *Movement Disorders*, *27*(1), 79–83. http://dx.doi.org/10.1002/mds.23939.
Gazibara, T., Stankovic, I., Tomic, A., Svetel, M., Tepavcevic, D. K., Kostic, V. S., & Pekmezovic, T. (2013). Validation and cross-cultural adaptation of the Self-Assessment Disability Scale in patients with Parkinson's disease in Serbia. *Journal of Neurology*, *260*(8), 1970–1977. http://dx.doi.org/10.1007/s00415-013-6906-2.
Gibb, W. R., & Lees, A. J. (1988). The relevance of the Lewy body to the pathogenesis of idiopathic Parkinson's disease. *Journal of Neurology, Neurosurgery, and Psychiatry*, *51*(6), 745–752.
Giladi, N., & Nieuwboer, A. (2008). Understanding and treating freezing of gait in parkinsonism, proposed working definition, and setting the stage. *Movement Disorders*, *23*(Suppl. 2), S423–S425. http://dx.doi.org/10.1002/mds.21927.
Giladi, N., Shabtai, H., Simon, E. S., Biran, S., Tal, J., & Korczyn, A. D. (2000). Construction of freezing of gait questionnaire for patients with Parkinsonism. *Parkinsonism & Related Disorders*, *6*(3), 165–170.
Giladi, N., Tal, J., Azulay, T., Rascol, O., Brooks, D. J., Melamed, E., … Tolosa, E. (2009). Validation of the freezing of gait questionnaire in patients with Parkinson's disease. *Movement Disorders*, *24*(5), 655–661. http://dx.doi.org/10.1002/mds.21745.
Ginis, P., Nieuwboer, A., Dorfman, M., Ferrari, A., Gazit, E., Canning, C. G., … Mirelman, A. (2016). Feasibility and effects of home-based smartphone-delivered automated feedback training for gait in people with Parkinson's disease: A pilot randomized controlled trial. *Parkinsonism & Related Disorders*, *22*, 28–34. http://dx.doi.org/10.1016/j.parkreldis.2015.11.004.
Godinho, C., Domingos, J., Cunha, G., Santos, A. T., Fernandes, R. M., Abreu, D., … Ferreira, J. J. (2016). A systematic review of the characteristics and validity of monitoring technologies to assess Parkinson's disease. *Journal of Neuroengineering and Rehabilitation*, *13*, 24. http://dx.doi.org/10.1186/s12984-016-0136-7.
Goetz, C. G., Fahn, S., Martinez-Martin, P., Poewe, W., Sampaio, C., Stebbins, G. T., … LaPelle, N. (2007). Movement Disorder Society-sponsored revision of the Unified Parkinson's Disease Rating Scale (MDS-UPDRS): Process, format, and clinimetric testing plan. *Movement Disorders*, *22*(1), 41–47. http://dx.doi.org/10.1002/mds.21198.
Goetz, C. G., Nutt, J. G., & Stebbins, G. T. (2008). The Unified Dyskinesia Rating Scale: Presentation and clinimetric profile. *Movement Disorders*, *23*(16), 2398–2403. http://dx.doi.org/10.1002/mds.22341.

Goetz, C. G., Nutt, J. G., Stebbins, G. T., & Chmura, T. A. (2009). Teaching program for the Unified Dyskinesia Rating Scale. *Movement Disorders*, *24*(9), 1296–1298. http://dx.doi.org/10.1002/mds.22563.

Goetz, C. G., Poewe, W., Rascol, O., Sampaio, C., Stebbins, G. T., Counsell, C., … Seidl, L. (2004). Movement Disorder Society Task Force report on the Hoehn and Yahr staging scale: Status and recommendations. *Movement Disorders*, *19*(9), 1020–1028. http://dx.doi.org/10.1002/mds.20213.

Goetz, C. G., Stebbins, G. T., Chmura, T. A., Fahn, S., Poewe, W., & Tanner, C. M. (2010). Teaching program for the Movement Disorder Society-sponsored revision of the Unified Parkinson's Disease Rating Scale: (MDS-UPDRS). *Movement Disorders*, *25*(9), 1190–1194. http://dx.doi.org/10.1002/mds.23096.

Goetz, C. G., Stebbins, G. T., Chung, K. A., Hauser, R. A., Miyasaki, J. M., Nicholas, A. P., … Ge, S. (2013). Which dyskinesia scale best detects treatment response? *Movement Disorders*, *28*(3), 341–346. http://dx.doi.org/10.1002/mds.25321.

Goetz, C. G., Stebbins, G. T., Shale, H. M., Lang, A. E., Chernik, D. A., Chmura, T. A., … Dorflinger, E. E. (1994). Utility of an objective dyskinesia rating scale for Parkinson's disease: Inter- and intrarater reliability assessment. *Movement Disorders*, *9*(4), 390–394. http://dx.doi.org/10.1002/mds.870090403.

Goetz, C. G., Stebbins, G. T., Theeuwes, A., Stocchi, F., Ferreira, J. J., van de Witte, S., & Bronzova, J. (2011). Temporal stability of the Unified Dyskinesia Rating Scale. *Movement Disorders*, *26*(14), 2556–2559. http://dx.doi.org/10.1002/mds.23931.

Goetz, C. G., Stebbins, G. T., & Tilley, B. C. (2012). Calibration of unified Parkinson's disease rating scale scores to Movement Disorder Society-unified Parkinson's disease rating scale scores. *Movement Disorders*, *27*(10), 1239–1242. http://dx.doi.org/10.1002/mds.25122.

Goetz, C. G., Stebbins, G. T., Wolff, D., DeLeeuw, W., Bronte-Stewart, H., Elble, R., … Taylor, C. B. (2009). Testing objective measures of motor impairment in early Parkinson's disease: Feasibility study of an at-home testing device. *Movement Disorders*, *24*(4), 551–556. http://dx.doi.org/10.1002/mds.22379.

Goetz, C. G., Tilley, B. C., Shaftman, S. R., Stebbins, G. T., Fahn, S., Martinez-Martin, P., … Movement Disorder Society UPDRS Revision Task Force. (2008). Movement Disorder Society-sponsored revision of the Unified Parkinson's Disease Rating Scale (MDS-UPDRS): Scale presentation and clinimetric testing results. *Movement Disorders*, *23*(15), 2129–2170. http://dx.doi.org/10.1002/mds.22340.

Griffiths, R. I., Kotschet, K., Arfon, S., Xu, Z. M., Johnson, W., Drago, J., … Horne, M. K. (2012). Automated assessment of bradykinesia and dyskinesia in Parkinson's disease. *Journal of Parkinson's Disease*, *2*(1), 47–55. http://dx.doi.org/10.3233/JPD-2012-11071.

Gros, P., Mery, V. P., Lafontaine, A. L., Robinson, A., Benedetti, A., Kimoff, R. J., & Kaminska, M. (2015). Diagnosis of obstructive sleep apnea in Parkinson's disease patients: Is unattended portable monitoring a suitable tool? *Journal of Parkinson's Disease*, *2015*, 258418. http://dx.doi.org/10.1155/2015/258418.

Günther, R., Richter, N., Sauerbier, A., Chaudhuri, K. R., Martinez-Martin, P., Storch, A., & Hermann, A. (2016). Non-motor symptoms in patients suffering from motor neuron diseases. *Frontiers in Neurology*, 7, 117.

Haubenberger, D., Abbruzzese, G., Bain, P. G., Bajaj, N., Benito-Leon, J., Bhatia, K. P., … Elble, R. J. (2016). Transducer-based evaluation of tremor. *Movement Disorders*, *31*(9), 1327–1336. http://dx.doi.org/10.1002/mds.26671.

Hauser, R. A., Friedlander, J., Zesiewicz, T. A., Adler, C. H., Seeberger, L. C., O'Brien, C. F., … Factor, S. A. (2000). A home diary to assess functional status in patients with Parkinson's disease with motor fluctuations and dyskinesia. *Clinical Neuropharmacology*, *23*(2), 75–81.

Hellwig, B., Mund, P., Schelter, B., Guschlbauer, B., Timmer, J., & Lucking, C. H. (2009). A longitudinal study of tremor frequencies in Parkinson's disease and essential tremor. *Clinical Neurophysiology, 120*(2), 431–435. http://dx.doi.org/10.1016/j.clinph.2008.11.002.

Hemmerle, A. M., Herman, J. P., & Seroogy, K. B. (2012). Stress, depression and Parkinson's disease. *Experimental Neurology, 233*(1), 79–86. http://dx.doi.org/10.1016/j.expneurol.2011.09.035.

Hentz, J. G., Mehta, S. H., Shill, H. A., Driver-Dunckley, E., Beach, T. G., & Adler, C. H. (2015). Simplified conversion method for unified Parkinson's disease rating scale motor examinations. *Movement Disorders, 30*(14), 1967–1970. http://dx.doi.org/10.1002/mds.26435.

Hoehn, M. M., & Yahr, M. D. (1967). Parkinsonism: Onset, progression and mortality. *Neurology, 17*(5), 427–442.

Hoff, J. I., Wagemans, E. A., & van Hilten, B. J. (2001). Ambulatory objective assessment of tremor in Parkinson's disease. *Clinical Neuropharmacology, 24*(5), 280–283.

Homann, C. N., Suppan, K., Wenzel, K., Giovannoni, G., Ivanic, G., Horner, S., … Hartung, H. P. (2000). The Bradykinesia Akinesia Incoordination Test (BRAIN TEST), an objective and user-friendly means to evaluate patients with parkinsonism. *Movement Disorders, 15*(4), 641–647.

Horne, M. K., McGregor, S., & Bergquist, F. (2015). An objective fluctuation score for Parkinson's disease. *PLoS One, 10*(4). e0124522. http://dx.doi.org/10.1371/journal.pone.0124522.

Hossen, A., Muthuraman, M., Al-Hakim, Z., Raethjen, J., Deuschl, G., & Heute, U. (2013). Discrimination of Parkinsonian tremor from essential tremor using statistical signal characterization of the spectrum of accelerometer signal. *Bio-Medical Materials and Engineering, 23*(6), 513–531. http://dx.doi.org/10.3233/BME-130773.

Hudson, C. J., Seeman, P., & Seeman, M. V. (2014). Parkinson's disease: Low-dose haloperidol increases dopamine receptor sensitivity and clinical response. *Parkinson's Disease, 2014*, 684973.

Iluz, T., Gazit, E., Herman, T., Sprecher, E., Brozgol, M., Giladi, N., … Hausdorff, J. M. (2014). Automated detection of missteps during community ambulation in patients with Parkinson's disease: A new approach for quantifying fall risk in the community setting. *Journal of Neuroengineering and Rehabilitation, 11*, 48. http://dx.doi.org/10.1186/1743-0003-11-48.

Jang, W., Han, J., Park, J., Kim, J. S., Cho, J. W., Koh, S. B., … Kim, H. T. (2013). Waveform analysis of tremor may help to differentiate Parkinson's disease from drug-induced parkinsonism. *Physiological Measurement, 34*(3), N15–N24. http://dx.doi.org/10.1088/0967-3334/34/3/N15.

Jankovic, J., McDermott, M., Carter, J., Gauthier, S., Goetz, C., Golbe, L., et al. (1990). Variable expression of Parkinson's disease: A base-line analysis of the DATATOP cohort. The Parkinson Study Group. *Neurology, 40*(10), 1529–1534.

Jenkinson, C., Fitzpatrick, R., Peto, V., Greenhall, R., & Hyman, N. (1997). The PDQ-8: Development and validation of a short-form Parkinson's disease questionnaire. *Psychology and Health, 12*, 805–814.

Jitkritsadakul, O., Jagota, P., & Bhidayasiri, R. (2015). Postural instability, the absence of sexual intercourse in the past month, and loss of libido are predictors of sexual dysfunction in Parkinson's disease. *Parkinsonism & Related Disorders, 21*(1), 61–67. http://dx.doi.org/10.1016/j.parkreldis.2014.11.003.

Katzenschlager, R., Schrag, A., Evans, A., Manson, A., Carroll, C. B., Ottaviani, D., … Hobart, J. (2007). Quantifying the impact of dyskinesias in PD: The PDYS-26: a patient-based outcome measure. *Neurology, 69*(6), 555–563. http://dx.doi.org/10.1212/01.wnl.0000266669.18308.af.

Keezer, M. R., Wolfson, C., & Postuma, R. B. (2016). Age, gender, comorbidity, and the MDS-UPDRS: Results from a population-based study. *Neuroepidemiology*, *46*(3), 222–227. http://dx.doi.org/10.1159/000444021.

Keijsers, N. L., Horstink, M. W., & Gielen, S. C. (2003a). Automatic assessment of levodopa-induced dyskinesias in daily life by neural networks. *Movement Disorders*, *18*(1), 70–80. http://dx.doi.org/10.1002/mds.10310.

Keijsers, N. L., Horstink, M. W., & Gielen, S. C. (2003b). Movement parameters that distinguish between voluntary movements and levodopa-induced dyskinesia in Parkinson's disease. *Human Movement Science*, *22*(1), 67–89.

Klawans, H. L., Jr., & Garvin, J. S. (1969). Treatment of parkinsonism with L-dopa (study of 105 patients). *Diseases of the Nervous System*, *30*(11), 737–746.

Klenk, J., Srulijes, K., Schatton, C., Schwickert, L., Maetzler, W., Becker, C., & Synofzik, M. (2016). Ambulatory activity components deteriorate differently across neurodegenerative diseases: A cross-sectional sensor-based study. *Neurodegenerative Diseases*, *16*(5–6), 317–323. http://dx.doi.org/10.1159/000444802.

Klingelhoefer, L., Rizos, A., Sauerbier, A., McGregor, S., Martinez-Martin, P., Reichmann, H., … Chaudhuri, K. R. (2016). Night-time sleep in Parkinson's disease—The potential use of Parkinson's KinetiGraph: A prospective comparative study. *European Journal of Neurology*, *23*(8), 1275–1288. http://dx.doi.org/10.1111/ene.13015.

Kluger, B. M., Herlofson, K., Chou, K. L., Lou, J. S., Goetz, C. G., Lang, A. E., … Friedman, J. (2016). Parkinson's disease-related fatigue: A case definition and recommendations for clinical research. *Movement Disorders*, *31*(5), 625–631. http://dx.doi.org/10.1002/mds.26511.

Kocer, A., & Oktay, A. B. (2016). Nintendo Wii assessment of Hoehn and Yahr score with Parkinson's disease tremor. *Technology and Health Care*, *24*(2), 185–191. http://dx.doi.org/10.3233/thc-151124.

Koh, S. B., Kim, J. W., Ma, H. I., Ahn, T. B., Cho, J. W., Lee, P. H., … Baik, J. S. (2012). Validation of the korean-version of the nonmotor symptoms scale for Parkinson's disease. *Journal of Clinical Neurology*, *8*(4), 276–283. http://dx.doi.org/10.3988/jcn.2012.8.4.276.

Koop, M. M., Andrzejewski, A., Hill, B. C., Heit, G., & Bronte-Stewart, H. M. (2006). Improvement in a quantitative measure of bradykinesia after microelectrode recording in patients with Parkinson's disease during deep brain stimulation surgery. *Movement Disorders*, *21*(5), 673–678. http://dx.doi.org/10.1002/mds.20796.

Kotschet, K., Johnson, W., McGregor, S., Kettlewell, J., Kyoong, A., O'Driscoll, D. M., … Horne, M. K. (2014). Daytime sleep in Parkinson's disease measured by episodes of immobility. *Parkinsonism & Related Disorders*, *20*(6), 578–583. http://dx.doi.org/10.1016/j.parkreldis.2014.02.011.

Lang, A., & Fahn, S. (1989). Assessment of Parkinson's disease. In T. L. Munsat (Ed.), *Quantification of neurologic deficit* (pp. 285–309). Boston: Butterworths.

LaRocca, N. (n.d). Statistical and methodological considerations in scale construction. In T.L. Mansat (Ed.), *Quantification of neurologic deficit*. Boston: Butterworths.

Larsen, T. A., Calne, S., & Calne, D. B. (1984). Assessment of Parkinson's disease. *Clinical Neuropharmacology*, 7(2), 165–169.

Leentjens, A. F., Dujardin, K., Pontone, G. M., Starkstein, S. E., Weintraub, D., & Martinez-Martin, P. (2014). The Parkinson Anxiety Scale (PAS): Development and validation of a new anxiety scale. *Movement Disorders*, *29*(8), 1035–1043. http://dx.doi.org/10.1002/mds.25919.

Lees, A. J., Blackburn, N. A., & Campbell, V. L. (1988). The nighttime problems of Parkinson's disease. *Clinical Neuropharmacology*, *11*(6), 512–519.

LeMoyne, R., & Mastroianni, T. (2015). Use of smartphones and portable media devices for quantifying human movement characteristics of gait, tendon reflex response, and

Parkinson's disease hand tremor. *Methods in Molecular Biology, 1256*, 335–358. http://dx.doi.org/10.1007/978-1-4939-2172-0_23.

Lieber, B., Taylor, B. E., Appelboom, G., McKhann, G., & Connolly, E. S., Jr. (2015). Motion sensors to assess and monitor medical and surgical management of Parkinson disease. *World Neurosurgery, 84*(2), 561–566. http://dx.doi.org/10.1016/j.wneu.2015.03.024.

Lieberman, A., Dziatolowski, W., Gopinathan, G., Kupersmith, M., Neophytides, A., & Korein, J. (1980). Evaluation of Parkinson's disease. In M. Goldstein, D. B. Calne, A. Lieberman, & M. D. Thorner (Eds.), *Ergot compounds and brain function: Neuroendocrine and neuropsychiatric aspects* (pp. 277–286). New York: Raven Press.

Ling, H., Massey, L. A., Lees, A. J., Brown, P., & Day, B. L. (2012). Hypokinesia without decrement distinguishes progressive supranuclear palsy from Parkinson's disease. *Brain, 135*(Pt. 4), 1141–1153. http://dx.doi.org/10.1093/brain/aws038.

Lopane, G., Mellone, S., Chiari, L., Cortelli, P., Calandra-Buonaura, G., & Contin, M. (2015). Dyskinesia detection and monitoring by a single sensor in patients with Parkinson's disease. *Movement Disorders, 30*(9), 1267–1271. http://dx.doi.org/10.1002/mds.26313.

Lord, S., Godfrey, A., Galna, B., Mhiripiri, D., Burn, D., & Rochester, L. (2013). Ambulatory activity in incident Parkinson's: More than meets the eye? *Journal of Neurology, 260*(12), 2964–2972. http://dx.doi.org/10.1007/s00415-013-7037-5.

Louter, M., Maetzler, W., Prinzen, J., van Lummel, R. C., Hobert, M., Arends, J. B., … Liepelt-Scarfone, I. (2015). Accelerometer-based quantitative analysis of axial nocturnal movements differentiates patients with Parkinson's disease, but not high-risk individuals, from controls. *Journal of Neurology, Neurosurgery, and Psychiatry, 86*(1), 32–37. http://dx.doi.org/10.1136/jnnp-2013-306851.

Maetzler, W., Domingos, J., Srulijes, K., Ferreira, J. J., & Bloem, B. R. (2013). Quantitative wearable sensors for objective assessment of Parkinson's disease. *Movement Disorders, 28*(12), 1628–1637. http://dx.doi.org/10.1002/mds.25628.

Manson, A. J., Brown, P., O'Sullivan, J. D., Asselman, P., Buckwell, D., & Lees, A. J. (2000). An ambulatory dyskinesia monitor. *Journal of Neurology, Neurosurgery, and Psychiatry, 68*(2), 196–201.

Marinus, J., Visser, M., Stiggelbout, A. M., Rabey, J. M., Martinez-Martin, P., Bonuccelli, U., … van Hilten, J. J. (2004). A short scale for the assessment of motor impairments and disabilities in Parkinson's disease: The SPES/SCOPA. *Journal of Neurology, Neurosurgery, and Psychiatry, 75*(3), 388–395.

Marinus, J., Visser, M., van Hilten, J. J., Lammers, G. J., & Stiggelbout, A. M. (2003a). Assessment of sleep and sleepiness in Parkinson disease. *Sleep, 26*(8), 1049–1054.

Marinus, J., Visser, M., Verwey, N. A., Verhey, F. R., Middelkoop, H. A., Stiggelbout, A. M., & van Hilten, J. J. (2003b). Assessment of cognition in Parkinson's disease. *Neurology, 61*(9), 1222–1228.

Marras, C., & Lang, A. (2013). Parkinson's disease subtypes: Lost in translation? *Journal of Neurology, Neurosurgery, and Psychiatry, 84*(4), 409–415. http://dx.doi.org/10.1136/jnnp-2012-303455.

Marsden, C. D., & Schachter, M. (1981). Assessment of extrapyramidal disorders. *British Journal of Clinical Pharmacology, 11*(2), 129–151.

Martinez Manzanera, O., Elting, J. W., van der Hoeven, J. H., & Maurits, N. M. (2016). Tremor detection using parametric and non-parametric spectral estimation methods: A comparison with clinical assessment. *PLoS One, 11*(6), e0156822. http://dx.doi.org/10.1371/journal.pone.0156822.

Martinez-Martin, P. (1987). Parametros evolutivos en la enfermedad de Parkinson. Madrid: Universidad Complutense.

Martinez-Martin, P., Benito-Leon, J., Burguera, J. A., Castro, A., Linazasoro, G., Martinez-Castrillo, J. C., … Frades, B. (2005). The SCOPA-Motor Scale for assessment

of Parkinson's disease is a consistent and valid measure. *Journal of Clinical Epidemiology*, *58*(7), 674–679. http://dx.doi.org/10.1016/j.jclinepi.2004.09.014.
Martinez-Martin, P., Chaudhuri, K. R., Rojo-Abuin, J. M., Rodriguez-Blazquez, C., Alvarez-Sanchez, M., Arakaki, T., … Goetz, C. G. (2015). Assessing the non-motor symptoms of Parkinson's disease: MDS-UPDRS and NMS Scale. *European Journal of Neurology*, *22*(1), 37–43. http://dx.doi.org/10.1111/ene.12165.
Martinez-Martin, P., & Forjaz, M. J. (2006). Metric attributes of the unified Parkinson's disease rating scale 3.0 battery: Part I, feasibility, scaling assumptions, reliability, and precision. *Movement Disorders*, *21*(8), 1182–1188. http://dx.doi.org/10.1002/mds.20916.
Martinez-Martin, P., Forjaz, M. J., Cubo, E., Frades, B., & de Pedro Cuesta, J. (2006). Global versus factor-related impression of severity in Parkinson's disease: A new clinimetric index (CISI-PD). *Movement Disorders*, *21*(2), 208–214. http://dx.doi.org/10.1002/mds.20697.
Martinez-Martin, P., Garcia Urra, D., del Ser Quijano, T., Balseiro Gomez, J., Gomez Utrero, E., Pineiro, R., & Andres, M. T. (1997). A new clinical tool for gait evaluation in Parkinson's disease. *Clinical Neuropharmacology*, *20*(3), 183–194.
Martinez-Martin, P., Gil-Nagel, A., Gracia, L. M., Gomez, J. B., Martinez-Sarries, J., & Bermejo, F. (1994). Unified Parkinson's Disease Rating Scale characteristics and structure. The Cooperative Multicentric Group. *Movement Disorders*, *9*(1), 76–83. http://dx.doi.org/10.1002/mds.870090112.
Martinez-Martin, P., Gil-Nagel, A., Morlan Gracia, L., Balseiro Gomez, J., Martinez-Sarries, F. J., Bermejo, F., … Burguera, J. A. (1995). Intermediate scale for assessment of Parkinson's disease. Characteristics and structure. *Parkinsonism & Related Disorders*, *1*(2), 97–102.
Martinez-Martin, P., & Hernandez, B. (2012). The Q10 questionnaire for detection of wearing-off phenomena in Parkinson's disease. *Parkinsonism & Related Disorders*, *18*(4), 382–385. http://dx.doi.org/10.1016/j.parkreldis.2011.12.011.
Martinez-Martin, P., Rodriguez-Blazquez, C., Abe, K., Bhattacharyya, K. B., Bloem, B. R., Carod-Artal, F. J., … Chaudhuri, K. R. (2009a). International study on the psychometric attributes of the non-motor symptoms scale in Parkinson disease. *Neurology*, *73*(19), 1584–1591. http://dx.doi.org/10.1212/WNL.0b013e3181c0d416.
Martinez-Martin, P., Rodriguez-Blazquez, C., Alvarez-Sanchez, M., Arakaki, T., Bergareche-Yarza, A., Chade, A., … Goetz, C. G. (2013). Expanded and independent validation of the Movement Disorder Society-Unified Parkinson's Disease Rating Scale (MDS-UPDRS). *Journal of Neurology*, *260*(1), 228–236. http://dx.doi.org/10.1007/s00415-012-6624-1.
Martinez-Martin, P., Rodriguez-Blazquez, C., Forjaz, M. J., & de Pedro, J. (2009b). The clinical impression of severity index for Parkinson's disease: International validation study. *Movement Disorders*, *24*(2), 211–217. http://dx.doi.org/10.1002/mds.22320.
Martinez-Martin, P., Rodriguez-Blazquez, C., Kurtis, M. M., Chaudhuri, K. R., & NMSS Validation Group. (2011). The impact of non-motor symptoms on health-related quality of life of patients with Parkinson's disease. *Movement Disorders*, *26*(3), 399–406. http://dx.doi.org/10.1002/mds.23462.
Martinez-Martin, P., Rojo-Abuin, J. M., Rodriguez-Violante, M., Serrano-Duenas, M., Garretto, N., & Martinez-Castrillo, J. C. (2016). Analysis of four scales for global severity evaluation in Parkinson's disease. *npj Parkinson's Disease*, *2*, 1600–1607.
Martinez-Martin, P., Schapira, A. H., Stocchi, F., Sethi, K., Odin, P., MacPhee, G., … Chaudhuri, K. R. (2007). Prevalence of nonmotor symptoms in Parkinson's disease in an international setting; study using nonmotor symptoms questionnaire in 545 patients. *Movement Disorders*, *22*(11), 1623–1629. http://dx.doi.org/10.1002/mds.21586.
Martinez-Martin, P., Tolosa, E., Hernandez, B., & Badia, X. (2008). Validation of the "QUICK" questionnaire—A tool for diagnosis of "wearing-off" in patients with

Parkinson's disease. *Movement Disorders, 23*(6), 830–836. http://dx.doi.org/10.1002/mds.21944.

Martino, D., Tamburini, T., Zis, P., Rosoklija, G., Abbruzzese, G., Ray-Chaudhuri, K., … Avanzino, L. (2016). An objective measure combining physical and cognitive fatigability: Correlation with subjective fatigue in Parkinson's disease. *Parkinsonism & Related Disorders, 32*, 80–86. http://dx.doi.org/10.1016/j.parkreldis.2016.08.021.

McDowell, F., Lee, J. E., Swift, T., Sweet, R. D., Ogsbury, J. S., & Kessler, J. T. (1970). Treatment of Parkinson's syndrome with L dihydroxyphenylalanine (levodopa). *Annals of Internal Medicine, 72*(1), 29–35.

McRae, C., Diem, G., Vo, A., O'Brien, C., & Seeberger, L. (2000). Schwab & England: Standardization of administration. *Movement Disorders, 15*(2), 335–336.

Merola, A., Romagnolo, A., Rosso, M., Lopez-Castellanos, J. R., Wissel, B. D., Larkin, S., … Espay, A. J. (2016). Orthostatic hypotension in Parkinson's disease: Does it matter if asymptomatic? *Parkinsonism & Related Disorders, 33*, 65–71. http://dx.doi.org/10.1016/j.parkreldis.2016.09.013.

Montero-Odasso, M., Oteng-Amoako, A., Speechley, M., Gopaul, K., Beauchet, O., Annweiler, C., & Muir-Hunter, S. W. (2014). The motor signature of mild cognitive impairment: Results from the gait and brain study. *The Journals of Gerontology. Series A, Biological Sciences and Medical Sciences, 69*(11), 1415–1421. http://dx.doi.org/10.1093/gerona/glu155.

Moore, S. T., MacDougall, H. G., & Ondo, W. G. (2008). Ambulatory monitoring of freezing of gait in Parkinson's disease. *Journal of Neuroscience Methods, 167*(2), 340–348. http://dx.doi.org/10.1016/j.jneumeth.2007.08.023.

Moore, S. T., Yungher, D. A., Morris, T. R., Dilda, V., MacDougall, H. G., Shine, J. M., … Lewis, S. J. (2013). Autonomous identification of freezing of gait in Parkinson's disease from lower-body segmental accelerometry. *Journal of Neuroengineering and Rehabilitation, 10*, 19. http://dx.doi.org/10.1186/1743-0003-10-19.

Morris, T. R., Cho, C., Dilda, V., Shine, J. M., Naismith, S. L., Lewis, S. J., & Moore, S. T. (2012). A comparison of clinical and objective measures of freezing of gait in Parkinson's disease. *Parkinsonism & Related Disorders, 18*(5), 572–577. http://dx.doi.org/10.1016/j.parkreldis.2012.03.001.

Movement Disorder Society Task Force on Rating Scales for Parkinson's Disease. (2003). The Unified Parkinson's Disease Rating Scale (UPDRS): Status and recommendations. *Movement Disorders, 18*(7), 738–750. PMID: 12815652.

Nieuwboer, A., Rochester, L., Herman, T., Vandenberghe, W., Emil, G. E., Thomaes, T., & Giladi, N. (2009). Reliability of the new freezing of gait questionnaire: Agreement between patients with Parkinson's disease and their carers. *Gait & Posture, 30*(4), 459–463. http://dx.doi.org/10.1016/j.gaitpost.2009.07.108.

Niwa, F., Kuriyama, N., Nakagawa, M., & Imanishi, J. (2011). Circadian rhythm of rest activity and autonomic nervous system activity at different stages in Parkinson's disease. *Autonomic Neuroscience, 165*(2), 195–200. http://dx.doi.org/10.1016/j.autneu.2011.07.010.

Nutt, J. G., Bloem, B. R., Giladi, N., Hallett, M., Horak, F. B., & Nieuwboer, A. (2011). Freezing of gait: Moving forward on a mysterious clinical phenomenon. *Lancet Neurology, 10*(8), 734–744. http://dx.doi.org/10.1016/S1474-4422(11)70143-0.

Ossig, C., Antonini, A., Buhmann, C., Classen, J., Csoti, I., Falkenburger, B., … Storch, A. (2016). Wearable sensor-based objective assessment of motor symptoms in Parkinson's disease. *Journal of Neural Transmission (Vienna), 123*(1), 57–64. http://dx.doi.org/10.1007/s00702-015-1439-8.

O'Sullivan, S. S., Williams, D. R., Gallagher, D. A., Massey, L. A., Silveira-Moriyama, L., & Lees, A. J. (2008). Nonmotor symptoms as presenting complaints in Parkinson's disease: A clinicopathological study. *Movement Disorders, 23*(1), 101–106. http://dx.doi.org/10.1002/mds.21813.

Ou, R., Yang, J., Cao, B., Wei, Q., Chen, K., Chen, X., … Shang, H. (2016). Progression of non-motor symptoms in Parkinson's disease among different age populations: A two-year follow-up study. *Journal of the Neurological Sciences*, *360*, 72–77. http://dx.doi.org/10.1016/j.jns.2015.11.047.

Ozinga, S. J., Machado, A. G., Miller Koop, M., Rosenfeldt, A. B., & Alberts, J. L. (2015). Objective assessment of postural stability in Parkinson's disease using mobile technology. *Movement Disorders*, *30*(9), 1214–1221. http://dx.doi.org/10.1002/mds.26214.

Pagonabarraga, J., Kulisevsky, J., Llebaria, G., Garcia-Sanchez, C., Pascual-Sedano, B., & Gironell, A. (2008). Parkinson's disease-cognitive rating scale: A new cognitive scale specific for Parkinson's disease. *Movement Disorders*, *23*(7), 998–1005. http://dx.doi.org/10.1002/mds.22007.

Pal, G., & Goetz, C. G. (2013). Assessing bradykinesia in parkinsonian disorders. *Frontiers in Neurology*, *4*, 54. http://dx.doi.org/10.3389/fneur.2013.00054.

Papapetropoulos, S. S. (2012). Patient diaries as a clinical endpoint in Parkinson's disease clinical trials. *CNS Neuroscience and Therapeutics*, *18*(5), 380–387. http://dx.doi.org/10.1111/j.1755-5949.2011.00253.x.

Papapetropoulos, S., Jagid, J. R., Sengun, C., Singer, C., & Gallo, B. V. (2008). Objective monitoring of tremor and bradykinesia during DBS surgery for Parkinson disease. *Neurology*, *70*(15), 1244–1249. http://dx.doi.org/10.1212/01.wnl.0000308936.27780.94.

Peto, V., Jenkinson, C., Fitzpatrick, R., & Greenhall, R. (1995). The development and validation of a short measure of functioning and well being for individuals with Parkinson's disease. *Quality of Life Research*, *4*(3), 241–248.

Petrinovich, L., & Hardyck, C. (1964). Behavioral changes in Parkinson patients following surgery. A factor analytic study. *Journal of Chronic Diseases*, *17*, 225–240.

Politis, M., Wu, K., Molloy, S., G Bain, P., Chaudhuri, K. R., & Piccini, P. (2010). Parkinson's disease symptoms: The patient's perspective. *Movement Disorders*, *25*(11), 1646–1651. http://dx.doi.org/10.1002/mds.23135.

Prakash, K. M., Nadkarni, N. V., Lye, W. K., Yong, M. H., Chew, L. M., & Tan, E. K. (2015). A longitudinal study of non-motor symptom burden in Parkinson's disease after a transition to expert care. *Parkinsonism & Related Disorders*, *21*(8), 843–847. http://dx.doi.org/10.1016/j.parkreldis.2015.04.017.

Rabey, J. M., Bass, H., Bonuccelli, U., Brooks, D., Klotz, P., Korczyn, A. D., … Van Hilten, B. (1997). Evaluation of the Short Parkinson's Evaluation Scale: A new friendly scale for the evaluation of Parkinson's disease in clinical drug trials. *Clinical Neuropharmacology*, *20*(4), 322–337.

Rahimi, F., Samotus, O., Lee, J., & Jog, M. (2015). Effective management of upper limb Parkinsonian Tremor by incobotulinumtoxinA injections using sensor-based biomechanical patterns. *Tremor and Other Hyperkinetic Movements (New York, N.Y.)*, *5*, 348. http://dx.doi.org/10.7916/D8BP0270.

Ray Chaudhuri, K., Rojo, J. M., Schapira, A. H., Brooks, D. J., Stocchi, F., Odin, P., … Martinez-Martin, P. (2013). A proposal for a comprehensive grading of Parkinson's disease severity combining motor and non-motor assessments: Meeting an unmet need. *PLoS One*, *8*(2), e57221. http://dx.doi.org/10.1371/journal.pone.0057221.

Reddy, P., Martinez-Martin, P., Brown, R. G., Chaudhuri, K. R., Lin, J. P., Selway, R., … Samuel, M. (2014). Perceptions of symptoms and expectations of advanced therapy for Parkinson's disease: Preliminary report of a Patient-Reported Outcome tool for Advanced Parkinson's disease (PRO-APD). *Health and Quality of Life Outcomes*, *12*, 11. http://dx.doi.org/10.1186/1477-7525-12-11.

Rocchi, C., Pierantozzi, M., Galati, S., Chiaravalloti, A., Pisani, V., Prosperetti, C., … Stefani, A. (2015). Autonomic function tests and MIBG in Parkinson's disease: Correlation to disease duration and motor symptoms. *CNS Neuroscience and Therapeutics*, *21*(9), 727–732. http://dx.doi.org/10.1111/cns.12437.

Sanchez-Ferro, A., Elshehabi, M., Godinho, C., Salkovic, D., Hobert, M. A., Domingos, J., ... Maetzler, W. (2016). New methods for the assessment of Parkinson's disease (2005 to 2015): A systematic review. *Movement Disorders*, *31*(9), 1283–1292. http://dx.doi.org/10.1002/mds.26723.

Santens, P., & de Noordhout, A. M. (2006). Detection of motor and non-motor symptoms of end-of dose wearing-off in Parkinson's disease using a dedicated questionnaire: A Belgian multicenter survey. *Acta Neurologica Belgica*, *106*(3), 137–141.

Schrag, A., Spottke, A., Quinn, N. P., & Dodel, R. (2009). Comparative responsiveness of Parkinson's disease scales to change over time. *Movement Disorders*, *24*(6), 813–818. http://dx.doi.org/10.1002/mds.22438.

Schwab, R. S. (1960). Progression and prognosis in Parkinson's disease. *The Journal of Nervous and Mental Disease*, *130*, 556–566.

Schwab, R. S., & England, A. (1969). Projection technique for evaluating surgey in Parkinson's disease. In F. J. Gillingham & I. M. L. Donaldson (Eds.), *Third Symposium on Parkinson's disease* (pp. 152–157). Edinburgh: E. and S. Livingstone.

Sellami, L., Kacem, I., Nasri, A., Djebara, M. B., Sidhom, Y., Gargouri, A., & Gouider, R. (2016). Evaluation of an Arabic version of the non-motor symptoms scale in Parkinson's disease. *Neurological Sciences*, *37*(6), 963–968. http://dx.doi.org/10.1007/s10072-016-2525-x.

Seppi, K., Weintraub, D., Coelho, M., Perez-Lloret, S., Fox, S. H., Katzenschlager, R., ... Sampaio, C. (2011). The movement disorder society evidence-based medicine review update: Treatments for the non-motor symptoms of Parkinson's disease. *Movement Disorders*, *26*(Suppl. 3), S42–S80. http://dx.doi.org/10.1002/mds.23884.

Shine, J. M., Moore, S. T., Bolitho, S. J., Morris, T. R., Dilda, V., Naismith, S. L., & Lewis, S. J. (2012). Assessing the utility of Freezing of Gait Questionnaires in Parkinson's Disease. *Parkinsonism Related Disorders*, *18*(1), 25–29.

Shulman, L. M., Armstrong, M., Ellis, T., Gruber-Baldini, A., Horak, F., Nieuwboer, A., ... Martinez-Martin, P. (2016). Disability rating scales in Parkinson's disease: Critique and recommendations. *Movement Disorders*, *31*(10), 1455–1465. http://dx.doi.org/10.1002/mds.26649.

Silva de Lima, A. L., Hahn, T., de Vries, N. M., Cohen, E., Bataille, L., Little, M. A., ... Faber, M. J. (2016). Large-scale wearable sensor deployment in parkinson's patients: The Parkinson@Home Study Protocol. *Journal of Medical Internet Research, Research Protocols*, *5*(3). e172http://dx.doi.org/10.2196/resprot.5990.

Simuni, T., Long, J. D., Caspell-Garcia, C., Coffey, C. S., Lasch, S., Tanner, C. M., ... Marek, K. (2016). Predictors of time to initiation of symptomatic therapy in early Parkinson's disease. *Annals of Clinical Translational Neurology*, *3*(7), 482–494. http://dx.doi.org/10.1002/acn3.317.

Snijders, A. H., Weerdesteyn, V., Hagen, Y. J., Duysens, J., Giladi, N., & Bloem, B. R. (2010). Obstacle avoidance to elicit freezing of gait during treadmill walking. *Movement Disorders*, *25*(1), 57–63. http://dx.doi.org/10.1002/mds.22894.

Sommerauer, M., Werth, E., Poryazova, R., Gavrilov, Y. V., Hauser, S., & Valko, P. O. (2015). Bound to supine sleep: Parkinson's disease and the impact of nocturnal immobility. *Parkinsonism & Related Disorders*, *21*(10), 1269–1272. http://dx.doi.org/10.1016/j.parkreldis.2015.08.010.

Speelman, A. D., van Nimwegen, M., Bloem, B. R., & Munneke, M. (2014). Evaluation of implementation of the ParkFit program: A multifaceted intervention aimed to promote physical activity in patients with Parkinson's disease. *Physiotherapy*, *100*(2), 134–141. http://dx.doi.org/10.1016/j.physio.2013.05.003.

Sringean, J., Taechalertpaisarn, P., Thanawattano, C., & Bhidayasiri, R. (2016a). How well do Parkinson's disease patients turn in bed? Quantitative analysis of nocturnal hypokinesia using multisite wearable inertial sensors. *Parkinsonism & Related Disorders*, *23*, 10–16. http://dx.doi.org/10.1016/j.parkreldis.2015.11.003.

Sringean, J., Taechalertpaisarn, P., Thanawattano, C., & Bhidayasiri, R. (2016b). When is the worst period of nocturnal hypokinesia in Parkinson's disease? A sensor-based analysis. *Movement Disorders*, *31*(Suppl. 2), S680.

Stacy, M., Bowron, A., Guttman, M., Hauser, R., Hughes, K., Larsen, J. P., … Stocchi, F. (2005). Identification of motor and nonmotor wearing-off in Parkinson's disease: Comparison of a patient questionnaire versus a clinician assessment. *Movement Disorders*, *20*(6), 726–733. http://dx.doi.org/10.1002/mds.20383.

Stacy, M. A., Murphy, J. M., Greeley, D. R., Stewart, R. M., Murck, H., & Meng, X. (2008). The sensitivity and specificity of the 9-item Wearing-off Questionnaire. *Parkinsonism & Related Disorders*, *14*(3), 205–212. http://dx.doi.org/10.1016/j.parkreldis.2007.07.013.

Stallibrass, C., Sissons, P., & Chalmers, C. (2002). Randomized controlled trial of the Alexander technique for idiopathic Parkinson's disease. *Clinical Rehabilitation*, *16*(7), 695–708.

Stamford, J. A., Schmidt, P. N., & Friedl, K. E. (2015). What engineering technology could do for quality of life in Parkinson's disease: A review of current needs and opportunities. *IEEE Journal of Biomedical and Health Informatics*, *19*(6), 1862–1872. http://dx.doi.org/10.1109/JBHI.2015.2464354.

Stebbins, G. T., & Goetz, C. G. (1998). Factor structure of the Unified Parkinson's Disease Rating Scale: Motor examination section. *Movement Disorders*, *13*(4), 633–636. http://dx.doi.org/10.1002/mds.870130404.

Stebbins, G. T., Goetz, C. G., Burn, D. J., Jankovic, J., Khoo, T. K., & Tilley, B. C. (2013). How to identify tremor dominant and postural instability/gait difficulty groups with the movement disorder society unified Parkinson's disease rating scale: Comparison with the unified Parkinson's disease rating scale. *Movement Disorders*, *28*(5), 668–670. http://dx.doi.org/10.1002/mds.25383.

Stevens, S. (1959). Measurement, psychophysics and utility. In C. W. Churchman & P. Ratoosh (Eds.), *Measurement: Definitions and theories* (pp. 18–63). New York: John Wiley.

Stone, A. A., Shiffman, S., Schwartz, J. E., Broderick, J. E., & Hufford, M. R. (2002). Patient non-compliance with paper diaries. *BMJ*, *324*(7347), 1193–1194.

Storch, A., Schneider, C. B., Klingelhofer, L., Odin, P., Fuchs, G., Jost, W. H., … Ebersbach, G. (2015). Quantitative assessment of non-motor fluctuations in Parkinson's disease using the Non-Motor Symptoms Scale (NMSS). *Journal of Neural Transmission (Vienna)*, *122*(12), 1673–1684. http://dx.doi.org/10.1007/s00702-015-1437-x.

Storch, A., Schneider, C. B., Wolz, M., Sturwald, Y., Nebe, A., Odin, P., … Ebersbach, G. (2013). Nonmotor fluctuations in Parkinson disease: Severity and correlation with motor complications. *Neurology*, *80*(9), 800–809. http://dx.doi.org/10.1212/WNL.0b013e318285c0ed.

Taylor Tavares, A. L., Jefferis, G. S., Koop, M., Hill, B. C., Hastie, T., Heit, G., & Bronte-Stewart, H. M. (2005). Quantitative measurements of alternating finger tapping in Parkinson's disease correlate with UPDRS motor disability and reveal the improvement in fine motor control from medication and deep brain stimulation. *Movement Disorders*, *20*(10), 1286–1298. http://dx.doi.org/10.1002/mds.20556.

Teravainen, H., & Calne, D. (1980). Quantitative assessment of parkinsonian deficits. In U. K. Rinne, M. Klinger, & G. Stamm (Eds.), *Parkinson's disease—Current progress, problems, and management* (pp. 145–164). Amsterdam: Elsevier.

Thanawattano, C., Pongthornseri, R., Anan, C., Dumnin, S., & Bhidayasiri, R. (2015). Temporal fluctuations of tremor signals from inertial sensor: A preliminary study in differentiating Parkinson's disease from essential tremor. *Biomedical Engineering Online*, *14*(1), 101. http://dx.doi.org/10.1186/s12938-015-0098-1.

Thielgen, T., Foerster, F., Fuchs, G., Hornig, A., & Fahrenberg, J. (2004). Tremor in Parkinson's disease: 24-hr monitoring with calibrated accelerometry. *Electromyography and Clinical Neurophysiology*, *44*(3), 137–146.

Tomlinson, C. L., Patel, S., Meek, C., Herd, C. P., Clarke, C. E., Stowe, R., … Ives, N. (2013). Physiotherapy versus placebo or no intervention in Parkinson's disease. *The Cochrane Database of Systematic Reviews*, *9*, CD002817. http://dx.doi.org/10.1002/14651858.CD002817.pub4.

Toosizadeh, N., Mohler, J., Lei, H., Parvaneh, S., Sherman, S., & Najafi, B. (2015). Motor performance assessment in Parkinson's disease: Association between objective in-clinic, objective in-home, and subjective/semi-objective measures. *PLoS One*, *10*(4). e0124763. http://dx.doi.org/10.1371/journal.pone.0124763.

Trenkwalder, C., Kies, B., Rudzinska, M., Fine, J., Nikl, J., Honczarenko, K., … Recover Study, G. (2011). Rotigotine effects on early morning motor function and sleep in Parkinson's disease: A double-blind, randomized, placebo-controlled study (RECOVER). *Movement Disorders*, *26*(1), 90–99. http://dx.doi.org/10.1002/mds.23441.

Tzallas, A. T., Tsipouras, M. G., Rigas, G., Tsalikakis, D. G., Karvounis, E. C., Chondrogiorgi, M., … Fotiadis, D. I. (2014). PERFORM: A system for monitoring, assessment and management of patients with Parkinson's disease. *Sensors (Basel)*, *14*(11), 21329–21357. http://dx.doi.org/10.3390/s141121329.

van der Kolk, N. M., van Nimwegen, M., Speelman, A. D., Munneke, M., Backx, F. J., Donders, R., … Bloem, B. R. (2014). A personalized coaching program increases outdoor activities and physical fitness in sedentary Parkinson patients; a post-hoc analysis of the ParkFit trial. *Parkinsonism & Related Disorders*, *20*(12), 1442–1444. http://dx.doi.org/10.1016/j.parkreldis.2014.10.004.

van Hilten, B., Hoff, J. I., Middelkoop, H. A., van der Velde, E. A., Kerkhof, G. A., Wauquier, A., … Roos, R. A. (1994). Sleep disruption in Parkinson's disease. Assessment by continuous activity monitoring. *Archives of Neurology*, *51*(9), 922–928.

van Uem, J. M., Maier, K. S., Hucker, S., Scheck, O., Hobert, M. A., Santos, A. T., … Maetzler, W. (2016). Twelve-week sensor assessment in Parkinson's disease: Impact on quality of life. *Movement Disorders*, *31*(9), 1337–1338. http://dx.doi.org/10.1002/mds.26676.

Verbaan, D., van Rooden, S. M., Benit, C. P., van Zwet, E. W., Marinus, J., & van Hilten, J. J. (2011). SPES/SCOPA and MDS-UPDRS: Formulas for converting scores of two motor scales in Parkinson's disease. *Parkinsonism & Related Disorders*, *17*(8), 632–634. http://dx.doi.org/10.1016/j.parkreldis.2011.05.022.

Visser, M., Marinus, J., Stiggelbout, A. M., & Van Hilten, J. J. (2004). Assessment of autonomic dysfunction in Parkinson's disease: The SCOPA-AUT. *Movement Disorders*, *19*(11), 1306–1312. http://dx.doi.org/10.1002/mds.20153.

Visser, M., Verbaan, D., van Rooden, S. M., Stiggelbout, A. M., Marinus, J., & van Hilten, J. J. (2007). Assessment of psychiatric complications in Parkinson's disease: The SCOPA-PC. *Movement Disorders*, *22*(15), 2221–2228. http://dx.doi.org/10.1002/mds.21696.

Walker, J. E., Albers, J. W., Tourtellotte, W. W., Henderson, W. G., Potvin, A. R., & Smith, A. (1972). A qualitative and quantitative evaluation of amantadine in the treatment of Parkinson's disease. *Journal of Chronic Diseases*, *25*(3), 149–182.

Webster, D. D. (1968). Critical analysis of the disability in Parkinson's disease. *Modern Treatment*, *5*(2), 257–282.

Weintraut, R., Karadi, K., Lucza, T., Kovacs, M., Makkos, A., Janszky, J., & Kovacs, N. (2016). Lille apathy rating scale and MDS-UPDRS for screening apathy in Parkinson's disease. *Journal of Parkinson's Disease*, *6*(1), 257–265. http://dx.doi.org/10.3233/jpd-150726.

Weiss, A., Brozgol, M., Dorfman, M., Herman, T., Shema, S., Giladi, N., & Hausdorff, J. M. (2013). Does the evaluation of gait quality during daily life provide insight into fall risk? A novel approach using 3-day accelerometer recordings. *Neurorehabilitation and Neural Repair*, *27*(8), 742–752. http://dx.doi.org/10.1177/1545968313491004.

Weiss, A., Herman, T., Giladi, N., & Hausdorff, J. M. (2014). Objective assessment of fall risk in Parkinson's disease using a body-fixed sensor worn for 3 days. *PLoS One*, *9*(5). e96675. http://dx.doi.org/10.1371/journal.pone.0096675.
Weiss, A., Herman, T., Giladi, N., & Hausdorff, J. M. (2015). New evidence for gait abnormalities among Parkinson's disease patients who suffer from freezing of gait: Insights using a body-fixed sensor worn for 3 days. *Journal of Neural Transmission*, *122*(3), 403–410. http://dx.doi.org/10.1007/s00702-014-1279-y.
Wharrad, H. J., & Jefferson, D. (2000). Distinguishing between physiological and essential tremor using discriminant and cluster analyses of parameters derived from the frequency spectrum. *Human Movement Science*, *19*(3), 319–339.
Wile, D. J., Ranawaya, R., & Kiss, Z. H. (2014). Smart watch accelerometry for analysis and diagnosis of tremor. *Journal of Neuroscience Methods*, *230*, 1–4. http://dx.doi.org/10.1016/j.jneumeth.2014.04.021.
Wong, W. Y., Wong, M. S., & Lo, K. H. (2007). Clinical applications of sensors for human posture and movement analysis: A review. *Prosthetics and Orthotics International*, *31*(1), 62–75. http://dx.doi.org/10.1080/03093640600983949.

CHAPTER SEVEN

Biomarkers of Parkinson's Disease: An Introduction

Nataliya Titova*[,1], Mubasher A. Qamar[†,‡,§], K. Ray Chaudhuri[†,‡,§]
*Federal State Budgetary Educational Institution of Higher Education "N.I. Pirogov Russian National Research Medical University" of the Ministry of Healthcare of the Russian Federation, Moscow, Russia
[†]National Parkinson Foundation International Centre of Excellence, Kings College and Kings College Hospital, London, United Kingdom
[‡]Maurice Wohl Clinical Neuroscience Institute, Kings College, London, United Kingdom
[§]National Institute for Health Research (NIHR) Mental Health Biomedical Research Centre (BRC) and Dementia Unit at South London and Maudsley NHS Foundation Trust, London, United Kingdom
[1]Corresponding author: e-mail address: nattitova@yandex.ru

Contents

Abstract

The development of biomarkers is of great importance in Parkinson's disease (PD) as it may contribute to confirmation and support of the diagnosis, tracking of progression, and prediction of the natural history of PD. Biomarkers also help in the identification of targets for treatment and measuring the efficacy of interventions. Biomarkers are, therefore, crucial to understanding the pathophysiology of PD, the second commonest neurodegenerative disorder in the world. Modern understanding of PD suggests that it is a multipeptide, multiorgan disorder presenting with a heterogeneous clinical condition, both motor and nonmotor. Biomarkers need to reflect this neuropathological and clinical heterogeneity of PD. In this review, we outline some key advances in the field of clinical, genetic, neuroimaging, and tissue-based biomarkers proposed or used for PD. The individual sections will be covered in relevant chapters and our review is largely a primer aimed to alert readers to the current state of the various biomarkers proposed for PD. In doing so, we have also underlined the important role multimodal rather than single biomarkers could play in our future understanding of PD.

International Review of Neurobiology, Volume 132
ISSN 0074-7742
http://dx.doi.org/10.1016/bs.irn.2017.03.003

1. INTRODUCTION

A biomarker is defined as a tool or a collection of tools that can objectively measure multitude of events which provides information on the normal, pathological, or pharmacological processes taking place during the course of a disorder. The Biomarkers Definitions Working Group have met and attempted to define biomarkers as "a characteristic that is objectively measured and evaluated as an indicator of normal biological processes, pathogenic processes or pharmacological responses to a therapeutic intervention" (Biomarkers Definitions Working Group, 2001). Biomarkers are needed for Parkinson's disease (PD) to address several issues (Table 1), some of which remain key unmet needs and a challenge for research.

2. THE TYPES OF BIOMARKERS

Several forms of biomarkers have been described and validated. These include clinical symptoms (comprising of motor and nonmotor symptoms

Table 1 The Need and Potential Utility for Biomarkers in Parkinson's Research

To confirm and support diagnosis
Motor diagnosis
Possibly prodromal diagnosis
To track progression of disease
Motor progression
Nonmotor progression
Holistic progression
To predict trajectory of disease
Early vs advanced/complex PD vs palliative stages of PD (Fig. 1)
To identify targets for treatment
Motor subtypes
Nonmotor subtypes
Individualized precision medicine
To address the efficacy of interventions
Outcome measures (clinical, imaging, biochemical)

(NMS) and/or relevant validated scales that chart progression of PD), genetics, neuroimaging (central and peripheral nervous system), and biochemical (tissue-derived) assessments. These are listed in Table 2.

Biomarkers could also be classified as per Sharma et al. (2013) who proposed the following groupings:

- In vivo (neuroimaging, neurophysiology (muscle action potential), polysomnography)
- In vitro (biochemical/genetics from tissue samples)
- Pathological (α-synuclein, dopamine transporter loss, iron accumulation)
- Neurobehavioral (depression, fatigue, cognition)
- Clinical (Table 2)

The role of biomarkers has become crucial to better define and understand PD which is no longer considered a motor disease alone. PD is now regarded as a syndrome characterized by a preprodromal stage progressing to the motor syndrome of PD followed by a palliative stage (Antonini et al., 2015; Jellinger, 2015; Titova, Padmakumar, Lewis, & Chaudhuri, 2016) (Fig. 1). Pathophysiology of PD includes multiple neurotransmitter dysfunction, dopaminergic and nondopaminergic deficits, and a complex medley of molecular mechanisms causing widespread (central and peripheral nervous system) neuronal degeneration with Lewy body deposition (Braak et al., 2003; Halliday, Holton, Revesz, & Dickson, 2011; Halliday, Lees, & Stern, 2011; Titova et al., 2016). It is now widely appreciated that, owing to the heterogeneity of PD, single biomarkers may not be useful and a multimodal approach with motor and NMS-driven biomarkers is required (Chaudhuri, 2016). For instance, availability of robust biomarkers for the different stages of PD as shown in Fig. 1 would allow development of precision and "stage-specific" therapies. Such an approach is likely to support basic scientists as well as translational research and clinicians to effectively diagnose, follow, and understand the motor and nonmotor syndrome of PD, currently an unmet need.

The syndromic nature of PD is further exemplified by four dominant neurotransmitter dysfunctions of varying severity (Fig. 2) which underpins the condition and is likely to express clinically as nonmotor subtypes of PD (Sauerbier, Jenner, Todorova, & Chaudhuri, 2016). Valid biomarkers for PD, therefore, need to reflect the heterogeneity of underlying pathophysiology. Recent evidence from a 2-year follow-up study of de novo PD suggests that single and cognitive biomarkers may not be adequate. Thirty possible biomarkers were examined in this study and the authors conclude that a multimodal approach, with clinical, biochemical, and laboratory-based biomarkers, is needed (Mollenhauer et al., 2016).

Table 2 A List of Proposed and Possibly Relevant Clinical, Biochemical, and Genetic Biomarkers

Type of Biomarker	Effect	Key References
Clinical		
Prodromal NMS		Schrag, Horsfall, Walters, Noyce, and Petersen (2015)
RBD	Progression to α-synucleinopathy	Postuma, Gagnon, and Montplaisir (2013)
REM sleep behavior events	PSG evidence of RBD	Sixel-Döring, Trautmann, Mollenhauer, and Trenkwalder (2014)
Late-onset hyposmia/anosmia	Progression to PD	Jennings, Siderowf, Stern, and Marek (2013)
Episodic major depression	Prodromal PD feature	Jennings et al. (2013) and Sauerbier and Chaudhuri (2015)
Constipation	Higher risk of developing PD	
Excessive daytime somnolence	Higher risk of developing PD	
Fatigue	Higher risk of developing PD	Kang, Ma, Lim, Hwang, and Kim (2013)
Abnormal color vision/visual perception	Higher risk of developing PD	Diederich et al. (2010)
Erectile dysfunction	Higher risk of developing PD	Gao et al. (2007)
Pain (often unilateral)	Pain often evident on side first affected at motor PD diagnosis	Lin, Wu, Chang, Chiang, and Lin (2013)
Cognitive impairment	Recent evidence from PPMI cohort	Chahine et al. (2016)

Motor symptoms		
Tremor	Could be prodromal	Schrag et al. (2015)
Postural instability	Prodromal and advancing motor PD	Delenclos, Jones, McLean, and Uitti (2016) and Schrag et al. (2015)
Dyskinesias	Advancing motor PD	
Micrographia	May be evident in prodromal stage	
Scales		
UPDRS	Well established for motor progression	
Scopa Autonomic	Evidence from DeNoPa study	Mollenhauer et al. (2016)
PD NMS scale	Evidence from DeNoPa study	
Genetics (proposed)		
GBA	5%–10% PD	Beavan et al. (2015)
LRRK2 (G2019S mutation)	Accounts for 2%–3% of all PD	Klein and Schlossmacher (2007) and Houlden and Singleton (2012)
α-syn (SNCA), Parkin, PINK1, DJ-1	Weak evidence	
Biochemical		
Blood based		Chahine, Stern, and Chen-Plotkin (2014)
α-Synuclein	Unclear and depends on oligomeric vs total and phosphorylated Both ↑ and ↓ reported	Chahine et al. (2014)

Continued

Table 2 A List of Proposed and Possibly Relevant Clinical, Biochemical, and Genetic Biomarkers—cont'd

Type of Biomarker	Effect	Key References
DJ-1	Studies suggest not useful for diagnosis even after quality control	Chahine et al. (2014) and Shi, Zabetian, et al. (2010)
Uric acid and serum urate	CEP 1347 trial (PRECEPT) cohort-based data show hazard ratio for receiving dopaminergic therapy declined with ↑ serum urate. Correlation with striatal beta CIT uptake	Cipriani, Chen, and Schwarzschild (2010)
EGF	↓ Values linked to cognitive performance	Chahine et al. (2014) and Pellecchia et al. (2013)
Apo A1	Proposed unbiased biomarker ↑ may reduce risk of developing PD and predictor of UPDRS III score Links with statins that ↑ Apo A1	Chahine et al. (2014), Gao, Simon, Schwarzschild, and Ascherio (2012), and Lee et al. (2013)
Cerebrospinal fluid based		Kroksveen, Opsahl, Aye, Ulvik, and Berven (2011)
α-Synuclein	Variations between total ↓ and oligomeric ↑ and phosphorylated ↑	Sharma et al. (2013)
DJ-1	↓	
GBA activity	↓	
Aß-42	↓ Levels of t-tau, p-tau Link with NMS including cognitive	Savica, Grossardt, Bower, Ahlskog, and Rocca (2013)
Neurofilaments	Maybe useful in differential diagnosis between PD and MSA	
α-Synuclein RT-QuIC	A real-time quaking-induced conversion RT-QuIC-based assay which can detect α-synuclein aggregation in cerebrospinal fluid	Fairfoul et al. (2016)

Other tissues		
Submandibular gland	Peripheral evidence of α-synuclein deposition	Adler et al. (2016)
Skin biopsy	Cutaneous α-synuclein deposition	Gibbons, Garcia, Wang, Shih, and Freeman (2016)
Colonic biopsy	Phosphorylated α-synuclein deposition across the myenteric plexus, submucosal layer, as well as the mucosal nerve fibers of the intestine	Shannon et al. (2012)
Urine	8-Hydroxydeoxyguanosine, a measure of oxidative stress	Sato, Mizuno, and Hattori (2005)
	Phosphorylated LRRK2 predicts phenotype with cognitive impairment	Shi, Huber, and Zhang (2010)
Saliva	Genetic testing (GBA, LRRK2)	Klein and Schlossmacher (2007) and Houlden and Singleton (2012)
Feces (fecal microbiota)	Significant differences and ↓ of "protective" gut microbiota composition in PD vs controls. However, consistency needs further confirmation	Scheperjans (2016)

None are robust in isolation. Multimodal validity is being tested. Neuroimaging is discussed elsewhere.
α-syn (SNCA), α-synuclein; *Aβ-42*, A beta containing amyloid; *AMSA*, multiple system atrophy; *Apo A1*, apolipoprotein A1; *CIT*, 2β-carbomethoxy-3β-(4-iodophenyl)tropane; *DeNoPa*, the de novo Parkinson's cohort; *EGF*, epidermal growth factor; *GBA*, glucocerebrosidase; *LRRK2*, leucine-rich repeat kinase 2; *NMS*, nonmotor symptoms; *PD*, Parkinson's disease; *PPMI*, Parkinson's progressive markers initiative; *PSG*, polysomnography; *RBD*, REM sleep behavior disorder; *REM*, rapid eye movement; *UPDRS*, Unified Parkinson's Disease Rating Scales.

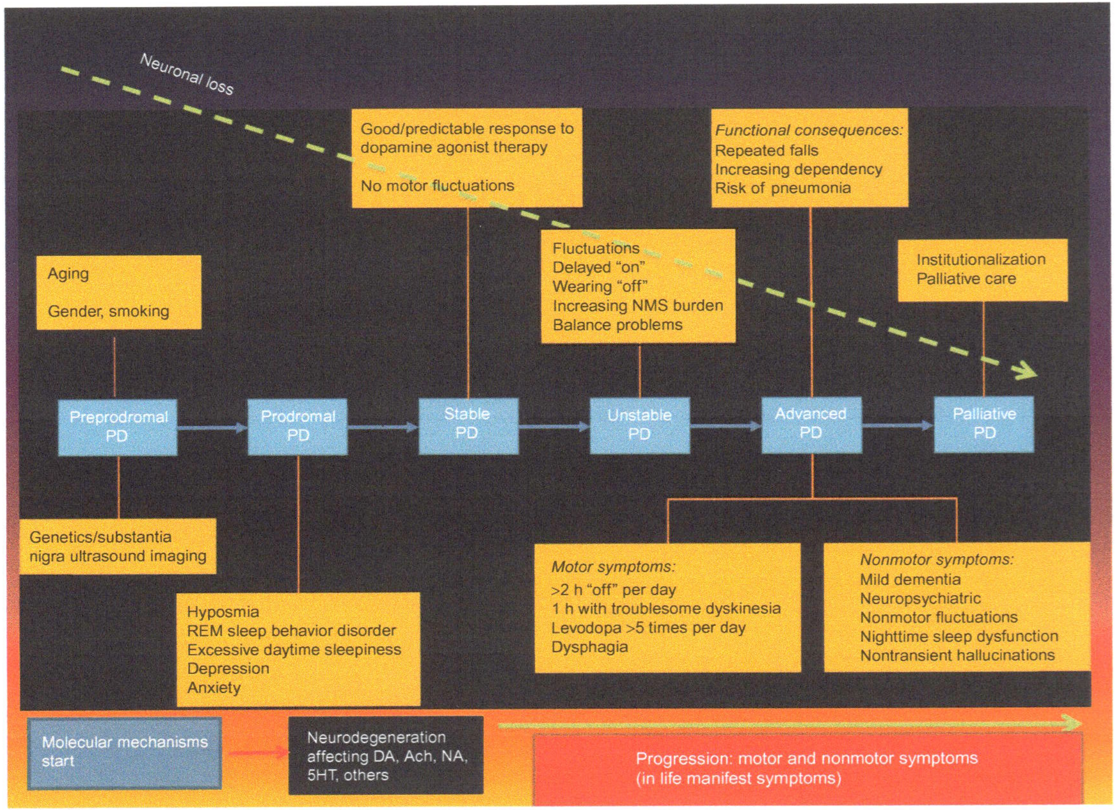

Fig. 1 The proposed natural history pattern of Parkinson's disease. It is to be noted that the neuronal loss in PD is unlikely to follow a linear pattern (as suggested in the figure) and the relevant line is a schematic representation. *Ach*, acetylcholine; *DA*, dopamine; *NA*, noradrenaline; *5HT*, serotonin. *Adapted from Chaudhuri, K. R., & Fung, V. S. C. (2016).* Fast facts: Parkinson's disease *(4th ed.) (p. 9). Oxford: Health Press Limited.*

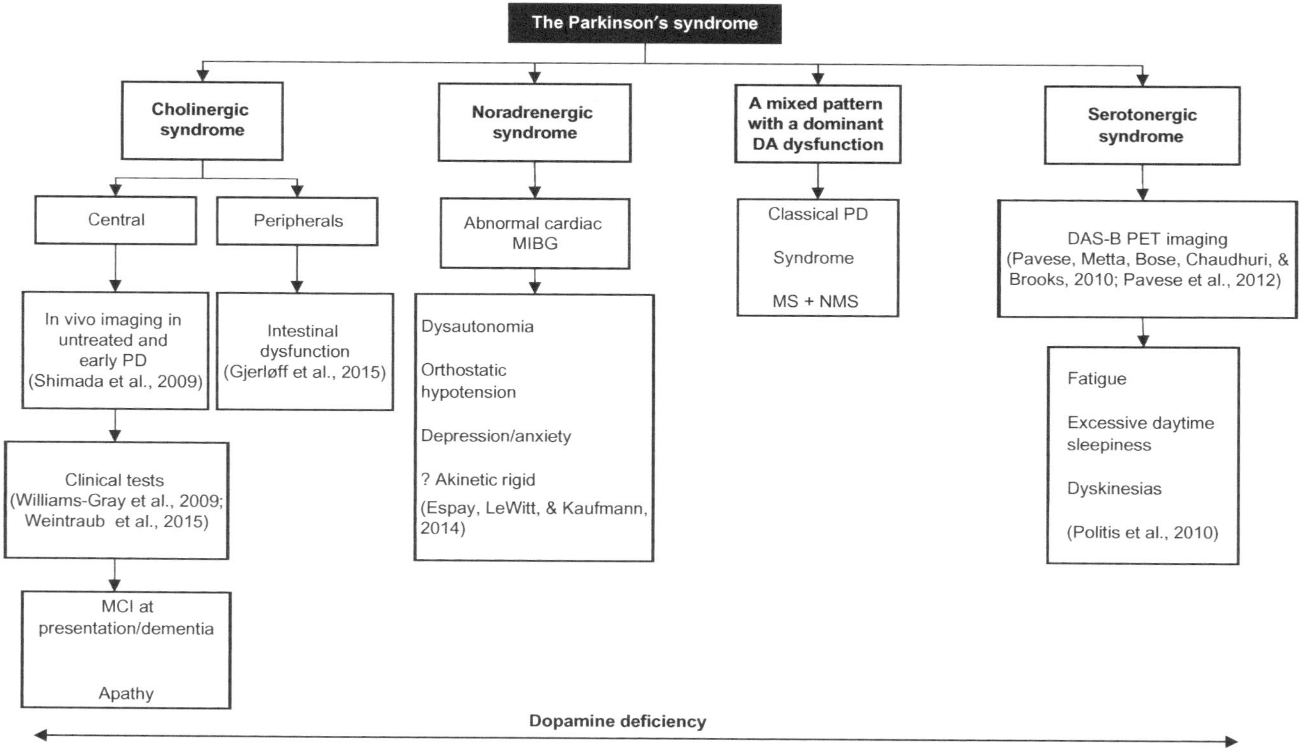

Fig. 2 The multineurotransmitter basis of Parkinson's disease and the need for multimodal biomarkers that reflect the heterogeneity of the Parkinson's syndrome. *Taken from Titova, N., Padmakumar, C., Lewis, S. J., & Chaudhuri, K. R. (2016). Parkinson's: A syndrome rather than a disease?* Journal of Neural Transmission *(in press).*

3. NEUROIMAGING

Neuroimaging techniques and modalities can generate high-resolution data and are now used commonly to support and validate the clinical diagnosis of PD (Pavese & Brooks, 2009). Magnetic resonance imaging (MRI) and transcranial sonography (TCS) are commonly available and less expensive which can noninvasively track pathways of molecular targets that are of relevance to the parkinsonian neurodegenerative process. Examples will include the use of MRI with T2-weighted fluid-attenuated inversion recovery sequences which can detect nigral or basal forebrain degeneration in PD. Using diffusion tensor imaging, MRI can also show subcortical white matter degeneration. Voxel-based morphometry is also a useful MRI technique. TCS can show increased nigral iron deposition in susceptible healthy older individuals (Mahlknecht, Seppi, & Poewe, 2015). Single-photon emission tomography and positron emission tomography (PET) are more expensive and are usually used with cyclotron-generated radioactive metabolic tracers to assess function at a receptor level and can also be used as surrogate marker for diagnosis, monitoring disease severity as well as progression. Imaging the dopaminergic system is the key approach in PD, although imaging other neurotransmitter systems is becoming increasingly relevant (Fig. 2). Furthermore, dopamine-based neuroimaging strategies can also be selectively combined with a range of clinical scales, symptoms, and biochemical markers to increase the diagnostic certainty of PD.

4. NEUROINFLAMMATION

In PD, postmortem studies as well as specific imaging using PET and tissue sampling suggest that neuroinflammation and microglial activation are common and could even occur in the prodromal stage (Hirsch & Hunot, 2009; Moehle & West, 2015). Tissue-based cytokines have been proposed as biomarkers and indeed have been linked to depression, anxiety, as well as cognitive dysfunction (Bufalino, Hepgul, Aguglia, & Pariante, 2013).

A detailed discussion of all proposed biomarkers is beyond the scope of this chapter and will be covered in relevant cognition, neuroimaging, and nonmotor chapters. For detailed discussion, we would like to refer the readers to a few excellent current reviews cited in Biomarkers Definitions Working Group (2001), Sharma et al. (2013), Chahine et al. (2014), and Miller and O'Callaghan (2015). A number of prospective cohort studies have now been initiated to address the role of clinical, genetic, and other biomarkers and their value in clinical practice. These include the PD biomarker program, the Parkinson's progression markers initiative, the Kassel DeNoPa cohort study, and the Parkinson's NMS longitudinal study (NILS) among others and are likely to report on the value of multimodal biomarker approach to PD in future.

5. THE FUTURE

As this review suggests, a single biomarker is unlikely to be successful for PD. In the last decade, new techniques such as proteomics, metabolomics, as well as transcriptomics have emerged. These tools can perform mass analyses and identify small changes in protein function, track metabolites, and identify RNA profiles in a variety of tissues and fluids from healthy and affected people. Genetic and clinical biomarkers continue to evolve particularly with the emergence of the concept of discrete motor and nonmotor subtypes of PD (Sauerbier et al., 2016). Functional imaging targeting nondopaminergic pathways in the brain and periphery will add to the range of biomarkers available for future. In addition, in clinical practice milestones of PD need to be better signposted by biomarkers. For instance, in future, the concept of "advanced" PD may be designated by a range of clinical, biochemical, and imaging biomarkers. Such studies are currently under way. The value of a multimodal biomarker approach has been illustrated in the study by Mollenhauer et al. (2016) and is likely to become the method of choice for tracking and managing a complex heterogeneous condition such as PD.

ACKNOWLEDGMENTS

We acknowledge the help of Prof. Maria Stamelou and Prof. Kailash Bhatia.

REFERENCES

Adler, C. H., Dugger, B. N., Hentz, J. G., Hinni, M. L., Lott, D. G., Driver-Dunckley, E., et al. (2016). Peripheral synucleinopathy in early Parkinson's disease: Submandibular gland needle biopsy findings. *Movement Disorders*, *31*(2), 250–256.

Antonini, A., Odin, P., Kleinman, L., Skalicky, A., Marshall, E., Sail, K., et al. (2015). Implementing a Delphi panel to improve understanding of patient characteristics of advanced Parkinson's disease. *Movement Disorders*, *30*. Poster No 1186. Presented at the 19th International Congress of Parkinson's Disease and Movement Disorders, June 14–18, 2015, San Diego, CA.

Beavan, M., McNeill, A., Proukakis, C., Hughes, D. A., Mehta, A., & Schapira, A. H. (2015). Evolution of prodromal clinical markers of Parkinson disease in a GBA mutation-positive cohort. *JAMA Neurology*, *72*(2), 201–208.

Biomarkers Definitions Working Group. (2001). Biomarkers and surrogate endpoints: Preferred definitions and conceptual framework. *Clinical Pharmacology and Therapeutics*, *69*(3), 89–95.

Braak, H., Del Tredici, K., Rub, U., de Vos, R. A., Jansen Steur, E. N., & Braak, E. (2003). Staging of brain pathology related to sporadic Parkinson's disease. *Neurobiology of Aging*, *24*(2), 197–211.

Bufalino, C., Hepgul, N., Aguglia, E., & Pariante, C. M. (2013). The role of immune genes in the association between depression and inflammation: A review of recent clinical studies. *Brain, Behavior, and Immunity*, *31*, 31–47.

Chahine, L. M., Stern, M. B., & Chen-Plotkin, A. (2014). Blood-based biomarkers for Parkinson's disease. *Parkinsonism & Related Disorders*, *20*(Suppl. 1), S99–103.

Chahine, L. M., Weintraub, D., Hawkins, K. A., Siderowf, A., Eberly, S., Oakes, D., et al. (2016). Cognition in individuals at risk for Parkinson's: Parkinson associated risk syndrome (PARS) study findings. *Movement Disorders*, *31*(1), 86–94.

Chaudhuri, K. R. (2016). Progression and biomarkers for Parkinson disease: Merging motor with nonmotor symptoms. *Neurology*, *87*(2), 128–129.

Cipriani, S., Chen, X., & Schwarzschild, M. A. (2010). Urate: A novel biomarker of Parkinson's disease risk, diagnosis and prognosis. *Biomarkers in Medicine*, *4*(5), 701–712.

Delenclos, M., Jones, D. R., McLean, P. J., & Uitti, R. J. (2016). Biomarkers in Parkinson's disease: Advances and strategies. *Parkinsonism & Related Disorders*, *22*(Suppl. 1), S106–S110.

Diederich, N. J., Pieri, V., Hipp, G., Rufra, O., Blyth, S., & Vaillant, M. (2010). Discriminative power of different nonmotor signs in early Parkinson's disease. A case-control study. *Movement Disorders*, *25*(7), 882–887.

Espay, A. J., LeWitt, P. A., & Kaufmann, H. (2014). Norepinephrine deficiency in Parkinson's disease: The case for noradrenergic enhancement. *Movement Disorders*, *29*(14), 1710–1719.

Fairfoul, G., McGuire, L. I., Pal, S., Ironside, J. W., Neumann, J., Christie, S., et al. (2016). Alpha-synuclein RT-QuIC in the CSF of patients with alpha-synucleinopathies. *Annals of Clinical and Translational Neurology*, *3*(10), 812–818.

Gao, X., Chen, H., Schwarzschild, M. A., Glasser, D. B., Logroscino, G., Rimm, E. B., et al. (2007). Erectile function and risk of Parkinson's disease. *American Journal of Epidemiology*, *166*(12), 1446–1450.

Gao, X., Simon, K. C., Schwarzschild, M. A., & Ascherio, A. (2012). Prospective study of statin use and risk of Parkinson disease. *Archives of Neurology*, *69*(3), 380–384.

Gibbons, C. H., Garcia, J., Wang, N., Shih, L. C., & Freeman, R. (2016). The diagnostic discrimination of cutaneous alpha-synuclein deposition in Parkinson disease. *Neurology*, *87*(5), 505–512.

Gjerløff, T., Fedorova, T., Knudsen, K., Munk, O. L., Nahimi, A., Jacobsen, S., et al. (2015). Imaging acetylcholinesterase density in peripheral organs in Parkinson's disease with 11C-donepezil PET. *Brain*, *138*(Pt. 3), 653–663.

Halliday, G. M., Holton, J. L., Revesz, T., & Dickson, D. W. (2011b). Neuropathology underlying clinical variability in patients with synucleinopathies. *Acta Neuropathologica*, *122*(2), 187–204.

Halliday, G., Lees, A., & Stern, M. (2011a). Milestones in Parkinson's disease—Clinical and pathologic features. *Movement Disorders*, *26*(6), 1015–1021.

Hirsch, E. C., & Hunot, S. (2009). Neuroinflammation in Parkinson's disease: A target for neuroprotection? *The Lancet Neurology*, *8*(4), 382–397.

Houlden, H., & Singleton, A. B. (2012). The genetics and neuropathology of Parkinson's disease. *Acta Neuropathologica, 124*(3), 325–338.

Jellinger, K. A. (2015). Neuropathobiology of non-motor symptoms in Parkinson disease. *Journal of Neural Transmission (Vienna, Austria: 1996), 122*(10), 1429–1440.

Jennings, D., Siderowf, M., Stern, M., & Marek, K. (2013). Evaluating phenoconversion to PD in the PARS prodromal cohort. *Movement Disorders, 29*(Suppl), S59–S60.

Kang, S. Y., Ma, H. I., Lim, Y. M., Hwang, S. H., & Kim, Y. J. (2013). Fatigue in drug-naïve Parkinson's disease. *European Neurology, 70*(1–2), 59–64.

Klein, C., & Schlossmacher, M. G. (2007). Parkinson disease, 10 years after its genetic revolution: Multiple clues to a complex disorder. *Neurology, 69*(22), 2093–2104.

Kroksveen, A. C., Opsahl, J. A., Aye, T. T., Ulvik, R. J., & Berven, F. S. (2011). Proteomics of human cerebrospinal fluid: Discovery and verification of biomarker candidates in neurodegenerative diseases using quantitative proteomics. *Journal of Proteomics, 74*(4), 371–388.

Lee, Y. C., Lin, C. H., Wu, R. M., Lin, M. S., Lin, J. W., Chang, C. H., et al. (2013). Discontinuation of statin therapy associates with Parkinson disease: A population-based study. *Neurology, 81*(5), 410–416.

Lin, C. H., Wu, R. M., Chang, H. Y., Chiang, Y. T., & Lin, H. H. (2013). Preceding pain symptoms and Parkinson's disease: A nationwide population-based cohort study. *European Journal of Neurology, 20*(10), 1398–1404.

Mahlknecht, P., Seppi, K., & Poewe, W. (2015). The concept of prodromal Parkinson's disease. *Journal of Parkinson's Disease, 5*(4), 681–697.

Miller, D. B., & O'Callaghan, J. P. (2015). Biomarkers of Parkinson's disease: Present and future. *Metabolism, 64*(3 Suppl. 1), S40–S46.

Moehle, M. S., & West, A. B. (2015). M1 and M2 immune activation in Parkinson's disease: Foe and ally? *Neuroscience, 302*, 59–73.

Mollenhauer, B., Zimmermann, J., Sixel-Doring, F., Focke, N. K., Wicke, T., Ebentheuer, J., et al. (2016). Monitoring of 30 marker candidates in early Parkinson disease as progression markers. *Neurology, 87*(2), 168–177.

Pavese, N., & Brooks, D. J. (2009). Imaging neurodegeneration in Parkinson's disease. *Biochimica et Biophysica Acta, 1792*(7), 722–729.

Pavese, N., Metta, V., Bose, S. K., Chaudhuri, K. R., & Brooks, D. J. (2010). Fatigue in Parkinson's disease is linked to striatal and limbic serotonergic dysfunction. *Brain, 133*(11), 3434–3443.

Pavese, N., Simpson, B. S., Metta, V., Ramlackhansingh, A., Chaudhuri, K. R., & Brooks, D. J. (2012). [^{18}F]FDOPA uptake in the raphe nuclei complex reflects serotonin transporter availability. A combined [^{18}F]FDOPA and [^{11}C]DASB PET study in Parkinson's disease. *Neuroimage, 59*(2), 1080–1084.

Pellecchia, M. T., Santangelo, G., Picillo, M., Pivonello, R., Longo, K., Pivonello, C., et al. (2013). Serum epidermal growth factor predicts cognitive functions in early, drug-naive Parkinson's disease patients. *Journal of Neurology, 260*(2), 438–444.

Politis, M., Wu, K., Loane, C., Kiferle, L., Molloy, S., Brooks, D. J., et al. (2010). Staging of serotonergic dysfunction in Parkinson's disease: An in vivo 11C-DASB PET study. *Neurobiology of Disease, 40*(1), 216–221.

Postuma, R. B., Gagnon, J.-F., & Montplaisir, J. Y. (2013). REM sleep behavior disorder and prodromal neurodegeneration—Where are we headed? *Tremor and Other Hyperkinetic Movements, 3*. pii: tre-03-134-2929-1.

Sato, S., Mizuno, Y., & Hattori, N. (2005). Urinary 8-hydroxydeoxyguanosine levels as a biomarker for progression of Parkinson disease. *Neurology, 64*(6), 1081–1083.

Sauerbier, A., & Chaudhuri, K. R. (2015). Nonmotor symptoms in Parkinson's disease. In J. Jankovic, & E. Tolosa (Eds.), *Parkinson's Disease and Movement Disorders* (6th Revised ed.). Lippincott Williams and Wilkins.

Sauerbier, A., Jenner, P., Todorova, A., & Chaudhuri, K. R. (2016). Non motor subtypes and Parkinson's disease. *Parkinsonism & Related Disorders*, *22*(Suppl. 1), S41–S46.

Savica, R., Grossardt, B. R., Bower, J. H., Ahlskog, J. E., & Rocca, W. A. (2013). Incidence and pathology of synucleinopathies and tauopathies related to parkinsonism. *JAMA Neurology*, *70*(7), 859–866.

Scheperjans, F. (2016). Can microbiota research change our understanding of neurodegenerative diseases? *Neurodegenerative Disease Management*, *6*(2), 81–85.

Schrag, A., Horsfall, L., Walters, K., Noyce, A., & Petersen, I. (2015). Prediagnostic presentations of Parkinson's disease in primary care: A case-control study. *The Lancet Neurology*, *14*(1), 57–64.

Shannon, K. M., Keshavarzian, A., Mutlu, E., Dodiya, H. B., Daian, D., Jaglin, J. A., et al. (2012). Alpha-synuclein in colonic submucosa in early untreated Parkinson's disease. *Movement Disorders*, *27*(6), 709–715.

Sharma, S., Moon, C. S., Khogali, A., Haidous, A., Chabenne, A., Ojo, C., et al. (2013). Biomarkers in Parkinson's disease (recent update). *Neurochemistry International*, *63*(3), 201–229.

Shi, M., Huber, B. R., & Zhang, J. (2010a). Biomarkers for cognitive impairment in Parkinson disease. *Brain Pathology (Zurich, Switzerland)*, *20*(3), 660–671.

Shi, M., Zabetian, C. P., Hancock, A. M., Ginghina, C., Hong, Z., Yearout, D., et al. (2010b). Significance and confounders of peripheral DJ-1 and alpha-synuclein in Parkinson disease. *Neuroscience Letters*, *480*(1), 78–82.

Shimada, H., Hirano, S., Shinotoh, H., Aotsuka, A., Sato, K., Tanaka, N., et al. (2009). Mapping of brain acetylcholinesterase alterations in Lewy body disease by PET. *Neurology*, *73*(4), 273–278.

Sixel-Döring, F., Trautmann, E., Mollenhauer, B., & Trenkwalder, C. (2014). Rapid eye movement sleep behavioral events: A new marker for neurodegeneration in early Parkinson disease? *Sleep*, *37*(3), 431–438.

Titova, N., Padmakumar, C., Lewis, S. J., & Chaudhuri, K. R. (2016). Parkinson's: A syndrome rather than a disease? *Journal of Neural Transmission*. in press. http://dx.doi.org/10.1007/s00702-016-1667-6.

Weintraub, D., Simuni, T., Caspell-Garcia, C., Coffey, C., Lasch, S., Siderowf, A., et al. (2015). Parkinson's Progression Markers Initiative. Cognitive performance and neuropsychiatric symptoms in early, untreated Parkinson's disease. *Movement Disorders*, *30*(7), 919–927.

Williams-Gray, C. H., Evans, J. R., Goris, A., Foltynie, T., Ban, M., Robbins, T. W., et al. (2009). The distinct cognitive syndromes of Parkinson's disease: 5 year follow-up of the CamPaIGN cohort. *Brain*, *132*(Pt. 11), 2958–2969.

CHAPTER EIGHT

Genetics of Parkinson's Disease: Genotype–Phenotype Correlations

Christos Koros[1], Athina Simitsi[1], Leonidas Stefanis[2]
National and Kapodistrian University of Athens Medical School, "Attikon" Hospital, Athens, Greece
[2]Corresponding author: e-mail address: lstefanis@bioacademy.gr

Contents

Abstract

Since the first discovery of a specific genetic defect in the *SNCA* gene, encoding for α-synuclein, as a causative factor for Parkinson's disease 20 years ago, a multitude of other genes have been linked to this disease in rare cases with Mendelian inheritance. Furthermore, the genetic contribution to the much more common sporadic disease has been demonstrated through case control association studies and, more recently, genome-wide association studies. Interestingly, some of the genes with Mendelian inheritance, such as *SNCA*, are also relevant to the sporadic disease, suggesting common pathogenetic mechanisms. In this review, we place an emphasis on Mendelian forms, and in particular genetic defects which present predominantly with Parkinsonism. We provide details into the particular phenotypes associated with each genetic defect, with a particular emphasis on nonmotor symptoms. For genetic defects for whom a sufficient number of patients has been assessed, there are evident genotype–phenotype correlations. However, it should be noted that patients with the same causative mutation may present with distinctly divergent phenotypes. This phenotypic variability may be due to genetic, epigenetic or environmental factors.

[1] These authors have contributed equally to this manuscript.

International Review of Neurobiology, Volume 132
ISSN 0074-7742
http://dx.doi.org/10.1016/bs.irn.2017.01.009

From a clinical and genetic point of view, it will be especially interesting in the future to identify genetic factors that modify disease penetrance, the age of onset or other specific phenotypic features.

1. INTRODUCTION

Since the discovery, 20 years ago, of Polymeropoulos et al. (1997) that a mutation in the *SNCA* gene encoding for α-synuclein was responsible for Parkinson's disease (PD), there have been enormous advances in the field of PD genetics, with numerous genetic defects linked to the disease, usually in relatively rare familial cases. The genetic make-up has also been linked to the much more common sporadic disease, through case–control and genome-wide association studies (GWAS). This has led to important advances in the understanding of PD pathogenesis, and the potential for disease-modifying therapies. In this review, we will restrict the analysis mostly to the clinical presentation of the various monogenic forms of the disease, in an attempt to disentangle commonalities and differences and to provide genotype–phenotype correlations. We will not provide a detailed analysis of the hits identified through GWAS, the biochemical pathways involved, or the implications of these findings for PD pathogenesis or treatment, as these are provided in recent excellent reviews (Hernandez, Reed, & Singleton, 2016; Kalinderi, Bostantjopoulou, & Fidani, 2016). We will furthermore restrict our analysis only to genes which have been conclusively demonstrated to be linked to PD and give rise predominantly to Parkinsonism.

2. MONOGENIC FORMS WITH A PICTURE LARGELY RESTRICTED TO PARKINSONISM

2.1 Autosomal Dominant Forms

2.1.1 SNCA

The discovery of the p.A53T mutation in the alpha-synuclein (SNCA) gene highlighted the importance of alpha-synuclein in PD pathogenesis (Golbe et al., 1996; Polymeropoulos et al., 1997). Since 1997, a number of additional, albeit rare, missense SNCA mutations, all inherited in autosomal dominant fashion, have been reported (reviewed in Hernandez et al., 2016; Petrucci, Ginevrino, & Valente, 2016). The basic hypothesis is that such mutations, or the multiplication mutations to be mentioned below, lead to a dominant gain of function that relates to the aggregation potential of the protein, acting deleteriously at the level of the synapse, and the lysosomal/endosomal compartment (Vekrellis, Xilouri, Emmanouilidou, Rideout, & Stefanis, 2011). The p.A53T mutation was first described in the large Italian Contursi kindred and in a number of Greek PD families harboring the same haplotype due to a common founder effect (Golbe et al., 1996; Polymeropoulos et al., 1997). The p.A53T mutation was subsequently reported in patients of Greek or Italian background in the United States, Australia, or Germany (Berg et al., 2005; Spira, Sharpe, Halliday, Cavanagh, & Nicholson, 2001) and in a limited number of unrelated cases from Sweden, Poland, Korea, and China (Choi et al., 2008; Ki et al., 2007; Michell, Barker, Raha, & Raha-Chowdhury, 2005; Puschmann et al., 2009; Xiong et al., 2016). The phenotypic spectrum of the p.A53T mutation presents marked intrafamilial and interfamilial variability (Kasten & Klein, 2013; Papadimitriou et al., 1999; Ricciardi et al., 2016). The average onset age is 46 years. The disease is about 80%–90% penetrant (Papadimitriou et al., 2016, 1999). Overall, mutation carriers have a similar, but more aggressive course than idiopathic PD (iPD). Motor features are classic for iPD, but resting tremor is likely less common (Bostantjopoulou et al., 2001; Bozi et al., 2014; Papapetropoulos et al., 2001). The disease course is often accelerated, as we recently showed through a prospective assessment of 30 symptomatic and asymptomatic p.A53T SNCA carriers for a 2-year period (Papadimitriou et al., 2016). Motor symptoms are L-dopa responsive, at least initially, and an early occurrence of motor complications can be observed (Bostantjopoulou et al., 2001; Kasten & Klein, 2013; Markopoulou et al., 2008). Nonmotor features are also prominent, as exemplified by olfactory and autonomic dysfunction, mainly in terms of severe orthostatic hypotension. RBD or depression are not obligate manifestations (Papadimitriou et al., 2016). Other rare features such as myoclonus or central hypoventilation have been reported (Spira et al., 2001). Cognitive decline is variable, but dementia usually occurs within 5–7 years of disease onset (Bostantjopoulou et al., 2001; Markopoulou, Wszolek, & Pfeiffer, 1995, Markopoulou et al., 2008; Papadimitriou et al., 2016; Papapetropoulos et al., 2003; Spira et al., 2001). A DLB presentation has been described (Morfis & Cordato, 2006). Although the pattern of dementia is consistent with PDD, certain cases exhibit atypical features: a Swedish patient developed, within a few years of disease onset, prominent language dysfunction, resembling primary progressive aphasia (Puschmann et al., 2009). We recently reported an atypical presentation at onset of frontotemporal dementia (FTD) with behavioral dysregulation and speech-related problems, in two Greek p.A53T carriers, expanding the phenotypic spectrum (Bougea et al., 2016). In these cases, there was marked frontotemporoparietal atrophy typical of FTD, unlike the normal brain MRI associated previously with the p.A53T mutation (Bougea et al., 2016). In the few dopaminergic imaging studies performed, p.A53T mutation carriers exhibit a rather symmetric loss of radioligand uptake when compared to sporadic PD (Bostantjopoulou, Katsarou, Gerasimou, Costa, & Gotzamani-Psarrakou, 2008; Samii et al., 1999). It is of special interest to assess a possible premotor phase in asymptomatic p.A53T carriers. In our study, retrospective assessment suggested that RBD and olfactory dysfunction could antedate motor symptoms (Papadimitriou et al., 2016), while Ricciardi et al. (2016) reported hyposmia and dopaminergic deficit in an asymptomatic carrier.

Other SNCA point mutations are very rare. The p.E46K mutation has been reported in a family of Spanish Basque origin (Zarranz et al., 2004). Affected patients exhibit a rather severe phenotype with high penetrance. Dementia with LB phenotype and autonomic dysregulation is typical of the full blown disease. Symptoms initiate between 50 and 65 years, and dementia ensues within a few years, although there is quite some variability. Neuropsychological evaluation demonstrated that posterior cortical dysfunction might be a distinct early feature of the cognitive impairment (Somme et al., 2011). In another family reported more recently, motor and nonmotor manifestations were substantially more benign (Pimentel et al., 2015). p.E46K symptomatic and asymptomatic carriers have marked cardiac sympathetic denervation (Tijero et al., 2013).

In carriers of the p.A30P mutation, found in a German family, the clinical phenotype was similar to that of iPD with onset around 60 years, an incomplete penetrance and a more benign course. Nonmotor symptoms were not reported except for cognitive decline, which was present in two out of four affected individuals (Krüger et al., 1998). PET studies showed striatal presynaptic dopaminergic alterations consistent with sporadic PD. Furthermore, neuropsychological testing provided evidence for cognitive impairment as a frequent and early symptom (Krüger et al., 2001).

The p.H50Q SNCA mutation has been reported in families with an English ancestry. In one family, the proband manifested rather typical PD motor manifestations at the age of 60 and mild cognitive decline along with apathy 4 years later. The interval between symptom initiation and death was 12 years. His mother had a more rapid course of PDD over 5 years (Appel-Cresswell et al., 2013). Another case of p.H50Q-related late onset PD exhibited dementia 9 years after disease onset (Proukakis et al., 2013).

Another newly described mutation, p.G51D, has been described in a number of families with different ethnic background (Kiely et al., 2013, 2015; Lesage et al., 2013; Tokutake et al., 2014) and can have a pleiotropic atypical presentation and course, including very early age of onset at age 19 in one case, and pyramidal tract findings, myoclonus, and seizures. Psychiatric symptoms, dementia, and autonomic dysfunction are usually, but not invariably present. An early onset form of motor PD without atypical features was reported in a Finnish family with a p.A53E SNCA mutation (Martikainen, Päivärinta, Hietala, & Kaasinen, 2015; Pasanen et al., 2014).

Apart from point mutations, SNCA gene multiplications are also responsible for inherited PD in families with several affected members. The severity of clinical symptoms correlates with the SNCA copy number, with triplications cases exhibiting more disabling deficits and an earlier disease onset (gene dose effect). SNCA triplication results in severe PD with concomitant cognitive decline and was initially described in the Iowa kindred (Gwinn et al., 2011; Singleton et al., 2003). Additional nonmotor symptoms include RBD and psychiatric manifestations, namely severe depression. Marked weight loss, dysautonomia, and fatigue can precede motor onset. The average onset age is around 40, and the time interval from onset to death 7 years. Dementia is a cardinal feature of SNCA triplication cases, occurring early in the disease course, with cognitive deficits consistent with PDD (Ferese et al., 2015; Fuchs et al., 2007; Gwinn et al., 2011; Olgiati et al., 2015). Brain imaging revealed frontoparietal atrophy and a severe striatal dopaminergic deficit (Olgiati et al., 2015).

SNCA locus duplications are more common and characterized by variable, and generally milder, clinical features, and a decreased penetrance. There have been reports of both familial and sporadic cases harboring the duplication. Moreover, unaffected carriers at advanced ages have been identified, thus suggesting reduced penetrance. The clinical outcome is largely heterogeneous with a benign form of typical late onset motor involvement resembling sporadic PD on the one end and a devastating course mimicking SNCA gene triplication on the other (Chartier-Harlin et al., 2004; Ibáñez et al., 2004; Nishioka et al., 2006; Ross et al., 2008). The average age at onset is 50 years and the interval from onset to death 15 years (Kasten & Klein, 2013). Nonmotor symptoms, including depression, psychosis, and dysautonomia, were present in approximately half of the reported cases. In a Japanese study, symptomatic patients showed abnormal olfactory function and polysomnography (Nishioka et al., 2009). Kara and coauthors described a family exhibiting parkinsonism and FTD with marked anxiety and features of obsessive–compulsive disorder (Kara et al., 2014). Another duplication carrier from Japan presented a bizarre phenotype with head-shaking movements (Itokawa et al., 2013).

Overall, there are certain similarities, but also specific clinical patterns associated with each of the SNCA mutations. Certainly, more in depth phenotypic analysis is needed in larger numbers of patients and asymptomatic carriers to solidify this impression. The picture, with certain notable exceptions mentioned above, is generally that of a classical LB disease; it should be noted however that neuropathological studies suggest some differences from iPD, in particular for certain mutations, such as the p.A53T and the p.G51D or p.A53E, with more prominent alpha-synuclein neuritic pathology and Tau aggregation in the former, and oligodendroglial inclusions in the latter (Duda et al., 2002; Kiely et al., 2013, 2015; Pasanen et al., 2014). The phenotypic spectrum can be wide even among members of the same family, ranging from nonmanifestation to a severe, devastating disease with atypical features. It will be very interesting to assess whether genetic modifying factors account for the clinical heterogeneity of SNCA mutation carriers.

GWAS, in which SNCA is consistently the most significant hit (Hernandez et al., 2016; Nalls et al., 2014), have cemented the role of alpha-synuclein in sporadic iPD, and thus genetic synucleinopathies, which by and large, despite the caveats mentioned above, are more severe forms of synucleinopathies, are clearly relevant to iPD.

2.1.2 LRRK2

Missense mutations in the *LRRK2* (leucine-rich repeat kinase 2) gene, located within the PARK8 locus, were first reported independently by two groups in PD patients by positional cloning (Paisan-Ruiz et al., 2004; Zimprich et al., 2004). In both cases, mutations segregated with the disease in families with autosomal dominant inheritance. Since that time, additional rare coding variants of *LRRK2* have been identified, although only six are definitively considered pathogenic mutations. These are p. R1441G/C/H (Paisan-Ruiz et al., 2004; Zabetian et al., 2005; Zimprich et al., 2004), p.G2019S (Di Fonzo et al., 2005; Gilks et al., 2005; Hernandez et al., 2005), p.Y1699C (Paisan-Ruiz et al., 2004; Zimprich et al., 2004), and p.I2020T (Funayama et al., 2005; Zimprich et al., 2004). We have recently assessed in cellular systems the functional consequences of three LRRK2 variants, p.A211V, p.K544E, and p.T1410M, identified in Greek PD patients (Bozi et al., 2014; Xiromerisiou et al., 2007), and found that all three confer neurotoxicity through similar mechanisms with those of the established LRRK2 mutations, suggesting that they may be pathogenic (Melachroinou et al., 2016), although clearly additional genetic data are needed to support this. The p.G2019S substitution is by far the most common mutation, and, in a large worldwide study, accounted for an extraordinary 4% of familial cases and 1% of sporadic cases (Healy et al., 2008). Furthermore, familial and sporadic LRRK2-associated PD appear quite similar to classic iPD (see below). Thus, of the forms of genetic PD identified to date, LRRK2-associated PD appears to be the one that is phenotypically closer to iPD (Khan et al., 2005), and p.G2019S *LRRK2* is the most common single mutation linked to PD worldwide.

The LRRK2 gene encodes for a very large protein with multiple functional domains. Arguably the most important one contains a kinase domain, and LRRK2 kinase activity is closely linked to its neurotoxic potential, and may be a therapeutic target. Given the genetic data, a dominant gain of function conferred by the *LRRK2* mutations is assumed. Various functions have been attributed to LRRK2, but probably the most relevant ones relate to its role in vesicular trafficking, through phosphorylation of Rab GTPases, function which appears to be aberrantly activated by disease-associated mutants (Roosen & Cookson, 2016).

It has to be noted that the frequency of *LRRK2* mutations is very variable depending on the geographical region ascertained, as it is very dependent on ethnicity. For example, a very high proportion of familial and even sporadic cases with the p.G2019S mutation has been identified in Ashkenazi Jews and North African Arabs (Lesage et al., 2006; Ozelius et al., 2006), whereas the percentage is very low in familial PD in other regions, such as Greece (Bozi et al., 2014; Xiromerisiou et al., 2007) or the Far East (Tan et al., 2005). The origin of the G2019 mutation is likely a founder effect that occurred thousands of years ago in the Near East and/or North Africa, accounting for a common haplotype shared by most carriers of European, Jewish, and North African ancestry; independent founder effects may account for two other less common haplotypes (Lesage et al., 2010). In Asia, the major genetic determinant that links *LRRK2* to PD is the presence of two coding substitutions, G2385R and R1628P, acting as genetic risk factors, by each increasing by about twofold the risk of developing PD (Li et al., 2007; Ross et al., 2008). The link of LRRK2 to sporadic PD at the population level has been cemented through GWAS (Hernandez et al., 2016; Nalls et al., 2014).

The issue of penetrance of *LRRK2* mutations has been contentious. The fact that many carriers worldwide are identified as cases of sporadic PD, while the p.G2019S mutation in particular can be detected in up to 2% of controls in populations where p.G2019S is a common cause of familial PD (Healy et al., 2008; Lesage et al., 2006; Ozelius et al., 2006), suggests that penetrance is incomplete. For the p.G2019S mutation, lifetime penetrance estimates range widely, from about 25% to 80%, likely due to methodological issues (Healy et al., 2008; Lesage et al., 2006; Marder et al., 2015; Ozelius et al., 2006; Trinh et al., 2014). Some consider the presence of a *LRRK2* mutation more a risk factor than a genetic determinant; however, it is more useful to consider it as an autosomal dominant trait with reduced penetrance. It is interesting to consider whether genetic modifiers could influence disease manifestation and severity. A very recent study reported that genetic variability with the *DNM3* gene influences substantially the age of onset in p.G2019S carriers (Trinh et al., 2016).

The clinical phenotype in *LRRK2*-associated PD is, as mentioned, quite similar to iPD. In a very large international study, *LRRK2* mutation carriers manifested a more benign motor course and maintenance of cognitive abilities, as ascertained by the MMSE, compared to iPD (Healy et al., 2008). Motor complications however appeared to occur more readily in *LRRK2* mutation carriers. In further studies, the improved motor profile relative to iPD has not been always confirmed (Alcalay et al., 2013; Nabli et al., 2015), and it has been suggested that an akinetic-rigid phenotype and affectation of the lower limbs are more common among *LRRK2* mutation carriers (Alcalay et al., 2013). Testing of general cognitive abilities was similar between the two groups (Alcalay et al., 2013), but *LRRK2* mutation carriers had better performance on tests of attention, executive function, and language (Alcalay et al., 2015). A number of studies have shown that olfaction is impaired in LRRK2-associated PD, but this occurs less often that in iPD (Gaig et al., 2014; Healy et al., 2008; Ruiz-Martínez et al., 2011; Saunders-Pullman et al., 2014). Furthermore, RBD, based on questionnaires or polysomnography, appears to be uncommon (Ehrminger et al., 2015; Pont-Sunyer et al., 2015; Saunders-Pullman et al., 2015). Autonomic dysfunction, based on the scale assessments, appeared to be similar to iPD (Gaig et al., 2014), while MIBG scintigraphy showed slightly preserved heart noradrenergic innervation in *LRRK2* carriers (Ruiz-Martínez et al., 2011). Thus, the general impression is that *LRRK2* mutation carriers have a slightly more benign form of the disease, encompassing both motor and nonmotor features, without any apparent atypical aspects. However, there are scattered case reports of *LRRK2* mutation carriers presenting with atypical phenotypes, such as corticobasal degeneration, progressive aphasia, progressive supranuclear palsy (PSP), or choreoathetosis (Borroni et al., 2013; Chen-Plotkin et al., 2008; Spanaki, Latsoudis, & Plaitakis, 2006). Whether different LRRK2 mutations may have disparate clinical manifestations is just beginning to be assessed (Marras et al., 2016).

A puzzling aspect of LRRK2 cases is that, although a lot of evidence suggests a close pathogenetic link of the LRRK2 protein to α-synuclein, only a proportion of autopsy cases have demonstrated findings consistent with a synucleinopathy; other pathologies include pure nigral degeneration, tauopathy, or ubiquitin-positive inclusions. Thus, the only common denominator in such cases is nigrostriatal degeneration. The p.G2019S mutation appears to be more frequently associated with diffuse LB pathology, which correlated with clinical symptoms of dementia and orthostatic hypotension, suggesting more widespread clinical involvement (Kalia et al., 2015). The pleiotropic pathology suggests that LRRK2 mutations cause disease through mechanisms acting upstream of protein aggregation of various types.

2.1.3 GBA

It is now well established that the most common genetic substrate for PD are *GBA1* gene mutations. The *GBA1* gene encodes the lysosomal enzyme Glucocerebrosidase (GCase), which cleaves the sphingolipid glucosylceramide into glucose and ceramide. About 300 different GBA mutations have been found, many of them resulting in a significant loss of GCase activity (Montfort, Chabás, Vilageliu, & Grinberg, 2004). *GBA1* gene mutations in a homozygous or compound heterozygous state cause Gaucher's disease (GD), the most common lysosomal storage disease (Grabowski, 2008). The recognition of the relation between *GBA1* mutations and parkinsonism began with clinical observations of patients with GD who also developed parkinsonian symptoms (Goker-Alpan et al., 2008; Machaczka, Rucinska, Skotnicki, & Jurczak, 1999; Tayebi et al., 2001, 2003), consequently with studies concerning relatives of patients with GD who had an increased incidence of PD (Halperin, Elstein, & Zimran, 2006) and finally established in 2009 with a large, worldwide multicenter association study (Sidransky et al., 2009). There is a wide variation in the proportion of PD patients who harbor GBA mutations and in the odds ratio

(OR) for disease such mutations confer, ranging from close to 1 to up to 30, depending on the population studied (Sidransky et al., 2009). The mean OR is about 5–6. GBA-associated PD (GBA-PD) is especially frequent among Askenazi Jews (AJ), accounting for 15% of cases with PD (Sidransky et al., 2009). In a study we performed in a Greek sporadic PD population OR was between 3 and 4, and about 10% of patients were GBA-PD (Moraitou et al., 2011). GBA-PD are more likely to have a positive family history, but most patients with GBA-PD have sporadic disease, consistent with the reduced penetrance of *GBA1* mutations (Asselta et al., 2014; Neumann, Bras, Deas, et al., 2009; Winder-Rhodes et al., 2013).

The exact mechanism by which GBA1 mutations leads to PD is still unclear. Many theories have been developed, including the accumulation of α-synuclein, impaired lysosomal function and endoplasmic reticulum (ER)-associated stress. There is a debate whether a loss or gain of function is involved, although most findings suggest the former (Sardi, Cheng, & Shihabuddin, 2015; Xilouri, Brekk, & Stefanis, 2016). The association with α-synuclein appears particularly relevant, as autopsy studies have consistently detected widespread synucleinopathy in GBA-PD.

A number of studies have assessed motor and nonmotor features of GBA-PD and compared them to noncarriers with PD. GBA mutations predispose to a younger age of onset of PD which occurs about 1.7–6.0 years earlier than in noncarriers (Aharon-Peretz, Rosenbaum, & Gershoni-Baruch, 2004; Asselta et al., 2014; Clark, Ross, Wang, et al., 2007; Gan-Or, Giladi, Rozovski, et al., 2008; Moraitou et al., 2011; Sidransky et al., 2009; Tan, Tong, Fook-Chong, et al., 2007). This finding is further strengthened when looking at PD patients with early onset PD (EOPD) in whom GBA mutations were at least twice as common as compared to late onset cases (Moraitou et al., 2011; Nichols, Pankratz, Marek, et al., 2009). Regarding the nature and severity of motor symptoms in GBA-PD, there are contradictory findings. In the large multicenter analysis by Sidransky et al. (2009), the profile of symptoms of GBA-PD and noncarriers was similar in general, although mutation carriers were associated with a significantly lower frequency of asymmetric onset, bradykinesia, resting tremor, and rigidity, but not postural instability. Brockmann et al. (2015), on the other hand, performed a prospective 3-year longitudinal study with more detailed outcome measures, but in a single center setting, and found that PD-GBA carriers, albeit younger and with an earlier age at onset vs noncarriers, had more rapid progression of motor deficits, as assessed by UPDRS

III and H&Y staging, and higher mortality rates. They suggested that the worsened profile of GBA-PD occurred after the first few years of the disease, which then assumed an accelerated course. Wang et al. (2014) also found that PD-GBA carriers had worse motor function that noncarriers based on total UPDRS and UPDRS-II, while PD-GBA were found to have developed motor complications earlier in their disease course. However, this latter finding was not confirmed by other studies (Oeda et al., 2015).

Regarding cognition, Alcalay et al. (2012) showed that GBA-PD with early age of onset had a worse score at MMSE compared to age-matched noncarriers, and met criteria for dementia more often. Brockmann et al. (2015) showed, using the MOCA, that cognitive impairment was more frequent and severe in GBA-PD with a classical age of onset compared to age- and sex-matched controls; furthermore, longitudinal intragroup analyses showed a more rapid trajectory of cognitive impairment in GBA-PD. Therefore, in these studies, and despite the different ages assessed, the result was identical: cognitive function is worse in GBA-PD compared to noncarriers. This was confirmed in a large PD cohort, with a greater risk for dementia in GBA-PD compared to noncarriers (Cilia et al., 2016). In the large multicenter study of Sidransky et al. (2009), a greater proportion of cognitive changes in GBA-PD was also reported. GBA carriers may have a particularly pronounced impairment in visual memory tasks, and this selective defect may enable their identification (Zokaei et al., 2014).

Regarding psychiatric symptoms, Swan et al. found that GBA-PD had increased odds of depression and anxiety compared to PD noncarriers, and that this difference was more pronounced in men (Swan et al., 2016). Brockmann et al. (2011) reported that PD-GBA carriers had higher scores for depression, anxiety, and apathy, when compared to noncarriers. Oeda et al. (2015) showed that GBA-PD developed psychosis significantly earlier than those without mutations, and Neumann et al. (2009) that visual hallucinations were present in almost half of GBA-PD.

Regarding sleep abnormalities, GBA-PD patients are consistently reported to have a higher risk of RBD compared to iPD (Beavan et al., 2015; Gan-Or et al., 2015). As far as olfactory function is concerned, all studies, albeit with a small total number of patients, report significant olfactory deficits in GBA-PD, that are at least as prominent as in iPD, and may even be more pronounced, although this issue requires further study (Brockmann et al., 2011; Goker-Alpan et al., 2008; Saunders-Pullman et al., 2010). Regarding effects on the autonomic nervous system, Brockmann et al.

(2011) evaluated autonomic dysfunction using items 9–12 of the Unified Multiple System Atrophy Rating Scale and found that severity of distinct autonomic disturbances (orthostatic symptoms, urinary function, sexual function, and bowel function) was more prominent in GBA-PD vs iPD.

GD has three clinical types and accordingly GBA mutations are categorized as mild (those that cause GDI) and severe (those that cause GDII and III). Genotype–phenotype correlations have shown that severe mutations (e.g., L444P) are associated with an increased PD risk, earlier age at onset and greater cognitive dysfunction compared to mild mutations (e.g., N370S) (Gan-Or et al., 2015). In another study (Cilia et al., 2016), 67 mild vs 56 severe GBA mutations carriers were compared, and the carriers of severe mutations had greater risk for dementia compared to mild ones, but similar mortality risk. In a recent study, Arkadir et al. (2016), trying to overcome biases deriving from ethnic dependent differences in allele frequencies, examined and genotyped the parents of GD I patients who were compound heterozygotes for one mild and one severe GBA mutation, and who also reported PD in one of their parents. They found that 10/13 PD parents had a severe mutation and only 3/10 carried a mild mutation, result that was statistically significant. This study strengthens the notion of an increased PD risk in severe mutation carriers compared to mild ones, and, by inference, suggests that haploinsufficiency, i.e., partial loss of function, may be the responsible mechanism.

GBA1 mutations are also commonly found in DLB. Geiger et al. (2016) performed exome sequencing in 111 pathologically confirmed Caucasian DLB patients from North America, and found 13% with *GBA1* pathogenic mutations. This finding was confirmed in Ashkenazi Jewish DLB patients by Shiner et al. (2016), where one in three patients was a carrier of a *GBA1* mutation and had a more severe clinical syndrome compared to noncarriers.

Overall, GBA-PD appears to represent a more severe form of PD, especially regarding nonmotor features. As such, this clinical profile matches quite well that of genetic synucleinopathies and suggests common pathogenetic mechanisms. This notion is reinforced by similar neuropathological findings.

2.1.4 VPS35

Mutations in the gene encoding for the VPS35 protein represent another confirmed cause of monogenic PD, and are of special interest, as affected carriers manifest, in a similar fashion to LRRK2 carriers, rather typical

PD features, except for an earlier age of onset in some cases. In the first reports, the mutation p.D620N was identified by exome sequencing in large pedigrees of Austrian and Swiss origin with multiple affected members; the manner of inheritance is autosomal dominant, and penetrance appears high, but is likely incomplete. Mean age of onset appears to be around 50 (Struhal et al., 2014; Vilarino-Guell et al., 2011; Zimprich et al., 2011). In a more detailed clinical report, PD patients carriers of this mutation showed features typical of iPD: absence of atypical signs, excellent levodopa response, impaired olfaction in about half of the subjects, generally normal cognition, except for a minority of subjects with mild cognitive impairment, and scarce neuropsychiatric features (Struhal et al., 2014). Classic motor features and absence of prominent nonmotor features in seven manifesting carriers of the p.D620N mutation were also identified in a worldwide search for pathogenic VPS35 mutations (Sharma et al., 2012). Apart from some large pedigrees identified, this mutation appears to be very rare worldwide, although it can sometimes be identified in seemingly sporadic patients (Kumar et al., 2012). Pathogenicity for some other rare variants of the gene has not been confirmed. Overall, manifesting carriers of the p.D620N VPS35 mutation represent a relatively homogeneous picture with a rather benign disease course, although certainly more studies on affected cases are needed to cement this impression; this may prove difficult, due to the rarity of the mutation. Interestingly, in one of the cases from the Swiss family where a partial neuropathological assessment was performed, there was no widespread synucleinopathy present (Wider et al., 2008); even though the study only assessed parts of the cortex and basal ganglia, the apparent lack of diffuse synucleinopathy appears to match the relatively restricted disease manifestations. In terms of pathophysiology, mutations in VPS35 highlight the involvement of vesicular recycling in PD pathogenesis, as the VPS35 protein forms part of the retromer complex, involved in recycling of proteins from the endosomes to the trans-Golgi network, thus regulating their intracellular localization and stability (Mohan & Mellick, 2016).

2.2 Autosomal Recessive Forms

2.2.1 Parkin

Mutations in the gene encoding for Parkin are the most common identified genetic cause of EOPD (defined as PD with AAO below 40, or, in some cases, 50), and were first found to occur in Japanese patients with juvenile autosomal recessive PD (ARPD) (Kitada et al., 1998). Genetic changes are often copy number variants (CNVs), especially deletions, but can also be missense or nonsense mutations. It is clear that this condition represents a loss of function. Parkin is an E3 ligase, participating in the degradation of specific substrates through the ubiquitin-proteasome system (UPS). The critical function linked to PD is not certain, but the evidence suggests involvement of Parkin at the level of mitochondria, in the process of proper removal of damaged mitochondria through autophagy, termed mitophagy (van der Merwe, Jalali Sefid Dashti, Christoffels, Loos, & Bardien, 2015).

Mutations in *Parkin* are identified in about 40%–50% of cases with EOPD and AR inheritance, and in about 10%–20% of EOPD without family history. Distribution is worldwide, although frequencies may vary. Although most cases present with EOPD, some may present later in life as in iPD (Khan et al., 2003; Kubo, Hattori, & Mizuno, 2006). There is substantial phenotypic heterogeneity even within single families, especially regarding age at onset, and penetrance may be incomplete (Koentjoro, Park, Ha, & Sue, 2012). The clinical picture is characterized by a benign course with slow progression, excellent response to levodopa or anticholinergic medication, common presentation as dystonia, especially in the lower extremities, early involvement of gait and balance, and frequent emergence of dyskinesias and motor fluctuations. Sleep benefit is characteristic, and exercise-induced dystonia may occur, creating an issue of differential diagnosis with dopa-responsive dystonia (DRD) (Khan et al., 2003; Kubo et al., 2006). Psychiatric manifestations, including psychosis, depression, and panic attacks occur commonly, sometimes antedating motor symptoms. However, cognition is normal even after very long disease duration (Khan et al., 2003), and this has been confirmed in comparative studies with iPD (Alcalay et al., 2014). Interestingly, DAT-SPECT indicates that dopaminergic innervation to the caudate nucleus is affected to a greater extent than in iPD in Parkin mutation carriers (Khan et al., 2003). Occasional patients with *Parkin* mutations present with additional atypical features, such as pyramidal or cerebellar dysfunction, severe autonomic failure, or peripheral neuropathy (Khan et al., 2003).

Regarding other nonmotor features, Parkin-related PD is generally associated with a decreased incidence of nonmotor symptomatology, based on the NMS questionnaire, compared to iPD; only anxiety was more frequent in Parkin-related PD (Kägi et al., 2010). More specifically, studies present concrete evidence that olfaction is preserved in Parkin homozygous/compound heterozygotes (Alcalay et al., 2011; Khan et al., 2004; Malek et al., 2016). Although it had been reported that autonomic dysfunction, mostly in the form of urinary urgency, occurs often in Parkin-related PD (Khan et al., 2003), a more recent study which used a structured SCOPA-AUT questionnaire reported a very low burden of autonomic symptoms in Parkin-related PD compared to iPD. In the same study, MIBG scintigraphy revealed relative preservation of heart noradrenergic innervation in Parkin-related PD compared to iPD (Tijero et al., 2015), consistent with other studies (Orimo et al., 2005). RBD is encountered quite frequently in Parkin-related PD and this does not appear to be different from iPD (Kumru et al., 2004; Limousin et al., 2009). Interestingly, in one study restless legs syndrome was reported to occur more commonly in *Parkin* carriers than in iPD (Limousin et al., 2009).

A hotly debated issue is whether heterozygote Parkin mutations are linked to PD (Klein, Lohmann-Hedrich, Rogaeva, Schlossmacher, & Lang, 2007; Kubo et al., 2006; Lincoln et al., 2003; Valente & Ferraris, 2007). This is based on the fact of a seemingly autosomal dominant character of inheritance in occasional families, and in the slight increase (1.5–2.5-fold) of the prevalence of Parkin rare variants in most case control studies among PD patients relative to controls. Many factors could be at play: haploinsufficiency, a dominant gain of function or a dominant negative effect, the presence of additional unidentified mutations either within the Parkin gene (in trans), or within other genes, or the conference of enhanced risk that could be further modulated by other genetic/environmental factors. We have encountered a similar situation in our study in Greece, where we identified three Parkin heterozygote carriers with PD; two of the cases fit well within the spectrum of Parkin-related PD (Bozi et al., 2014). The link could be mutation dependent. In a recent study, Huttenlocher et al. (2015) reported a significant association with the disease only for heterozygote CNVs, and not for point mutation heterozygote carriers. The CNV effect was buttressed by a metaanalysis of published reports (Huttenlocher et al., 2015). The general picture that emerges is that affected heterozygotes manifest a clinical picture more compatible with iPD than with homozygous/compound heterozygote carriers, and therefore *Parkin* heterozygosity, especially at advanced ages, may be considered an incidental finding or, at best, a risk factor for the disease, especially if it involves CNVs. This may not apply to select individuals with very EOPD or to rare families with apparent autosomal dominant inheritance.

Pathology in classical Parkin-related PD reveals selective neuronal loss in substantia nigra and locus ceruleus, without LBs. However, select rare cases have been reported with LBs. This may relate to the lack of complete inactivation of Parkin, to the more advanced age of such subjects, and even to the presence of incidental LB disease (Doherty & Hardy, 2013; Doherty et al., 2013). In any case, the general picture that emerges is the lack of significant synuclein pathology and the restricted nature of neuronal loss, leading to the term "nigral cytopathy" (Ahlskog, 2009).

2.2.2 *PINK1*

After *Parkin*, *PINK1* mutations appear to represent the second most common cause of EOPD worldwide, accounting for 1%–5% of cases, although there is substantial variation depending on the ethnic background. Missense, nonsense, splice mutations, or small deletions or insertions are encountered, either in a compound heterozygote or homozygous state, and can be detected either in families with autosomal inheritance or, more frequently, in sporadic cases (Marongiu et al., 2008; Valente et al., 2004). It is clear that this represents a loss-of-function mitochondrial disease, as PINK1 is a kinase localized to the mitochondria. Its exact role remains uncertain, but it appears to be involved in the pathway of mitophagy, acting upstream of Parkin, while it may also have a role in the proper function of mitochondrial complex I (Voigt, Berlemann, & Winklhofer, 2016).

Regarding the patients' phenotype, Ishihara-Paul et al. (2008) reported on a large number of carriers of homozygote *PINK1* missense mutations in familial and nonfamilial cases in Tunisia. Such cases were quite frequent (15% in familial and 2.5% in nonfamilial cases) and differed from noncarriers, who were assessed in parallel, in a number of factors: the earlier age of onset (mean AAO < 40), the initial presentation, which was less frequently associated with tremor and more often with problems in gait and balance, the more frequent designation as akinetic-rigid syndrome on examination, and, most importantly, with a more benign clinical course. Cognition was not assessed, and dystonia as initial symptom was present only in a small minority of *PINK1* mutation carriers. Marongiu et al. (2008) provided a similarly comprehensive comparative report in Italian patients. They found that the 10 identified *PINK1* homozygote/compound heterozygote mutation carriers differed from other PD patients in earlier age of onset, more benign course, better response to levodopa therapy, more frequent gait trouble on examination and disease onset with lower limb problems, and enhanced dyskinesias. Notably, dementia was not present in any of the PINK1 patients, despite a mean disease duration of 18 years, and Parkin-like features such as dystonia or sleep benefits were not different from controls. This contrasts with other studies which have found that such features may be occasionally present in PINK1 patients, although no comparison with noncarriers was performed (Bonifati et al., 2005; Doostzadeh, Tetrud, Allen-Auerbach, Langston, & Schüle, 2007). Regarding other nonmotor features, it is interesting to note that patients with *PINK1* mutations manifest quite significant hyposmia (Doostzadeh et al., 2007; Eggers et al., 2010; Ferraris et al., 2009); some may also show autonomic dysfunction (Albanese et al., 2005; Quattrone et al., 2008), although the number of studied patients is small. RBD does not appear to occur, even in advanced cases (Tuin et al., 2008). Furthermore, quite a few affected subjects manifest psychiatric symptoms, such as anxiety, affective disorders, or psychosis that may even antedate motor symptoms (Marongiu et al., 2008; Samaranch et al., 2010; Steinlechner et al., 2007).

The issue of the relevance of heterozygote mutations in *PINK1* to PD is hotly debated, as in the case with *Parkin*, mentioned above; overall, it appears that heterozygote status confers only a very slight risk of developing PD (Abou-Sleiman et al., 2006; Klein et al., 2007; Marongiu et al., 2008; Valente & Ferraris, 2007). In a new twist, Puschmann et al. (2016) have recently reported that the p.G411S *PINK1* mutation is significantly more common in PD patients compared to controls, acts in families as an autosomal dominant trait, and confers a dominant negative function, impairing the kinase function of the wild-type allele. It appears therefore that this complex issue may relate to the particular *PINK1* mutation.

The only neuropathological study in a PINK1 PD patient was performed in a 39-year old with typical features of PINK1-related PD, which included psychiatric manifestations (Samaranch et al., 2010). The subject carried a c.1488 + 1G > A splicing mutation and exon 7 deletion. Somewhat surprisingly, neurodegeneration was restricted exclusively to the substantia nigra and did not involve the locus ceruleus or other brain regions. Importantly, a restricted pattern of synucleinopathy was observed, that only involved to a relatively small extent the substantia nigra, other brainstem areas and the nucleus basalis of Myenert. Thus, this case appears distinct neuropathologically both from iPD- and Parkin-associated PD.

2.2.3 *DJ-1*

A rare autosomal recessive form of EOPD is due to mutations in the *DJ-1* gene, encoding for a protein which has a role in the antioxidant response, and may participate in common biochemical pathways with PINK-1 and Parkin (Bonifati et al., 2003; van der Merwe et al., 2015). A homozygous deletion spanning a large extent of the gene was first identified in a genetic isolate from the Netherlands, while a homozygous point mutation, p.L166P, was identified in an Italian kindred (Bonifati et al., 2003). Additional mutations, either small deletions or missense mutations, in a compound heterozygous or homozygous form, have been identified in further studies, but they are exceedingly rare, even among subjects with EOPD, comprising about 1% of such cases. Although not thoroughly assessed, the phenotype resembles quite closely that usually seen in Parkin-related PD: absence of atypical features, early age of onset, very good response to dopaminergic treatment, slow progression, frequent occurrence of focal dystonia, prominent motor complications upon treatment, and psychiatric symptoms, especially anxiety, frequently antedating motor symptoms; due to the rarity of *DJ-1* mutations, whether other nonmotor symptoms are present in mutation carriers has not been systematically assessed (Abou-Sleiman, Healy, Quinn, Lees, & Wood, 2003; Bonifati et al., 2002; Dekker et al., 2003; Macedo et al., 2009; van Duijn et al., 2001). This homogeneous picture is based on very few reports worldwide and is counterbalanced by certain cases where the clinical picture is drastically different: Annesi et al. (2005) reported on three brothers from an Italian family with a homozygous point mutation in *DJ-1* (p.E163K), affected with a very severe form of Parkinsonism-dementia-motor neuron disease, while a more recent report described a Portuguese patient with a homozygous p.L172Q mutation who developed Parkinsonism at age 22, that was poorly responsive to levodopa; moreover, his picture was complicated, apart from dystonia, by prominent bulbar signs, and the late appearance of pyramidal tract signs and dementia (Taipa et al., 2016). Interestingly enough, this is the only reported DJ-1 case for whom neuropathological data are available, showing, apart from the expected severe affectation of the substantia nigra and locus coeruleus, widespread synucleinopathy reminiscent of that seen in sporadic PD; there were however some atypical features, such as preservation of the dorsal motor nucleus of the vagus, moderate affectation of the basal ganglia, and the presence of α-synuclein-immunoreactive axonal spheroids. Generalization of these neuropathological findings to other cases with *DJ-1* mutations should be interpreted with caution, given the divergent clinical picture in this case. Clearly, autopsy studies in cases with a more classical clinical picture of DJ-1-associated PD are sorely needed.

2.2.4 *VPS13C*

A very recent discovery provides another interesting piece in the puzzle of ARPD manifesting as a synucleinopathy. Lesage et al. (2016) searched a population of EOPD patients with consanguinity with next-generation sequencing (NGS) in order to identify novel genetic variants linked to the disease; they identified a total of three unrelated subjects with point mutations in the gene encoding for VPS13C. Common features in all three subjects were the rapid progression of the motor phenotype and the emergence of severe cognitive dysfunction; two out of three subjects also had dystonia and pyramidal tract features. Interestingly, neuropathology in one subject showed diffuse deposition of α-synuclein, accounting for the quite severe cognitive phenotype. Of note, *VPS13C* had previously been linked to PD through a metaanalysis of GWAS data, suggesting that it may play a role in iPD as well (Hernandez et al., 2016; Nalls et al., 2014). Although the reported cases are very few, it does appear that this loss-of-function condition leads to a clinical and neuropathological picture more like a diffuse synucleinopathy and, in this respect, resembles more genetic synucleinopathies linked to SNCA mutations. Interestingly, in cellular studies that were performed, VPS13C appeared to oppose the function of Parkin/Pink-1 on mitophagy, suggesting that either excess or inadequate mitophagy may be deleterious.

3. MONOGENIC FORMS WITH ADDITIONAL CLINICAL FEATURES

A group of genetic disorders with autosomal recessive inheritance manifest as a main feature a pallido-pyramidal syndrome, a combination of pyramidal tract dysfunction and parkinsonism, suboptimally responsive to levodopa, with disease onset in childhood. These cases are often accompanied by mental retardation or dementia, dystonia, impaired saccadic eye movements, and other atypical signs. There are sometimes signs of brain iron accumulation on imaging (Lai, Lin, & Wu, 2012; Paisán-Ruiz et al., 2010; Schneider et al., 2010). Prototypical among these disorders is the Kufor–Rakeb syndrome, which is characterized, in addition to the above, by frank supranuclear gaze palsy and myoclonus (Lai et al., 2012; Najim al-Din, Wriekat, Mubaidin, Dasouki, & Hiari, 1994). This syndrome is due to homozygous or compound heterozygote mutations in the *ATP13A2* gene, which encodes for a lysosomal P-type ATPase (Ramirez et al., 2006; Santoro et al., 2011). Homozygous or compound heterozygous mutations in the gene PLA2G6, encoding for a phospholipase A2, likely involved in cell and mitochondrial membrane stability, can cause a pallido-pyramidal syndrome, but also, when manifesting very early in life, neuroaxonal dystrophy, or, somewhat later in life, a phenotype of neurodegeneration with brain iron accumulation (NBIA) (Khateeb et al., 2006; Morgan et al., 2006; Paisan-Ruiz et al., 2009; Yoshino et al., 2010). Interestingly, such patients on autopsy demonstrate widespread synucleinopathy and occasionally Tau deposits (Paisán-Ruiz et al., 2012). Homozygous or compound heterozygote mutations in the gene *FBXO7*, encoding for an adaptor protein involved in substrate degradation through the UPS, and likely participating together with Parkin in mitophagy (Zhao et al., 2011; Zhou, Sathiyamoorthy, Angeles, & Tan, 2016), can also lead to a pallido-pyramidal syndrome (Di Fonzo et al., 2009; Shojaee et al., 2008). Although mutations in these three genes, when manifesting in childhood, usually cause a pallido-pyramidal syndrome, when manifesting later in life, can be more benign and reminiscent of more classical EOPD; this may be especially true for *FBXO7* (Malakouti-Nejad et al., 2014; Paisán-Ruiz et al., 2010; Shi et al., 2011).

Mutations in two additional genes can cause, when transmitted in an autosomal recessive fashion, a picture similar to the complicated phenotype of the pallido-pyramidal syndrome. A homozygous p.R258Q mutation was identified in the gene *SYNJ1*, encoding for Synaptojanin 1, which has a role in postendocytic recycling of synaptic vesicles, in a few cases with severe EOPD. Bulbar signs and postural instability were prominent, as well as a relative lack of response to levodopa, whose use however was limited by severe motor complications (Krebs et al., 2013; Quadri et al., 2013). RBD and autonomic dysfunction do not appear to be part of the clinical picture in these cases (De Rosa et al., 2016). Homozygous mutations in *DNAJC6*, encoding for auxilin, involved in calthrin-mediated endocytosis, were associated with a spectrum of phenotypes ranging from the typical pallido-pyramidal syndrome to more restricted juvenile Parkinsonism (Edvardson et al., 2012; Koroglu, Baysal, Cetinkaya, Karasoy, & Tolun, 2013). As is the case for the first three genes, it appears that *DNAJ6* mutations may manifest as more typical EOPD, perhaps because the involved mutations do not lead to a total loss of auxilin (Olgiati et al., 2016). Along these lines, there is a suggestion that identified mutations in the genes involved in the pallido-pyramidal syndrome, when present in a heterozygote state, may lead to EOPD through haploinsufficiency (Di Fonzo et al., 2007).

Overall, these genetic defects cause a complicated juvenile PD, but may enter in the differential diagnosis of EOPD. The identified genes are implicated in processes such as vesicle trafficking and mitochondrial and lysosomal functions that are also relevant to the monogenic defects associated with adult onset PD.

4. INVOLVEMENT OF GENES LINKED TO THE DOPAMINE BIOSYNTHESIS PATHWAY

Given the importance of dopamine in PD, it is appropriate to consider separately the role of genetic defects in the dopamine biosynthesis pathway. DRD manifests at a young age, is often accompanied by Parkinsonism and is almost always due to autosomal dominant mutations in the *GCH1* gene, encoding for GTP cyclohydrolase 1, a cofactor for dopamine biosynthesis; mutations in other components of the dopamine biosynthetic pathway, such as in the *TH* (tyrosine hydroxylase) gene can also occur. It has long been known that the DRD phenotype may overlap with that of EOPD, especially Parkin-related PD. More recently, it has been appreciated that within certain DRD families there are individuals with a typical PD phenotype; in fact, these individuals, who, in contrast to their DRD relatives, have an abnormal DAT scan, are invariably also carriers of *GCH1* mutations, suggesting that PD is due to this genetic defect (Mencacci et al., 2014); furthermore, a large association study showed that rare variants within the *GCH1* gene are more common in iPD compared to controls (Mencacci et al., 2014), while *GCH1* has also emerged as a PD-related gene on GWAS (Nalls et al., 2014). Further families with cooccurrence of DRD and PD cases due to *GCH1* mutations have been identified (Lewthwaite et al., 2015), although in sporadic PD populations *GCH1* mutations are very rare (Rengmark, Pihlstrøm, Linder, Forsgren, & Toft, 2016). In a population of Greek subjects with high probability for a genetic factor underlying the disease, we failed to identify in a heterozygous state a founder mutation in the *TH* gene, which, in a homozygous state, leads to a severe TH deficiency syndrome, again suggesting that at a population level the effects of mutations in the dopamine biosynthesis pathway are likely to be small (Pons et al., 2016).

5. GWAS AND LOWLY SIMPLE CASE CONTROL ASSOCIATION STUDIES

As mentioned in Section 1, this review does not aim to provide the reader with a list of susceptibility loci linked to the disease. This can be found in more detail elsewhere (e.g., Nalls et al., 2014; review by Hernandez et al., 2016). It should however be noted that large GWAS and further analyses based on these data have cemented the idea of a substantial genetic contribution to sporadic PD. Multiple susceptibility loci for sporadic PD have been identified, and many of them have been confirmed in independent studies, although, in other cases, they seem to be population specific. Links of *SNCA*, *GBA*, *VPS13C*, *GCH1*, and *LRRK2* to sporadic disease through GWAS have already been mentioned earlier.

From the point of view of the magnitude of the effect and the pathogenic pathways involved, loci linked to *MTAP* (Tau) and the HLA complex appear the most relevant, although how they could be linked to PD pathogenesis remains unclear. An additional GWAS hit that is of interest, due to its relation to GCase, is the *SCARB2* gene, encoding for the protein LIMP2, which acts as a GCase transporter. Interestingly, we had previously identified disease-associated haplotypes within *SCARB2* as part of an association study performed in the Greek population (Michelakakis et al., 2012), suggesting that even in the GWAS era targeted association studies may provide useful and valid information. This point is obviously relevant to the case of *GBA* as well.

6. CONCLUSION

This review has highlighted genetic defects linked to PD, and in particular focused on the phenotypes conferred by monogenic forms of the disease. For the forms where a sufficient amount of information is available, a broad genotype–phenotype correlation can be established (see Table 1). The comparative analysis in the table serves to demonstrate certain interesting points, for example phenotypes of Parkin and PINK1 mutation carriers have certain differences. Noted within this review however is the issue of marked phenotypic variability even within families with the same genetic defect. Such variability may take the form of lack of disease manifestation in obligate carriers, atypical presentations with additional features, extreme variations in age of onset or disease severity. It will be important in such cases to perform a complete panel of genetic testing to exclude additional genetic defects in PD-causing genes, and in genes leading to other neurodegenerative conditions. This will be most easily achieved through NGS. A challenge for the future will be to identify, at least for the most common forms, additional genetic modifying factors that influence phenotypes. In this regard, the study of Trinh et al. (2016), which has identified genetic variations within the DNM3 gene to be associated with age of onset of p.G2019S LRRK2 mutation carriers, the most common worldwide genetic defect linked to PD, represents an important step.

Table 1 Genotype–Phenotype Correlations for Genetic Defects Linked to PD for Whom Sufficient Numbers of Cases Are Available

	Penetrance	Mean Age at Onset	Severity (Relative to iPD)	L-Dopa Response (Relative to iPD)	Motor Complications (Relative to iPD)	Dementia	Autonomic Dysfunction	RBD	Hyposmia	Psychiatric	Additional Features	Atypical Features
p.A53T SNCA	80%–90%	46	↑	↔	↔	++	++	+	++	+		FTD; DLB
SNCA duplication	40%–50%	50	↔	↔	↔	+	+	+	+	+		FTD
SNCA triplication	100%	40	↑	↔	↔	+++	++	+	+	++ (depression)	Severe Weight loss	
LRRK2	25%–80% (likely closer to the former)	50s	Slightly ↓	↔	↔	±	+	±	±	±		Clinical tauopathy
GBA	OR of 5–6	40s–early 50s	↑	↔	↔	+/++	++	++	++	+	DLB	
Parkin	Nearly complete	JPD or EOPD	↓	↑	↑	–	±	+ (late)	–	++ (can be early)	Dystonia at onset; sleep benefit legs/gait affected early	PPS
PINK1	Nearly complete	EOPD	↓	↑	↑	–	–	–	+	++ (can be early)	Legs/gait affected early	JPD; cognitive deterioration

OR: Odds ratio; *JPD*: juvenile PD (age at onset < 20); *EOPD*: early onset PD (age at onset 20–40 or 50); *FTD*: frontotemporal dementia phenotype; *PPS*: pallido-pyramidal syndrome; *LB*: dementia with Lewy bodies; *RBD*: REM sleep behavior disorder.

REFERENCES

Abou-Sleiman, P. M., Healy, D. G., Quinn, N., Lees, A. J., & Wood, N. W. (2003). The role of pathogenic DJ-1 mutations in Parkinson's disease. *Annals of Neurology*, *54*, 283–286.

Abou-Sleiman, P. M., Muqit, M. M., McDonald, N. Q., Yang, Y. X., Gandhi, S., Healy, D. G., et al. (2006). A heterozygous effect for PINK1 mutations in Parkinson's disease? *Annals of Neurology*, *60*, 414–419.

Aharon-Peretz, J., Rosenbaum, H., & Gershoni-Baruch, R. (2004). Mutations in the glucocerebrosidase gene and Parkinson's disease in Ashkenazi Jews. *New England Journal of Medicine*, *351*, 1972–1977.

Ahlskog, J. E. (2009). Parkin and PINK1 parkinsonism may represent nigral mitochondrial cytopathies distinct from Lewy body Parkinson's disease. *Parkinsonism & Related Disorders*, *15*, 721–727.

Albanese, A., Valente, E. M., Romito, L. M., Bellacchio, E., Elia, A. E., & Dallapiccola, B. (2005). The PINK1 phenotype can be indistinguishable from idiopathic Parkinson disease. *Neurology*, *64*, 1958–1960.

Alcalay, R. N., Caccappolo, E., Mejia-Santana, H., Tang, M., Rosado, L., Orbe Reilly, M., et al. (2012). Cognitive performance of GBA mutation carriers with early-onset PD: The CORE-PD study. *Neurology*, *78*, 1434–1440.

Alcalay, R. N., Caccappolo, E., Mejia-Santana, H., Tang, M. X., Rosado, L., Orbe Reilly, M., et al. (2014). Cognitive and motor function in long-duration PARKIN-associated Parkinson disease. *JAMA Neurology*, *71*, 62–67.

Alcalay, R. N., Mejia-Santana, H., Mirelman, A., Saunders-Pullman, R., Raymond, D., Palmese, C., et al. (2015). Neuropsychological performance in LRRK2 G2019S carriers with Parkinson's disease. *Parkinsonism & Related Disorders*, *21*, 106–110.

Alcalay, R. N., Mirelman, A., Saunders-Pullman, R., Tang, M. X., Mejia Santana, H., Raymond, D., et al. (2013). Parkinson disease phenotype in Ashkenazi Jews with and without LRRK2 G2019S mutations. *Movement Disorders*, *28*, 1966–1971.

Alcalay, R. N., Siderowf, A., Ottman, R., Caccappolo, E., Mejia-Santana, H., Tang, M. X., et al. (2011). Olfaction in Parkin heterozygotes and compound heterozygotes: The CORE-PD study. *Neurology*, *76*, 319–326.

Annesi, G., Savettieri, G., Pugliese, P., D'Amelio, M., Tarantino, P., Ragonese, P., La Bella, V., et al. (2005). DJ-1 mutations and parkinsonism-dementia-amyotrophic lateral sclerosis complex. *Annals of Neurology*, *58*, 803–807.

Appel-Cresswell, S., Vilarino-Guell, C., Encarnacion, M., Sherman, H., Yu, I., Shah, B., et al. (2013). Alpha-synuclein p.H50Q, a novel pathogenic mutation for Parkinson's disease. *Movement Disorders*, *28*, 811–813.

Arkadir, D., Dinur, T., Mullin, S., Mehta, A., Baris, H. N., Alcalay, R. N., et al. (2016). Trio approach reveals higher risk of PD in carriers of severe vs. mild GBA mutations. *Blood Cells Molecular Disease*, 30272–30278. pii: S1079-9796 (e-pub ahead of print).

Asselta, R., Rimoldi, V., Siri, C., Cilia, R., Guella, I., Tesei, S., et al. (2014). Glucocerebrosidase mutations in primary parkinsonism. *Parkinsonism & Related Disorders*, *20*, 1215–1220.

Beavan, M., McNeill, A., Proukakis, C., Hughes, D. A., Mehta, A., & Schapira, A. H. (2015). Evolution of prodromal clinical markers of Parkinson disease in a GBA mutation-positive cohort. *JAMA Neurology*, *72*, 201–208.

Berg, D., Niwar, M., Maass, S., Zimprich, A., Möller, J. C., Wuellner, U., et al. (2005). Alpha-synuclein and Parkinson's disease: Implications from the screening of more than 1,900 patients. *Movement Disorders*, *20*, 1191–1194.

Bonifati, V., Breedveld, G. J., Squitieri, F., Vanacore, N., Brustenghi, P., Harhangi, B. S., et al. (2002). Localization of autosomal recessive early-onset parkinsonism to chromosome 1p36 (PARK7) in an independent dataset. *Annals of Neurology*, *51*, 253–256.

Bonifati, V., Rizzu, P., van Baren, M. J., Schaap, O., Breedveld, G. J., Krieger, E., et al. (2003). Mutations in the DJ-1 gene associated with autosomal recessive early-onset parkinsonism. *Science, 299*, 256–259.

Bonifati, V., Rohé, C. F., Breedveld, G. J., Fabrizio, E., De Mari, M., Tassorelli, C., et al. (2005). Early-onset parkinsonism associated with PINK1 mutations: Frequency, genotypes, and phenotypes. *Neurology, 65*, 87–95.

Borroni, B., Cotelli, M. S., Marchina, E., Filosto, M., Premi, E., & Padovani, A. (2013). Choreo-athetosis in LRRK2 R1441C mutation: Expanding the clinical phenotype. *Clinical Neurology Neurosurgery, 115*, 2217–2218.

Bostantjopoulou, S., Katsarou, Z., Gerasimou, G., Costa, D. C., & Gotzamani-Psarrakou, A. (2008). (123)I-FP-CIT SPET striatal uptake in parkinsonian patients with the alpha-synuclein (G209A) mutation A. *Hellenic Journal of Nuclear Medicine, 11*, 157–159.

Bostantjopoulou, S., Katsarou, Z., Papadimitriou, A., Veletza, V., Hatzigeorgiou, G., & Lees, A. (2001). Clinical features of parkinsonian patients with the alpha-synuclein (G209A) mutation. *Movement Disorders, 16*, 1007–1013.

Bougea, A., Koros, C., Stamelou, M., Simitsi, A., Papagiannakis, N., Antonelou, R., et al. (2016). Frontotemporal dementia as the presenting phenotype of p.A53T mutation carriers in the alpha-synuclein gene. *Parkinsonism & Related Disorders, 35*, 82–87. http://dx.doi.org/10.1016/j.parkreldis.2016.12.002. pii: S1353-8020(16)30470-9.

Bozi, M., Papadimitriou, D., Antonellou, R., Moraitou, M., Maniati, M., Vassilatis, D. K., et al. (2014). Genetic assessment of familial and early-onset Parkinson's disease in a Greek population. *European Journal of Neurology, 21*, 963–968.

Brockmann, K., Srulijes, K., Hauser, A. K., Schulte, C., Csoti, I., Gasser, T., et al. (2011). GBA-associated PD presents with nonmotor characteristics. *Neurology, 77*, 276–280.

Brockmann, K., Srulijes, K., Pflederer, S., Hauser, A. K., Schulte, C., Maetzler, W., et al. (2015). GBA-associated Parkinson's disease: Reduced survival and more rapid progression in a prospective longitudinal study. *Movement Disorders, 30*, 407–411.

Chartier-Harlin, M. C., Kachergus, J., Roumier, C., Mouroux, V., Douay, X., Lincoln, S., et al. (2004). Alpha-synuclein locus duplication as a cause of familial Parkinson's disease. *Lancet, 364*, 1167–1169.

Chen-Plotkin, A. S., Yuan, W., Anderson, C., McCarty Wood, E., Hurtig, H. I., Clark, C. M., et al. (2008). Corticobasal syndrome and primary progressive aphasia as manifestations of LRRK2 gene mutations. *Neurology, 70*, 521–527.

Choi, J. M., Woo, M. S., Ma, H. I., Kang, S. Y., Sung, Y. H., Yong, S. W., et al. (2008). Analysis of PARK genes in a Korean cohort of early-onset Parkinson disease. *Neurogenetics, 9*, 263–269.

Cilia, R., Tunesi, S., Marotta, G., Cereda, E., Siri, C., Tesei, S., et al. (2016). Survival and dementia in GBA-associated Parkinson's disease: The mutation matters. *Annals of Neurology, 80*, 662–673.

Clark, L. N., Ross, B. M., Wang, Y., et al. (2007). Mutations in the glucocerebrosidase gene are associated with early-onset Parkinson disease. *Neurology, 69*, 1270–1277.

De Rosa, A., Pellegrino, T., Pappatà, S., Lieto, M., Bonifati, V., Palma, V., et al. (2016). Non-motor symptoms and cardiac innervation in SYNJ1-related parkinsonism. *Parkinsonism & Related Disorders, 23*, 102–105.

Dekker, M., Bonifati, V., van Swieten, J., Leenders, N., Galjaard, R. J., Snijders, P., et al. (2003). Clinical features and neuroimaging of PARK7-linked parkinsonism. *Movement Disorders, 18*, 751–757.

Di Fonzo, A., Chien, H. F., Socal, M., Giraudo, S., Tassorelli, C., Iliceto, G., et al. (2007). ATP13A2 missense mutations in juvenile parkinsonism and young onset Parkinson disease. *Neurology, 68*, 1557–1562.

Di Fonzo, A., Dekker, M. C., Montagna, P., Baruzzi, A., Yonova, E. H., Correia Guedes, L., et al. (2009). FBXO7 mutations cause autosomal recessive, early-onset parkinsonian-pyramidal syndrome. *Neurology, 72*, 240–245.

Di Fonzo, A., Rohe, C. F., Ferreira, J., Chien, H. F., Vacca, L., Stocchi, F., et al. (2005). A frequent LRRK2 gene mutation associated with autosomal dominant Parkinson's disease. *Lancet, 365*, 412–415.

Doherty, K. M., & Hardy, J. (2013). Parkin disease and the Lewy body conundrum. *Movement Disorders, 28*, 702–704.

Doherty, K. M., Silveira-Moriyama, L., Parkkinen, L., Healy, D. G., Farrell, M., Mencacci, N. E., et al. (2013). Parkin disease: A clinicopathologic entity? *JAMA Neurology, 70*, 571–579.

Doostzadeh, J., Tetrud, J. W., Allen-Auerbach, M., Langston, J. W., & Schüle, B. (2007). Novel features in a patient homozygous for the L347P mutation in the PINK1 gene. *Parkinsonism & Related Disorders, 13*, 359–361.

Duda, J. E., Giasson, B. I., Mabon, M. E., Miller, D. C., Golbe, L. I., Lee, V. M., et al. (2002). Concurrence of alpha-synuclein and tau brain pathology in the Contursi kindred. *Acta Neuropathologica, 104*, 7–11.

Edvardson, S., Cinnamon, Y., Ta-Shma, A., Shaag, A., Yim, Y. I., & Zenvirt, S. (2012). A deleterious mutation in DNAJC6 encoding the neuronal-specific clathrinuncoating co-chaperone auxilin, is associated with juvenile parkinsonism. *PLoS One, 7*, e36458.

Eggers, C., Schmidt, A., Hagenah, J., Brüggemann, N., Klein, J. C., Tadic, V., et al. (2010). Progression of subtle motor signs in PINK1 mutation carriers with mild dopaminergic deficit. *Neurology, 74*, 1798–1805.

Ehrminger, M., Leu-Semenescu, S., Cormier, F., Corvol, J. C., Vidailhet, M., Debellemaniere, E., et al. (2015). Sleep aspects on video-polysomnography in LRRK2 mutation carriers. *Movement Disorders, 30*, 1839–1843.

Ferese, R., Modugno, N., Campopiano, R., Santilli, M., Zampatti, S., Giardina, E., et al. (2015). Four copies of SNCA responsible for autosomal dominant Parkinson's disease in Two Italian siblings. *Parkinson's Disease, 2015*, 546462.

Ferraris, A., Ialongo, T., Passali, G. C., Pellecchia, M. T., Brusa, L., Laruffa, M., et al. (2009). Olfactory dysfunction in Parkinsonism caused by PINK1 mutations. *Movement Disorders, 24*, 2350–2357.

Fuchs, J., Nilsson, C., Kachergus, J., Munz, M., Larsson, E. M., Schüle, B., et al. (2007). Phenotypic variation in a large Swedish pedigree due to SNCA duplication and triplication. *Neurology, 68*, 916–922.

Funayama, M., Hasegawa, K., Ohta, E., Kawashima, N., Komiyama, M., Kowa, H., et al. (2005). An LRRK2 mutation as a cause for the parkinsonism in the original PARK8 family. *Annals of Neurology, 57*, 918–921.

Gaig, C., Vilas, D., Infante, J., Sierra, M., García-Gorostiaga, I., Buongiorno, M., et al. (2014). Nonmotor symptoms in LRRK2 G2019S associated Parkinson's disease. *PLoS One, 9*, e108982

Gan-Or, Z., Amshalom, I., Kilarski, L. L., Bar-Shira, A., Gana-Weisz, M., Mirelman, A., et al. (2015). Differential effects of severe vs mild GBA mutations on Parkinson disease. *Neurology, 84*, 880–887.

Gan-Or, Z., Giladi, N., Rozovski, U., et al. (2008). Genotype–phenotype correlations between GBA mutations and Parkinson disease risk and onset. *Neurology, 70*, 2277–2283.

Gan-Or, Z., Mirelman, A., Postuma, R. B., Arnulf, I., Bar-Shira, A., Dauvilliers, Y., et al. (2015). GBA mutations are associated with rapid Eye movement sleep behavior disorder. *Annals of Clinical Translational Neurology, 2*, 941–945.

Geiger, J. T., Ding, J., Crain, B., Pletnikova, O., Letson, C., Dawson, T. M., et al. (2016). Next-generation sequencing reveals substantial genetic contribution to dementia with Lewy bodies. *Neurobiology of Disease, 94*, 55–62.

Gilks, W. P., Abou-Sleiman, P. M., Gandhi, S., Jain, S., Singleton, A., Lees, A. J., et al. (2005). A common LRRK2 mutation in idiopathic Parkinson's disease. *Lancet, 365*, 415–416.

Goker-Alpan, O., Lopez, G., Vithayathil, J., Davis, J., Hallett, M., & Sidransky, E. (2008). The spectrum of parkinsonian manifestations associated with glucocerebrosidase mutations. *Archives of Neurology, 65*, 1353–1357.

Golbe, L. I., Di Iorio, G., Sanges, G., Lazzarini, A. M., La Sala, S., Bonavita, V., et al. (1996). Clinical genetic analysis of Parkinson's disease in the Contursi kindred. *Annals of Neurology, 40*, 767–775.

Grabowski, G. A. (2008). Phenotype, diagnosis and treatment of Gaucher's disease. *Lancet, 372*, 1263–1271.

Gwinn, K., Devine, M. J., Jin, L. W., Johnson, J., Bird, T., Muenter, M., et al. (2011). Clinical features, with video documentation, of the original familial Lewy body parkinsonism caused by α-synuclein triplication (Iowa kindred). *Movement Disorders, 26*, 2134–2136.

Halperin, A., Elstein, D., & Zimran, A. (2006). Increased incidence of Parkinson disease among relatives of patients with Gaucher disease. *Blood Cells Molecular Disease, 36*, 426–428.

Healy, D. G., Falchi, M., O'Sullivan, S. S., Bonifati, V., Durr, A., Bressman, S., et al. (2008). Phenotype, genotype, and worldwide genetic penetrance of LRRK2-associated Parkinson's disease: A case–control study. *Lancet Neurology, 7*, 583–590.

Hernandez, D. G., Paisan-Ruiz, C., McInerney-Leo, A., Jain, S., Meyer-Lindenberg, A., Evans, E. W., et al. (2005). Clinical and positron emission tomography of Parkinson's disease caused by LRRK2. *Annals of Neurology, 57*, 453–456.

Hernandez, D. G., Reed, X., & Singleton, A. B. (2016). Genetics in Parkinson disease: Mendelian versus non-mendelian inheritance. *Journal of Neurochemistry, 139*(Suppl. 1), 59–74.

Huttenlocher, J., Stefansson, H., Steinberg, S., Helgadottir, H. T., Sveinbjörnsdóttir, S., Riess, O., et al. (2015). Heterozygote carriers for CNVs in PARK2 are at increased risk of Parkinson's disease. *Human Molecular Genetics, 24*, 5637–5643.

Ibáñez, P., Bonnet, A. M., Débarges, B., Lohmann, E., Tison, F., Pollak, P., et al. (2004). Causal relation between alpha-synuclein gene duplication and familial Parkinson's disease. *Lancet, 364*, 1169–1171.

Ishihara-Paul, L., Hulihan, M. M., Kachergus, J., Upmanyu, R., Warren, L., Amouri, R., et al. (2008). PINK1 mutations and parkinsonism. *Neurology, 71*, 896–902.

Itokawa, K., Sekine, T., Funayama, M., Tomiyama, H., Fukui, M., Yamamoto, T., et al. (2013). A case of α-synuclein gene duplication presenting with head-shaking movements. *Movement Disorders, 28*, 384–387.

Kägi, G., Klein, C., Wood, N. W., Schneider, S. A., Pramstaller, P. P., Tadic, V., et al. (2010). Nonmotor symptoms in Parkin gene-related parkinsonism. *Movement Disorders, 25*, 1279–1284.

Kalia, L. V., Lang, A. E., Hazrati, L. N., Fujioka, S., Wszolek, Z. K., Dickson, D. W., et al. (2015). Clinical correlations with Lewy body pathology in LRRK2-related Parkinson disease. *JAMA Neurology, 72*, 100–105.

Kalinderi, K., Bostantjopoulou, S., & Fidani, L. (2016). The genetic background of Parkinson's disease: Current progress and future prospects. *Acta Neurologica Scandinavica, 134*, 314–326.

Kara, E., Kiely, A. P., Proukakis, C., Giffin, N., Love, S., Hehir, J., et al. (2014). A 6.4 Mb duplication of the α-synuclein locus causing frontotemporal dementia and Parkinsonism: Phenotype–genotype correlations. *JAMA Neurology, 71*, 1162–1171.

Kasten, M., & Klein, C. (2013). The many faces of alpha-synuclein mutations. *Movement Disorders, 28*, 697–701.

Khan, N. L., Graham, E., Critchley, P., Schrag, A. E., Wood, N. W., Lees, A. J., et al. (2003). Parkin disease: A phenotypic study of a large case series. *Brain, 126*, 1279–1292.

Khan, N. L., Jain, S., Lynch, J. M., Pavese, N., Abou-Sleiman, P., Holton, J. L., et al. (2005). Mutations in the gene LRRK2 encoding dardarin (PARK8) cause familial Parkinson's disease: Clinical, pathological, olfactory and functional imaging and genetic data. *Brain, 128*, 2786–2796.

Khan, N. L., Katzenschlager, R., Watt, H., Bhatia, K. P., Wood, N. W., Quinn, N., et al. (2004). Olfaction differentiates parkin disease from early-onset parkinsonism and Parkinson disease. *Neurology, 62*, 1224–1226.

Khateeb, S., Flusser, H., Ofir, R., Shelef, I., Narkis, G., Vardi, G., et al. (2006). PLA2G6 mutation underlies infantile neuroaxonal dystrophy. *American Journal of Human Genetics*, *79*, 942–948.

Ki, C. S., Stavrou, E. F., Davanos, N., Lee, W. Y., Chung, E. J., Kim, J. Y., et al. (2007). The Ala53Thr mutation in the alpha-synuclein gene in a Korean family with Parkinson disease. *Clinical Genetics*, *71*, 471–473.

Kiely, A. P., Asi, Y. T., Kara, E., Limousin, P., Ling, H., Lewis, P., et al. (2013). α-Synucleinopathy associated with G51D SNCA mutation: A link between Parkinson's disease and multiple system atrophy? *Acta Neuropathologica*, *125*, 753–769.

Kiely, A. P., Ling, H., Asi, Y. T., Kara, E., Proukakis, C., Schapira, A. H., et al. (2015). Distinct clinical and neuropathological features of G51D SNCA mutation cases compared with SNCA duplication and H50Q mutation. *Molecular Neurodegeneration*, *10*, 41.

Kitada, T., Asakawa, S., Hattori, N., Matsumine, H., Yamamura, Y., Minoshima, S., et al. (1998). Mutations in the parkin gene cause autosomal recessive juvenile parkinsonism. *Nature*, *392*, 605–608.

Klein, C., Lohmann-Hedrich, K., Rogaeva, E., Schlossmacher, M. G., & Lang, A. E. (2007). Deciphering the role of heterozygous mutations in genes associated with parkinsonism. *Lancet Neurology*, *6*, 652–662.

Koentjoro, B., Park, J. S., Ha, A. D., & Sue, C. M. (2012). Phenotypic variability of parkin mutations in single kindred. *Movement Disorders*, *27*, 1299–1303.

Koroglu, C., Baysal, L., Cetinkaya, M., Karasoy, H., & Tolun, A. (2013). DNAJC6 is responsible for juvenile Parkinsonism with phenotypic variability. *Parkinsonism & Related Disorders*, *19*, 320–324.

Krebs, C. E., Karkheiran, S., Powell, J. C., Cao, M., Makarov, V., Darvish, H., et al. (2013). The Sac1 domain of SYNJ1 identified mutated in a family with early-onset progressive Parkinsonism with generalized seizures. *Human Mutations*, *34*, 1200–1207.

Krüger, R., Kuhn, W., Müller, T., Woitalla, D., Graeber, M., Kösel, S., et al. (1998). Ala30Pro mutation in the gene encoding alpha-synuclein in Parkinson's disease. *Nature Genetics*, *18*, 106–108.

Krüger, R., Schöls, L., Müller, T., Kuhn, W., Woitalla, D., Przuntek, H., et al. (2001). Evaluation of the gamma-synuclein gene in German Parkinson's disease patients. *Neuroscience Letters*, *310*, 191–193.

Kubo, S., Hattori, N., & Mizuno, Y. (2006). Recessive Parkinson's disease. *Movement Disorders*, *21*, 885–893.

Kumar, K. R., Weissbach, A., Heldmann, M., Kasten, M., Tunc, S., Sue, C. M., et al. (2012). Frequency of the D620N mutation in VPS35 in Parkinson disease. *Archives of Neurology*, *69*, 1360–1364.

Kumru, H., Santamaria, J., Tolosa, E., Valldeoriola, F., Muñoz, E., Marti, M. J., et al. (2004). Rapid eye movement sleep behavior disorder in parkinsonism with parkin mutations. *Annals of Neurology*, *56*, 599–603.

Lai, H. J., Lin, C. H., & Wu, R. M. (2012). Early-onset autosomal-recessive parkinsonian-pyramidal syndrome. *Acta Neurologica Taiwan*, *21*, 99–107.

Lesage, S., Anheim, M., Letournel, F., Bousset, L., Honoré, A., Rozas, N., et al. (2013). G51D α-synuclein mutation causes a novel parkinsonian-pyramidal syndrome. *Annals of Neurology*, *73*, 459–471.

Lesage, S., Drouet, V., Majounie, E., Deramecourt, V., Jacoupy, M., Nicolas, A., et al. (2016). Loss of VPS13C function in autosomal-recessive parkinsonism causes mitochondrial dysfunction and increases PINK1/parkin-dependent mitophagy. *The American Journal of Human Genetics*, *98*, 500–513.

Lesage, S., Durr, A., Tazir, M., Lohmann, E., Leutenegger, A. L., Janin, S., et al. (2006). LRRK2 G2019S as a cause of Parkinson's disease in North African Arabs. *New England Journal of Medicine*, *354*, 422–423.

Lesage, S., Patin, E., Condroyer, C., Leutenegger, A. L., Lohmann, E., Giladi, N., et al. (2010). Parkinson's disease-related LRRK2 G2019S mutation results from independent mutational events in humans. *Human Molecular Genetics, 19*, 1998–2004.

Lewthwaite, A. J., Lambert, T. D., Rolfe, E. B., Olgiati, S., Quadri, M., Simons, E. J., et al. (2015). Novel GCH1 variant in Dopa-responsive dystonia and Parkinson's disease. *Parkinsonism & Related Disorders, 21*, 394–397.

Li, C., Ting, Z., Qin, X., Ying, W., Li, B., Guo Qiang, L., et al. (2007). The prevalence of LRRK2 Gly2385Arg variant in Chinese Han population with Parkinson's disease. *Movement Disorders, 22*, 2439–2443.

Limousin, N., Konofal, E., Karroum, E., Lohmann, E., Theodorou, I., Dürr, A., et al. (2009). Restless legs syndrome, rapid eye movement sleep behavior disorder, and hypersomnia in patients with two Parkin mutations. *Movement Disorders, 24*, 1970–1976.

Lincoln, S. J., Maraganore, D. M., Lesnick, T. G., Bounds, R., de Andrade, M., Bower, J. H., et al. (2003). Parkin variants in North American Parkinson's disease: Cases and controls. *Movement Disorders, 18*, 1306–1311.

Macedo, M. G., Verbaan, D., Fang, Y., van Rooden, S. M., Visser, M., Anar, B., et al. (2009). Genotypic and phenotypic characteristics of Dutch patients with early onset Parkinson's disease. *Movement Disorders, 24*, 196–203.

Machaczka, M., Rucinska, M., Skotnicki, A. B., & Jurczak, W. (1999). Parkinson's syndrome preceding clinical manifestation of Gaucher's disease. *American Journal of Hematology, 61*, 216–217.

Malakouti-Nejad, M., Shahidi, G. A., Rohani, M., Shojaee, S. M., Hashemi, M., Klotzle, B., et al. (2014). Identification of p.Gln858* in ATP13A2 in two EOPD patients and presentation of their clinical features. *Neuroscience Letters, 577*, 106–111.

Malek, N., Swallow, D. M., Grosset, K. A., Lawton, M. A., Smith, C. R., Bajaj, N. P., et al. (2016). Olfaction in Parkin single and compound heterozygotes in a cohort of young onset Parkinson's disease patients. *Acta Neurologica Scandinavica, 134*, 271–276.

Marder, K., Wang, Y., Alcalay, R. N., Mejia-Santana, H., Tang, M. X., Lee, A., et al. (2015). Age-specific penetrance of LRRK2 G2019S in the Michael J. Fox Ashkenazi Jewish LRRK2 Consortium. *Neurology, 85*, 89–95.

Markopoulou, K., Dickson, D. W., McComb, R. D., Wszolek, Z. K., Katechalidou, L., Avery, L., et al. (2008). Clinical, neuropathological and genotypic variability in SNCA A53T familial Parkinson's disease. Variability in familial Parkinson's disease. *Acta Neuropathologica, 116*, 25–35.

Markopoulou, K., Wszolek, Z. K., & Pfeiffer, R. F. (1995). A Greek-American kindred with autosomal dominant, levodopa-responsive parkinsonism and anticipation. *Annals of Neurology, 38*, 373–378.

Marongiu, R., Ferraris, A., Ialongo, T., Michiorri, S., Soleti, F., Ferrari, F., et al. (2008). PINK1 heterozygous rare variants: Prevalence, significance and phenotypic spectrum. *Human Mutation, 29*, 565.

Marras, C., Alcalay, R. N., Caspell-Garcia, C., Coffey, C., Chan, P., Duda, J. E., et al. (2016). Motor and nonmotor heterogeneity of LRRK2-related and idiopathic Parkinson's disease. *Movement Disorders, 31*, 1192–1202.

Martikainen, M. H., Päivärinta, M., Hietala, M., & Kaasinen, V. (2015). Clinical and imaging findings in Parkinson disease associated with the A53E SNCA mutation. *Neurology Genetics, 1*, e27.

Melachroinou, K., Leandrou, E., Valkimadi, P. E., Memou, A., Hadjigeorgiou, G., Stefanis, L., et al. (2016). Activation of FADD-dependent neuronal death pathways as a predictor of pathogenicity for LRRK2 mutations. *PLoS One, 11*, e0166053.

Mencacci, N. E., Isaias, I. U., Reich, M. M., Ganos, C., Plagnol, V., Polke, J. M., et al. (2014). Parkinson's disease in GTP cyclohydrolase 1 mutation carriers. *Brain, 137*, 2480–2492.

Michelakakis, H., Xiromerisiou, G., Dardiotis, E., Bozi, M., Vassilatis, D., Kountra, P. M., et al. (2012). Evidence of an association between the scavenger receptor class B member 2 gene and Parkinson's disease. *Movement Disorders, 27*, 400–405.
Michell, A. W., Barker, R. A., Raha, S. K., & Raha-Chowdhury, R. (2005). A case of late onset sporadic Parkinson's disease with an A53T mutation in alpha-synuclein. *Journal of Neurology, Neurosurgery, and Psychiatry, 76*, 596–597.
Mohan, M., & Mellick, G. D. (2016). Role of the VPS35 D620N mutation in Parkinson's disease. *Parkinsonism & Related Disorders*. pii: S1353-8020(16)30469-2 (e-pub ahead of print).
Montfort, M., Chabás, A., Vilageliu, L., & Grinberg, D. (2004). Functional analysis of 13 GBA mutant alleles identified in Gaucher disease patients: Pathogenic changes and "modifier" polymorphisms. *Human Mutations, 23*, 567–575.
Moraitou, M., Hadjigeorgiou, G., Monopolis, I., Dardiotis, E., Bozi, M., Vassilatis, D., et al. (2011). β-Glucocerebrosidase gene mutations in two cohorts of Greek patients with sporadic Parkinson's disease. *Molecular Genetics Metabolism, 104*, 149–152.
Morfis, L., & Cordato, D. J. (2006). Dementia with Lewy bodies in an elderly Greek male due to alpha-synuclein gene mutation. *Journal of Clinical Neuroscience, 13*, 942–944.
Morgan, N. V., Westaway, S. K., Morton, J. E., Gregory, A., Gissen, P., Sonek, S., et al. (2006). PLA2G6, encoding a phospholipase A2, is mutated in neurodegenerative disorders with high brain iron. *Nature Genetics, 38*, 752–754.
Nabli, F., Ben Sassi, S., Amouri, R., Duda, J. E., Farrer, M. J., & Hentati, F. (2015). Motor phenotype of LRRK2-associated Parkinson's disease: A Tunisian longitudinal study. *Movement Disorders, 30*, 253–258.
Najim al-Din, A. S., Wriekat, A., Mubaidin, A., Dasouki, M., & Hiari, M. (1994). Pallido-pyramidal degeneration, supranuclear upgaze paresis and dementia: Kufor–Rakeb syndrome. *Acta Neurologica Scandinavica, 89*, 347–352.
Nalls, M. A., Pankratz, N., Lill, C. M., Do, C. B., Hernandez, G., Saad, M., et al. (2014). Large-scale meta-analysis of genome-wide association data identifies six new risk loci for Parkinson's disease. *Nature Genetics, 46*, 989–993.
Neumann, J., Bras, J., Deas, E., et al. (2009). Glucocerebrosidase mutations in clinical and pathologically proven Parkinson's disease. *Brain, 132*, 1783–1794.
Nichols, W. C., Pankratz, N., Marek, D. K., et al. (2009). Mutations in GBA are associated with familial Parkinson disease susceptibility and age at onset. *Neurology, 72*, 310–316.
Nishioka, K., Hayashi, S., Farrer, M. J., Singleton, A. B., Yoshino, H., Imai, H., et al. (2006). Clinical heterogeneity of alpha-synuclein gene duplication in Parkinson's disease. *Annals of Neurology, 59*, 298–309.
Nishioka, K., Ross, O. A., Ishii, K., Kachergus, J. M., Ishiwata, K., Kitagawa, M., et al. (2009). Expanding the clinical phenotype of SNCA duplication carriers. *Movement Disorders, 24*, 1811–1819.
Oeda, T., Umemura, A., Mori, Y., Tomita, S., Kohsaka, M., Park, K., et al. (2015). Impact of glucocerebrosidase mutations on motor and nonmotor complications in Parkinson's disease. *Neurobiology of Aging, 36*, 3306–3313.
Olgiati, S., Quadri, M., Fang, M., Rood, J. P., Saute, J. A., Chien, H. F., et al. (2016). DNAJC6 mutations associated with early-onset Parkinson's disease. *Annals of Neurology, 79*, 244–256.
Olgiati, S., Thomas, A., Quadri, M., Breedveld, G. J., Graafland, J., Eussen, H., et al. (2015). Early-onset parkinsonism caused by alpha-synuclein gene triplication: Clinical and genetic findings in a novel family. *Parkinsonism & Related Disorders, 21*, 981–986.
Orimo, S., Amino, T., Yokochi, M., Kojo, T., Uchihara, T., Takahashi, A., et al. (2005). Preserved cardiac sympathetic nerve accounts for normal cardiac uptake of MIBG in PARK2. *Movement Disorders, 20*, 1350–1353.
Ozelius, L. J., Senthil, G., Saunders-Pullman, R., Ohmann, E., Deligtisch, A., Tagliati, M., et al. (2006). LRRK2 G2019S as a cause of Parkinson's disease in Ashkenazi Jews. *New England Journal of Medicine, 354*, 424–425.

Paisan-Ruiz, C., Bhatia, K. P., Li, A., Hernandez, D., Davis, M., Wood, N. W., et al. (2009). Characterization of PLA2G6 as a locus for dystonia-parkinsonism. *Annals of Neurology*, *65*, 19–23.

Paisán-Ruiz, C., Guevara, R., Federoff, M., Hanagasi, H., Sina, F., Elahi, E., et al. (2010). Early-onset L-dopa-responsive parkinsonism with pyramidal signs due to ATP13A2, PLA2G6, FBXO7 and spatacsin mutations. *Movement Disorders*, *25*, 1791–1800.

Paisan-Ruiz, C., Jain, S., Evans, E. W., Gilks, W. P., Simon, J., van der Brug, M., et al. (2004). Cloning of the gene containing mutations that cause PARK8-linked Parkinson's disease. *Neuron*, *44*, 595–600.

Paisán-Ruiz, C., Li, A., Schneider, S. A., Holton, J. L., Johnson, R., Kidd, D., et al. (2012). Widespread Lewy body and tau accumulation in childhood and adult onset dystonia-parkinsonism cases with PLA2G6 mutations. *Neurobiology of Aging*, *33*, 814–823.

Papadimitriou, D., Antonelou, R., Miligkos, M., Maniati, M., Papagiannakis, N., & Bostantjopoulou, S. (2016). Motor and nonmotor features of carriers of the p.A53T alpha-synuclein mutation: A longitudinal study. *Movement Disorders*, *31*, 1226–1230.

Papadimitriou, A., Veletza, V., Hadjigeorgiou, G. M., Patrikiou, A., Hirano, M., & Anastasopoulos, I. (1999). Mutated alpha-synuclein gene in two Greek kindreds with familial PD: Incomplete penetrance? *Neurology*, *52*, 651–654.

Papapetropoulos, S., Ellul, J., Paschalis, C., Athanassiadou, A., Papadimitriou, A., & Papapetropoulos, T. (2003). Clinical characteristics of the alpha-synuclein mutation (G209A)-associated Parkinson's disease in comparison with other forms of familial Parkinson's disease in Greece. *European Journal of Neurology*, *10*, 281–286.

Papapetropoulos, S., Paschalis, C., Athanassiadou, A., Papadimitriou, A., Ellul, J., Polymeropoulos, M. H., et al. (2001). Clinical phenotype in patients with alpha-synuclein Parkinson's disease living in Greece in comparison with patients with sporadic Parkinson's disease. *Journal of Neurology, Neurosurgery, and Psychiatry*, *70*, 662–665.

Pasanen, P., Myllykangas, L., Siitonen, M., Raunio, A., Kaakkola, S., Lyytinen, J., et al. (2014). Novel α-synuclein mutation A53E associated with atypical multiple system atrophy and Parkinson's disease-type pathology. *Neurobiology of Aging*, *35*. 2180.e1–5.

Petrucci, S., Ginevrino, M., & Valente, E. M. (2016). Phenotypic spectrum of alpha-synuclein mutations: New insights from patients and cellular models. *Parkinsonism & Related Disorders*, *22*, S16–S20.

Pimentel, M. M., Rodrigues, F. C., Leite, M. A., Campos Júnior, M., Rosso, A. L., Nicaretta, D. H., et al. (2015). Parkinson disease: α-synuclein mutational screening and new clinical insight into the p.E46K mutation. *Parkinsonism & Related Disorders*, *21*, 586–589.

Polymeropoulos, M. H., Lavedan, C., Leroy, E., Ide, S. E., Dehejia, A., Dutra, A., et al. (1997). Mutation in the alpha-synuclein gene identified in families with Parkinson's disease. *Science*, *276*, 2045–2047.

Pons, R., Kekou, K., Antonellou, R., Svingou, M., Kanavakis, E., & Stefanis, L. (2016). Analysis of a founder mutation in the TH gene in a cohort of Greek patients with Parkinson's disease. *Movement Disorders*, *31*, 1753–1754.

Pont-Sunyer, C., Iranzo, A., Gaig, C., Fernández-Arcos, A., Vilas, D., Valldeoriola, F., et al. (2015). Sleep disorders in parkinsonian and nonparkinsonian LRRK2 mutation carriers. *PLoS One*, *10*, e0132368.

Proukakis, C., Dudzik, C. G., Brier, T., MacKay, D. S., Cooper, J. M., Millhauser, G. L., et al. (2013). A novel α-synuclein missense mutation in Parkinson disease. *Neurology*, *80*, 1062–1064.

Puschmann, A., Fiesel, F. C., Caulfield, T. R., Hudec, R., Ando, M., Truban, D., et al. (2016). Heterozygous PINK1 p.G411S increases risk of Parkinson's disease via a dominant-negative mechanism. *140*, 98–117. pii: aww261.

Puschmann, A., Ross, O. A., Vilariño-Güell, C., Lincoln, S. J., Kachergus, J. M., Cobb, S. A., et al. (2009). A Swedish family with de novo alpha-synuclein A53T mutation: Evidence for early cortical dysfunction. *Parkinsonism & Related Disorders*, *15*, 627–632.

Quadri, M., Fang, M., Picillo, M., Olgiati, S., Breedveld, G. J., Graafland, J., et al. (2013). Mutation in the SYNJ1 gene associated with autosomal recessive, early-onset Parkinsonism. *Human Mutations*, *34*, 1208–1215.

Quattrone, A., Bagnato, A., Annesi, G., Novellino, F., Morgante, L., Savettieri, G., et al. (2008). Myocardial 123metaiodobenzylguanidine uptake in genetic Parkinson's disease. *Movement Disorders*, *23*, 21–27.

Ramirez, A., Heimbach, A., Gründemann, J., Stiller, B., Hampshire, D., Cid, L. P., et al. (2006). Hereditary parkinsonism with dementia is caused by mutations in ATP13A2, encoding a lysosomal type 5 P-type ATPase. *Nature Genetics*, *38*, 1184–1191.

Rengmark, A., Pihlstrøm, L., Linder, J., Forsgren, L., & Toft, M. (2016). Low frequency of GCH1 and TH mutations in Parkinson's disease. *Parkinsonism & Related Disorders*, *29*, 109–111.

Ricciardi, L., Petrucci, S., Di Giuda, D., Serra, L., Spanò, B., Sensi, M., et al. (2016). The contursi family 20 years later: Intrafamilial phenotypic variability of the SNCA p.A53T mutation. *Movement Disorders*, *31*, 257–258.

Roosen, D. A., & Cookson, M. R. (2016). LRRK2 at the interface of autophagosomes, endosomes and lysosomes. *Molecular Neurodegeneration*, *11*, 73.

Ross, O. A., Braithwaite, A. T., Skipper, L. M., Kachergus, J., Hulihan, M. M., Middleton, F. A., et al. (2008). Genomic investigation of alpha-synuclein multiplication and parkinsonism. *Annals of Neurology*, *63*, 743–750.

Ross, O. A., Wu, Y. R., Lee, M. C., Funayama, M., Chen, M. L., Soto, A. I., et al. (2008). Analysis of Lrrk2 R1628P as a risk factor for Parkinson's disease. *Annals of Neurology*, *64*, 88–92.

Ruiz-Martínez, J., Gorostidi, A., Goyenechea, E., Alzualde, A., Poza, J. J., Rodríguez, F., et al. (2011). Olfactory deficits and cardiac 123I-MIBG in Parkinson's disease related to the LRRK2 R1441G and G2019S mutations. *Movement Disorders*, *26*, 2026–2031.

Samaranch, L., Lorenzo-Betancor, O., Arbelo, J. M., Ferrer, I., Lorenzo, E., Irigoyen, J., et al. (2010). PINK1-linked parkinsonism is associated with Lewy body pathology. *Brain*, *133*, 1128–1142.

Samii, A., Markopoulou, K., Wszolek, Z. K., Sossi, V., Dobko, T., Mak, E., et al. (1999). PET studies of parkinsonism associated with mutation in the alpha-synuclein gene. *Neurology*, *53*, 2097–2102.

Santoro, L., Breedveld, G. J., Manganelli, F., Di Fonzo, A., Oostra, B. A., & Bonifati, V. (2011). Novel ATP13A2 (PARK9) homozygous mutation in a family with marked phenotype variability. *Neurogenetics*, *12*, 33–39.

Sardi, S. P., Cheng, S. H., & Shihabuddin, L. S. (2015). Gaucher-related synucleinopathies: The examination of sporadic neurodegeneration from a rare (disease) angle. *Progress in Neurobiology*, *125*, 47–62.

Saunders-Pullman, R., Alcalay, R. N., Mirelman, A., Wang, C., Luciano, M. S., Ortega, R. A., et al. (2015). REM sleep behavior disorder, as assessed by questionnaire, in G2019S LRRK2 mutation PD and carriers. *Movement Disorders*, *30*, 1834–1839.

Saunders-Pullman, R., Hagenah, J., Dhawan, V., Stanley, K., Pastores, G., Sathe, S., et al. (2010). Gaucher disease ascertained through a Parkinson's center: Imaging and clinical characterization. *Movement Disorders*, *25*, 1364–1372.

Saunders-Pullman, R., Mirelman, A., Wang, C., Alcalay, R. N., San Luciano, M., Ortega, R., et al. (2014). Olfactory identification in LRRK2 G2019S mutation carriers: A relevant marker? *Annals of Clinical and Translational Neurology*, *1*, 670–678.

Schneider, S. A., Paisan-Ruiz, C., Quinn, N. P., Lees, A. J., Houlden, H., Hardy, J., et al. (2010). ATP13A2 mutations (PARK9) cause neurodegeneration with brain iron accumulation. *Movement Disorders, 25*, 979–984.

Sharma, M., Ioannidis, J. P., Aasly, J. O., Annesi, G., Brice, A., Bertram, L., et al. (2012). A multi-centre clinico-genetic analysis of the VPS35 gene in Parkinson disease indicates reduced penetrance for disease-associated variants. *Journal of Medical Genetics, 49*, 721–726.

Shi, C. H., Tang, B. S., Wang, L., Lv, Z. Y., Wang, J., Luo, L. Z., et al. (2011). PLA2G6 gene mutation in autosomal recessive early-onset parkinsonism in a Chinese cohort. *Neurology, 77*, 75–81.

Shiner, T., Mirelman, A., Gana Weisz, M., Bar-Shira, A., Ash, E., Cialic, R., et al. (2016). High frequency of GBA gene mutations in dementia with Lewy bodies among Ashkenazi Jews. *JAMA Neurology, 3*, 1448–1453.

Shojaee, S., Sina, F., Banihosseini, S. S., Kazemi, M. H., Kalhor, R., Shahidi, G. A., et al. (2008). Genomewide linkage analysis of a Parkinsonian-pyramidal syndrome pedigree by 500 K SNP arrays. *American Journal of Human Genetics, 82*, 1375–1384.

Sidransky, E., Nalls, M. A., Aasly, J. O., Aharon-Peretz, J., Annesi, G., Barbosa, E. R., et al. (2009). Multicenter analysis of glucocerebrosidase mutations in Parkinson's disease. *New England Journal of Medicine, 361*, 1651–1661.

Singleton, A. B., Farrer, M., Johnson, J., Singleton, A., Hague, S., Kachergus, J., et al. (2003). alpha-Synuclein locus triplication causes Parkinson's disease. *Science, 302*, 841.

Somme, J. H., Gomez-Esteban, J. C., Molano, A., Tijero, B., Lezcano, E., & Zarranz, J. J. (2011). Initial neuropsychological impairments in patients with the E46K mutation of the α-synuclein gene (PARK 1). *Journal of Neurological Sciences, 310*, 86–89.

Spanaki, C., Latsoudis, H., & Plaitakis, A. (2006). LRRK2 mutations on crete: R1441H associated with PD evolving to PSP. *Neurology, 67*, 1518–1519.

Spira, P. J., Sharpe, D. M., Halliday, G., Cavanagh, J., & Nicholson, G. A. (2001). Clinical and pathological features of a Parkinsonian syndrome in a family with an Ala53Thr alpha-synuclein mutation. *Annals of Neurology, 49*, 313–319.

Steinlechner, S., Stahlberg, J., Völkel, B., Djarmati, A., Hagenah, J., Hiller, A., et al. (2007). Co-occurrence of affective and schizophrenia spectrum disorders with PINK1 mutations. *Journal of Neurology, Neurosurgery & Psychiatry, 78*, 532–535.

Struhal, W., Presslauer, S., Spielberger, S., Zimprich, A., Auff, E., Bruecke, T., et al. (2014). VPS35 Parkinson's disease phenotype resembles the sporadic disease. *Journal of Neural Transmission (Vienna), 121*, 755–759.

Swan, M., Doan, N., Ortega, R. A., Barrett, M., Nichols, W., Ozelius, L., et al. (2016). Neuropsychiatric characteristics of GBA-associated Parkinson disease. *Journal of Neurological Sciences, 370*, 63–69.

Taipa, R., Pereira, C., Reis, I., Alonso, I., Bastos-Lima, A., Melo-Pires, M., et al. (2016). DJ-1 linked parkinsonism (PARK7) is associated with Lewy body pathology. *Brain, 139*, 1680–1687.

Tan, E. K., Shen, H., Tan, L. C., Farrer, M., Yew, K., Chua, E., et al. (2005). The G2019S LRRK2 mutation is uncommon in an Asian cohort of Parkinson's disease patients. *Neuroscience Letters, 384*, 327–329.

Tan, E. K., Tong, J., Fook-Chong, S., et al. (2007). Glucocerebrosidase mutations and risk of Parkinson disease in Chinese patients. *Archives of Neurology, 64*, 1056–1058.

Tayebi, N., Callahan, M., Madike, V., Stubblefield, B. K., Orvisky, E., Krasnewich, D., et al. (2001). Gaucher disease and parkinsonism: A phenotypic and genotypic characterization. *Molecular Genetics Metabolism, 73*, 313–321.

Tayebi, N., Walker, J., Stubblefield, B., Orvisky, E., LaMarca, M. E., Wong, K., et al. (2003). Gaucher disease with parkinsonian manifestations: Does glucocerebrosidase deficiency contribute to a vulnerability to parkinsonism? *Molecular Genetics Metabolism, 79*, 104–109.

Tijero, B., Gabilondo, I., Lezcano, E., Teran-Villagrá, N., Llorens, V., Ruiz-Martinez, J., et al. (2015). Autonomic involvement in Parkinsonian carriers of PARK2 gene mutations. *Parkinsonism & Related Disorders, 21*, 717–722.

Tijero, B., Gómez-Esteban, J. C., Lezcano, E., Fernández-González, C., Somme, J., Llorens, V., et al. (2013). Cardiac sympathetic denervation in symptomatic and asymptomatic carriers of the E46K mutation in the α synuclein gene. *Parkinsonism & Related Disorders, 19*, 95–100.

Tokutake, T., Ishikawa, A., Yoshimura, N., Miyashita, A., Kuwano, R., Nishizawa, M., et al. (2014). Clinical and neuroimaging features of patient with early-onset Parkinson's disease with dementia carrying SNCA p.G51D mutation. *Parkinsonism & Related Disorders, 20*, 262–264.

Trinh, J., Amouri, R., Duda, J. E., Morley, J. F., Read, M., Donald, A., et al. (2014). Comparative study of Parkinson's disease and leucine-rich repeat kinase 2 p.G2019S parkinsonism. *Neurobiology of Aging, 35*, 1125–1131.

Trinh, J., Gustavsson, E. K., Vilariño-Güell, C., Bortnick, S., Latourelle, J., McKenzie, M. B., et al. (2016). DNM3 and genetic modifiers of age of onset in LRRK2 Gly2019Ser parkinsonism: A genome-wide linkage and association study. *Lancet Neurology, 15*, 1248–1256.

Tuin, I., Voss, U., Kessler, K., Krakow, K., Hilker, R., Morales, B., et al. (2008). Sleep quality in a family with hereditary parkinsonism (PARK6). *Sleep Medicine, 9*, 684–688.

Valente, E. M., Abou-Sleiman, P. M., Caputo, V., Muqit, M. M., Harvey, K., Gispert, S., et al. (2004). Hereditary early-onset Parkinson's disease caused by mutations in PINK1. *Science, 304*, 1158–1160.

Valente, E. M., & Ferraris, A. (2007). Heterozygous mutations in genes causing parkinsonism: Monogenic disorders go complex. *Lancet Neurology, 6*, 576–578.

van der Merwe, C., Jalali Sefid Dashti, Z., Christoffels, A., Loos, B., & Bardien, S. (2015). Evidence for a common biological pathway linking three Parkinson's disease-causing genes: Parkin, PINK1 and DJ-1. *European Journal of Neuroscience, 41*, 1113–1125.

van Duijn, C. M., Dekker, M. C., Bonifati, V., Galjaard, R. J., Houwing-Duistermaat, J. J., Snijders, P. J., et al. (2001). Park7, a novel locus for autosomal recessive early-onset parkinsonism, on chromosome 1p36. *The American Journal of Human Genetics, 69*, 629–634.

Vekrellis, K., Xilouri, M., Emmanouilidou, E., Rideout, H. J., & Stefanis, L. (2011). Pathological roles of α-synuclein in neurological disorders. *Lancet Neurology, 10*, 1015–1025.

Vilarino-Guell, C., Wider, C., Ross, O. A., Dachsel, J. C., Kachergus, J. M., Lincoln, S. J., et al. (2011). VPS35 mutations in Parkinson disease. *American Journal of Human Genetics, 89*, 162–167.

Voigt, A., Berlemann, L. A., & Winklhofer, K. F. (2016). The mitochondrial kinase PINK1: Functions beyond mitophagy. *Journal of Neurochemistry, 139*, 232–239.

Wang, C., Cai, Y., Gu, Z., Ma, J., Zheng, Z., Tang, B. S., et al. (2014). Clinical profiles of Parkinson's disease associated with common leucine-rich repeat kinase 2 and glucocerebrosidase genetic variants in Chinese individuals. *Neurobiology of Aging, 35*, 725.e1–6.

Wider, C., Skipper, L., Solida, A., Brown, L., Farrer, M., Dickson, D., et al. (2008). Autosomal dominant dopa-responsive parkinsonism in a multigenerational Swiss family. *Parkinsonism & Related Disorders, 14*, 465–470.

Winder-Rhodes, S. E., Evans, J. R., Ban, M., Mason, S. L., Williams-Gray, H., Foltynie, T., et al. (2013). Glucocerebrosidase mutations influence the natural history of Parkinson's disease in a community-based incident cohort. *Brain, 136*, 392–399.

Xilouri, M., Brekk, O. R., & Stefanis, L. (2016). Autophagy and Alpha-Synuclein: Relevance to Parkinson's Disease and Related Synucleopathies. *Movement Disorders*, *31*, 178–192.

Xiong, W. X., Sun, Y. M., Guan, R. Y., Luo, S. S., Chen, C., An, Y., et al. (2016). The heterozygous A53T mutation in the alpha-synuclein gene in a Chinese Han patient with Parkinson disease: Case report and literature review. *Journal of Neurology*, *263*, 1984–1992.

Xiromerisiou, G., Hadjigeorgiou, G. M., Gourbali, V., Johnson, J., Papakonstantinou, I., Papadimitriou, A., et al. (2007). Screening for SNCA and LRRK2 mutations in Greek sporadic and autosomal dominant Parkinson's disease: Identification of two novel LRRK2 variants. *European Journal of Neurology*, *14*, 7–11.

Yoshino, H., Tomiyama, H., Tachibana, N., Ogaki, K., Li, Y., Funayama, M., et al. (2010). Phenotypic spectrum of patients with PLA2G6 mutation and PARK14-linked parkinsonism. *Neurology*, *75*, 1356–1361.

Zabetian, C. P., Samii, A., Mosley, A. D., Roberts, J. W., Leis, B. C., Yearout, D., et al. (2005). A clinic-based study of the LRRK2 gene in Parkinson disease yields new mutations. *Neurology*, *65*, 741–744.

Zarranz, J. J., Alegre, J., Gómez-Esteban, J. C., Lezcano, E., Ros, R., Ampuero, I., et al. (2004). The new mutation, E46K, of alpha-synuclein causes Parkinson and Lewy body dementia. *Annals of Neurology*, *55*, 164–173.

Zhao, T., De Graaff, E., Breedveld, G. J., Loda, A., Severijnen, L. A., Wouters, C. H., et al. (2011). Loss of nuclear activity of the FBXO7 protein in patients with parkinsonian-pyramidal syndrome (PARK15). *PLoS One*, *6*, e16983.

Zhou, Z. D., Sathiyamoorthy, S., Angeles, D. C., & Tan, E. K. (2016). Linking F-box protein 7 and parkin to neuronal degeneration in Parkinson's disease (PD). *Molecular Brain*, *9*, 41.

Zimprich, A., Benet-Pages, A., Struhal, W., Graf, E., Eck, S. H., Offman, M. N., et al. (2011). A mutation in VPS35, encoding a subunit of the retromer complex, causes late-onset Parkinson disease. *American Journal of Human Genetics*, *89*, 168–175.

Zimprich, A., Biskup, S., Leitner, P., Lichtner, P., Farrer, M., Lincoln, S., et al. (2004). Mutations in LRRK2 cause autosomal-dominant parkinsonism with pleomorphic pathology. *Neuron*, *44*, 601–607.

Zokaei, N., McNeill, A., Proukakis, C., Beavan, M., Jarman, P., Korlipara, P., et al. (2014). Visual short-term memory deficits associated with GBA mutation and Parkinson's disease. *Brain*, *37*, 2303–2311.

CHAPTER NINE

Imaging in Parkinson's Disease

Marios Politis[1], Gennaro Pagano, Flavia Niccolini
Neurodegeneration Imaging Group, Institute of Psychiatry, Psychology and Neuroscience (IoPPN), King's College London, London, United Kingdom
[1]Corresponding author: e-mail address: marios.politis@kcl.ac.uk

Contents

Abstract

Parkinson's disease (PD) is a chronic neurodegenerative disease characterized by the loss of nigrostriatal dopaminergic neurons and aggregation of misfolded α-synuclein in Lewy bodies. The underlying mechanisms of neurodegeneration in PD are still unknown, and there are no disease-modifying treatments to slow the neurodegenerative processes. There is an urgent need to identify biomarkers that are able to monitor disease progression and assess the development and efficacy of novel disease-modifying drugs. Over the past years, neuroimaging techniques such as magnetic resonance imaging (MRI), single-photon emission computed tomography (SPECT), and positron emission tomography (PET) have provided important advances in our understanding of PD. MRI provides information about structural and functional organization of the brain, while SPECT and PET can detect molecular changes in the brain. Here, we review the current neuroimaging literature in sporadic and genetic PD, which have contributed to our understanding of the physiopathological mechanisms of the disease.

1. IDIOPATHIC PARKINSON'S DISEASE: INTRODUCTION

Several neuroimaging techniques have been deployed over the past decades, to help understanding the pathophysiology of Parkinson's disease (PD) and to provide us with biological indicators for early diagnosis and response to treatment (Pagano, Niccolini, Fusar-Poli, & Politis, 2017; Pagano, Niccolini, & Politis, 2016a, 2016b). Neuroimaging techniques such

International Review of Neurobiology, Volume 132
ISSN 0074-7742
http://dx.doi.org/10.1016/bs.irn.2017.02.015

as magnetic resonance imaging (MRI) have played a critical role in assessing structural and functional changes in the brain, which can be related to the pathophysiology and clinical manifestations of PD. Single-photon emission computed tomography (SPECT) and positron emission tomography (PET) are molecular noninvasive imaging techniques for the quantitative and qualitative imaging of biological functions (Phelps, 2000). The distribution and kinetic profiles of compounds targeting specific biological molecules in tissue reflect specific biological functions in the living body. Here, we review the findings from neuroimaging studies, which have contributed in the understanding of the pathophysiological mechanisms underlying PD.

1.1 Molecular Imaging

1.1.1 Dopaminergic System

The main pathological hallmark of PD is the progressive loss of dopamine neurons in the substantia nigra *pars compacta* and the loss of dopaminergic neurotransmission in the denervated areas of the forebrain, above all in the striatum (Jellinger, 1991; Samii, Nutt, & Ransom, 2004). The loss of dopaminergic neurons in PD results in a decrease in the excitatory activity of the D1 *direct* (striatonigral) pathway and an increase in the inhibitory activity of the D2 *indirect* (striatopallidal) pathway; this enhances the activity of nigral neurons, resulting in decreased motor response and subsequent manifestation of some classic PD symptoms (Hamani & Lozano, 2003). PET with radioligands targeting presynaptic and postsynaptic dopaminergic markers has been extensively employed to aid with the early diagnosis of PD, track disease progression, and investigate motor and nonmotor correlates of PD (Politis, 2014).

Six selective SPECT radioligands targeting dopamine transporter (DAT), [^{123}I]-β-CIT, [^{123}I]-FP-β-CIT, [^{123}I]-IPT, [^{123}I]-Altropane, [^{123}I]-β-PE2I, and [^{99}Tcm]-TRODAT-1, have been used to assess presynaptic dopamine reuptake availability in PD (Politis, 2014; Roussakis, Piccini, & Politis, 2013). DAT-SPECT is useful for the differential diagnosis between PD and nondegenerative parkinsonism, such as drug-induced parkinsonism, essential tremor (ET), dystonic tremor, or psychogenic parkinsonism. [^{123}I]-FP-CIT DAT-SPECT showed high accuracy in the differential diagnosis of PD vs drug-induced parkinsonism (Cuberas-Borrós et al., 2011; Diaz-Corrales, Sanz-Viedma, Garcia-Solis, Escobar-Delgado, & Mir, 2010; Loberboym et al., 2006). Lower [^{123}I]-FP-CIT binding in the putamen was found in PD patients compared to patients with ET or drug-induced parkinsonism (Cuberas-Borrós et al., 2011).

Dopaminergic degeneration of DAT is an age-related process; however, it is much faster in PD than in physiological aging (Winogrodzka et al., 2001). Pathology and clinical symptoms of PD progress gradually starting as unilateral and progressively affecting both sides (Larsen et al., 2008). DAT-SPECT has been proven to be an objective tool for monitoring PD progression. [^{123}I]-β-CIT, [^{123}I]-FP-CIT SPECT, [^{123}I]-IPT, and [^{99}Tcm]-TRODAT-1 DAT-SPECT have been used to evaluate disease progression in PD (Marek et al., 2001; Tatsch et al., 1997; Weng et al., 2004; Winogrodzka et al., 2001, 2003). [^{123}I]-β-CIT SPECT have been used in a group of 50 early-stage PD patients showing an average decrease of 8% in the whole striatum (8% in the putamen and 4% in the caudate) at 12-month follow-up (Winogrodzka et al., 2003). Sequential SPECT scans using [^{123}I]-β-CIT demonstrated a decline in striatal uptake of 11.2% per year in PD patients, compared with 0.8% per year in controls (Marek et al., 2001). [^{123}I]-FP-CIT SPECT showed consistent results with an annual decrease in striatal binding ratios of 8% (Winogrodzka et al., 2001). Also, [^{123}I]-IPT SPECT and [^{99}Tcm]-TRODAT-1 uptake in the striatum showed a progressive decline with the progression of the disease (Tatsch et al., 1997; Weng et al., 2004), and lower striatal uptake correlated with increased motor symptoms severity as measured by the Unified PD Rating Scale part III (UPDRS-III) and Hoehn and Yahr (H&Y) stage (Tatsch et al., 1997; Weng et al., 2004).

There are several PET radioligands available for measuring presynaptic dopaminergic markers such as DAT ([^{11}C]CFT, [^{11}C]PE2I, [^{11}C]RTI32, [^{11}C]MP), dopa decarboxylases (DDC; [^{18}F]dopa), and vesicular monoamine transporter type 2 (VMAT-2; [^{11}C]DTBZ, [^{18}F]DBTZ), which can be used to provide a measure of integrity of dopaminergic function in PD. [^{18}F]dopa PET has shown that early-stage PD patients displayed a rapid progression of dopaminergic denervation in the putamen with a posterior-to-anterior gradient and a side-to-side asymmetry between the less and more affected striatal structures (Hilker, Schweitzer, et al., 2005; Hilker, Thomas, et al., 2005; Nandhagopal et al., 2009). In advanced stages, dopaminergic degeneration becomes slower, and although the gradient is maintained, the degree of asymmetry diminishes (Hilker, Schweitzer, et al., 2005; Hilker, Thomas, et al., 2005; Nandhagopal et al., 2009). The mean annual decline in [^{18}F]dopa uptake ranges from 8% to 12% in the putamen and from 4% to 6% in the caudate and it is considerably more than the decline typical of aging (Nurmi et al., 2001; Pavese, Rivero-Bosch, Lewis, Whone, & Brooks, 2011). Moreover, presynaptic dopaminergic

PET imaging has been used to estimate the duration of preclinical PD and it has shown 30%–55% loss of putamen dopaminergic function at the time of symptom onset (de la Fuente-Fernández et al., 2011; Hilker, Schweitzer, et al., 2005; Hilker, Thomas, et al., 2005; Lee, 2000). [^{11}C]DTBZ PET imaging estimated a preclinical state lasting up to 17 years, and [^{11}C]MP PET has shown a period of up to 13 years in patients with PD who were diagnosed at just over 50 years of age. Several studies have shown a correlation between decreased putamen [^{18}F]dopa uptake severity of bradykinesia and rigidity in PD patients (Brooks et al., 2003; Vingerhoets, Schulzer, Calne, & Snow, 1997).

To date, two radioligands, [^{11}C]SCH23390 and [^{11}C]NNC112, have been developed to image dopamine D1 receptors (D1R) (Halldin et al., 1986; Slifstein et al., 2007). [^{11}C]SCH23390 PET has shown no changes in striatal and cortical D1R density in both early-stage de novo (Rinne, Laihinen, et al., 1991; Rinne, Myllykylä, Lönnberg, & Marjamäki, 1991) and levodopa-treated (Ouchi et al., 1999) PD patients. No differences were found in dopamine D1R binding between PD patients with L-dopa-induced dyskinesias (LIDs) and those who were stable responders to levodopa treatment (Turjanski, Lees, & Brooks, 1997). Moreover, executive dysfunction was not associated with striatal and cortical dopamine D1R density as measured by [^{11}C]NNC112 PET, whereas decreases in putamen [^{18}F]dopa uptake predicted performance on executive tasks (Cropley et al., 2008). These findings may be hindered by the lack of specific binding of [^{11}C]SCH23390 and [^{11}C]NNC112 displayed high affinity to the serotoninergic 5-HT_{2A} receptors (Catafau et al., 2010; Ekelund et al., 2007).

PET imaging of dopamine D2 receptor (D2R) expression can be performed by using both dopamine antagonists, such as [^{11}C]raclopride, [^{11}C]NMSP, and [^{18}F]DMFP along with dopamine agonist radioligands ([^{11}C]NPA and [^{11}C]MNPA). Among these radioligands, the most widely used is [^{11}C]raclopride. Increases in D2R availability can occur at the early stages of the disease with reported elevations of [^{11}C]raclopride binding in the putamen of de novo PD patients (Rinne et al., 1993, 1995; Turjanski et al., 1997). Moreover, striatal decreases in [^{18}F]dopa uptake correlated with higher [^{11}C]raclopride binding in early de novo PD patients, suggesting that upregulation of D2R may be a compensatory mechanism in response to synaptic dopamine depletion (Sawle, Playford, Brooks, Quinn, & Frackowiak, 1993). However, as the disease progresses this compensatory upregulation may fail and D2R availability decreases back to normal levels or less in comparison to healthy subjects (Antonini, Schwarz, Oertel, Pogarell, &

Leenders, 1997; Brooks et al., 1992; Dentresangle et al., 1999). Moreover, long-term downregulation of striatal dopamine D2R binding may be induced by chronic dopaminergic therapy (Antonini et al., 1997). D2R availability was reduced by 16% in the caudate of levodopa-treated patients compared to de novo PD patients, and there were no differences in mean caudate and putamen D2R binding between dyskinetic and nondyskinetic PD patients (Turjanski et al., 1997). PET investigations of dopamine D3 receptor (D3R) have also been of current interest because of its potential involvement in psychiatric and motor complications in PD. PET with [^{11}C]PHNO, a radioligand with preferential affinity for D3R over D2R (Rabiner et al., 2009), showed bilaterally decreased [^{11}C]PHNO but not [^{11}C]raclopride binding in the D3-rich ventral striatum, and globus pallidus and [^{11}C]PHNO/[^{11}C]raclopride ratio correlated with motor deficits and depressive symptoms (Boileau et al., 2009). Changes in dopamine receptors are not only restricted to the striatal areas. [^{11}C]raclopride PET showed that D2R binding was significantly reduced in the hypothalamus of PD patients, suggesting a role of hypothalamus in the development of PD nonmotor symptoms (Politis, Piccini, Pavese, Koh, & Brooks, 2008). In advanced PD patients, PET with [^{11}C]FLB457, an extrastriatal D2R radioligand, showed 17%–40% decreases in cortical areas, whereas extrastriatal D2R availability was not significantly different in early PD (Kaasinen et al., 2000). A longitudinal [^{11}C]FLB457 PET study demonstrated 6%–11% annual decline in extrastriatal D2R availability in PD patients (Kaasinen et al., 2003).

[^{11}C]raclopride competes with endogenous dopamine for D2R binding, allowing an indirect measure of synaptic dopamine levels based on changes in D2 receptor availability, and it is estimated that a 10% reduction in D2 receptor binding by ^{11}C-raclopride reflects a fivefold increase in synaptic dopamine levels (Breier et al., 1997). There is a rapid reduction in [^{11}C] raclopride binding following administration of levodopa (Tedroff et al., 1996) or a methamphetamine (Piccini et al., 2003) challenge in PD patients. Following methamphetamine challenge, advanced PD patients could still induce significant endogenous dopamine release in the putamen, which reflected motor symptoms improvement, although dopamine release was significantly smaller than those observed in healthy subjects (Piccini et al., 2003). Altered synaptic dopamine release may play a role in the pathogenesis of motor complications such as LIDs. Using [^{11}C]raclopride PET, it has been demonstrated that 1 h after levodopa administration, dopamine levels in the putamen were three times higher in the group of PD patients with motor fluctuations than PD patients with stable response to levodopa (de la Fuente-Fernandez, Lim, et al., 2001; de la Fuente-Fernandez, Lu, et al., 2001; de la Fuente-Fernandez, Ruth, et al., 2001). However, 4 h after levodopa challenge, PD patients with motor fluctuations showed major reductions in putaminal dopamine levels, whereas in PD patients with a stable response to levodopa, putaminal dopamine levels remained unchanged (de la Fuente-Fernandez, Lim, et al., 2001; de la Fuente-Fernandez, Lu, et al., 2001; de la Fuente-Fernandez, Ruth, et al., 2001). These findings suggest that swings in striatal synaptic dopamine levels precede the occurrence of motor fluctuations in PD and that increased dopamine turnover might play a relevant role in levodopa-related motor complications. As the disease advances, PD patients lose their ability to regulate synaptic dopamine levels (de la Fuente-Fernandez et al., 2004). Following levodopa administration, mean caudate and putamen [^{11}C]raclopride binding were significantly lower compared to baseline and correlated with levodopa-induced improvements in UPDRS-III. Additionally, large putaminal [^{11}C]raclopride binding changes were associated with higher dyskinesia scores (Pavese et al., 2006). [^{11}C]raclopride PET has been used also to monitor response to transplantation of fetal ventral mesencephalic (fVM) tissue. Transplantation led to a restoration of both basal and drug-induced dopamine release to normal levels (Piccini et al., 1999, 2005; Politis, Loane, Wu, Brooks, & Piccini, 2011; Politis, Oertel, et al., 2011; Politis, Wu, Loane, Kiferle, et al., 2010; Politis, Wu, Loane, Quinn, et al., 2010; Politis, Wu, Loane, Turkheimer, et al., 2010; Politis & Piccini, 2012).

Altered dopamine release appears to play a role in PD impulse control disorders (ICD) and addictive behaviors. Following levodopa challenge, dopamine levels within the ventral striatum were significantly higher in PD patients with dopamine dysregulation syndrome (DDS) compared to those without DDS and correlated in the DDS cohort with them "wanting" but not "liking" the medication even if it produced unpleasant effects (Evans et al., 2006). [^{11}C]raclopride PET imaging has suggested that the development of ICDs is related to a drug-induced overstimulation of dopamine release in the ventral striatum (O'Sullivan et al., 2011; Steeves et al., 2009). Although no differences in D2R availability were observed at baseline and following levodopa challenge with neutral cues, PD patients with ICD showed greater decrease in ventral striatal [^{11}C]raclopride binding than those without ICD following exposure to reward-related cues (O'Sullivan et al., 2011). These findings suggest that as a result of neural sensitization in vulnerable individuals, reward-related cues are attributed with pathological incentive salience, leading to compulsive pursuit.

Activation of the nigrostriatal dopaminergic system appears to be relevant in determining placebo effect in PD. In the placebo group, reductions in striatal [^{11}C]raclopride binding were comparable to that observed in PD patients that received a therapeutic dose of apomorphine (de la Fuente-Fernandez, Lim, et al., 2001; de la Fuente-Fernandez, Lu, et al., 2001; de la Fuente-Fernandez, Ruth, et al., 2001). PD patients in the placebo group showed a decrease in [^{11}C]raclopride binding in the ventral striatum after placebo as compared to baseline. However, in contrast to the dorsal striatum, no differences in [^{11}C]raclopride binding were found between patients who experienced the reward and those who did not, suggesting that release of dopamine in the ventral striatum is related to the expectation of reward and not to the reward itself (de la Fuente-Fernandez et al., 2002).

1.1.2 Serotonergic System

Serotonergic system plays an important role in modulating cognition, emotion, and motor behavior and its dysfunction may contribute to the motor and nonmotor symptoms observed in PD (Pagano, Niccolini, Fusar-Poli, et al., 2017; Pagano, Niccolini, & Politis, 2016a, 2016b; Politis & Niccolini, 2015).

PET radioligands tagging serotonin targets have been used to assess the serotonergic system in PD patients (Politis & Niccolini, 2015; Schrag & Politis, 2016). [^{11}C]DASB, which binds to 5-HT transporter (SERT), is the most widely serotonergic radioligand used to image the serotonergic system (Wilson et al., 2000). PET with [^{11}C]DASB has shown global reductions of SERT density at different stages of the PD, which did not correlate with disease duration, motor disability, or chronic exposure to dopamine replacement therapy (Politis, Wu, Loane, Kiferle, et al., 2010; Politis, Wu, Loane, Quinn, et al., 2010; Politis, Wu, Loane, Turkheimer, et al., 2010). The pattern of serotonergic dysfunction in PD is different from that observed for dopaminergic system which greatly affects the posterior putamen (Brooks et al., 1990; Nurmi et al., 2000).

Serotonergic system may play an important role in the development of motor symptoms such as tremor. PET with [^{11}C]WAY100635, a selective marker of 5-HT_{1A} receptors, found that the midbrain raphe 5-HT_{1A} binding was reduced by 27% in PD patients compared to healthy controls and there was a significant correlation between reductions in midbrain raphe 5-HT_{1A} binding and the severity of tremor (Doder, Rabiner, Turjanski, Lees, & Brooks, 2003). PD patients with tremor-dominant phenotype had significant reductions in [^{11}C]DASB binding in caudate, putamen, raphe nuclei, thalamus, and Brodmann areas 4 and 10 compared with those who had akinetic-rigid PD and with a group of normal controls (Loane et al., 2013). Loss of SERT binding in caudate, putamen, and raphe nuclei in patients with tremor-dominant PD correlated with the severity of postural and action tremor, providing evidence for the role of presynaptic serotonergic terminal dysfunction in the development of tremor in PD (Loane et al., 2013).

Striatal serotonergic neurons are able to take up, convert exogenous levodopa into dopamine, and subsequently release it from the serotonergic terminals (Maeda, Nagata, Yoshida, & Kannari, 2005; Ng, Chase, & Kopin, 1970; Tanaka et al., 1999). This feature is of great interest in advanced stages of PD when the majority of the striatal dopaminergic terminals degenerated, and serotonin terminals might play a role in handling striatal synaptic dopamine concentrations following levodopa treatment. An in vivo [^{11}C]DASB PET study showed that although PD patients with LIDs had no difference in serotonergic terminal density compared with those who had a stable response to levodopa, similar levodopa doses induced markedly higher striatal synaptic dopamine concentrations in PD patients with LIDs compared with those with stable responses to levodopa (Politis, Wu, Loane, Brooks, et al., 2014; Politis, Wu, Loane, Quinn, et al., 2014). When buspirone, a 5-HT$_{1A}$ agonist, was administered before levodopa, it reduced the levodopa-evoked striatal synaptic dopamine increases and attenuated LIDs. Moreover, PD patients with LIDs who exhibited greater decreases in synaptic dopamine after buspirone pretreatment had higher levels of serotonergic terminal functional integrity (Politis, Wu, Loane, Brooks, et al., 2014; Politis, Wu, Loane, Quinn, et al., 2014). When PD patients with LIDs were divided into two groups depending on LIDs severity, buspirone-associated modulation of dopamine levels was greater in PD patients with milder LIDs compared to those with more severe LIDs (Politis, Wu, Loane, Brooks, et al., 2014; Politis, Wu, Loane, Quinn, et al., 2014). Overall the findings from this study provide the first human evidence for the role of striatal serotonergic ternimals in LIDs pathophysiology and support the development of selective 5-HT$_{1A}$ agonists for use as antidyskinetic agents in PD. Serotonin terminals are also involved in graft-induced dyskinesias (GIDs), which are involuntary movements when "off" dopaminergic drugs occurring after transplantation of fVM tissue (Kefalopoulou et al., 2014; Politis, Loane, et al., 2011; Politis, Oertel, et al., 2011; Politis, Wu, Loane, Kiferle, et al., 2010; Politis, Wu, Loane, Quinn, et al., 2010; Politis, Wu, Loane, Turkheimer, et al., 2010). [^{11}C]DASB and [^{18}F]dopa

PET studies have shown that three PD patients who received striatal transplantation with fVM tissue and exhibited GIDs had excessive graft-derived serotonergic innervation and high serotonin-to-dopamine terminal ratio (Politis, Loane, et al., 2011; Politis, Oertel, et al., 2011; Politis, Wu, Loane, Kiferle, et al., 2010; Politis, Wu, Loane, Quinn, et al., 2010; Politis, Wu, Loane, Turkheimer, et al., 2010). Administration of small, repeated doses of buspirone, was able to attenuate GIDs possibly by attenuating the abnormal serotonin terminal-derived dopamine release (Loane & Politis, 2012; Politis, 2010, 2011; Politis, Loane, et al., 2011; Politis, Oertel, et al., 2011; Politis, Wu, Loane, Kiferle, et al., 2010; Politis, Wu, Loane, Quinn, et al., 2010; Politis, Wu, Loane, Turkheimer, et al., 2010).

Serotonergic dysfunction has been implicated also in the pathogenesis of several PD nonmotor symptoms. [^{11}C]DASB PET studies have reported relative increases of SERT binding in limbic structures of depressed PD patients (Boileau et al., 2008; Politis, Wu, Loane, Kiferle, et al., 2010; Politis, Wu, Loane, Quinn, et al., 2010; Politis, Wu, Loane, Turkheimer, et al., 2010). Depressed PD patients had significantly increased [^{11}C]DASB binding in the amygdala, hypothalamus, caudal raphe nuclei, and posterior cingulate cortex compared to nondepressed PD patients which correlated with the severity of depressive symptoms (Politis, Wu, Loane, Kiferle, et al., 2010; Politis, Wu, Loane, Quinn, et al., 2010; Politis, Wu, Loane, Turkheimer, et al., 2010). These findings provide support for the use of agents acting on SERT for the treatment of PD depression.

SERT dysfunction has been also associated with body mass index (BMI) changes in PD patients (Politis, Loane, et al., 2011; Politis, Oertel, et al., 2011). PD patients with abnormal BMI changes over a 12-month period showed significantly increase of [^{11}C]DASB binding in rostral raphe nuclei, hypothalamus, caudate nucleus, and ventral striatum compared to those with no significant weight alterations (Politis, Loane, et al., 2011; Politis, Oertel, et al., 2011). Thus, BMI changes are associated to increased SERT availability in rostral raphe nuclei and its connections to limbic and cognitive areas. Serotonergic dysfunction may have relevance in the development of fatigue symptoms in PD. PD patients with fatigue had 66%–83% significant reductions in [^{11}C]DASB binding in the putamen, caudate nucleus, ventral striatum, thalamus, cingulate, and amygdala, compared to the PD patients without fatigue (Pavese, Metta, Bose, Chaudhuri, & Brooks, 2010). Serotonergic system is involved in the regulation of sleep, and its dysfunction could have relevance to the development of sleep problems in PD. Abnormalities in serotonin neurotransmission could be involved in the neural mechanisms underlying the development of visual hallucinations and psychosis in PD. PET with [^{18}F]setoperone, a selective 5-HT_{2A} receptor radioligand, showed increased 5-HT_{2A} binding in ventral visual pathway, dorsolateral prefrontal cortex, medial orbitofrontal cortex, and insula of PD patients with visual hallucinations (Ballanger et al., 2010). Moreover, pimavanserin, a selective 5-HT_{2A} antagonist/inverse agonist, has been recently approved by the FDA for treating the delusions and hallucinations associated with psychosis in PD (Cummings et al., 2014). Although transplanted PD patients showed improvement in their motor symptoms, they still suffered from nonmotor symptoms such as depression, fatigue, visual hallucinations, and sleep problems (Politis & Piccini, 2012). [^{11}C] DASB PET indicated decreased SERT binding in raphe nuclei and several brain regions receiving serotonergic projections in these PD patients, suggesting ongoing degeneration of serotonergic neurons despite the surgical-induced improvement in dopaminergic function (Politis & Piccini, 2012).

1.1.3 Cholinergic System

Although cholinergic interneurons represent only 1%–2% of the striatal neural population, they play a key role in the functional and structural remodeling of striatocortical circuits by enhancing both dopamine and GABA release and modulating striatal output (Schliebs & Arendt, 2011; Zhou, Wilson, & Dani, 2002). PET with selective radioligands targeting functional components of the cholinergic system, such as acetylcholinesterase (AChE), the nicotinic acetylcholine receptor (nAChR), and the muscarinic acetylcholine receptor (mAChR), has led to significant advances in the understanding of the neurobiology and pathophysiology of PD.

Evidence from postmortem studies indicates that both presynaptic and postsynaptic cholinergic markers are decreased in PD patients with and without dementia (Perry et al., 1993; Quik, Bordia, Forno, & McIntosh, 2004; Rinne, Laihinen, et al., 1991; Rinne, Myllykylä, et al., 1991; Schmaljohann et al., 2006; Shiozaki et al., 1999). Two selective SPECT radioligands, [^{123}I]-QNB and [^{123}I]-5IA, have been used to assess postsynaptic cholinergic system availability of M1 mAChR and $\alpha4\beta2$ nAChR, respectively (Colloby et al., 2005; Fujita et al., 2006; Isaias et al., 2014; Lorenz et al., 2014; Oishi et al., 2007). SPECT studies using [^{123}I]-5IA showed in early cognitively normal PD patients significantly higher nAChR density in the putamen, the insular cortex, and the supplementary motor area and lower in the caudate nucleus, the orbitofrontal cortex, and the middle temporal gyrus. Disease duration positively correlated with nAChR density in the putamen ipsilateral but not contralateral to the clinically most affected side (Isaias et al., 2014). Advanced PD patients without dementia showed a widespread nAChR decrease, ranging between 10% and 25%, in cortical and subcortical areas (Fujita et al., 2006; Lorenz et al., 2014; Oishi et al., 2007), and a significant correlation was found between cognitive dysfunction and cortical nAChR uptakes (Lorenz et al., 2014).

Two selective AChE radioligands: [^{11}C]PMP and [^{11}C]MP4A have been used to assess presynaptic cholinergic system integrity in PD patients (Iyo et al., 1997; Namba et al., 1998). PET studies using [^{11}C]MP4A and [^{11}C]PMP have demonstrated 11%–12% decreases in cortical and subcortical AChE activity in PD patients without dementia (Bohnen et al., 2006, 2012; Gilman et al., 2010; Shimada et al., 2009). Early de novo PD patients also showed significant 12% AChE losses in the medial occipital cortex, suggesting that loss of AChE activity occurs even in early stages of the disease (Shimada et al., 2009). However, differences in AChE activity between early and advanced PD patients were nonsignificant, suggesting that cholinergic dysfunction occurs early, but does not progress with the disease (Shimada et al., 2009). Cortical and thalamic cholinergic denervation as measured by [^{11}C]PMP PET were associated with increased falls, slower gait speed, and increased freezing of gait in PD patients, suggesting that cholinergic degeneration is a major factor leading to impaired postural control and gait dysfunction in PD (Bohnen et al., 2014, 2013, 2009).

Postsynaptic cholinergic function is also impaired in PD patients. Two PET studies with [^{11}C]NMPB, a marker for mAChR, demonstrated increased mAChR levels in the frontal cortex of PD patients which did not correlate with disease duration, motor, and cognitive symptoms severity (Asahina et al., 1995, 1998). The increased mAChR availability may represent denervation hypersensitivity caused by loss of the ascending cholinergic system in frontal areas.

Two PET studies have studied nAChR availability in PD patients using [^{18}F]2FA, a radioligand selective for $\alpha4\beta2$ nAChR (Kas et al., 2009; Meyer et al., 2009). Kas and colleagues (2009) found significant reduction in nAChR in the striatum and substantia nigra of nondemented PD patients, but no significant correlations were observed between decreased nAChR availability and disease duration and severity, dopaminergic medication intake, and [^{18}F]dopa uptake in PD patients. [^{18}F]2FA was decreased in several brain regions in PD patients, including the frontoparietal and anterior cingulate cortices, midbrain, pons, and cerebellum, with the highest reduction seen in the left parietal cortex (Meyer et al., 2009).

Dysfunction of the ascending cholinergic systems from the basal forebrain and brain stem and the associated loss of cholinergic neurotransmission in the cerebral cortex have been suggested as the underlying substrates of cognitive decline in dementia (Bartus, Dean, Beer, & Lippa, 1982). PET studies using [^{11}C]MP4A and [^{11}C]PMP have shown 20%–30% decreases in cortical AChE activity in PD with dementia (PDD) and dementia Lewy body (DLB) patients (Bohnen et al., 2006; Hilker, Schweitzer, et al., 2005; Hilker, Thomas, et al., 2005; Klein et al., 2010). Loss of cortical AChE activity as measured by [^{11}C]PMP correlated with worse performance in working memory and attention tests in PD patients (Bohnen et al., 2006). Moreover, in PDD patients, decreased striatal [^{18}F]dopa uptake correlated with cortical [^{11}C]MPA reduction, suggesting that cognitive decline in PD occurs when the disease spreads from nigral neurons to the cortex, leading to a cholinergic dysfunction in this region (Hilker, Schweitzer, et al., 2005; Hilker, Thomas, et al., 2005). Postsynaptic nAChR loss, as measured by [^{18}F]2FA PET, also correlated with depression and cognitive decline (Meyer et al., 2009).

With regards to other nonmotor symptoms, cholinergic denervation in neocortical, limbic, and thalamic regions was associated with rapid eye movement (REM) sleep behavior disorder (RBD) in PD (Kotagal et al., 2012).

It has been suggested that abnormal aggregation of α-synuclein in PD initially starts in the autonomic nerve endings of the gastrointestinal mucosa and then spreads in a prion-like fashion via the vagal nerve to the brain stem (Hawkes, Del Tredici, & Braak, 2007). Therefore, parasympathetic nervous system imaging could become an important biomarker for diagnosing prodromal disease. [^{11}C]donepezil PET has been recently validated for quantification of AChE density in peripheral organs (Gjerloff et al., 2014). In early-to-moderate stage PD patients, [^{11}C]donepezil binding was markedly decreased in the small intestine (−35%) and pancreas (−30%) compared with healthy controls, suggesting that systemic parasympathetic denervation can play a role in the pathogenesis of PD (Gjerløff et al., 2015).

1.1.4 Neuroinflammation

Microglia constitute 10%–20% of glial cells and represent the main form of immune defense in the central nervous system (CNS) (Kreutzberg, 1996). Following CNS injury, microglia become activated overexpress the 18-kDa translocator protein (TSPO) that is involved in the release of proinflammatory cytokines during inflammation and is present at very low levels in the normal healthy CNS (Banati, 2002). The upregulation of TSPO expression can be detected in vivo with PET and selective radioligands (Fujita et al., 2008; Ikoma et al., 2007; Oh et al., 2011; Owen et al., 2010, 2014; Su & Politis, 2012; Vas et al., 2008), and the most widely used TSPO radioligand to date is [^{11}C]PK11195 (Banati et al., 1999, 2000; Chauveau, Boutin, Van Camp, Dollé, & Tavitian, 2008). In early de novo PD patients, [^{11}C]PK11195 PET binding in the midbrain contralateral to the clinically affected side was significantly increased compared to a group of healthy controls and increased microglial activation was associated with putamen dopaminergic deficits and increased motor symptom severity (Ouchi et al., 2005). Moderate/advanced levodopa-treated PD patients showed widespread increases in [^{11}C]PK11195 binding in the pons, basal ganglia, and frontal and temporal cortical regions, which did not correlate with symptom severity and striatal dopaminergic deficits (Gerhard et al., 2006). Moreover, the levels of microglial activation remained stable over a period of 2 years (Gerhard et al., 2006). [^{11}C]PK11195 binding was also increased in the anterior and posterior cingulate, striatum, frontal, temporal, parietal, and occipital cortical regions in PDD patients (Edison et al., 2013) and in the substantia nigra, putamen, and several associative cortices of DLB patients (Iannaccone et al., 2013).

However, evaluation of microglial activation using [^{11}C]PK11195 is hampered by unfavorable radioligand characteristics (Chauveau et al., 2008). [^{11}C]PK11195 shows high level of nonspecific binding and a poor signal-to-noise ratio (Petit-Taboué et al., 1991), which complicates its quantification; moreover, test–retest data in control subjects showed only moderate intraindividual reproducibility (Jučaite et al., 2012). Second-generation TSPO radioligands for PET imaging provide a better quantification of microglial activation, although they present three patterns of binding affinity based on genetic polymorphism: high-affinity, mixed-affinity, and low-affinity binders (Owen et al., 2011) which require genotype screening before enrolling the subjects in the study. A recent study using the second-generation TSPO radioligand [^{18}F]FEPPA showed that striatal microglial activation was increased by 16% in both caudate nucleus and putamen of high-affinity binders but not in mixed-affinity binders PD patients compared to the group of healthy controls (Koshimori et al., 2015). The second-generation TSPO radioligand, [^{11}C]PBR28, was used to assess the efficacy of AZD3241, a selective and irreversible myeloperoxidase inhibitor, in reducing neuroinflammation in a small cohort of PD patients (Jucaite et al., 2015). This double-blind and placebo-controlled study showed that 8 weeks treatment with AZD3241 was able to decrease

[^{11}C]PBR28 binding across cortical and subcortical brain regions as compared to baseline (Jucaite et al., 2015).

Thus, microglial activation may contribute to the neurodegenerative processes in PD and drugs aiming to decrease neuroinflammation in the brain of PD patients may be aid in slowing down disease progression.

1.1.5 Misfolded Proteins

PD is neuropathologically characterized by Lewy body intracellular inclusions that are rich in α-synuclein (Harding & Halliday, 2001). However, extracellular Aβ-amyloid plaques and intracellular tau neurofibrillary tangle are also observed at autopsy in PD, PDD, and DLB patients (Horvath, Herrmann, Burkhard, Bouras, & Kövari, 2013; Jellinger & Attems, 2008; Jellinger, Seppi, Wenning, & Poewe, 2002).

PET studies with the thioflavin derivative ligand [^{11}C]Pittsburgh compound-B (PiB) and related clinically approved radiofluorinated tracers including [^{18}F]Florbetapir, [^{18}F]Florbetaben, and [^{18}F]Flutemetamol have investigated the role of amyloid deposition in PD, PDD, and DLB. Overall these studies found that amyloid deposition tends to be modest in PD with normal cognition occurring in about 0%–13% of PD patients (Edison et al., 2013, 2008; Foster et al., 2010; Gomperts et al., 2012, 2008; Johansson et al., 2008; Jokinen et al., 2010; Maetzler et al., 2009; Siderowf et al., 2014; Villemagne et al., 2011). Amyloid burden is generally low in PD subjects with mild cognitive impairment (MCI), and does not distinguish cognitively normal PD patients from PD-MCI (Foster et al., 2010; Gomperts et al., 2012, 2013; Petrou et al., 2012). PDD patients have higher incidence of cortical Aβ-amyloid deposition compared to healthy subjects, PD and PD-MCI, ranging from 0% to 80% (Edison et al., 2013, 2008; Foster et al., 2010; Gomperts et al., 2012, 2008; Jokinen et al., 2010; Maetzler et al., 2009, 2008). Amyloid burden in PDD patients is heterogeneous with cases of PDD, where amyloid deposition overlaps with the levels observed in healthy subjects and in PD patients (Edison et al., 2013, 2008; Foster et al., 2010; Gomperts et al., 2012, 2008; Jokinen et al., 2010; Maetzler et al., 2009, 2008) and other cases of PDD showing elevated cortical amyloid deposition in the Alzheimer's disease (AD) range (Edison et al., 2013, 2008; Foster et al., 2010; Gomperts et al., 2012; Jokinen et al., 2010; Maetzler et al., 2009, 2008; Shimada et al., 2013). In contrast, amyloid burden is usually elevated in DLB patients compared to healthy subjects and PD patients and the incidence ranges between 33% and 100% (Burke et al., 2011; Claassen, Lowe, Peller, Petersen, & Josephs, 2011; Edison et al.,

2008; Foster et al., 2010; Gomperts et al., 2012, 2008; Graff-Radford et al., 2012; Kantarci et al., 2012; Maetzler et al., 2009, 2008; Rowe et al., 2007; Siderowf et al., 2014; Villemagne et al., 2011).

Similarly to healthy subjects, apolipoprotein ε4 allele and older age are risk factors for increased cortical amyloid burden in DLB and PDD patients (Gomperts et al., 2012; Maetzler et al., 2009; Rowe et al., 2007). Global amyloid deposition has been associated to worse cognitive performance (Foster et al., 2010; Gomperts et al., 2013; Petrou et al., 2012; Villemagne et al., 2011), and the absence of cortical amyloid deposition was associated with a better response to ACh inhibitors (Burke et al., 2011). The clinical significance of amyloid burden in Lewy bodies diseases is still unclear, but it has been suggested that early and significant cortical amyloid burden may accelerate cognitive decline as a result of synergistic Aβ–α-synuclein neurotoxicity. A longitudinal PET study has shown that nondemented PD patients with higher amyloid burden have baseline progressed to cognitive impairment faster than those with lower amyloid burden over a period of 5 years (Gomperts et al., 2013). Thus, higher amyloid burden in cognitively normal PD patients may predict cognitive decline.

Moreover, postural instability and gait difficulty in PD patients was associated with increased neocortical [^{11}C]PiB retention, suggesting that cortical amyloidopathy may play a role on the etiology of balance and gait impairments (Müller et al., 2013).

A recent PET study using [^{18}F]T807 investigated tau deposition in DLB, PD with and without cognitive impairment (Gomperts et al., 2016). Cortical [^{18}F]T807 uptake was higher in the DLB and PD with cognitive impairment than healthy controls with in low-amyloid pathology, and higher uptake was observed in the inferolateral temporal and parietal/precuneus regions (Gomperts et al., 2016). Tau deposition was more variable in DLB patients and was lower in magnitude and extent in PD with cognitive impairment, whereas PD patients without cognitive impairment showed no evidence for tau deposition (Gomperts et al., 2016). These findings suggest that, beside α-synuclein, also tau pathology may play a role in determining cognitive dysfunction in Lewy body diseases.

1.1.6 Other Systems

1.1.6.1 Glutamate

Increased glutamatergic transmission may play a role in the pathogenesis of LIDs, and a PET study using [^{11}C]CNS51619, a marker of activated NMDA receptors, has shown increased [^{11}C]CNS5161 uptake in caudate, putamen, and precentral gyrus in PD patients with LIDs in ON condition (Ahmed et al., 2011). However, [^{11}C]CNS51619 uptake did not differ between PD patients with LIDs and those with stable response to levodopa when patients were scanned in OFF condition, suggesting that increased glutamatergic transmission may be involved in the development of LIDs (Ahmed et al., 2011).

1.1.6.2 Cannabinoid

Cannabinoid type 1 receptors (CB1Rs) are expressed in the basal ganglia where they regulate intracellular levels of cAMP by interacting with Gi/o and Gs proteins in the *direct* and *indirect* pathways, respectively (Glass, Dragunow, & Faull, 1997; Herkenham et al., 1991; Mailleux & Vanderhaeghen, 1992; Martín et al., 2008). A PET study using [^{18}F]MK-9470 has shown significant decreases in CB1R levels in the substantia nigra of early de novo and advanced PD patients with and without LIDs (van Laere et al., 2012). However, no differences were found in regional CB1R availability between advanced PD patients with and without LIDs and regional CB1R levels were not associated with LIDs severity (van Laere et al., 2012). Further studies using higher selective CB1R PET radioligands are needed in order to further elucidate the role of these receptors in the pathophysiology of PD.

1.1.6.3 Opioid

All three opioid receptors (μ, κ, and δ) are involved in regulating dopaminergic signaling in the basal ganglia (Samadi, Bedard, & Rouillard, 2006). Two PET studies using [^{11}C]diprenorphine, a nonselective opioid receptor antagonist, have investigated cortical and subcortical opioid receptor availability in PD patients (Burn et al., 1995; Piccini, Weeks, & Brooks, 1997). Burn and colleagues (1995) found no differences in striatal opioid receptor levels between PD patients and healthy controls, whereas mean striatal opioid receptor binding was significant decreased in patients with progressive supranuclear palsy (PSP)–Richardson compared to PD patients and healthy controls. When comparing PD patients with and without LIDs, Piccini and colleagues (1997) found reduced striatal, thalamic, and cingulate and increased prefrontal opioid binding in PD patients with LIDs. However, there were no correlations between [^{11}C]diprenorphine binding and PD severity, disease duration, or duration of levodopa treatment (Piccini et al., 1997). Thus, the role of opioid receptors in the pathophysiology of

PD and its complication remains unclear and further PET studies using more selective opioid radioligands could aid in elucidating the role of the opioid system in PD.

1.1.6.4 Adenosine

Adenosine modulates dopaminergic signaling by acting on A_{2A} adenosine receptors (A_{2A}Rs). These receptors are mainly expressed in the striatopallidal medium spiny neurons (*indirect* pathway) where they stimulate adenylate cyclase and interact with dopamine D2R negatively at the level of second messengers (Fredholm & Svenningsson, 2003). Two PET studies using [^{11}C]TMSX and [^{11}C]SCH442,416, both markers of A_{2A}Rs, have shown increased striatal A_{2A}Rs in PD patients with LIDs (Mishina et al., 2011; Ramlackhansingh et al., 2011). Moreover, in de novo PD patients, [^{11}C]TMSX binding was significantly decreased in the putamen but not in the caudate on the most affected side and A_{2A}Rs availability was increased in the putamen following antiparkinsonian therapy (Mishina et al., 2011). These findings suggest that increased striatal A_{2A}R availability is involved in the pathophysiology of LIDs, and at the early stage of the disease A_{2A}R in the putamen may compensate for in the putamen compensate for the asymmetrical decrease of dopamine.

1.1.6.5 Phosphodiesterases

Phosphodiesterases (PDEs) are intracellular enzyme that modulate the activation of G-proteins through the hydrolysis of cyclic nucleotides, such as cAMP and cGMP, and play an important role in cell signal transduction (Fujishige, Kotera, & Omori, 1999). Among PDEs family, PDE10A is expressed almost exclusively in the striatum (Coskran et al., 2006; Lakics, Karran, & Boess, 2010), where it modulates cAMP/PKA/DARPP-32 signaling cascade thus having a key role in the regulation of striatal output and in promoting neuronal survival (Girault, 2012; Nishi et al., 2008). Using [^{11}C]IMA107 PET, our group has recently investigated PDE10A expression in 24 levodopa-treated moderate to advanced PD patients (Niccolini, Foltynie, et al., 2015; Niccolini, Haider, et al., 2015). PD patients showed lower [^{11}C]IMA107 binding in the caudate, putamen, and pallidum compared to healthy controls. Longer PD duration and higher UPDRS-III motor scores correlated with lower [^{11}C]IMA107 binding in the caudate, putamen, and pallidum (Niccolini, Foltynie, et al., 2015; Niccolini, Haider, et al., 2015). Higher Unified Dyskinesia Rating Scale (UDysRS) scores in those PD patients with levodopa-induced dyskinesias correlated with lower [^{11}C]IMA107 binding in the caudate and putamen. These findings provide evidence for the role of PDE10A in the development of PD motor symptoms and complications. Positive evidence on the role of PDE10A in movement disorders comes from recent genetic studies on PDE10A gene mutations (Diggle et al., 2016; Mencacci et al., 2016). Patients with homozygous (Diggle et al., 2016) and heterozygous (Mencacci et al., 2016) PDE10A mutation present with benign childhood-onset chorea that may be followed by adult-onset levodopa-responsive parkinsonism (Mencacci et al., 2016). Moreover, PET molecular studies using [^{11}C]IMA107, [^{18}F]MNI-659, and [^{18}F]JNJ42259152 have shown 30%–70% reduction of striatal PDE10A in Huntington's disease gene-expansion carriers (HDGECs) (Pagano, Niccolini, Fusar-Poli, et al., 2017; Pagano, Niccolini, & Politis, 2016a, 2016b) spanning from far-onset premanifest stages (Niccolini, Foltynie, et al., 2015; Niccolini, Haider, et al., 2015) to early manifest (Russell et al., 2014, 2016) and advanced (Ahmad et al., 2014) manifest HDGECs. Thus, PDE10A activity is critical for the control of movements and for neuronal survival and could serve as a novel therapeutic target for manipulation with pharmacotherapy in the neuropathological salient circuits, which promote neuronal survival and control of movements.

1.1.6.6 Sigma 1 Receptors

Sigma 1 receptor (S1R) is considered a marker of the mitochondrion-associated endoplasmic reticulum (ER) membrane involved in the regulation mitochondrial activity via Ca^{2+} influx (Hayashi & Su, 2007). S1R plays a role in a wide variety of cellular functions, including regulation of ion channels, synaptogenesis, and neuronal plasticity (Hayashi & Su, 2007; Renaudo, L'Hoste, Guizouarn, Borgèse, & Soriani, 2007). S1R functions as a molecular chaperone in the ER, which facilitates the proper folding of newly synthesized proteins, but also prevents accumulation of misfolded proteins such as α-synuclein, suggesting that S1R plays a key role in cellular survival (Hayashi & Su, 2007). Moreover, preclinical studies have shown that S1R stimulates striatal dopamine synthesis in rats (Booth & Baldessarini, 1991; Chaki, Okuyama, Ogawa, & Tomisawa, 1998). A small PET study using [^{11}C]SA4503, a S1R agonist, has demonstrated marked decreases of S1R levels in the anterior putamen on the most affected side of in six PD patients providing preliminary evidence for the involvement of S1R in PD (Mishina et al., 2005).

1.2 Magnetic Resonance Imaging

1.2.1 Volumetric MRI

Gray matter (GM) changes have been assessed with voxel-based morphometry and cortical thickness analyses in PD.

Structural MRI studies have mainly focussed on regional GM changes associated with cognitive impairment in PD patients. The general consensus suggests widespread cortical atrophy in PDD, although it is less severe compared to AD and DLB (Beyer, Larsen, & Aarsland, 2007; Burton, McKeith, Burn, Williams, & O'Brien, 2004). Cortical atrophy progresses linearly across the cognitive stages in PD and affects temporal, frontal, parietal (Beyer et al., 2007; Burton et al., 2004; Melzer et al., 2012; Pagonabarraga et al., 2013; Tam, Burton, McKeith, Burn, & O'Brien, 2005; Weintraub et al., 2011; Zarei et al., 2013), and less commonly, occipital regions (Burton et al., 2004). Subcortical GM changes can also occur in PDD and affect mainly the hippocampus (Apostolova et al., 2010; Camicioli et al., 2003; Junque et al., 2005; Zarei et al., 2013), thalamus (Burton et al., 2004), putamen (Burton et al., 2004), amygdala (Junque et al., 2005; Zarei et al., 2013), and the caudate (Apostolova et al., 2010; Burton et al., 2004). Regional atrophy in temporal, parietal, and frontal cortices (Melzer et al., 2012; Pagonabarraga et al., 2013; Pereira et al., 2014; Segura et al., 2014; Weintraub et al., 2011) and thalamus (Mak, Bergsland, Dwyer, Zivadinov, & Kandiah, 2014) and hippocampus (Weintraub et al., 2011) has been observed in PD-MCI.

Longitudinal assessment using brain boundary shift integral demonstrated higher rates of global atrophy in PDD (1.12%) compared to nondemented PD patients (0.31%) and control subjects (0.34%) (Burton, McKeith, Burn, & O'Brien, 2005). Additionally, longitudinal analyses of cortical thinning patterns showed that frontal cortical thinning could be a risk factor for the development of PDD (Compta et al., 2013). Nondemented PD patients also presented a more aggressive rate of cortical thinning with a bilateral frontotemporal pattern than healthy subjects (Compta et al., 2013; Ibarretxe-Bilbao et al., 2012; Mak et al., 2015).

Cortical thinning in the parietotemporal association cortex was also associated with longer disease duration, severity of motor symptoms, and in specific with worse bradykinesia and axial motor deficits but not with rigidity and tremor (Lyoo, Ryu, & Lee, 2011). Increased cortical thickness in the right inferior frontal sulcus was observed in PD patients with LIDs supporting the role of the prefrontal cortex in the pathophysiology of LID (Cerasa, Morelli, et al., 2013). Moreover, early-onset dyskinetic patients showed increased volume in substantia nigra and red nucleus, whereas late-onset dyskinetic patients were characterized by abnormal GM increase in the supplementary motor area (Cerasa, Salsone, et al., 2013).

Mood disorders were also associated with cortical and subcortical changes in PD patients (Carriere et al., 2014; Huang et al., 2016). Surface-based morphometric analysis showed that depressed PD patients had significant cortical thickness in the orbitofrontal regions and insula compared to nondepressed PD patients (Huang et al., 2016), and apathy in PD patients was associated with atrophy of the left nucleus accumbens (Carriere et al., 2014). PD patients who experienced visual hallucinations had significant loss of GM volume in the lingual gyrus and superior parietal lobe compared to healthy controls and PD patients without visual hallucinations (Ramírez-Ruiz et al., 2007). PD patients with probable RBD showed volume loss in the pontomesencephalic tegmentum, medullary reticular formation, hypothalamus, thalamus, putamen, amygdala, and anterior cingulate cortex compared to healthy controls and PD patients without RBD (Boucetta et al., 2016). Structural cortical and subcortical changes in mesocortical and limbic reward-related areas have been observed in PD patients with ICDs. These changes consist in volume loss in nucleus accumbens, caudate, hippocampus, and amygdala (Biundo et al., 2015; Pellicano et al., 2015) as well as increased thickening of anterior cingulate, frontal pole, and orbitofrontal cortices in PD patients with ICDs (Pellicano et al., 2015; Tessitore et al., 2016). These patterns of cortical and subcortical GM changes may be due to maladaptive synaptic plasticity under nonphysiological dopaminergic in patients with a preexisting vulnerability to impulsivity.

1.2.2 Iron Deposition and Neuromelanin

Iron accumulation in the brain can be detected in brain nuclei using sequences sensitive to local magnetic field in homogeneities, such as T2 and T2*, and susceptibility-weighted imaging (SWI) which combines T2* and phase information, increasing the sensitivity to iron (Haacke et al., 2009).

PD patients showed increased iron deposition in the substantia nigra *pars compacta*, putamen, and globus pallidus (Kosta, Argyropoulou, Markoula, & Konitsiotis, 2006) and substantia nigra *pars compacta* and red nucleus correlated with higher UPDRS scores (Lewis et al., 2013; Wallis et al., 2008). Over a 3-year follow-up, increased R2* in the substantia nigra correlated with the worsening of motor symptoms of PD, suggesting that R2* may be a biomarker of disease progression in PD (Ulla et al., 2013). Association between high R2* signal and LIDs has yielded inconsistent results either showing a positive (Bunzeck et al., 2013) or no correlations (Wieler, Gee, & Martin, 2015) between iron deposition and motor complications. Early-onset PD patients showed a higher field-dependent R2 increases in the substantia nigra, putamen, and pallidum, which decreases as the disease progresses, suggesting that dysregulation of iron metabolism occurs in PD (Bartzokis et al., 1999).

SWI studies showed lower levels of phase radians in the substantia nigra *pars compacta* as well as in the caudate nuclei and red nucleus, with higher phase shift in substantia nigra *pars compacta* and basal ganglia, were found in PD patients, indicating an increased iron content which correlated with UPDRS scores (Martin-Bastida et al., 2017; Zhang et al., 2009, 2010).

Nigrosomes are small clusters of dopaminergic cells within the substantia nigra exhibiting calbindin D_{28K} negativity on immunohistochemical staining (Damier, Hirsch, Agid, & Graybiel, 1999). Nigrosome-1 is located in the posterior third of the substantia nigra *pars compacta* and presents high signal on SWI sequences. The healthy nigrosome-1 appears as a "swallow tail" on 3T-SWI sequences, this feature is lost in PD (Blazejewska et al., 2013; Schwarz et al., 2014). Thus, assessing substantia nigra on SWI sequences for the typical "swallow tail" appearance may be an easy applicable 3T MRI diagnostic tool for nigral degeneration in PD.

Neuromelanin is produced by the noradrenergic neurons and is mainly expressed in the neurons of substantia nigra *pars compacta*, ventral tegmental area, and locus coeruleus (Bazelon, Fenichel, & Randall, 1967). T1-weighted "neuromelanin-sensitive" MRI sequences have been developed to identify and characterize the substantia nigra *pars compacta* and locus coeruleus in vivo in PD (Ohtsuka et al., 2013; Sasaki et al., 2006). Loss of neuromelanin-related signal intensity in the substantia nigra *pars compacta* was observed in PD patients and correlated H&Y stages (Kashihara, Shinya, & Higaki, 2011; Matsuura et al., 2013; Schwarz et al., 2011). Additionally, neuromelanin-rich volumes loss follow a specific spatial pattern starting from posterior part of the substantia nigra *pars compacta* and as the disease progresses, including the anterior part of the substantia nigra *pars compacta* and locus coeruleus (Schwarz, Xing, Tomar, Bajaj, & Auer, 2016). Neuromelanin-rich volumes loss in the substantia nigra *pars compacta* significantly correlated with disease severity, as measured by the UPDRS (Schwarz et al., 2016).

1.2.3 Structural Connectivity

Diffusion-weighted imaging and diffusion tensor imaging (DTI) represent advanced morphological approaches useful to detect changes in white matter (WM) integrity (Le Bihan, 2003). The most common finding in many DTI studies was a reduction in fractional anisotropy (FA) in the substantia nigra of PD patients (Chan et al., 2007; Du et al., 2011; Péran et al., 2010; Vaillancourt et al., 2009; Yoshikawa, Nakata, Yamada, & Nakagawa, 2004), and the reduction in FA values in the substantia nigra was inversely correlated with the severity of the clinical symptoms of PD patient (Chan et al., 2007). Extranigral WM changes have been observed in PD patients. Whole-brain DTI approach has detected distinct pattern of microstructural abnormalities in the thalamus, motor, premotor, supplementary motor cortical areas, and somatosensory areas, which correlated with the severity of motor symptoms (Zhan et al., 2012). PD patients with freezing of gait had extensive WM damage in the intrahemispheric cortical areas, motor-related corticofugal, and several basal ganglia WM tracts projecting to motor, sensory, and cognitive frontal regions in the brain (Vercruysse et al., 2015). PD patients with hyposmia or anosmia showed a reduced FA in the WM adjacent to gyrus rectus bilaterally compared to healthy subjects and PD patients without olfactory dysfunction (Ibarretxe-Bilbao et al., 2010). WM tissue loss has been found in cognitive impaired PD patients (Agosta et al., 2014). FA reduction in the bilateral posterior cingulate bundles was found in PDD patients compared with cognitively normal PD patients and significant correlations between these microstructural changes and cognitive parameters were also detected (Matsui et al., 2007). Executive dysfunction, language, and attentional performance in PD were associated with WM abnormalities within frontal connecting tracts (Zheng et al., 2014). Attention domain additionally recruited regions widespread throughout the brain, with the most significant correlation identified in cingulate gyrus, whereas memory impairment mainly involved mean diffusivity alterations within the fornix (Zheng et al., 2014). DTI studies may be useful also in differentiating PD from other atypical parkinsonism such as multiple system atrophy and PSP where WM abnormalities were seen also in the brain stem and cerebellum (Blain et al., 2006; Ito et al., 2007).

1.2.4 Functional Connectivity

Functional connectivity can be assessed with resting-state functional MRI (rs-fMRI), which measure the blood oxygenation level-dependent signal when subjects are positioned in the scanner in an awake-state without performing any particular task.

Seed-based rs-fMRI studies have shown that advanced PD had reduced functional connectivity between the striatum and several regions, including the thalamus, midbrain, pons, and cerebellum, and the degree of these abnormalities were associated with UPDRS scores (Hacker, Perlmutter, Criswell, Ances, & Snyder, 2012). Changes in functional connectivity with increased functional connectivity in the globus pallidus-cerebello-thalamic circuit were also observed in tremor-dominant PD patients (Helmich, Janssen, Oyen, Bloem, & Toni, 2011). A longitudinal study showed progressive functional connectivity disruption in the posterior cortical areas over a period of 3 years, which correlated with cognitive decline in PD patients (Olde Dubbelink et al., 2014). Several rs-fMRI studies have applied network-based method in PD patients and shown alterations to motor networks (Tessitore et al., 2012). PD patients compared with controls had decreased functional connectivity between posterior putamen with cingulate motor area, postcentral gyrus, and inferior parietal cortex, and increased functional connectivity between anterior putamen and inferior parietal cortex, and in PD patients the precentral gyrus was connected with posterior putamen, while the inferior parietal cortex connected with the anterior putamen (Helmich et al., 2010). These findings suggest that compensatory alterations within the corticostriatal network occur in PD with increased connectivity in the anterior putamen in comparison with the posterior putamen, consistent with the posterior putamen's earlier and greater dopaminergic dysfunction in PD (Brooks & Pavese, 2011). In addition to striatal network, increased functional connectivity between the subthalamic nucleus and cortex in PD has also been observed (Fernandez-Seara et al., 2015; Kahan et al., 2014). PDD patients showed selective disruption of corticostriatal connectivity (Seibert, Murphy, Kaestner, & Brewer, 2012), specifically, the connectivity of the so-called default mode network, was disrupted in PD patients with cognitive deficits (Disbrow et al., 2014; Gorges et al., 2015). Abnormal prefrontal limbic network connectivity was found in depressed PD patients (Luo et al., 2014; Surdhar et al., 2012), and PD patients with depression showed disrupted functional connectivity between the median cingulate cortex and precuneus, prefrontal cortex, and cerebellum (Hu et al., 2015). Visual hallucinations in PD were associated with functional abnormalities in the occipital corticostriatal network (Meppelink et al., 2009; Yao et al., 2015). Abnormal functional connectivity within the neural network centered on the inferior frontal cortex was found in PD patients with LIDs (Cerasa et al., 2015; Herz et al., 2015, 2016).

1.2.5 Task-Related Functional MRI

Several task-related fMRI studies have investigated brain activity in patients with PD in order to elucidate pathophysiological mechanisms underlying PD symptoms and complications. The most frequently studied tasks in PD neuroimaging have been motor tasks (finger and hand). Overall these studies showed decreased activation in the right posterior putamen but increased activation in left superior parietal lobule (Herz, Eickhoff, Lokkegaard, & Siebner, 2014). Inconsistent results were yielded by studies investigating functional brain activation in ON vs OFF dopaminergic medication condition. Some studies reported increased and others decreased activation of the presupplementary motor area, putamen, and middle frontal gyrus in PD patients (Herz et al., 2014).

Additional fMRI studies have investigated brain activation using different tasks such as motor or motor sequence learning (Burciu et al., 2015; Gonzalez-Garcia et al., 2011; Herz et al., 2015; Jahanshahi et al., 2010; Ko et al., 2013; Mure et al., 2012; Van Nuenen et al., 2009; Weiss et al., 2015; Wu, Long, et al., 2011; Wu, Wang, et al., 2011), selection (MacDonald et al., 2011), affective face processing (Anders et al., 2012), virtual reality gait (Shine et al., 2013), visuomotor tracking (Palmer, Li, Wang, & McKeown, 2010), and visual tasks that can identify patients with hallucinations (Shine et al., 2014). fMRI studies investigated also the neural visual-cue response in PD with ICD (Loane et al., 2015; Politis et al., 2013). PD patients with hypersexuality following exposure to sexual cues showed significantly increased sexual desire and hedonic responses and enhanced activations in the ventral striatum, and cingulate and orbitofrontal cortices compared with the PD control patients (Politis et al., 2013). When the hypersexuality PD patients were OFF medication, the functional imaging data showed decreases in activation during the presentation of sexual cues relative to rest. These deactivations were not observed when the patients were ON medication, suggesting that dopamine drugs may release inhibition within local neuronal circuits in the cerebral cortex that may contribute to compulsive sexual behavior (Politis et al., 2013). Following drug cue exposure, also PD DDS felt significantly more ON medication and this correlated with significant increases in reward-related regions, suggesting that visual stimuli are sufficient to elicit behavioral response (Loane et al., 2015).

2. CONCLUSIONS AND FUTURE DIRECTIONS

SPECT, PET molecular, and MR imaging have provided a new insight into PD pathophysiology showing that the pathological processes in PD are not only confined within the dopaminergic system as there is a more diffuse pathology involving other, nondopaminergic systems. Among these imaging modalities, PET has the potential to provide a unique tool for the direct evaluation of human in vivo neurochemistry and has become an indispensable part of CNS drug development. Despite the several efforts, a radioligand able to bind to intracellular α-synuclein aggregates has not yet been developed. The development of such biomarker will have widespread application in understanding the pathophysiology, monitoring the progression and response to treatment of PD and other Lewy bodies diseases.

ACKNOWLEDGMENTS

M.P. research is supported by Parkinson's UK, Lily and Edmond J. Safra Foundation, Michael J. Fox Foundation (MJFF) for Parkinson's research, and KCL's NIHR Biomedical Research Unit. G.P. research is supported by Lily and Edmond J. Safra Foundation.

Potential Conflicts of Interest. No potential conflict of interest relevant to this article was reported.

REFERENCES

Agosta, F., Canu, E., Stefanova, E., Sarro, L., Tomic, A., Spica, V., et al. (2014). Mild cognitive impairment in Parkinson's disease is associated with a distributed pattern of brain white matter damage. *Human Brain Mapping*, *35*, 1921–1929.

Ahmad, R., Bourgeois, S., Postnov, A., Schmidt, M. E., Bormans, G., Van Laere, K., et al. (2014). PET imaging shows loss of striatal PDE10A in patients with Huntington disease. *Neurology*, *82*(3), 279–281.

Ahmed, I., Bose, S., Pavese, N., Ramlackhansingh, A., Turkheimer, F., Hotton, G., et al. (2011). Glutamate NMDA receptor dysregulation in Parkinson's disease with dyskinesias. *Brain*, *134*, 979–986.

Anders, S., Sack, B., Pohl, A., Münte, T., Pramstaller, P., Klein, C., et al. (2012). Compensatory premotor activity during affective face processing in subclinical carriers of a single mutant Parkin allele. *Brain*, *135*, 1128–1140.

Antonini, A., Schwarz, J., Oertel, W. H., Pogarell, O., & Leenders, K. L. (1997). Long-term changes of striatal dopamine D2 receptors in patients with Parkinson's disease: A study with positron emission tomography and [11C]raclopride. *Movement Disorders*, *12*(1), 33–38.

Apostolova, L. G., Beyer, M., Green, A. E., Hwang, K. S., Morra, J. H., Chou, Y. Y., et al. (2010). Hippocampal, caudate, and ventricular changes in Parkinson's disease with and without dementia. *Movement Disorders*, *25*, 687–695.

Asahina, M., Shinotoh, H., Hirayama, K., Suhara, T., Shishido, F., Inoue, O., et al. (1995). Hypersensitivity of cortical muscarinic receptors in Parkinson's disease demonstrated by PET. *Acta Neurologica Scandinavica, 91*(6), 437–443.
Asahina, M., Suhara, T., Shinotoh, H., Inoue, O., Suzuki, K., & Hattori, T. (1998). Brain muscarinic receptors in progressive supranuclear palsy and Parkinson's disease: A positron emission tomographic study. *Journal of Neurology, Neurosurgery, and Psychiatry, 65*(2), 155–163.
Ballanger, B., Strafella, A. P., van Eimeren, T., Zurowski, M., Rusjan, P. M., Houle, S., et al. (2010). Serotonin 2A receptors and visual hallucinations in Parkinson disease. *Archives of Neurology, 67*(4), 416–421.
Banati, R. B. (2002). Visualising microglial activation in vivo. *Glia, 40*, 206–217.
Banati, R. B., Goerres, G. W., Myers, R., Gunn, R. N., Turkheimer, F. E., Kreutzberg, G. W., et al. (1999). [11C](R)-PK11195 positron emission tomography imaging of activated microglia in vivo in Rasmussen's encephalitis. *Neurology, 53*, 2199–2203.
Banati, R. B., Newcombe, J., Gunn, R. N., Cagnin, A., Turkheimer, F., Heppner, F., et al. (2000). The peripheral benzodiazepine binding site in the brain in multiple sclerosis: Quantitative in vivo imaging of microglia as a measure of disease activity. *Brain, 123*, 2321–2337.
Bartus, R. T., Dean, R. L., 3rd., Beer, B., & Lippa, A. S. (1982). The cholinergic hypothesis of geriatric memory dysfunction. *Science (New York, NY), 217*, 408–414.
Bartzokis, G., Cummings, J. L., Markham, C. H., Marmarelis, P. Z., Treciokas, L. J., Tishler, T. A., et al. (1999). MRI evaluation of brain iron in earlier- and later-onset Parkinson's disease and normal subjects. *Magnetic Resonance Imaging, 17*, 213–222.
Bazelon, M., Fenichel, G. M., & Randall, J. (1967). Studies on neuromelanin. I. A melanin system in the human adult brainstem. *Neurology, 17*(5), 512–519.
Beyer, M. K., Larsen, J. P., & Aarsland, D. (2007). Gray matter atrophy in Parkinson disease with dementia and dementia with Lewy bodies. *Neurology, 69*, 747–754.
Biundo, R., Weis, L., Facchini, S., Formento-Dojot, P., Vallelunga, A., Pilleri, M., et al. (2015). Patterns of cortical thickness associated with impulse control disorders in Parkinson's disease. *Movement Disorders, 30*(5), 688–695.
Blain, C. R., Barker, G. J., Jarosz, J. M., Coyle, N. A., Landau, S., Brown, R. G., et al. (2006). Measuring brain stem and cerebellar damage in parkinsonian syndromes using diffusion tensor MRI. *Neurology, 67*, 2199–2205.
Blazejewska, A. I., Schwarz, S. T., Pitiot, A., Stephenson, M. C., Lowe, J., Bajaj, N., et al. (2013). Visualization of nigrosome 1 and its loss in PD: Pathoanatomical correlation and in vivo 7T MRI. *Neurology, 81*, 534–540.
Bohnen, N. I., Frey, K. A., Studenski, S., Kotagal, V., Koeppe, R. A., Constantine, G. M., et al. (2014). Extra-nigral pathological conditions are common in Parkinson's disease with freezing of gait: An in vivo positron emission tomography study. *Movement Disorders, 29*(9), 1118–1124.
Bohnen, N. I., Frey, K. A., Studenski, S., Kotagal, V., Koeppe, R. A., Scott, P. J., et al. (2013). Gait speed in Parkinson disease correlates with cholinergic degeneration. *Neurology, 81*(18), 1611–1616.
Bohnen, N. I., Kaufer, D. I., Hendrickson, R., Ivanco, L. S., Lopresti, B. J., Constantine, G. M., et al. (2006). Cognitive correlates of cortical cholinergic denervation in Parkinson's disease and parkinsonian dementia. *Journal of Neurology, 253*, 242–247.
Bohnen, N. I., Müller, M. L., Koeppe, R. A., Studenski, S. A., Kilbourn, M. A., Frey, K. A., et al. (2009). History of falls in Parkinson disease is associated with reduced cholinergic activity. *Neurology, 73*(20), 1670–1676.
Bohnen, N. I., Müller, M. L., Kotagal, V., Koeppe, R. A., Kilbourn, M. R., Gilman, S., et al. (2012). Heterogeneity of cholinergic denervation in Parkinson's disease without dementia. *Journal of Cerebral Blood Flow and Metabolism, 32*(8), 1609–1617.

Boileau, I., Guttman, M., Rusjan, P., Adams, J. R., Houle, S., Tong, J., et al. (2009). Decreased binding of the D3 dopamine receptor-preferring ligand [11C]-PHNO in drug-naive Parkinson's disease. *Brain*, *132*(Pt. 5), 1366–1375.

Boileau, I., Warsh, J. J., Guttman, M., Saint-Cyr, J. A., McCluskey, T., Rusjan, P., et al. (2008). Elevated serotonin transporter binding in depressed patients with Parkinson's disease: A preliminary PET study with [11C]DASB. *Movement Disorders*, *23*, 1776–1780.

Booth, R. G., & Baldessarini, R. J. (1991). (+)-6,7-Benzomorphan sigma ligands stimulate dopamine synthesis in rat corpus striatum tissue. *Brain Research*, *557*, 349–352.

Boucetta, S., Salimi, A., Dadar, M., Jones, B. E., Collins, D. L., & Dang-Vu, T. T. (2016). Structural brain alterations associated with rapid eye movement sleep behavior disorder in Parkinson's disease. *Scientific Reports*, *6*, 26782.

Breier, A., Su, T. P., Saunders, R., Carson, R. E., Kolachana, B. S., de Bartolomeis, A., et al. (1997). Schizophrenia is associated with elevated amphetamine-induced synaptic dopamine concentrations: Evidence from a novel positron emission tomography method. *Proceedings of the National Academy of Sciences of the United States of America*, *94*(6), 2569–2574.

Brooks, D. J., Frey, K. A., Marek, K. L., Oakes, D., Paty, D., Prentice, R., et al. (2003). Assessment of neuroimaging techniques as biomarkers of the progression of Parkinson's disease. *Experimental Neurology*, *184*, S68–S79.

Brooks, D. J., Ibanez, V., Saule, G. V., Playford, E. D., Quinn, N., Mathias, C. J., et al. (1992). Striatal D2 receptor status in patients with Parkinson's disease, striatonigral degeneration and progressive supranuclear palsy, measured with 11C-raclopride and positron emission tomography. *Annals of Neurology*, *31*, 184–192.

Brooks, D. J., Ibanez, V., Sawle, G. V., Quinn, N., Lees, A. J., Mathias, C. J., et al. (1990). Differing patterns of striatal 18F-dopa uptake in Parkinson's disease, multiplesystem atrophy and progressive supranuclear palsy. *Annals of Neurology*, *28*, 547–555.

Brooks, D. J., & Pavese, N. (2011). Imaging biomarkers in Parkinson's disease. *Progress in Neurobiology*, *95*(4), 614–628.

Bunzeck, N., Singh-Curry, V., Eckart, C., Weiskopf, N., Perry, R. J., Bain, P. G., et al. (2013). Motor phenotype and magnetic resonance measures of basal ganglia iron levels in Parkinson's disease. *Parkinsonism & Related Disorders*, *19*, 1136–1142.

Burciu, R. G., Ofori, E., Shukla, P., Planetta, P. J., Snyder, A. F., Li, H., et al. (2015). Distinct patterns of brain activity in progressive supranuclear palsy and Parkinson's disease. *Movement Disorders*, *30*(9), 1248–1258.

Burke, J. F., Albin, R. L., Koeppe, R. A., Giordani, B., Kilbourn, M. R., Gilman, S., et al. (2011). Assessment of mild dementia with amyloid and dopamine terminal positron emission tomography. *Brain*, *134*, 1647–1657.

Burn, D. J., Rinne, J. O., Quinn, N. P., Lees, A. J., Marsden, C. D., & Brooks, D. J. (1995). Striatal opioid receptor binding in Parkinson's disease, striatonigral degeneration and Steele-Richardson-Olszewski syndrome A [^{11}C]diprenoiphine PET study. *Brain*, *118*, 951–958.

Burton, E. J., McKeith, I. G., Burn, D. J., & O'Brien, J. T. (2005). Brain atrophy rates in Parkinson's disease with and without dementia using serial magnetic resonance imaging. *Movement Disorders*, *20*, 1571–1576.

Burton, E. J., McKeith, I. G., Burn, D. J., Williams, E. D., & O'Brien, J. T. (2004). Cerebral atrophy in Parkinson's disease with and without dementia: A comparison with Alzheimer's disease, dementia with Lewy bodies and controls. *Brain*, *127*, 791–800.

Camicioli, R., Moore, M. M., Kinney, A., Corbridge, E., Glassberg, K., & Kaye, J. A. (2003). Parkinson's disease is associated with hippocampal atrophy. *Movement Disorders*, *18*, 784–790.

Carriere, N., Besson, P., Dujardin, K., Duhamel, A., Defebvre, L., Delmaire, C., et al. (2014). Apathy in Parkinson's disease is associated with nucleus accumbens atrophy: A magnetic resonance imaging shape analysis. *Movement Disorders*, *29*, 897–903.

Catafau, A. M., Searle, G. E., Bullich, S., Gunn, R. N., Rabiner, E. A., Herance, R., et al. (2010). Imaging cortical dopamine D1 receptors using [11C]NNC112 and ketanserin blockade of the 5-HT 2A receptors. *Journal of Cerebral Blood Flow and Metabolism, 30*(5), 985–993.

Cerasa, A., Donzuso, G., Morelli, M., Mangone, G., Salsone, M., Passamonti, L., et al. (2015). The motor inhibition system in Parkinson's disease with levodopa-induced dyskinesias. *Movement Disorders, 30*, 1912–1920.

Cerasa, A., Morelli, M., Augimeri, A., Salsone, M., Novellino, F., Gioia, M. C., et al. (2013). Prefrontal thickening in PD with levodopa-induced dyskinesias: New evidence from cortical thickness measurement. *Parkinsonism & Related Disorders, 19*(1), 123–125.

Cerasa, A., Salsone, M., Morelli, M., Pugliese, P., Arabia, G., Gioia, C. M., et al. (2013). Age at onset influences neurodegenerative processes underlying PD with levodopa-induced dyskinesias. *Parkinsonism & Related Disorders, 19*(10), 883–888.

Chaki, S., Okuyama, S., Ogawa, S., & Tomisawa, K. (1998). Regulation of NMDA-induced [3H]dopamine release from rat hippocampal slices through sigma-1 binding sites. *Neurochemistry International, 33*, 29–34.

Chan, L.-L., Rumpel, H., Yap, K., Lee, E., Loo, H.-V., Ho, G.-L., et al. (2007). Case control study of diffusion tensor imaging in Parkinson's disease. *Journal of Neurology, Neurosurgery, and Psychiatry, 78*, 1383–1386.

Chauveau, F., Boutin, H., Van Camp, N., Dollé, F., & Tavitian, B. (2008). Nuclear imaging of neuroinflammation: A comprehensive review of [11C]PK11195 challengers. *European Journal of Nuclear Medicine and Molecular Imaging, 35*, 2304–2319.

Claassen, D. O., Lowe, V. J., Peller, P. J., Petersen, R. C., & Josephs, K. A. (2011). Amyloid and glucose imaging in dementia with Lewy bodies and multiple systems atrophy. *Parkinsonism & Related Disorders, 17*, 160–165.

Colloby, S. J., Williams, E. D., Burn, D. J., Lloyd, J. J., McKeith, I. G., & O'Brien, J. T. (2005). Progression of dopaminergic degeneration in dementia with Lewy bodies and Parkinson's disease with and without dementia assessed using 123I-FP-CIT SPECT. *European Journal of Nuclear Medicine and Molecular Imaging, 32*(10), 1176–1185.

Compta, Y., Pereira, J. B., Ríos, J., Ibarretxe-Bilbao, N., Junque, C., Bargallo, N., et al. (2013). Combined dementia-risk biomarkers in Parkinson's disease: A prospective longitudinal study. *Parkinsonism & Related Disorders, 19*, 717–724.

Coskran, T. M., Morton, D., Menniti, F. S., Adamowicz, W. O., Kleiman, R. J., Ryan, A. M., et al. (2006). Immunohistochemical localization of phosphodiesterase 10A in multiple mammalian species. *The Journal of Histochemistry and Cytochemistry, 54*, 1205–1213.

Cropley, V. L., Fujita, M., Bara-Jimenez, W., Brown, A. K., Zhang, X. Y., Sangare, J., et al. (2008). Pre- and post-synaptic dopamine imaging and its relation with frontostriatal cognitive function in Parkinson disease: PET studies with [11C]NNC 112 and [18F] FDOPA. *Psychiatry Research, 163*(2), 171–182.

Cuberas-Borrós, G., Lorenzo-Bosquet, C., Aguadé-Bruix, S., Hernández-Vara, J., Pifarré-Montaner, P., Miquel, F., et al. (2011). Quantitative evaluation of striatal I-123-FP-CIT uptake in essential tremor and parkinsonism. *Clinical Nuclear Medicine, 36*(11), 991–996.

Cummings, J., Isaacson, S., Mills, R., Williams, H., Chi-burris, K., Corbett, A., et al. (2014). Pimavanserin for patients with Parkinson's disease psychosis: A randomised, placebo-controlled phase 3 trial. *The Lancet, 383*, 533–540.

Damier, P., Hirsch, E. C., Agid, Y., & Graybiel, A. M. (1999). The substantia nigra of the human brain. I. Nigrosomes and the nigral matrix, a compartmental organization based on calbindin D(28 K) immunohistochemistry. *Brain: A Journal of Neurology, 122*(Pt. 8), 1421–1436.

de la Fuente-Fernandez, R., Lim, A. S., Sossi, V., Holden, J. E., Calne, D. B., Ruth, T. J., et al. (2001). Apomorphine-induced changes in synaptic dopamine levels: Positron

emission tomography evidence for presynaptic inhibition. *Journal of Cerebral Blood Flow and Metabolism, 21*, 1151–1159.
de la Fuente-Fernandez, R., Lu, J. Q., Sossi, V., Jivan, S., Schulzer, M., Holden, J. E., et al. (2001). Biochemical variations in the synaptic levels of dopamine precede motor fluctuations in Parkinson's disease: PET evidence of increased dopamine turnover. *Annals of Neurology, 49*, 298–303.
de la Fuente-Fernandez, R., Phillips, A. G., Zamburlini, M., Sossi, V., Calne, D. B., Ruth, T. J., et al. (2002). Dopamine release in human ventral striatum and expectation of reward. *Behavioural Brain Research, 136*(2), 359–363.
de la Fuente-Fernandez, R., Ruth, T. J., Sossi, V., Schulzer, M., Calne, D. B., & Stoessl, A. J. (2001). Expectation and dopamine release: Mechanisms of the placebo effect in Parkinson's disease. *Science, 293*, 1164–1166.
de la Fuente-Fernández, R., Schulzer, M., Kuramoto, L., Cragg, J., Ramachandiran, N., Au, W. L., et al. (2011). Age-specific progression of nigrostriatal dysfunction in Parkinson's disease. *Annals of Neurology, 69*, 803–810.
de la Fuente-Fernandez, R., Sossi, V., Huang, Z., Furtado, S., Lu, Q. R., Calne, D. B., et al. (2004). Levodopa-induced changes in synaptic dopamine levels increase with progression of Parkinson's disease: Implications for dyskinesias. *Brain, 127*, 2747–2754.
Dentresangle, C., Veyre, L., le Bars Pierre, C., Lavenne, F., Pollak, P., Guerin, J., et al. (1999). Striatal D2 dopamine receptor status in Parkinson's disease: An [^{18}F]dopa and [^{11}C]raclopride PET study. *Movement Disorders, 14*(6), 1025–1030.
Diaz-Corrales, F. J., Sanz-Viedma, S., Garcia-Solis, D., Escobar-Delgado, T., & Mir, P. (2010). Clinical features and I123-FP-CIT SPECT imaging in drug-induced parkinsonism and Parkinson's disease. *European Journal of Nuclear Medicine and Molecular Imaging, 37*(3), 556–564.
Diggle, C. P., Sukoff Rizzo, S. J., Popiolek, M., Hinttala, R., Schülke, J. P., Kurian, M. A., et al. (2016). Biallelic mutations in PDE10A lead to loss of striatal PDE10A and a hyperkinetic movement disorder with onset in infancy. *American Journal of Human Genetics, 98*(4), 735–743.
Disbrow, E. A., Carmichael, O., He, J., Lanni, K. E., Dressler, E. M., Zhang, L., et al. (2014). Resting state functional connectivity is associated with cognitive dysfunction in non-demented people with Parkinson's disease. *Journal of Parkinson's Disease, 4*, 453–465.
Doder, M., Rabiner, E. A., Turjanski, N., Lees, A. J., & Brooks, D. J. (2003). Tremor in Parkinson's disease and serotonergic dysfunction: An 11C-WAY 100635 PET study. *Neurology, 60*, 601–605.
Du, G., Lewis, M. M., Styner, M., Shaffer, M. L., Sen, S., Yang, Q. X., et al. (2011). Combined R2* and diffusion tensor imaging changes in the substantia nigra in Parkinson's disease. *Movement Disorders, 26*, 1627–1632.
Edison, P., Ahmed, I., Fan, Z., Hinz, R., Gelosa, G., Ray Chaudhuri, K., et al. (2013). Microglia, amyloid, and glucose metabolism in Parkinson's disease with and without dementia. *Neuropsychopharmacology, 38*(6), 938–949.
Edison, P., Rowe, C. C., Rinne, J. O., Ng, S., Ahmed, I., Kemppainen, N., et al. (2008). Amyloid load in Parkinson's disease dementia and Lewy body dementia measured with [11C]PIB positron emission tomography. *Journal of Neurology, Neurosurgery, and Psychiatry, 79*, 1331–1338.
Ekelund, J., Slifstein, M., Narendran, R., Guillin, O., Belani, H., et al. (2007). In vivo DA D(1) receptor selectivity of NNC 112 and SCH 23390. *Molecular Imaging and Biology, 9*(3), 117–125.
Evans, A. H., Pavese, N., Lawrence, A. D., Tai, F. Y., Appel, S., Doder, M., et al. (2006). Compulsive drug use linked to sensitized ventral striatal dopamine transmission. *Annals of Neurology, 59*, 852–858.
Fernandez-Seara, M. A., Mengual, E., Vidorreta, M., Castellanos, G., Irigoyen, J., Erro, E., et al. (2015). Resting state functional connectivity of the subthalamic nucleus in

Parkinson's disease assessed using arterial spin-labeled perfusion fMRI. *Human Brain Mapping, 36*, 1937–1950.

Foster, E. R., Campbell, M. C., Burack, M. A., Hartlein, J., Flores, H. P., Cairns, N. J., et al. (2010). Amyloid imaging of Lewy body-associated disorders. *Movement Disorders, 25*, 2516–2523.

Fredholm, B. B., & Svenningsson, P. (2003). Adenosine-dopamine interactions: Development of a concept and some comments on therapeutic possibilities. *Neurology, 61*, S5–S9.

Fujishige, K., Kotera, J., & Omori, K. (1999). Striatum- and testis-specific phosphodiesterase PDE10A isolation and characterization of a rat PDE10A. *European Journal of Biochemistry, 266*, 1118–1127.

Fujita, M., Ichise, M., Zoghbi, S. S., Liow, J. S., Ghose, S., Vines, D. C., et al. (2006). Widespread decrease of nicotinic acetylcholine receptors in Parkinson's disease. *Annals of Neurology, 59*, 174–177.

Fujita, M., Imaizumi, M., Zoghbi, S. S., Fujimura, Y., Farris, A. G., Suhara, T., et al. (2008). Kinetic analysis in healthy humans of a novel positron emission tomography radioligand to image the peripheral benzodiazepine receptor, a potential biomarker for inflammation. *NeuroImage, 40*, 43–52.

Gerhard, A., Pavese, N., Hotton, G., Turkheimer, F., Es, M., Hammers, A., et al. (2006). In vivo imaging of microglial activation with [11C](R)-PK11195 PET in idiopathic Parkinson's disease. *Neurobiology of Disease, 21*(2), 404–412.

Gilman, S., Koeppe, R. A., Nan, B., Wang, C. N., Wang, X., Junck, L., et al. (2010). Cerebral cortical and subcortical cholinergic deficits in parkinsonian syndromes. *Neurology, 74*(18), 1416–1423.

Girault, J. A. (2012). Integrating neurotransmission in striatal medium spiny neurons. *Advances in Experimental Medicine and Biology, 970*, 407–429.

Gjerløff, T., Fedorova, T., Knudsen, K., Munk, O. L., Nahimi, A., Jacobsen, S., et al. (2015). Imaging acetylcholinesterase density in peripheral organs in Parkinson's disease with 11C-donepezil PET. *Brain, 138*(Pt. 3), 653–663.

Gjerloff, T., Jakobsen, S., Nahimi, A., Munk, O. L., Bender, D., Alstrup, A. K., et al. (2014). In vivo imaging of human acetylcholinesterase density in peripheral organs using 11C-donepezil: Dosimetry, biodistribution, and kinetic analyses. *Journal of Nuclear Medicine, 55*, 1818–1824.

Glass, M., Dragunow, M., & Faull, R. L. M. (1997). Cannabinoid receptors in the human brain: A detailed anatomical and quantitative autoradiographic study in the fetal, neonatal and adult human brain. *Neuroscience, 77*, 299–318.

Gomperts, S. N., Locascio, J. J., Makaretz, S. J., Schultz, A., Caso, C., Vasdev, N., et al. (2016). Tau positron emission tomographic imaging in the Lewy body diseases. *JAMA Neurology, 73*(11), 1334–1341.

Gomperts, S. N., Locascio, J. J., Marquie, M., Santarlasci, A. L., Rentz, D. M., Maye, J., et al. (2012). Brain amyloid and cognition in Lewy body diseases. *Movement Disorders, 27*, 965–973.

Gomperts, S. N., Locascio, J. J., Rentz, D., Santarlasci, A., Marquie, M., Johnson, K. A., et al. (2013). Amyloid is linked to cognitive decline in patients with Parkinson disease without dementia. *Neurology, 80*, 85–91.

Gomperts, S. N., Rentz, D. M., Moran, E., Becker, J. A., Locascio, J. J., Klunk, W. E., et al. (2008). Imaging amyloid deposition in Lewy body diseases. *Neurology, 71*, 903–910.

Gonzalez-Garcia, N., Armony, J. L., Soto, J., Trejo, D., Alegria, M. A., & Drucker-Colin, R. (2011). Effects of rTMS on Parkinson's disease: A longitudinal fMRI study. *Journal of Neurology, 258*, 1268–1280.

Gorges, M., Muller, H. P., Lule, D., Pinkhardt, E. H., Ludolph, A. C., & Kassubek, J. (2015). To rise and to fall: Functional connectivity in cognitively normal and cognitively impaired patients with Parkinson's disease. *Neurobiology of Aging, 36*, 1727–1735.

Graff-Radford, J., Boeve, B. F., Pedraza, O., Ferman, T. J., Przybelski, S., Lesnick, T. G., et al. (2012). Imaging and acetylcholinesterase inhibitor response in dementia with Lewy bodies. *Brain, 135*, 2470–2477.

Haacke, E. M., Makki, M., Ge, Y., Maheshwari, M., Sehgal, V., Hu, J., et al. (2009). Characterizing iron deposition in multiple sclerosis lesions using susceptibility weighted imaging. *Journal of Magnetic Resonance Imaging, 29*, 537–544.

Hacker, C. D., Perlmutter, J. S., Criswell, S. R., Ances, B. M., & Snyder, A. Z. (2012). Resting state functional connectivity of the striatum in Parkinson's disease. *Brain, 135*(Pt. 12), 3699–3711.

Halldin, C., Stone-Elander, S., Farde, L., Ehrin, E., Fasth, K. J., Langstrom, B., et al. (1986). Preparation of 11C-labelled SCH 23390 for the in vivo study of dopamine D-1 receptors using positron emission tomography. *International Journal of Radiation Applications and Instrumentation Part A, 37*(10), 1039–1043.

Hamani, C., & Lozano, A. M. (2003). Physiology and pathophysiology of Parkinson's disease. *Annals of the New York Academy of Sciences, 991*, 15–21.

Harding, A. J., & Halliday, G. M. (2001). Cortical Lewy body pathology in the diagnosis of dementia. *Acta Neuropathologica, 102*(4), 355–363.

Hawkes, C. H., Del Tredici, K., & Braak, H. (2007). Parkinson's disease: A dual-hit hypothesis. *Neuropathology and Applied Neurobiology, 33*(6), 599–614.

Hayashi, T., & Su, T. P. (2007). Sigma-1 receptor chaperones at the ER-mitochondrion interface regulate Ca(2+) signaling and cell survival. *Cell, 131*, 596–610.

Helmich, R. C., Derikx, L. C., Bakker, M., Scheeringa, R., Bloem, B. R., & Toni, I. (2010). Spatial remapping of cortico-striatal connectivity in Parkinson's disease. *Cerebral Cortex, 20*(5), 1175–1186.

Helmich, R. C., Janssen, M. J., Oyen, W. J., Bloem, B. R., & Toni, I. (2011). Pallidal dysfunction drives a cerebellothalamic circuit into Parkinson tremor. *Annals of Neurology, 69*, 269–281.

Herkenham, M., Lynn, A. B., Johnson, M. R., Melvin, L. S., de Costa, B. R., & Rice, K. C. (1991). Characterization and localization of cannabinoid receptors in the rat brain: A quantitative in vitro autoradiographic study. *The Journal of Neuroscience, 11*, 563–583.

Herz, D. M., Eickhoff, S. B., Lokkegaard, A., & Siebner, H. R. (2014). Functional neuroimaging of motor control in Parkinson's disease: A meta-analysis. *Human Brain Mapping, 35*, 3227–3237.

Herz, D. M., Haagensen, B. N., Christensen, M. S., Madsen, K. H., Rowe, J. B., & Lokkegaard, A. (2015). Abnormal dopaminergic modulation of striato-cortical networks underlies levodopa-induced dyskinesias in humans. *Brain, 138*, 1658–1666.

Herz, D. M., Haagensen, B. N., Nielsen, S. H., Madsen, K. H., Lokkegaard, A., & Siebner, H. R. (2016). Resting-state connectivity predicts levodopa-induced dyskinesias in Parkinson's disease. *Movement Disorders, 31*, 521–529.

Hilker, R., Schweitzer, K., Coburger, S., Ghaemi, M., Weisenbach, S., Jacobs, A. H., et al. (2005). Nonlinear progression of Parkinson disease as determined by serial positron emission tomographic imaging of striatal fluorodopa F 18 activity. *Archives of Neurology, 62*, 378–382.

Hilker, R., Thomas, A. V., Klein, J. C., Weisenbach, S., Kalbe, E., Burghaus, L., et al. (2005). Dementia in Parkinson disease: Functional imaging of cholinergic and dopaminergic pathways. *Neurology, 65*, 1716–1722.

Horvath, J., Herrmann, F. R., Burkhard, P. R., Bouras, C., & Kövari, E. (2013). Neuropathology of dementia in a large cohort of patients with Parkinson's disease. *Parkinsonism & Related Disorders, 19*(10), 864–868.

Hu, X., Song, X., Li, E., Liu, J., Yuan, Y., Liu, W., et al. (2015). Altered resting-state brain activity and connectivity in depressed Parkinson's disease. *PLoS One, 10*, e131133.

Huang, P., Lou, Y., Xuan, M., Gu, Q., Guan, X., Xu, X., et al. (2016). Cortical abnormalities in Parkinson's disease patients and relationship to depression: A surface-based morphometry study. *Psychiatry Research, 250*, 24–28.

Iannaccone, S., Cerami, C., Alessio, M., Garibotto, V., Panzacchi, A., Olivieri, S., et al. (2013). In vivo microglia activation in very early dementia with Lewy bodies, comparison with Parkinson's disease. *Parkinsonism & Related Disorders*, *19*(1), 47–52.

Ibarretxe-Bilbao, N., Junque, C., Marti, M. J., Valldeoriola, F., Vendrell, P., & Bargallo, N. (2010). Olfactory impairment in Parkinson's disease and white matter abnormalities in central olfactory areas: A voxel-based diffusion tensor imaging study. *Movement Disorders*, *25*, 1888–1894.

Ibarretxe-Bilbao, N., Junque, C., Segura BBaggio, H. C., Marti, M. J., Valldeoriola, F., et al. (2012). Progression of cortical thinning in early Parkinson's disease. *Movement Disorders*, *27*, 1746–1753.

Ikoma, Y., Yasuno, F., Ito, H., Suhara, T., Ota, M., Toyama, H., et al. (2007). Quantitative analysis for estimating binding potential of the peripheral benzodiazepine receptor with [(11)C]DAA1106. *Journal of Cerebral Blood Flow and Metabolism*, *27*, 173–184.

Isaias, I. U., Spiegel, J., Brumberg, J., Cosgrove, K. P., Marotta, G., Oishi, N., et al. (2014). Nicotinic acetylcholine receptor density in cognitively intact subjects at an early stage of Parkinson's disease. *Frontiers in Aging Neuroscience*, *6*, 213.

Ito, M., Watanabe, H., Kawai, Y., Atsuta, N., Tanaka, F., & Naganawa, S. (2007). Usefulness of combined fractional anisotropy and apparent diffusion coefficient values for detection of involvement in multiple system atrophy. *Journal of Neurology, Neurosurgery, and Psychiatry*, *78*, 722–728.

Iyo, M., Namba, H., Fukushi, K., Shinotoh, H., Nagatsuka, S., Suhara, T., et al. (1997). Measurement of acetylcholinesterase by positron emission tomography in the brains of healthy controls and patients with Alzheimer's disease. *Lancet*, *349*, 1805–1809.

Jahanshahi, M., Jones, C. R. G., Zijlmans, J., Katsenschlager, R., Lee, L., Quinn, N., et al. (2010). Dopaminergic modulation of striato-frontal connectivityduring motor timing in Parkinson's disease. *Brain*, *133*, 727–745.

Jellinger, K. A. (1991). Pathology of Parkinson's disease. *Molecular and Chemical Neuropathology*, *3*, 153–197.

Jellinger, K. A., & Attems, J. (2008). Prevalence and impact of vascular and Alzheimer pathologies in Lewy body disease. *Acta Neuropathologica*, *115*(4), 427–436.

Jellinger, K. A., Seppi, K., Wenning, G. K., & Poewe, W. (2002). Impact of coexistent Alzheimer pathology on the natural history of Parkinson's disease. *Journal of Neural Transmission (Vienna)*, *109*(3), 329–339.

Johansson, A., Savitcheva, I., Forsberg, A., Engler, H., Långström, B., Nordberg, A., et al. (2008). [11C]-PIB imaging in patients with Parkinson's disease: Preliminary results. *Parkinsonism & Related Disorders*, *14*, 345–347.

Jokinen, P., Scheinin, N., Aalto, S., Någren, K., Savisto, N., Parkkola, R., et al. (2010). [11C]PIB-, [18F]FDG-PET and MRI imaging in patients with Parkinson's disease with and without dementia. *Parkinsonism & Related Disorders*, *16*, 666–670.

Jučaite, A., Cselényi, Z., Arvidsson, A., Ahlberg, G., Julin, P., Varnäs, K., et al. (2012). Kinetic analysis and test-retest variability of the radioligand [11C](R)-PK11195 binding to TSPO in the human brain—A PET study in control subjects. *EJNMMI Research*, *2*, 15.

Jucaite, A., Svenningsson, P., Rinne, J. O., Cselényi, Z., Varnäs, K., Johnström, P., et al. (2015). Effect of the myeloperoxidase inhibitor AZD3241 on microglia: A PET study in Parkinson's disease. *Brain*, *138*(Pt 9), 2687–2700.

Junque, C., Ramírez-Ruiz, B., Tolosa, E., Summerfield, C., Martí, M. J., Pastor, P., et al. (2005). Amygdalar and hippocampal MRI volumetric reductions in Parkinson's disease with dementia. *Movement Disorders*, *20*, 540–544.

Kaasinen, V., Någren, K., Hietala, J., Oikonen, V., Vilkman, H., Farde, L., et al. (2000). Extrastriatal dopamine D2 and D3 receptors in early and advanced Parkinson's disease. *Neurology*, *54*(7), 1482–1487.

Kaasinen, V., Aalto, S., Nagren, K., Hietala, J., Sonninen, P., & Rinne, J. O. (2003). Extrastriatal dopamine D(2) receptors in Parkinson's disease: A longitudinal study. *Journal of Neural Transmission*, *110*(6), 591–601.

Kahan, J., Urner, M., Moran, R., Flandin, G., Marreiros, A., Mancini, L., et al. (2014). Resting state functional MRI in Parkinson's disease: The impact of deep brain stimulation on 'effective' connectivity. *Brain*, *137*, 1130–1144.

Kantarci, K., Lowe, V. J., Boeve, B. F., Weigand, S. D., Senjem, M. L., Przybelski, S. A., et al. (2012). Multimodality imaging characteristics of dementia with Lewy bodies. *Neurobiology of Aging*, *33*, 2091–2105.

Kas, A., Bottlaender, M., Gallezot, J. D., Vidailhet, M., Villafane, G., Grégoire, M. C., et al. (2009). Decrease of nicotinic receptors in the nigrostriatal system in Parkinson's disease. *Journal of Cerebral Blood Flow & Metabolism*, *29*, 1601–1608.

Kashihara, K., Shinya, T., & Higaki, F. (2011). Neuromelanin magnetic resonance imaging of nigral volume loss in patients with Parkinson's disease. *Journal of Clinical Neuroscience*, *18*(8), 1093–1096.

Kefalopoulou, Z., Politis, M., Piccini, P., Mencacci, N., Bhatia, K., Jahanshahi, M., et al. (2014). Long-term clinical outcome of fetal cell transplantation for Parkinson disease: Two case reports. *JAMA Neurology*, *71*, 83–87.

Klein, J. C., Eggers, C., Kalbe, E., Weisenbach, S., Hohmann, C., Vollmar, S., et al. (2010). Neurotransmitter changes in dementia with Lewy bodies and Parkinson disease dementia in vivo. *Neurology*, *74*, 885–892.

Ko, J. H., Mure, H., Tang, C. C., Ma, Y., Dhawan, V., Spetsieris, P., et al. (2013). Parkinson's disease: Increased motor network activity in the absence of movement. *The Journal of Neuroscience*, *33*, 4540–4549.

Koshimori, Y., Ko, J. H., Mizrahi, R., Rusjan, P., Mabrouk, R., Jacobs, M. F., et al. (2015). Imaging striatal microglial activation in patients with Parkinson's disease. *PLoS One*, *10*(9), e0138721.

Kosta, P., Argyropoulou, M. I., Markoula, S., & Konitsiotis, S. (2006). MRI evaluation of the basal ganglia size and iron content in patients with Parkinson's disease. *Journal of Neurology*, *253*, 26–32.

Kotagal, V., Albin, R. L., Müller, M. L., Koeppe, R. A., Chervin, R. D., Frey, K. A., et al. (2012). Symptoms of rapid eye movement sleep behavior disorder are associated with cholinergic denervation in Parkinson disease. *Annals of Neurology*, *71*(4), 560–568.

Kreutzberg, G. W. (1996). Microglia: A sensor for pathological events in the CNS. *Trends in Neurosciences*, *19*, 312–318.

Lakics, V., Karran, E. H., & Boess, F. G. (2010). Quantitative comparison of phosphodiesterase mRNA distribution in human brain and peripheral tissues. *Neuropharmacology*, *59*(6), 367–374.

Larsen, J. P., Beiske, A. G., Bekkelund, S. I., Dietrichs, E., Tysnes, O. B., Vilming, S. T., et al. (2008). Motor symptoms in Parkinson's disease. *Tidsskrift for Den Norske Legeforening*, *128*, 2068–2071.

Le Bihan, D. (2003). Looking into the functional architecture of the brain with diffusion MRI. *Nature Reviews. Neuroscience*, *4*, 469–480.

Lee, C. S. (2000). In vivo positron emission tomographic evidence for compensatory changes in presynaptic dopaminergic nerve terminals in Parkinson's disease. *Annals of Neurology*, *47*, 493–503.

Lewis, M. M., Du, G., Kidacki, M., Patel, N., Shaffer, M. L., Mailman, R. B., et al. (2013). Higher iron in the red nucleus marks Parkinson's dyskinesia. *Neurobiology of Aging*, *34*, 1497–1503.

Loane, C., & Politis, M. (2012). Buspirone: What is it all about? *Brain Research*, *1461*, 111–118.

Loane, C., Wu, K., Bain, P., Brooks, D. J., Piccini, P., & Politis, M. (2013). Serotonergic loss in motorcircuitries correlates with severity of action-postural tremor in PD. *Neurology*, *80*, 1850–1855.

Loane, C., Wu, K., O'Sullivan, S. S., Lawrence, A. D., Woodhead, Z., Lees, A. J., et al. (2015). Psychogenic and neural visual-cue response in PD dopamine dysregulation syndrome. *Parkinsonism & Related Disorders*, *21*(11), 1336–1341.

Loberboym, M., Traves, T. A., Melamed, E., Lampl, Y., Hellman, M., & Djaldetti, R. (2006). [I123]-EP/CIT SPECT imaging for distinguishing drug-induced Parkinsonism from Parkinson's disease. *Movement Disorders*, *21*(4), 510–514.

Lorenz, R., Samnick, S., Dillmann, U., Schiller, M., Ong, M. F., Faßbender, K., et al. (2014). Nicotinic α4β2 acetylcholine receptors and cognitive function in Parkinson's disease. *Acta Neurologica Scandinavica*, *130*(3), 164–171.

Luo, C., Chen, Q., Song, W., Chen, K., Guo, X., & Yang, J. (2014). Resting-state fMRI study on drug-naive patients with Parkinson's disease and with depression. *Journal of Neurology, Neurosurgery, and Psychiatry*, *85*, 675–683.

Lyoo, C. H., Ryu, Y. H., & Lee, M. S. (2011). Cerebral cortical areas in which thickness correlates with severity of motor deficits of Parkinson's disease. *Journal of Neurology*, *258*(10), 1871–1876.

MacDonald, P. A., MacDonald, A. A., Seergobin, K. N., Tamjeedi, R., Ganjavi, H., Provost, J.-S., et al. (2011). The effect of dopamine therapy on ventral and dorsal striatum-mediated cognition in Parkinson's disease: Support from functional MRI. *Brain*, *134*, 1447–1463.

Maeda, T., Nagata, K., Yoshida, Y., & Kannari, K. (2005). Serotonergic hyperinnervation into the dopaminergic denervated striatum compensates for dopamine conversion from exogenously administered L-DOPA. *Brain Research*, *1046*, 230–233.

Maetzler, W., Liepelt, I., Reimold, M., Reischl, G., Solbach, C., Becker, C., et al. (2009). Cortical PIB binding in Lewy body disease is associated with Alzheimer-like characteristics. *Neurobiology of Disease*, *34*, 107–112.

Maetzler, W., Reimold, M., Liepelt, I., Solbach, C., Leyhe, T., Schweitzer, K., et al. (2008). [11C]PIB binding in Parkinson's disease dementia. *NeuroImage*, *39*, 1027–1033.

Mailleux, P., & Vanderhaeghen, J. J. (1992). Localization of cannabinoid receptor in the human developing and adult basal ganglia. Higher levels in the striatonigral neurons. *Neuroscience Letters*, *148*, 173–176.

Mak, E., Bergsland, N., Dwyer, M. G., Zivadinov, R., & Kandiah, N. (2014). Subcortical atrophy is associated with cognitive impairment in mild Parkinson disease: A combined investigation of volumetric changes, cortical thickness, and vertex-based shape analysis. *AJNR. American Journal of Neuroradiology*, *35*, 2257–2264.

Mak, E., Su, L., Williams, G. B., Firbank, M. J., Lawson, R. A., Yarnall, A. J., et al. (2015). Baseline and longitudinal grey matter changes in newly diagnosed Parkinson's disease: ICICLE-PD study. *Brain*, *138*(Pt. 10), 2974–2986.

Marek, K., Innis, R., van Dyck, C., Fussell, B., Early, M., Eberly, S., et al. (2001). [I123]β-CIT SPECT imaging assessment of the rate of Parkinson's disease progression. *Neurology*, *57*(11), 2089–2094.

Martín, A. B., Fernandez-Espejo, E., Ferrer, B., Gorriti, M. A., Bilbao, A., Navarro, M., et al. (2008). Expression and function of CB1 receptor in the rat striatum: Localization and effects on D1 and D2 dopamine receptor-mediated motor behaviors. *Neuropsychopharmacology*, *33*, 1667–1679.

Martin-Bastida, A., Lao-Kaim, N. P., Loane, C., Politis, M., Roussakis, A. A., Valle-Guzman, N., et al. (2017). Motor associations of iron accumulation in deep grey matter nuclei in Parkinson's disease: A cross-sectional study of iron-related magnetic resonance imaging susceptibility. *European Journal of Neurology*, *24*, 357–365.

Matsui, H., Nishinaka, K., Oda, M., Niikawa, H., Kubori, T., & Udaka, F. (2007). Dementia in Parkinson's disease: Diffusion tensor imaging. *Acta Neurologica Scandinavica*, *116*, 177–181.

Matsuura, K., Maeda, M., Yata, K., Ichiba, Y., Yamaguchi, T., Kanamaru, K., et al. (2013). Neuromelanin magnetic resonance imaging in Parkinson's disease and multiple system atrophy. *European Neurology*, *70*(1–2), 70–77.

Melzer, T. R., Watts, R., MacAskill, M. R., Pitcher, T. L., Livingston, L., Keenan, R. J., et al. (2012). Grey matter atrophy in cognitively impaired Parkinson's disease. *Journal of Neurology, Neurosurgery, and Psychiatry*, *83*, 188–194.

Mencacci, N. E., Kamsteeg, E. J., Nakashima, K., R'Bibo, L., Lynch, D. S., Balint, B., et al. (2016). De novo mutations in PDE10A cause childhood-onset chorea with bilateral striatal lesions. *American Journal of Human Genetics*, *98*(4), 763–771.

Meppelink, A. M., de Jong, B. M., Renken, R., Leenders, K. L., Cornelissen, F. W., & van Laar, T. (2009). Impaired visual processing preceding image recognition in Parkinson's disease patients with visual hallucinations. *Brain*, *132*, 2980–2993.

Meyer, P. M., Strecker, K., Kendziorra, K., Becker, G., Hesse, S., Woelpl, D., et al. (2009). Reduced α4β2*–nicotinic acetylcholine receptor binding and its relationship to mild cognitive and depressive symptoms in Parkinson disease. *Archives of General Psychiatry*, *66*, 866–877.

Mishina, M., Ishiwata, K., Ishii, K., Kitamura, S., Kimura, Y., Kawamura, K., et al. (2005). Function of sigma1 receptors in Parkinson's disease. *Acta Neurologica Scandinavica*, *112*, 103–107.

Mishina, M., Ishiwata, K., Naganawa, M., Kimura, Y., Kitamura, S., Suzuki, M., et al. (2011). Adenosine A2A receptors measured with [11C]TMSX PET in the striata of Parkinson's disease patients. *PLoS One*, *6*, e17338, 1–8.

Müller, M. L., Frey, K. A., Petrou, M., Kotagal, V., Koeppe, R. A., Albin, R. L., et al. (2013). β-Amyloid and postural instability and gait difficulty in Parkinson's disease at risk for dementia. *Movement Disorders*, *28*(3), 296–301.

Mure, H., Tang, C. C., Argyelan, M., Ghilardi, M.-F., Kaplitt, M. G., Dhawan, V., et al. (2012). Improved sequence learning with subthalamic nucleus deep brain stimulation: Evidence for treatment-specific network modulation. *The Journal of Neuroscience*, *32*, 2804–2813.

Namba, H., Iyo, M., Shinotoh, H., Nagatsuka, S., Fukushi, K., & Irie, T. (1998). Preserved acetylcholinesterase activity in aged cerebral cortex. *Lancet*, *351*, 881–882.

Nandhagopal, R., Kuramoto, L., Schulzer, M., Mak, E., Cragg, J., Lee, C. S., et al. (2009). Longitudinal progression of sporadic Parkinson's disease: A multi-tracer positron emission tomography study. *Brain*, *132*, 2970–2979.

Ng, K. Y., Chase, T. N., & Kopin, I. J. (1970). Drug-induced release of 3H-norepinephrine and 3H-serotonin from brain slices. *Nature*, *228*(5270), 468–469.

Niccolini, F., Foltynie, T., Reis Marques, T., Muhlert, N., Tziortzi, A. C., Searle, G. E., et al. (2015). Loss of phosphodiesterase 10A expression is associated with progression and severity in Parkinson's disease. *Brain*, *138*(Pt. 10), 3003–3015.

Niccolini, F., Haider, S., Reis Marques, T., Muhlert, N., Tziortzi, A. C., Searle, G. E., et al. (2015). Altered PDE10A expression detectable early before symptomatic onset in Huntington's disease. *Brain*, *138*(Pt. 10), 3016–3029.

Nishi, A., Kuroiwa, M., Miller, D. B., O'Callaghan, J. P., Bateup, H. S., Shuto, T., et al. (2008). Distinct roles of PDE4 and PDE10A in the regulation of cAMP/PKA signaling in the striatum. *The Journal of Neuroscience*, *28*(42), 10460–10471.

Nurmi, E., Ruottinen, H. M., Bergman, J., Haaparanta, M., Solin, O., Sonninen, P., et al. (2001). Rate of progression in Parkinson's disease: A 6-[18F]fluoro-L-dopa PET study. *Movement Disorders*, *16*, 608–615.

Nurmi, E., Ruottinen, H. M., Kaasinen, V., Bergman, J., Haaparanta, M., Solin, O., et al. (2000). Progression in Parkinson's disease: A positron emission tomography study with a dopamine transporter ligand [18F]CFT. *Annals of Neurology*, *47*, 804–808.

O'Sullivan, S. S., Wu, K., Politis, M., Lawrence, A. D., Evans, A. H., Bose, S. K., et al. (2011). Cue induced striatal dopamine release in Parkinson's disease associated impulsive-compulsive behaviours. *Brain*, *134*(Pt. 4), 969–978.

Oh, U., Fujita, M., Ikonomidou, V. N., Evangelou, I. E., Matsuura, E., Harberts, E., et al. (2011). Translocator protein PET imaging for glial activation in multiple sclerosis. *Journal of Neuroimmune Pharmacology*, *6*, 354–361.

Ohtsuka, C., Sasaki, M., Konno, K., Koide, M., Kato, K., Takahashi, J., et al. (2013). Changes in substantia nigra and locus coeruleus in patients with early-stage Parkinson's disease using neuromelanin-sensitive MR imaging. *Neuroscience Letters*, *541*, 93–98.

Oishi, N., Hashikawa, K., Yoshida, H., Ishizu, K., Ueda, M., Kawashima, H., et al. (2007). Quantification of nicotinic acetylcholine receptors in Parkinson's disease with 123I-5IA SPECT. *Journal of the Neurological Sciences*, *256*, 52–60.

Olde Dubbelink, K. T., Schoonheim, M. M., Deijen, J. B., Twisk, J. W., Barkhof, F., & Berendse, H. W. (2014). Functional connectivity and cognitive decline over 3 years in Parkinson disease. *Neurology*, *83*(22), 2046–2053.

Ouchi, Y., Kanno, T., Okada, H., Yoshikawa, E., Futatsubashi, M., Nobezawa, S., et al. (1999). Presynaptic and postsynaptic dopaminergic binding densities in the nigrostriatal and mesocortical systems in early Parkinson's disease: A double tracer positron emission tomography study. *Annals of Neurology*, *46*(5), 723–731.

Ouchi, Y., Yoshikawa, E., Sekine, Y., Futatsubashi, M., Kanno, T., Ogusu, T., et al. (2005). Microglial activation and dopamine terminal loss in early Parkinson's disease. *Annals of Neurology*, *57*(2), 168–175.

Owen, D. R., Guo, Q., Kalk, N. J., Colasanti, A., Kalogiannopoulou, D., Dimber, R., et al. (2014). Determination of [(11)C]PBR28 binding potential in vivo: A first human TSPO blocking study. *Journal of Cerebral Blood Flow and Metabolism*, *34*(6), 989–994.

Owen, D. R., Howell, O. W., Tang, S. P., Wells, L. A., Bennacef, I., Bergstrom, M., et al. (2010). Two binding sites for [3H]PBR28 in human brain: Implications for TSPO PET imaging of neuroinflammation. *Journal of Cerebral Blood Flow and Metabolism*, *30*, 1608–1618.

Owen, D. R., Yeo, A. J., Gunn, R. N., Song, K., Wadsworth, G., Lewis, A., et al. (2011). An 18-kDa translocator protein (TSPO) polymorphism explains differences in binding affinity of the PET radioligand PBR28. *Journal of Cerebral Blood Flow and Metabolism*, *32*, 1–5.

Pagano, G., Niccolini, F., Fusar-Poli, P., & Politis, M. (2017). Serotonin transporter in Parkinson's disease: A meta-analysis of PET studies. *Annals of Neurology*, *8*, 171–180. http://dx.doi.org/10.1002/ana.24859.

Pagano, G., Niccolini, F., & Politis, M. (2016a). Current status of PET imaging in Huntington's disease. *European Journal of Nuclear Medicine and Molecular Imaging*, *43*(6), 1171–1182.

Pagano, G., Niccolini, F., & Politis, M. (2016b). Imaging in Parkinson's disease. *Clinical Medicine (London, England)*, *16*(4), 371–375.

Pagonabarraga, J., Corcuera-Solano, I., Vives-Gilabert, Y., Llebaria, G., García-Sanchez, C., Pascual-Sedano, B., et al. (2013). Pattern of regional cortical thinning associated with cognitive deterioration in Parkinson's disease. *PLoS One*, *8*, e54980.

Palmer, S. J., Li, J., Wang, Z. J., & McKeown, M. J. (2010). Joint amplitude and connectivity compensatory mechanisms in Parkinson's disease. *Neuroscience*, *166*, 1110–1118.

Pavese, N., Evans, A. H., Tai, Y. F., Hotton, G., Brooks, D. J., Lees, A. J., et al. (2006). Clinical correlates of levodopa induced dopamine release in Parkinson's disease: A PET study. *Neurology*, *67*, 1612–1617.

Pavese, N., Metta, V., Bose, S. K., Chaudhuri, K. R., & Brooks, D. J. (2010). Fatigue in Parkinson's disease is linked to striatal and limbic serotonergic dysfunction. *Brain*, *133*, 3434–3443.

Pavese, N., Rivero-Bosch, M., Lewis, S. J., Whone, A. L., & Brooks, D. J. (2011). Progression of monoaminergic dysfunction in Parkinson's disease: A longitudinal 18F-dopa PET study. *NeuroImage, 56*, 1463–1468.

Pellicano, C., Niccolini, F., Wu, K., O'Sullivan, S. S., Lawrence, A. D., Lees, A. J., et al. (2015). Morphometric changes in the reward system of Parkinson's disease patients with impulse control disorders. *Journal of Neurology, 262*(12), 2653–2661.

Péran, P., Cherubini, A., Assogna, F., Piras, F., Quattrocchi, C., Peppe, A., et al. (2010). Magnetic resonance imaging markers of Parkinson's disease nigrostriatal signature. *Brain, 133*(11), 3423–3433.

Pereira, J. B., Svenningsson, P., Weintraub, D., Brønnick, K., Lebedev, A., Westman, E., et al. (2014). Initial cognitive decline is associated with cortical thinning in early Parkinson disease. *Neurology, 82*, 2017–2025.

Perry, E. K., Irving, D., Kerwin, J. M., McKeith, I. G., Thompson, P., Collerton, D., et al. (1993). Cholinergic transmitter and neurotrophic activities in Lewy body dementia: Similarity to Parkinson's and distinction from Alzheimer disease. *Alzheimer Disease & Associated Disorders, 7*, 69–79.

Petit-Taboué, M. C., Baron, J. C., Barré, L., Travère, J. M., Speckel, D., Camsonne, R., et al. (1991). Brain kinetics and specific binding of [11C]PK 11195 to omega 3 sites in baboons: Positron emission tomography study. *European Journal of Pharmacology, 200*, 347–351.

Petrou, M., Bohnen, N. I., Müller, M. L., Koeppe, R. A., Albin, R. L., & Frey, K. A. (2012). Aβ-amyloid deposition in patients with Parkinson disease at risk for development of dementia. *Neurology, 79*, 1161–1167.

Phelps, M. E. (2000). Positron emission tomography provides molecular imaging of biological processes. *Proceedings of the National Academy of Sciences of the United States of America, 97*, 9226–9233.

Piccini, P., Brooks, D. J., Bjorklund, A., Gunn, R. N., Grasby, P. M., Rimoldi, O., et al. (1999). Dopamine release from nigral transplants visualised in vivo in a Parkinson's patient. *Nature Neuroscience, 2*(12), 1047–1048.

Piccini, P., Pavese, N., & Brooks, D. J. (2003). Endogenous dopamine release after pharmacological challenges in Parkinson's disease. *Annals of Neurology, 53*(5), 647–653.

Piccini, P., Pavese, N., Hagell, P., Reiner, J., Bjorklund, A., Oertel, W. H., et al. (2005). Factors affecting the clinical outcome after neural transplantation in Parkinson's disease. *Brain, 128*(12), 2977–2986.

Piccini, P., Weeks, R. A., & Brooks, D. J. (1997). Alterations in opioid receptor binding in Parkinson's disease patients with levodopa-induced dyskinesias. *Annals of Neurology, 42*, 720–726.

Politis, M. (2010). Dyskinesias after neural transplantation in Parkinson's disease: What do we know and what is next? *BMC Medicine, 8*, 80.

Politis, M. (2011). Optimizing functional imaging protocols for assessing the outcome of fetal cell transplantation in Parkinson's disease. *BMC Medicine, 9*, 50.

Politis, M. (2014). Neuroimaging in Parkinson disease: From research setting to clinical practice. *Nature Reviews. Neurology, 10*, 708–722.

Politis, M., Loane, C., Wu, K., Brooks, D. J., & Piccini, P. (2011). Serotonergic mediated body mass index changes in Parkinson's disease. *Neurobiology of Disease, 43*, 609–615.

Politis, M., Loane, C., Wu, K., O'Sullivan, S. S., Woodhead, Z., Kiferle, L., et al. (2013). Neural response to visual sexual cues in dopamine treatment-linked hypersexuality in Parkinson's disease. *Brain, 136*(Pt. 2), 400–411.

Politis, M., & Niccolini, F. (2015). Serotonin in Parkinson's disease. *Behavioural Brain Research, 277*, 136–145.

Politis, M., Oertel, W. H., Wu, K., Quinn, N. P., Pogarell, O., Brooks, D. J., et al. (2011). Graft-induced dyskinesias in Parkinson's disease: High striatal serotonin/dopamine transporter ratio. *Movement Disorders, 26*, 1997–2003.

Politis, M., & Piccini, P. (2012). In vivo imaging of the integration and function of nigral grafts in clinical trials. *Progress in Brain Research, 200*, 199–220.

Politis, M., Piccini, P., Pavese, N., Koh, S. B., & Brooks, D. J. (2008). Evidence of dopamine dysfunction in the hypothalamus of patients with Parkinson's disease: An in vivo 11C-raclopride PET study. *Experimental Neurology, 214*, 112–116.

Politis, M., Wu, K., Loane, C., Brooks, D. J., Kiferle, L., Turkheimer, F. E., et al. (2014a). Serotonergic mechanisms responsible for levodopa-induced dyskinesias in Parkinson's disease patients. *The Journal of Clinical Investigation, 124*, 1340–1349.

Politis, M., Wu, K., Loane, C., Kiferle, L., Molloy, S., Brooks, D. J., et al. (2010a). Staging of sero-tonergic dysfunction in Parkinson's disease: An in vivo 11C-DASB PET study. *Neurobiology of Disease, 40*, 216–221.

Politis, M., Wu, K., Loane, C., Quinn, N. P., Brook, D. J., Oertel, W. H., et al. (2014b). Serotonin neuron loss and non motor symptoms continue in Parkinson's patients treated with dopamine grafts. *Science Translational Medicine, 4*, 128–141.

Politis, M., Wu, K., Loane, C., Quinn, N. P., Brooks, D. J., Rehncrona, S., et al. (2010b). Serotonergic neurons mediate dyskinesia side effects in Parkinson's patients with neural transplants. *Science Translational Medicine, 2*, 38–46.

Politis, M., Wu, K., Loane, C., Turkheimer, F. E., Molloy, S., Brooks, D. J., et al. (2010c). Depressive symptoms in PD correlate with higher 5-HTT binding in raphe and limbic structures. *Neurology, 75*, 1920–1927.

Quik, M., Bordia, T., Forno, L., & McIntosh, J. M. (2004). Loss of alpha-conotoxinMII- and A85380-sensitive nicotinic receptors in Parkinson's disease striatum. *Journal of Neurochemistry, 88*, 668–679.

Rabiner, E. A., Slifstein, M., Nobrega, J., Plisson, C., Huiban, M., Raymond, R., et al. (2009). In vivo quantification of regional dopamine-D3 receptor binding potential of [11C]PHNO: Studies in nonhuman primates and transgenic mice. *Synapse, 63*(9), 782–793.

Ramírez-Ruiz, B., Martí, M. J., Tolosa, E., Giménez, M., Bargalló, N., Valldeoriola, F., et al. (2007). Cerebral atrophy in Parkinson's disease patients with visual hallucinations. *European Journal of Neurology, 14*(7), 750–756.

Ramlackhansingh, A. F., Bose, S. K., Ahmed, I., Turkheimer, F. E., Pavese, N., & Brooks, D. J. (2011). Adenosine 2A receptor availability in dyskinetic and nondyskinetic patients with Parkinson disease. *Neurology, 76*, 1811–1816.

Renaudo, A., L'Hoste, S., Guizouarn, H., Borgèse, F., & Soriani, O. (2007). Cancer cell cycle modulated by a functional coupling between sigma-1 receptors and Cl- channels. *The Journal of Biological Chemistry, 282*, 2259–2267.

Rinne, J. O., Laihinen, A., Nagren, K., Bergman, J., Haaparanta, M., Solin, O., et al. (1991). Positron emission tomography of brain dopamine D-1 receptors with 11C-SCH23390 in Parkinson's disease. *Acta Radiologica. Supplementum, 376*, 152.

Rinne, J. O., Laihinen, A., Rinne, U. K., Nagren, K., Bergman, J., & Ruotsalainen, U. (1993). PET study on striatal dopamine D2 receptor changes during the progression of early Parkinson's disease. *Movement Disorders, 8*(2), 134–138.

Rinne, J. O., Laihinen, A., Ruottinen, H., Ruotsalainen, U., Nagren, K., Lehikoinen, P., et al. (1995). Increased density of dopamine D2 receptors in the putamen, but not in the caudate nucleus in early Parkinson's disease: A PET study with [11C]raclopride. *Journal of the Neurological Sciences, 132*(2), 156–161.

Rinne, J. O., Myllykylä, T., Lönnberg, P., & Marjamäki, P. (1991). A postmortem study of brain nicotinic receptors in Parkinson's and Alzheimer's disease. *Brain Research, 547*(1), 167–170.

Roussakis, A. A., Piccini, P., & Politis, M. (2013). Clinical utility of DaTscan™ (123I-ioflupane injection) in the diagnosis of parkinsonian syndromes. *Degenerative Neurological and Neuromuscular Disease, 3*, 33–39.

Rowe, C. C., Ng, S., Ackermann, U., Gong, S. J., Pike, K., Savage, G., et al. (2007). Imaging β-amyloid burden in aging and dementia. *Neurology*, *68*, 1718–1725.

Russell, D. S., Barret, O., Jennings, D. L., Friedman, J. H., Tamagnan, G. D., Thomae, D., et al. (2014). The phosphodiesterase 10 positron emission tomography tracer, [18F] MNI-659, as a novel biomarker for early Huntington disease. *JAMA Neurology*, *71*(12), 1520–1528.

Russell, D. S., Jennings, D. L., Barret, O., Tamagnan, G. D., Carroll, V. M., Caillé, F., et al. (2016). Change in PDE10 across early Huntington disease assessed by [18F]MNI-659 and PET imaging. *Neurology*, *86*(8), 748–754.

Samadi, P., Bedard, P. J., & Rouillard, C. (2006). Opioids and motor complications in Parkinson's disease. *Trends in Pharmacological Sciences*, *27*, 512–517.

Samii, A., Nutt, J. G., & Ransom, B. R. (2004). Parkinson's disease. *Lancet*, *363*(9423), 1783–1793.

Sasaki, M., Shibata, E., Tohyama, K., Takahashi, J., Otsuka, K., Tsuchiya, K., et al. (2006). Neuromelanin magnetic resonance imaging of locus ceruleus and substantia nigra in Parkinson's disease. *Neuroreport*, *17*(11), 1215–1218.

Sawle, G. V., Playford, E. D., Brooks, D. J., Quinn, N., & Frackowiak, R. S. (1993). Asymmetrical presynaptic and postsynaptic changes in the striatal dopamine projection in dopa naïve parkinsonism. Diagnostic implications of the D2 receptor status. *Brain*, *116*, 853–867.

Schliebs, R., & Arendt, T. (2011). The cholinergic system in aging and neuronal degeneration. *Behavioural Brain Research*, *221*, 555–563.

Schmaljohann, J., Gündisch, D., Minnerop, M., Bucerius, J., Joe, A., Reinhardt, M., et al. (2006). In vitro evaluation of nicotinic acetylcholine receptors with 2-[18F]F-A85380 in Parkinson's disease. *Nuclear Medicine and Biology*, *33*(3), 305–309.

Schrag, A., & Politis, M. (2016). Serotonergic loss underlying apathy in Parkinson's disease. *Brain*, *139*(Pt. 9), 2338–2339.

Schwarz, S. T., Afzal, M., Morgan, P. S., Bajaj, N., Gowland, P. A., & Auer, D. P. (2014). The 'swallow tail' appearance of the healthy nigrosome—A new accurate test of Parkinson's disease: A case–control and retrospective cross-sectional MRI study at 3T. *PLoS One*, *9*, e93814.

Schwarz, S. T., Rittman, T., Gontu, V., Morgan, P. S., Bajaj, N., & Auer, D. P. (2011). T1-weighted MRI shows stage-dependent substantia nigra signal loss in Parkinson's disease. *Movement Disorders*, *26*(9), 1633–1638.

Schwarz, S. T., Xing, Y., Tomar, P., Bajaj, N., & Auer, D. P. (2016). In vivo assessment of brainstem depigmentation in Parkinson disease: Potential as a severity marker for multicenter studies. *Radiology*, 7, 160662.

Segura, B., Baggio, H. C., Marti, M. J., Valldeoriola, F., Compta, Y., Garcia-Diaz, A. I., et al. (2014). Cortical thinning associated with mild cognitive impairment in Parkinson's disease. *Movement Disorders*, *29*, 1495–1503.

Seibert, T. M., Murphy, E. A., Kaestner, E. J., & Brewer, J. B. (2012). Interregional correlations in Parkinson disease and Parkinson-related dementia with resting functional MR imaging. *Radiology*, *263*, 226–234.

Shimada, H., Hirano, S., Shinotoh, H., Aotsuka, A., Sato, K., Tanaka, N., et al. (2009). Mapping of brain acetylcholinesterase alterations in Lewy body disease by PET. *Neurology*, *73*, 273–278.

Shimada, H., Shinotoh, H., Hirano, S., Miyoshi, M., Sato, K., Tanaka, N., et al. (2013). β-Amyloid in Lewy body disease is related to Alzheimer's disease-like atrophy. *Movement Disorders*, *28*(2), 169–175.

Shine, J. M., Halliday, G. M., Gilat, M., Matar, E., Bolitho, S. J., Carlos, M., et al. (2014). The role of dysfunctional attentional networks in visual misperceptionsin Parkinson's disease. *Human Brain Mapping*, *35*, 2206–2219.

Shine, J. M., Mata, E., Ward, P. B., Bolitho, S. J., Pearson, M., Naismith, S. L., et al. (2013). Differential neural activation patterns in patients with Parkinson's disease and freezing of gait in response to concurrent cognitive and motorload. *PLoS One*, *8*(1), e52602.

Shiozaki, K., Iseki, E., Uchiyama, H., Watanabe, Y., Haga, T., Kameyama, K., et al. (1999). Alterations of muscarinic acetylcholine receptor subtypes in diffuse Lewy body disease: Relation to Alzheimer's disease. *Journal of Neurology, Neurosurgery, and Psychiatry*, *67*, 209–213.

Siderowf, A., Pontecorvo, M. J., Shill, H. A., Mintun, M. A., Arora, A., Joshi, A. D., et al. (2014). PET imaging of amyloid with Florbetapir F 18 and PET imaging of dopamine degeneration with 18F-AV-133 (florbenazine) in patients with Alzheimer's disease and Lewy body disorders. *BMC Neurology*, *14*, 79.

Slifstein, M., Kegeles, L. S., Gonzales, R., Frankle, W. G., Xu, X., et al. (2007). [11C] NNC 112 selectivity for dopamine D1 and serotonin 5-HT(2A) receptors: A PET study in healthy human subjects. *Journal of Cerebral Blood Flow and Metabolism*, *27*(10), 1733–1741.

Steeves, T. D. L., Miyasaki, J., Zurowski, M., Lang, A. E., Pellecchia, G., van Elmeren, T., et al. (2009). Increased striatal dopamine release in parkinsonian patients with pathological gambling: A 11C-raclopride PET study. *Brain*, *132*, 1376–1385.

Su, P., & Politis, M. (2012). The role of microglia in neurodegenerative disease. In C. Kaur & L. Eng-Ang (Eds.), *Microglia: Biology, functions and roles in disease* (pp. 93–117). New York: Nova publishers.

Surdhar, I., Gee, M., Bouchard, T., Coupland, N., Malykhin, N., & Camicioli, R. (2012). Intact limbic-prefrontal connections and reduced amygdala volumes in Parkinson's disease with mild depressive symptoms. *Parkinsonism & Related Disorders*, *18*, 809–813.

Tam, C. W. C., Burton, E. J., McKeith, I. G., Burn, D. J., & O'Brien, J. T. (2005). Temporal lobe atrophy on MRI in Parkinson disease with dementia: A comparison with Alzheimer disease and dementia with Lewy bodies. *Neurology*, *64*, 861–865.

Tanaka, H., Kannari, K., Maeda, T., Tomiyama, M., Suda, T., & Matsunaga, M. (1999). Role of serotonergic neurons in L-DOPA-derived extracellular dopamine in the striatum of 6-OHDA-lesioned rats. *Neuroreport*, *10*, 631–634.

Tatsch, K., Schwarz, J., Mozley, P. D., Linke, R., Pogarell, O., Oertel, W. H., et al. (1997). Relationship between clinical features of Parkinson's disease and presynaptic dopamine transporter binding assessed with [I123]IPT and single-photon emission tomography. *European Journal of Nuclear Medicine*, *24*(4), 415–421.

Tedroff, J., Pederson, M., Aquilonius, S. M., Hartvig, P., Jacobsson, G., & Langstrom, B. (1996). Levodopa induced changes in synaptic dopamine in patients with Parkinson's disease as measured by 11C-raclopride displacement and PET. *Neurology*, *46*, 1430–1436.

Tessitore, A., Esposito, F., Vitale, C., Santangelo, G., Amboni, M., Russo, A., et al. (2012). Default-mode network connectivity in cognitively unimpaired patients with Parkinson disease. *Neurology*, *79*(23), 2226–2232.

Tessitore, A., Santangelo, G., De Micco, R., Vitale, C., Giordano, A., Raimo, S., et al. (2016). Cortical thickness changes in patients with Parkinson's disease and impulse control disorders. *Parkinsonism & Related Disorders*, *24*, 119–125.

Turjanski, N., Lees, A. J., & Brooks, D. J. (1997). In vivo studies on striatal dopamine D1 and D2 site binding in L-DOPA treated Parkinson's disease patients with and without dyskinesias. *Neurology*, *49*, 717–723.

Ulla, M., Bonny, J. M., Ouchchane, L., Rieu, I., Claise, B., & Durif, F. (2013). Is R2* a new MRI biomarker for the progression of Parkinson's disease? A longitudinal follow-up. *PLoS One*, *8*, e57904.

Vaillancourt, D. E., Spraker, M. B., Prodoehl, J., Abraham, I., Corcos, D. M., Zhou, X. J., et al. (2009). High-resolution diffusion tensor imaging in the substantia nigra of de novo Parkinson disease. *Neurology*, *72*, 1378–1384.

van Laere, K., Casteels, C., Lunskens, S., Goffin, K., Grachev, I. D., Bormans, G., et al. (2012). Regional changes in type 1 cannabinoid receptor availability in Parkinson's disease in vivo. *Neurobiology of Aging*, *33*, 620.

Van Nuenen, B. F. L., van Eimeren, T., van der Vegt, J. P. M., Buhmann, C., Klein, C., Bloem, B. R., et al. (2009). Mapping preclinical compensation in Parkinson's disease: An imaging genomics approach. *Movement Disorders*, *24*, S703–S710.

Vas, A., Shchukin, Y., Karrenbauer, V. D., Cselényi, Z., Kostulas, K., Hillert, J., et al. (2008). Functional neuroimaging in multiple sclerosis with radiolabelled glia markers: Preliminary comparative PET studies with [11C]vinpocetine and [11C]PK11195 in patients. *Journal of the Neurological Sciences*, *264*, 9–17.

Vercruysse, S., Leunissen, I., Vervoort, G., Vandenberghe, W., Swinnen, S., & Nieuwboer, A. (2015). Microstructural changes in white matter associated with freezing of gait in Parkinson's disease. *Movement Disorders*, *30*, 567–576.

Villemagne, V. L., Ong, K., Mulligan, R. S., Holl, G., Pejoska, S., Jones, G., et al. (2011). Amyloid imaging with 18F-florbetaben in Alzheimer disease and other dementias. *Journal of Nuclear Medicine*, *52*, 1210–1217.

Vingerhoets, F. J. G., Schulzer, M., Calne, D. B., & Snow, B. J. (1997). Which clinical sign of Parkinson's disease best reflects the nigrostriatal lesion? *Annals of Neurology*, *41*, 58–64.

Wallis, L. I., Paley, M. N., Graham, J. M., Grünewald, R. A., Wignall, E. L., Joy, H. M., et al. (2008). MRI assessment of basal ganglia iron deposition in Parkinson's disease. *Journal of Magnetic Resonance Imaging*, *28*, 1061–1067.

Weintraub, D., Doshi, J., Koka, D., Davatzikos, C., Siderowf, A. D., Duda, J. E., et al. (2011). Neurodegeneration across stages of cognitive decline in Parkinson disease. *Archives of Neurology*, *68*, 1562–1568.

Weiss, P. H., Herzog, J., Pötter-Nerger, M., Falk, D., Herzog, H., Deuschl, G., et al. (2015). Subthalamic nucleus stimulation improves parkinsonian gait viabrainstem locomotor centers. *Movement Disorders*, *30*(8), 1121–1125.

Weng, Y. H., Yen, T. C., Chen, M. C., Kao, P. F., Tzen, K. Y., Chen, R. S., et al. (2004). Sensitivity and specificity of (99m)Tc-TRODAT-1 SPECT imaging in differentiating patients with idiopathic Parkinson's disease from healthy subjects. *Journal of Nuclear Medicine*, *45*(3), 393–401.

Wieler, M., Gee, M., & Martin, W. R. (2015). Longitudinal midbrain changes in early Parkinson's disease: Iron content estimated from R2*/MRI. *Parkinsonism & Related Disorders*, *21*, 179–183.

Wilson, A. A., Ginovart, N., Schmidt, M., Meyer, J. H., Threlkeld, P. G., & Houle, S. (2000). Novel radiotracers for imaging the serotonin transporter by positron emission tomography: Synthesis, radiosynthesis, and in vitro and ex vitro evaluation of 11C labelled 2-(phenylthio) araalkylamines. *Journal of Medicinal Chemistry*, *43*, 3103–3110.

Winogrodzka, A., Bergmans, P., Booij, J., van Royen, E. A., Janssen, A. G., & Wolters, E. C. (2001). [123I]FP-CIT SPECT is a useful method to monitor the rate of dopaminergic degeneration in early-stage Parkinson's disease. *Journal of Neural Transmission (Vienna)*, *108*(8–9), 1011–1019.

Winogrodzka, A., Bergmans, P., Booij, J., van Royen, E. A., Stoof, J. C., & Wolters, E. C. (2003). [I123]β-CIT SPECT is a useful method for monitoring dopaminergic degeneration in early stage Parkinson's disease. *Journal of Neurology, Neurosurgery, and Psychiatry*, *74*(3), 294–298.

Wu, T., Long, X., Wang, L., Hallett, M., Zang, Y., Li, K., et al. (2011). Functionalconnectivity of cortical motor areas in the resting state in Parkinson's disease. *Human Brain Mapping*, *32*, 1443–1457.

Wu, T., Wang, L., Hallett, M., Chen, Y., Li, K., & Chan, P. (2011). Effective connectivityof brain networks during self-initiated movement in Parkinson's disease. *NeuroImage*, *55*, 204–215.

Yao, N., Pang, S., Cheung, C., Chang, R. S., Lau, K. K., Suckling, J., et al. (2015). Resting activity in visual and corticostriatal pathways in Parkinson's disease with hallucinations. *Parkinsonism & Related Disorders*, *21*, 131–137.
Yoshikawa, K., Nakata, Y., Yamada, K., & Nakagawa, M. (2004). Early pathological changes in the parkinsonian brain demonstrated by diffusion tensor MRI. *Journal of Neurology, Neurosurgery, and Psychiatry*, *75*, 481–484.
Zarei, M., Ibarretxe-Bilbao, N., Compta, Y., Hough, M., Junque, C., Bargallo, N., et al. (2013). Cortical thinning is associated with disease stages and dementia in Parkinson's disease. *Journal of Neurology, Neurosurgery, and Psychiatry*, *84*, 875–881.
Zhan, W., Kang, G. A., Glass, G. A., Zhang, Y., Shirley, C., Millin, R., et al. (2012). Regional alterations of brain microstructure in Parkinson's disease using diffusion tensor imaging. *Movement Disorders*, *27*, 90–97.
Zhang, W., Sun, S. G., Jiang, Y. H., Qiao, X., Sun, X., & Wu, Y. (2009). Determination of brain iron content in patients with Parkinson's disease using magnetic susceptibility imaging. *Neuroscience Bulletin*, *25*, 353–360.
Zhang, J., Zhang, Y., Wang, J., Cai, P., Luo, C., Qian, Z., et al. (2010). Characterizing iron deposition in Parkinson's disease using susceptibility-weighted imaging: An in vivo MR study. *Brain Research*, *1330*, 124–130.
Zheng, Z., Shemmassian, S., Wijekoon, C., Kim, W., Bookheimer, S. Y., & Pouratian, N. (2014). DTI correlates of distinct cognitive impairments in Parkinson's disease. *Human Brain Mapping*, *35*, 1325–1333.
Zhou, F. M., Wilson, C. J., & Dani, J. A. (2002). Cholinergic interneuron characteristics and nicotinic properties in the striatum. *Journal of Neurobiology*, *53*(4), 590–605.

CHAPTER TEN

Cerebrospinal Fluid Biomarkers of Cognitive Decline in Parkinson's Disease

Iskandar Johar*, Brit Mollenhauer[†,‡], Dag Aarsland[*,1]
*Institute of Psychiatry, Psychology and Neuroscience, King's College London, London, United Kingdom
[†]Paracelsus-Elena-Klinik, Kassel, Germany
[‡]University Medical Center, Göttingen, Germany
[1]Corresponding author: e-mail address: dag.aarsland@kcl.ac.uk

Contents

Abstract

Among the nonmotor symptoms in Parkinson's disease (PD), cognitive impairment is one of the most common and devastating. Over recent years, mild cognitive impairment (MCI) has become a recognized feature of PD (PD-MCI). The underlying mechanisms which influence onset, rate of decline, and conversion to dementia (PDD) are largely unknown. Adding to this uncertainty is the heterogeneity of cognitive domains affected. Currently there are no disease-modifying treatments that can slow or reverse this process. Identification of biomarkers that can predict rate and risk of cognitive decline is therefore an unmet need. Cerebrospinal fluid (CSF) is an ideal biomarker candidate as its constituents reflect the metabolic processes underlying the functioning of brain parenchyma. The pathological hallmark of PD is the presence of aggregated α-synuclein (α-Syn) in intracellular Lewy inclusions. In addition, there is concomitant Alzheimer's disease (AD) pathology. In AD, decreased CSF β-amyloid 1–42 (Aβ42) and increased CSF tau levels are predictive of future cognitive decline, setting a precedent for such studies to be carried out in PD. CSF studies in PD have focused on the classical AD biomarkers and α-Syn. Longitudinal studies indicate that low levels of

International Review of Neurobiology, Volume 132
ISSN 0074-7742
http://dx.doi.org/10.1016/bs.irn.2016.12.001

CSF Aβ42 are predictive of cognitive decline; however, results for tau and α-Syn were not consistent. This chapter summarizes recent findings of CSF biomarker studies and cognitive dysfunction in PD.

1. INTRODUCTION

Parkinson's disease (PD) is a neurodegenerative condition clinically characterized by the combination of motor symptoms—resting tremor, rigidity, bradykinesia, and postural instability. Nonmotor symptoms, in particular, cognitive decline in PD, are highly prevalent with cumulative incidence of dementia, reaching up to 80% in PD patients living more than 20 years (Aarsland, Zaccai, & Brayne, 2005). Although the average time from onset of PD to dementia is around 10 years, this is highly variable, with some patients developing dementia within the first 5 years or even earlier, whereas others may remain free of dementia for more than 20 years or never get demented. Over recent years, mild cognitive impairment (MCI) has become recognized as an important clinical manifestation of PD (PD-MCI), leading to the formulation of diagnostic criteria (Litvan et al., 2012). PD-MCI is common with point prevalence estimated to be as high as 40% (Aarsland, Bronnick, Larsen, Tysnes, & Alves, 2009; Yarnall et al., 2014). Individuals with PD-MCI are at increased risk of developing PD dementia (PDD), contributing to worsening disability, higher caregiver burden, and an increase in mortality (Aarsland et al., 2009; Schrag, Jahanshahi, & Quinn, 2000).

Treatment of cognitive dysfunction in PD is mainly symptomatic and supportive with no disease-modifying treatments that can affect or reverse disease course and prevent progression from PD-MCI to PDD. Identifying PD patients who are at risk of developing MCI and dementia in the early stages of disease progression will allow physicians to better assess the patient's prognosis and make informed decisions on the best course of management. Furthermore, early identification would allow for appropriate clinical trials to explore potential of novel neuroprotective or neurorestorative therapies and as secondary prevention efforts would be expected to have the most efficacious benefits early on in the disease. Given the need to stratify and predict patient risk of cognitive decline, along with the heterogeneity of cognitive domains affected including executive, function, memory, attention, and working memory (Caviness et al., 2007), the relationships between PD with cognitive dysfunction and imaging, biofluid, and genetic biomarkers have been studied in great detail.

Cerebrospinal fluid (CSF) has been extensively studied and is representative of cognitive decline in other neurodegenerative disorders due to its proximity to the central nervous system. The pathological hallmark of PD is the presence of presynaptic α-synuclein (α-Syn) aggregates (Schulz-Schaeffer, 2010) and Lewy bodies that are ubiquitin-positive and α-Syn-enriched intracytoplasmic neuronal inclusions in neocortical and limbic brain regions (Braak et al., 2003). There is overlap with Alzheimer's disease (AD) pathology—neurofibrillary tau tangles and amyloid-beta (Aβ) plaques frequently coexisting with evidence, suggesting that severity of amyloid plaque burden being associated with PDD (Compta et al., 2011). Postmortem studies have found Aβ plaques and neurofibrillary tau tangles in 50% of PDD patients (Irwin, Lee, & Trojanowski, 2013), and these are also present in PD-MCI (Jellinger, 2010). CSF is in direct contact with the extracellular space of the brain. It is estimated that 80% of CSF proteins are derived from direct filtration of peripheral blood once crossing the blood–brain barrier, while the remaining 20% are synthesized de novo from within neuronal cells (Reiber, 2003) and so reflect brain metabolism and neuronal health, mirroring many of the cellular and biochemical changes during the pathological process making CSF an excellent source for reliable biomarkers. In AD, CSF biomarkers can accurately predict which patients with MCI will develop AD (Olsson et al., 2016), setting a promising precedent for such studies to be carried out in PD. It is consequently of no surprise that CSF studies have mainly focused on AD biomarkers—β-amyloid 1–42 (Aβ42)—a fragment of the most common isoform of Aβ in plaques, total tau (t-tau), and tau protein phosphorylated at threonine-181 (p-tau). In AD, Aβ levels reflect amyloid plaque pathology, whereas t-tau and p-tau levels correspond to neuronal degeneration and tau tangle pathology, respectively, with the classical signature of AD showing low levels of Aβ42 and high levels of t-tau and p-tau (Olsson et al., 2016). Given the likely role of AD-type pathology for cognitive decline in PD, these CSF markers may also be relevant markers of cognitive decline in PD. In addition to the AD biomarkers, and potentially more specific for PD, α-Syn, both total (t-α-Syn) and, more recently, its oligomeric form (o-α-Syn) have also been investigated. The aim of this chapter is to examine the role of CSF biomarkers associated with cognitive dysfunction and as potential biomarkers in predicting risk of progression to PD-MCI and conversion to PDD.

2. β-AMYLOID 1–42

2.1 Cross-Sectional Studies

As diagnostic criteria for PD-MCI had only been established in 2012, early cross-sectional studies examined Aβ42 in PDD compared to PD with no dementia or healthy controls. Levels of CSF Aβ42 were found to be consistently lower in PDD compared to controls (Compta et al., 2015; Montine et al., 2010) and PD (Compta et al., 2009, 2015; Mollenhauer et al., 2006). Studies have associated low levels of Aβ42 with deficits in phonetic memory (Compta et al., 2009), attention, working memory (Leverenz et al., 2011), visual memory (Yarnall et al., 2014), verbal learning, delayed recall, and response inhibition (Stav et al., 2015). Other fragments of the Aβ peptide—Aβ38 and Aβ40—have also been investigated with one associating both Aβ38 and Aβ40 (Alves et al., 2010) and another correlating Aβ40 only (Yarnall et al., 2014) with memory deficits; however, this has not been replicated in other studies (Beyer et al., 2013; Stav et al., 2015).

Cross-sectional studies in PD-MCI individuals project a more varied picture, with three studies associating low levels of Aβ42 with PD-MCI (Montine et al., 2010; Skogseth et al., 2015; Yarnall et al., 2014) and two studies showing no association (Beyer et al., 2013; Yu et al., 2014). Overall, these studies in PDD and PD-MCI strongly associate low CSF Aβ42 levels and cognitive dysfunction in PD. However, due to the single-survey nature of cross-sectional studies, it is not possible to infer any predictive information on which PD individuals will go on to develop cognitive deficits. This requires a longitudinal design.

2.2 Longitudinal Studies

Nine studies assessed whether CSF Aβ42 levels could predict future cognitive decline using a prospective design. Of these, seven studies showed that Aβ42 was consistently associated with cognitive decline (Table 1). Interestingly, these findings were observed despite differences regarding outcome measures, CSF biomarker analysis methods, and neuropsychological tests between studies. Several studies examined for the rate of change from baseline to follow-up assessments on cognitive measures. Siderowf et al. (2010) published the first longitudinal study of 45 PD subjects and demonstrated that low CSF levels of Aβ42 at baseline correlated significantly with faster decline on the Mattis Dementia Rating Scale-2 after an interval of 18 months. Since then, a number of studies have linked low CSF Aβ42 levels with a more rapid rate of cognitive decline, using scales such as Alzheimer's Disease Assessment Scale Cognitive Subscale—specifically delayed recall (Hall et al., 2015), Mini-Mental State Examination (MMSE) (Parnetti et al., 2014), and the Montreal Cognitive Assessment (MoCA) (Fullard et al., 2016; Parnetti et al., 2014) with Fullard et al. using a composite measure of impaired olfaction in combination with low CSF Aβ42 to predict

Table 1 An Overview of Longitudinal Studies of Cerebrospinal Fluid Biomarker Candidates Predicting Cognitive Decline in Parkinson's Disease

Study	Cases and Controls	Follow-Up Duration (Years)	Disease Duration (Years)	MMSE at Baseline	Aβ42	t-Tau	p-Tau	Other Biomarkers	Summary Findings
Siderowf et al. (2010)	PD 45	1.5	11	DRS-2 133	↓ Aβ42	No association	No association	—	Low Aβ42 associated with more rapid cognitive decline measured by DRS-2
Compta et al. (2013)	PD 27	1.5	10	28	↓ Aβ42	No association	No association	—	Low Aβ42 associated with progression to PDD
Alves et al. (2014)	PD 104	5	De novo	28	↓ Aβ42	No association	No association	Aβ40, Aβ38	Low Aβ42 associated with progression to PDD. Aβ40 and Aβ38 not associated with cognitive decline
Parnetti et al. (2014)	PD 44 Control 25	3	3	27	↓ Aβ42	No association	No association	—	Low Aβ42 associated with more rapid cognitive decline measured by MMSE and MoCA
Liu et al. (2015)	PD 403	4.3	3.8	29	No association	No association	↑ p-Tau	—	High p-tau and p-tau/Aβ42 correlated with increased rate of cognitive decline measured by SRT-Total and SDMT

Continued

Table 1 An Overview of Longitudinal Studies of Cerebrospinal Fluid Biomarker Candidates Predicting Cognitive Decline in Parkinson's Disease—cont'd

Study	Cases and Controls	Follow-Up Duration (Years)	Disease Duration (Years)	MMSE at Baseline	Aβ42	t-Tau	p-Tau	Other Biomarkers	Summary Findings
Backstrom et al. (2015)	PD 99 Control 30	5–9	1.4	29	↓ Aβ42	No association	No association	NFL, HFABP	Low Aβ42 associated with progression to PDD. Combination of low Aβ42, high NFL, and HFABP predicted PDD with high accuracy
Terrelonge et al. (2016)	PD 341	2	0.6	—	↓ Aβ42	No association	No association	—	Low Aβ42 associated with cognitive impairment
Hall et al. (2015)	PD 42 Control 69	2	7	29	↓ Aβ42	No association	No association	NFL	Low Aβ42 associated with cognitive decline as measured by delayed recall in ADAS-Cog. NFL not predictive of cognitive decline
Hall et al. (2016)	PD 63 Control 21	2	5.5	29	No association	No association	Increase in p-tau	NFL, YKL-40	Increase in p-tau and YKL-40 correlated with worsening of cognitive function measured by letter fluency

Please see Table 2 for studies on α-synuclein. *NB*: Fullard et al. (2016) excluded from table as cohort used in the study was the same as Terrelonge et al. (2016).
Abbreviations: *PD*, Parkinson's disease; *PDD*, Parkinson's disease dementia; *ADAS-Cog*, Alzheimer's Disease Assessment Scale Cognitive Subscale; *MMSE*, Mini--Mental State Exam; *MoCA*, Montreal Cognitive Assessment; *DRS-2*, Mattis Dementia Rating Scale-2; *SRT-Total*, Selective Reminding Test-Total; *SDMT*, Symbol Digit Modalities Test; *NFL*, neurofilament light; *HFABP*, heart fatty acid-binding protein.

cognitive decline. Another study associated low baseline CSF Aβ42 and the development of PD with "cognitive impairment," defined as at least two out of six neuropsychological scores greater than 1.5 standard deviations below the standardized means based on healthy controls (Terrelonge, Marder, Weintraub, & Alcalay, 2016). Other studies used conversion from PD to PDD as an outcome measure. Three longitudinal studies associated low Aβ42 CSF levels at baseline with greater risk of developing PDD both in comparison to healthy controls (Backstrom et al., 2015) and PD patients without cognitive impairment (Alves et al., 2014; Compta et al., 2013). In contrast to Aβ42, although in only one study, Aβ38 and Aβ40 CSF levels were not predictive of cognitive decline in PD (Alves et al., 2014).

Overall, low levels of CSF Aβ42 are an independent predictor of cognitive decline in PD despite the variability in outcome measures and differing follow-up lengths. However, given the lack of consistent cognitive assessment tools used, it is not possible to identify which specific cognitive domains are associated with low CSF Aβ42. Further research on longitudinal studies should involve standardized cognitive assessments to elucidate this matter. Biological confounding factors that affect CSF Aβ42 levels need to be taken into consideration as it is not possible to attribute decreased CSF Aβ42 levels solely due to amyloid plaque pathology. Low levels of CSF Aβ42 are also observed in other neurodegenerative conditions where plaque formation is rare such as in Creutzfeldt–Jakob disease (CJD) (Otto et al., 2000), although the CSF profile of PD individuals with low Aβ42 and increased tau supports the hypothesis that AD copathology contributes to the development of cognitive impairment. There is evidence of an interaction between amyloid, α-Syn, and tau-pathology, indicating that they increase the aggregation of each other, although it was recently shown that α-Syn interacts with Aβ to inhibit plaque formation in vivo but the precise mechanism remains unknown (Bachhuber et al., 2015). Further research is needed to understand this interaction. Other factors may contribute to cognitive decline in PD, such as chronic cerebrovascular disease affecting brain parenchymal metabolism, CSF production, blood–brain barrier filtration rate, and permeability, thus altering CSF composition (Mollenhauer et al., 2015) or alternatively through novel undiscovered mechanisms.

3. T-TAU AND P-TAU

Several studies assessed whether CSF levels of t-tau and/or p-tau were associated with cognition in PD. The evidence in cross-sectional studies for tau as an indicator of cognitive decline in PD is less consistent than Aβ42, with some showing higher levels (Compta et al., 2009, 2015; Hall et al., 2012; Mollenhauer et al., 2006) and others showing no differences (Montine et al., 2010; Parnetti et al., 2008; Vranova et al., 2014) in CSF tau levels in PDD as compared to PD with no dementia or controls. A similar picture is seen in PD-MCI with one study showing higher levels of t-tau in comparison to PD and control (Yu et al., 2014) and other studies demonstrated no discernible differences between levels of both tau species compared to control (Beyer et al., 2013; Montine et al., 2010; Skogseth et al., 2015).

All nine longitudinal studies showed that CSF t-tau levels measured at baseline were not predictive of cognitive decline in PD (Table 1), although one study associated low Aβ42/t-tau with increased rate of decline in MMSE but not MoCA (Parnetti et al., 2014). While another study used a composite measure of olfaction and t-tau/Aβ42 and found that worse olfaction in combination with higher t-tau/Aβ42 ratio corresponded to a faster rate of decline in MoCA (Fullard et al., 2016). These nine studies also examined for p-tau with only two studies finding a significant association with p-tau and rate of cognitive decline (Hall et al., 2016; Liu et al., 2015). Liu et al. (2015) reported that high p-tau levels at baseline correlated with a more rapid decline in memory and executive function as measured by Selective Reminding Test-Total and Symbol Digit Modalities Test. In addition, the ratio of p-tau/Aβ42 was also associated with increased rate of decline in these same assessments. In one of the few studies of repeated CSF measurements to determine longitudinal biomarker trajectories in relation to cognitive decline, Hall et al. (2016) measured CSF levels of 63 PD patients at baseline and subsequently after 2 years. There was an increase in p-tau and t-tau over the 2 years compared to controls but only in the PD group with long disease duration (>5 years). Although an increase in CSF t-tau levels from baseline did not correspond to cognitive impairment, increasing CSF p-tau measurements over 2 years corresponded with a worsening of executive function as measured by letter fluency. Thus, CSF tau levels are not likely to be predictive of cognitive decline as all but two of the longitudinal studies failed to find a relationship. Furthermore, the addition of t-tau and p-tau with Aβ42 in a combined metric lessened the predictive effects of Aβ42 alone (Siderowf et al., 2010) but with majority sample sizes in the studies not exceeding 100, firm conclusions are not possible to make.

4. TOTAL α-SYN AND OLIGOMERIC α-SYN

A meta-analysis and a large multicenter cohort study indicated that low levels of CSF total α-synuclein (t-α-Syn) are observed in PD compared to controls (Gao et al., 2015; Kang et al., 2013). However, the association between t-α-Syn and cognitive impairment continues to be inconsistent (Table 2). Thirteen studies have explored this association, seven cross-sectional and six with longitudinal design. In PDD, several recent studies of t-α-Syn have been reported with the majority of cross-sectional studies showing significant overlap in single values of levels of t-α-Syn compared to controls (Buddhala et al., 2015; Hall et al., 2012; Hansson et al., 2014; Stav et al., 2015; Yarnall et al., 2014). Only two studies associated low levels of t-α-Syn with cognitive impairment as measured by deficits in composite cognition and executive-attention domain scores in a cohort of newly diagnosed untreated PD patients (Skogseth et al., 2015) and phonetic fluency (Compta et al., 2015). Results for longitudinal studies show a similar picture. Out of the seven longitudinal studies that assessed t-α-Syn, only two described positive associations between t-α-Syn and cognitive decline (Table 2). Both studies reported high levels of CSF t-α-Syn at baseline, predicting a more rapid cognitive decline (Hall et al., 2015; Stewart et al., 2014). Stewart et al. (2014) found that high levels of CSF t-α-Syn correlated with a faster decline in memory performance and visual memory as measured by Selective Reminding Test-Total and Delayed and the New Dot Test, respectively. Similarly, Hall et al. (2015) associated high levels of CSF t-α-Syn with worsening of cognitive processing speed as measured by A Quick Test of Cognitive Speed. There are several factors which could have influenced the contrasting results. Not much is known on confounding factors and reasons for large variation of single values. One possible explanation could be the differences in sample handling of CSF, i.e., variations in accounting for CSF hemoglobin concentration as a result of blood contamination which is key due to the high abundance of α-Syn in peripheral blood. Another explanation may be attributed to differences in disease stage and subsequent temporal variation of t-α-Syn. Average symptom duration in the studies varied: Skogseth et al. (2015): 4 months; Stewart et al. (2014): 4 years; and Hall et al. (2015): 7 years. As described in the previous section, Hall et al. (2016) carried out serial measurements of CSF levels and after 2 years found that in addition to tau, t-α-Syn levels were also increased in PD with longer disease duration compared to the PD with shorter disease

Table 2 Cerebrospinal Fluid Studies Examining Associations Between α-Synuclein and Cognition in Parkinson's Disease

Study	Type	Cases and Controls	Disease Duration (Years)	Average MMSE	t-α-Syn	o-α-Syn	Method	Summary Findings
Hall et al. (2012)	Cross sectional	PD 90 PDD 30 Control 107	—	29	+	–	Luminex	No differences in t-α-Syn between PDD and controls
Stewart et al. (2014)	Longitudinal	PDD 266	4	29	+	–	Luminex	High CSF t-α-Syn associated with more rapid cognitive decline measured by SRT-Total and Delayed and New Dot Test
Parnetti et al. (2014)	Longitudinal	PD 44 Control 25	3	27	+	+	ELISA	No association with t-α-Syn and o-α-Syn with cognitive decline measured by MMSE and MoCA
Yarnall et al. (2014)	Cross sectional	PD 126 PD-MCI 93 Control 99	0.5	PD 29 PD-MCI 28	+	–	ELISA	t-α-Syn levels not associated with cognitive impairment
Backstrom et al. (2015)	Longitudinal	PD 99	1.4	29	+	–	ELISA	No association with t-α-Syn and cognitive decline
Terrelonge et al. (2016)	Longitudinal	PD 341	0.6	—	+	–	ELISA	No association with t-α-Syn and cognitive decline
Hall et al. (2015)	Longitudinal	PD 42 Control 69	7	29	+	–	Luminex	High CSF t-α-Syn at baseline associated faster decline in cognitive processing speed measured by AQT

Skogseth et al. (2015)	Cross sectional	PD 414 Control 189	0.3	—	+	–	ELISA	Lower t-α-Syn associated with cognitive impairment measured by composite cognition score and executive-attention domain
Buddhala, Campbell, Perlmutter, and Kotzbauer (2015)	Cross sectional	PD 77 Control 33	5	—	+	–	ELISA	No association with t-α-Syn and cognitive impairment
Hansson et al. (2014)	Cross sectional	PDD 48 Control 98	—	24	+	+	Luminex t-α-Syn ELISA o-α-Syn	o-α-Syn levels are higher in PDD compared to controls. No association with cognition as measured by MMSE
Compta et al. (2015)	Cross sectional	PDD 20 PD 21 Control 13	PD 10 PDD 11	PD 28 PDD 18	+	+	ELISA	t-α-Syn associated with deficits in phonetic fluency. o-α-Syn levels are higher in PDD compared to control
Stav et al. (2015)	Cross sectional	PD 31 Control 34	2.5	29	+	–	MesoScale Discovery	No association with t-α-Syn and cognitive impairment
Hall et al. (2016)	Longitudinal	PD 63 Control 21	5.5	29	+	–	Luminex	No association with t-α-Syn and cognitive decline

Abbreviations: *PD*, Parkinson's disease; *PDD*, Parkinson's disease dementia; *PD-MCI*, Parkinson's disease mild cognitive impairment; *CSF*, cerebrospinal fluid; *MMSE*, Mini-Mental State Exam; *MoCA*, Montreal Cognitive Assessment; *SRT*, Selective Reminding Test; *AQT*, A Quick Test of Cognitive Speed.

duration group; however, this increase was not associated with cognitive decline. Nevertheless, the authors have proposed a two-phase model of CSF t-α-Syn levels reflecting disease duration, with t-α-Syn levels initially low in the earlier stages of PD likely due to intracellular accumulation of α-Syn and later, as PD progresses, t-α-Syn levels increase as a result of worsening neuronal damage. Other confounding factors may be due to the type of immunoassays used, differences in preanalytical handling, and sample processing. α-Syn undergoes a series of posttranslational modifications (Schmid, Fauvet, Moniatte, & Lashuel, 2013). For higher specificity it is crucial to identify possible disease-specific posttranslational modified forms in biofluids in PD patients. Several posttranslational modified forms of α-Syn have been identified in PD including ubiquitinated, phosphorylated, nitrated, and also oligomeric forms (Ohrfelt et al., 2011; Simonsen et al., 2016). Currently, there have been no cross-sectional or longitudinal studies of ubiquitinated, phosphorylated, and nitrated forms of α-Syn in PD and cognitive decline. Studies in CSF o-α-Syn levels in relation to cognition are very limited. o-α-Syn, in particular the prefibrillar o-α-Syn species, is thought be the major neurotoxic species (Conway et al., 2000; El-Agnaf, Walsh, & Allsop, 2003) with levels raised in PD compared to controls (Park, Cheon, Bae, Kim, & Kim, 2011; Tokuda et al., 2010). Cross-sectional studies show higher o-α-Syn levels in PDD compared to controls (Compta et al., 2015; Hansson et al., 2014). Only one longitudinal study has examined the role of o-α-Syn and found no relationship with cognitive decline but identified an increase in levels of o-α-Syn and decrease in t-α-Syn in the PD group compared to controls (Parnetti et al., 2014). Despite this, given the role of α-Syn in PD neuropathology, α-Syn and its posttranslational modified forms possibly present in other biological fluids continue to be an attractive biomarker for future studies. Very much analogous to AD and identifying various isoforms of Aβ which predict rate and risk of future cognitive decline, the development of new, more sensitive immunoassays for posttranslational modified forms of α-Syn, standardized analyzing techniques, and more longitudinal studies with serial CSF measurements may identify an α-Syn species with more prognostic yield with regard to cognitive decline.

5. OTHER CSF BIOMARKERS

Cross-sectional studies examining other CSF biomarkers have mainly focused on markers of inflammation and reactive oxygen species. In PDD, levels of both CSF C-reactive protein (Lindqvist et al., 2013), a marker of inflammation, and neurofilament light (NFL) (Hall et al., 2012)—an indicator of neuronal damage—were higher compared to PD and controls. CSF levels of cystatin C—proposed to inhibit Aβ aggregation (Mathews & Levy, 2016) and CSF uric acid, which has antioxidant properties—have been shown to be lower in PDD compared to controls and PD, respectively (Maetzler et al., 2010, 2011). PD-MCI is associated with higher levels of certain cytokines—interleukin-6 (IL-6), interleukin-1β (IL-1β), free radicals—hydroxyl (OH) and nitric oxide (NO) with lower levels of interferon-γ and tumor necrosis factor-α (TNF-α) compared to controls (Yu et al., 2014). Of note, levels of IL-6 were also higher in PD-MCI compared to PD and along with OH levels, correlating negatively with MoCA. Overall, it is known that neuroinflammation occurs in PD and might be a trigger for propagation of the disease (Hirsch, Vyas, & Hunot, 2012), but it is unlikely that this is PD specific as other neurodegenerative disorders such as Huntington's disease and progressive supranuclear palsy show evidence of neuroinflammatory processes (McGeer & McGeer, 2004).

Several of the longitudinal studies were examined for other CSF biomarkers (Table 1). CSF levels of NFL were not predictive of cognitive decline in PD (Hall et al., 2016, 2015). Interestingly, one study was able to predict conversion to PDD with high accuracy using a combination of high NFL, low Aβ42, and high heart fatty acid-binding protein (HFABP)—which plays a role in lipid metabolism and a marker of neurodegeneration with a sensitivity of 90% and specificity of 71% (Backstrom et al., 2015). Though originally discovered in the myocardium, HFABP distribution is widespread in other tissues especially the brain and has also been found to be elevated in other neurodegenerative conditions such as AD (Chiasserini et al., 2010) and CJD (Guillaume, Zimmermann, Burkhard, Hochstrasser, & Sanchez, 2003). Another study found that YKL-40, a marker of inflammation, increased over 2 years and correlated with a worsening in cognitive function as measured by letter fluency (Hall et al., 2016). Though promising, further research is required to expand on these findings, given the small number of studies. One potential avenue for future exploration are CSF markers of synaptic dysfunction. Alterations in synaptic function occur in PD (Pienaar, Burn, Morris, & Dexter, 2012). Pathological studies have shown that ZnT3, neurogranin (Ng), and SNAP25, markers of synaptic plasticity and function, are associated with cognition and PD (Bereczki et al., 2016; Whitfield et al., 2014). Preliminary studies on CSF synaptic protein levels in PD are currently ongoing and are promising candidates for future biomarker studies.

6. LUMBAR PUNCTURE SAFETY

CSF is regularly collected by lumbar puncture (LP). The most common adverse side effect of LP is post-LP headache, with prevalence estimated to be up to 32% (Armon & Evans, 2005) depending on the population, technique, and needle type used (Hammond, Wang, Bhulani, McArthur, & Levy, 2011). Several studies have examined the safety profile of carrying out LPs in the older population. Prevalence of post-LP headache in a memory clinic setting ranges from 3% to 9% (Blennow, Wallin, & Hager, 1993; Duits et al., 2016; Zetterberg et al., 2010). The largest and most systematic of these studies ($n=3868$) reported incidence of post-LP headache at 9%. In this study, all patients were systematically asked for complications (Duits et al., 2016), most likely explaining the higher post-LP headache rate. When performed with small-bore atraumatic (noncutting) spinal needles, post-LP headache rates drop to less than 2% (Peskind, Nordberg, Darreh-Shori, & Soininen, 2009; Peskind et al., 2005; Vidoni, Morris, Raider, & Burns, 2014) and are not related to the amount of CSF obtained during the procedure (Duits et al., 2016). Other infrequent complications include infection (<0.1%) (van de Beek, Drake, & Tunkel, 2010) and spinal hematomas (<0.1%) (Zetterberg et al., 2010).

It is clear that additional work on peripheral biomarkers in PD needs to be pursued. Studies for other fluid biomarkers have been discussed, and though promising, longitudinal studies are limited (Delgado-Alvarado, Gago, Navalpotro-Gomez, Jimenez-Urbieta, & Rodriguez-Oroz, 2016). Given the proximity of CSF and its relation to brain parenchyma, the excellent safety profile of LPs in an older population (when using small-bore atraumatic needles), and lack of cost compared to imaging modalities, CSF is an ideal biomarker and should be done routinely in clinical practice or research. This will allow for early diagnosis in differentiating different types of dementia, predicting risk of cognitive decline and further the development of novel CSF biomarkers not only in PD but also in other neurodegenerative conditions affecting cognition.

7. CONCLUSION

Identification, prediction, and treatment of cognitive dysfunction in PD is a priority, and to achieve this, we need to understand the biology underlying cognition and PD. There is now robust evidence, including several longitudinal studies, to conclude that low CSF Aβ42 is predictive of cognitive decline, and thus may have a role in clinical practice. Low CSF Aβ42 has also been shown to predict cognitive decline in a related disorder dementia with Lewy bodies (DLB) (Abdelnour et al., 2016), strengthening this conclusion. A subgroup of PD and perhaps DLB patients with low CSF Aβ42 may therefore benefit from immunotherapies targeting amyloid which are currently being trialed in AD. Although the evidence for α-Syn is inconsistent, with the elucidation of posttranslational α-Syn species including o-α-Syn and the ongoing development of newer and more sensitive immunoassays, it continues to hold much promise as a biomarker of cognitive decline. It is likely that a multimodal approach is necessary to identify PD patients at risk of cognitive decline and should include biochemical, imaging, and genetic biomarkers allowing for the accurate assessment of risk and prediction of future cognitive decline in PD.

REFERENCES

Aarsland, D., Bronnick, K., Larsen, J. P., Tysnes, O. B., & Alves, G. (2009). Cognitive impairment in incident, untreated Parkinson disease: The Norwegian ParkWest study. *Neurology*, *72*(13), 1121–1126. http://dx.doi.org/10.1212/01.wnl.0000338632.00552.cb.

Aarsland, D., Zaccai, J., & Brayne, C. (2005). A systematic review of prevalence studies of dementia in Parkinson's disease. *Movement Disorders*, *20*(10), 1255–1263. http://dx.doi.org/10.1002/mds.20527.

Abdelnour, C., van Steenoven, I., Londos, E., Blanc, F., Auestad, B., Kramberger, M. G., … Aarsland, D. (2016). Alzheimer's disease cerebrospinal fluid biomarkers predict cognitive decline in Lewy body dementia. *Movement Disorders*, *31*(8), 1203–1208. http://dx.doi.org/10.1002/mds.26668.

Alves, G., Bronnick, K., Aarsland, D., Blennow, K., Zetterberg, H., Ballard, C., … Mulugeta, E. (2010). CSF amyloid-beta and tau proteins, and cognitive performance, in early and untreated Parkinson's disease: The Norwegian ParkWest study. *Journal of Neurology, Neurosurgery, and Psychiatry*, *81*(10), 1080–1086. http://dx.doi.org/10.1136/jnnp.2009.199950.

Alves, G., Lange, J., Blennow, K., Zetterberg, H., Andreasson, U., Forland, M. G., … Pedersen, K. F. (2014). CSF Abeta42 predicts early-onset dementia in Parkinson disease. *Neurology*, *82*(20), 1784–1790. http://dx.doi.org/10.1212/wnl.0000000000000425.

Armon, C., & Evans, R. W. (2005). Addendum to assessment: Prevention of post-lumbar puncture headaches: Report of the Therapeutics and Technology Assessment Subcommittee of the American Academy of Neurology. *Neurology*, *65*(4), 510–512. http://dx.doi.org/10.1212/01.wnl.0000173034.96211.1b.

Bachhuber, T., Katzmarski, N., McCarter, J. F., Loreth, D., Tahirovic, S., Kamp, F., … Meyer-Luehmann, M. (2015). Inhibition of amyloid-beta plaque formation by alpha-synuclein. *Nature Medicine*, *21*(7), 802–807. http://dx.doi.org/10.1038/nm.3885.

Backstrom, D. C., Eriksson Domellof, M., Linder, J., Olsson, B., Ohrfelt, A., Trupp, M., … Forsgren, L. (2015). Cerebrospinal fluid patterns and the risk of future dementia in early, incident Parkinson disease. *JAMA Neurology*, *72*(10), 1175–1182. http://dx.doi.org/10.1001/jamaneurol.2015.1449.

Bereczki, E., Francis, P. T., Howlett, D., Pereira, J. B., Hoglund, K., Bogstedt, A., … Aarsland, D. (2016). Synaptic proteins predict cognitive decline in Alzheimer's disease and Lewy body dementia. *Alzheimer's & Dementia*, *12*(11), 1149–1158. http://dx.doi.org/10.1016/j.jalz.2016.04.005.

Beyer, M. K., Alves, G., Hwang, K. S., Babakchanian, S., Bronnick, K. S., Chou, Y. Y., … Apostolova, L. G. (2013). Cerebrospinal fluid Abeta levels correlate with structural brain changes in Parkinson's disease. *Movement Disorders*, *28*(3), 302–310. http://dx.doi.org/10.1002/mds.25282.

Blennow, K., Wallin, A., & Hager, O. (1993). Low frequency of post-lumbar puncture headache in demented patients. *Acta Neurologica Scandinavica*, *88*(3), 221–223.

Braak, H., Del Tredici, K., Rub, U., de Vos, R. A., Jansen Steur, E. N., & Braak, E. (2003). Staging of brain pathology related to sporadic Parkinson's disease. *Neurobiology of Aging*, *24*(2), 197–211.

Buddhala, C., Campbell, M. C., Perlmutter, J. S., & Kotzbauer, P. T. (2015). Correlation between decreased CSF alpha-synuclein and Abeta(1)(-)(4)(2) in Parkinson disease. *Neurobiology of Aging*, *36*(1), 476–484. http://dx.doi.org/10.1016/j.neurobiolaging.2014.07.043.

Caviness, J. N., Driver-Dunckley, E., Connor, D. J., Sabbagh, M. N., Hentz, J. G., Noble, B., … Adler, C. H. (2007). Defining mild cognitive impairment in Parkinson's disease. *Movement Disorders*, *22*(9), 1272–1277. http://dx.doi.org/10.1002/mds.21453.

Chiasserini, D., Parnetti, L., Andreasson, U., Zetterberg, H., Giannandrea, D., Calabresi, P., & Blennow, K. (2010). CSF levels of heart fatty acid binding protein are altered during early phases of Alzheimer's disease. *Journal of Alzheimer's Disease*, *22*(4), 1281–1288. http://dx.doi.org/10.3233/jad-2010-101293.

Compta, Y., Marti, M. J., Ibarretxe-Bilbao, N., Junque, C., Valldeoriola, F., Munoz, E., … Tolosa, E. (2009). Cerebrospinal tau, phospho-tau, and beta-amyloid and neuropsychological functions in Parkinson's disease. *Movement Disorders*, *24*(15), 2203–2210. http://dx.doi.org/10.1002/mds.22594.

Compta, Y., Parkkinen, L., O'Sullivan, S. S., Vandrovcova, J., Holton, J. L., Collins, C., … Revesz, T. (2011). Lewy- and Alzheimer-type pathologies in Parkinson's disease dementia: Which is more important? *Brain*, *134*(Pt. 5), 1493–1505. http://dx.doi.org/10.1093/brain/awr031.

Compta, Y., Pereira, J. B., Rios, J., Ibarretxe-Bilbao, N., Junque, C., Bargallo, N., … Marti, M. J. (2013). Combined dementia-risk biomarkers in Parkinson's disease: A prospective longitudinal study. *Parkinsonism & Related Disorders*, *19*(8), 717–724. http://dx.doi.org/10.1016/j.parkreldis.2013.03.009.

Compta, Y., Valente, T., Saura, J., Segura, B., Iranzo, A., Serradell, M., … Marti, M. J. (2015). Correlates of cerebrospinal fluid levels of oligomeric- and total-alpha-synuclein in premotor, motor and dementia stages of Parkinson's disease. *Journal of Neurology*, *262*(2), 294–306. http://dx.doi.org/10.1007/s00415-014-7560-z.

Conway, K. A., Lee, S. J., Rochet, J. C., Ding, T. T., Williamson, R. E., & Lansbury, P. T., Jr. (2000). Acceleration of oligomerization, not fibrillization, is a shared property of both alpha-synuclein mutations linked to early-onset Parkinson's disease: Implications for pathogenesis and therapy. *Proceedings of the National Academy of Sciences of the United States of America*, *97*(2), 571–576.

Delgado-Alvarado, M., Gago, B., Navalpotro-Gomez, I., Jimenez-Urbieta, H., & Rodriguez-Oroz, M. C. (2016). Biomarkers for dementia and mild cognitive impairment in Parkinson's disease. *Movement Disorders*, *31*(6), 861–881. http://dx.doi.org/10.1002/mds.26662.

Duits, F. H., Martinez-Lage, P., Paquet, C., Engelborghs, S., Lleo, A., Hausner, L., … Blennow, K. (2016). Performance and complications of lumbar puncture in memory clinics: Results of the multicenter lumbar puncture feasibility study. *Alzheimer's & Dementia*, *12*(2), 154–163. http://dx.doi.org/10.1016/j.jalz.2015.08.003.

El-Agnaf, O. M., Walsh, D. M., & Allsop, D. (2003). Soluble oligomers for the diagnosis of neurodegenerative diseases. *Lancet Neurology, 2*(8), 461–462.

Fullard, M. E., Tran, B., Xie, S. X., Toledo, J. B., Scordia, C., Linder, C., … Morley, J. F. (2016). Olfactory impairment predicts cognitive decline in early Parkinson's disease. *Parkinsonism & Related Disorders, 25*, 45–51. http://dx.doi.org/10.1016/j.parkreldis.2016.02.013.

Gao, L., Tang, H., Nie, K., Wang, L., Zhao, J., Gan, R., … Wang, L. (2015). Cerebrospinal fluid alpha-synuclein as a biomarker for Parkinson's disease diagnosis: A systematic review and meta-analysis. *The International Journal of Neuroscience, 125*(9), 645–654. http://dx.doi.org/10.3109/00207454.2014.961454.

Guillaume, E., Zimmermann, C., Burkhard, P. R., Hochstrasser, D. F., & Sanchez, J. C. (2003). A potential cerebrospinal fluid and plasmatic marker for the diagnosis of Creutzfeldt-Jakob disease. *Proteomics, 3*(8), 1495–1499. http://dx.doi.org/10.1002/pmic.200300478.

Hall, S., Ohrfelt, A., Constantinescu, R., Andreasson, U., Surova, Y., Bostrom, F., … Hansson, O. (2012). Accuracy of a panel of 5 cerebrospinal fluid biomarkers in the differential diagnosis of patients with dementia and/or parkinsonian disorders. *Archives of Neurology, 69*(11), 1445–1452. http://dx.doi.org/10.1001/archneurol.2012.1654.

Hall, S., Surova, Y., Ohrfelt, A., Blennow, K., Zetterberg, H., & Hansson, O. (2016). Longitudinal measurements of cerebrospinal fluid biomarkers in Parkinson's disease. *Movement Disorders, 31*(6), 898–905. http://dx.doi.org/10.1002/mds.26578.

Hall, S., Surova, Y., Ohrfelt, A., Zetterberg, H., Lindqvist, D., & Hansson, O. (2015). CSF biomarkers and clinical progression of Parkinson disease. *Neurology, 84*(1), 57–63. http://dx.doi.org/10.1212/wnl.0000000000001098.

Hammond, E. R., Wang, Z., Bhulani, N., McArthur, J. C., & Levy, M. (2011). Needle type and the risk of post-lumbar puncture headache in the outpatient neurology clinic. *Journal of the Neurological Sciences, 306*(1–2), 24–28. http://dx.doi.org/10.1016/j.jns.2011.04.004.

Hansson, O., Hall, S., Ohrfelt, A., Zetterberg, H., Blennow, K., Minthon, L., … El-Agnaf, O. M. (2014). Levels of cerebrospinal fluid alpha-synuclein oligomers are increased in Parkinson's disease with dementia and dementia with Lewy bodies compared to Alzheimer's disease. *Alzheimer's Research & Therapy, 6*(3), 25. http://dx.doi.org/10.1186/alzrt255.

Hirsch, E. C., Vyas, S., & Hunot, S. (2012). Neuroinflammation in Parkinson's disease. *Parkinsonism & Related Disorders, 18*(Suppl. 1), S210–S212. http://dx.doi.org/10.1016/s1353-8020(11)70065-7.

Irwin, D. J., Lee, V. M., & Trojanowski, J. Q. (2013). Parkinson's disease dementia: Convergence of alpha-synuclein, tau and amyloid-beta pathologies. *Nature Reviews. Neuroscience, 14*(9), 626–636. http://dx.doi.org/10.1038/nrn3549.

Jellinger, K. A. (2010). Neuropathology in Parkinson's disease with mild cognitive impairment. *Acta Neuropathologica, 120*(6), 829–830. http://dx.doi.org/10.1007/s00401-010-0755-1. author reply 831.

Kang, J. H., Irwin, D. J., Chen-Plotkin, A. S., Siderowf, A., Caspell, C., Coffey, C. S., … Shaw, L. M. (2013). Association of cerebrospinal fluid beta-amyloid 1-42, T-tau, P-tau181, and alpha-synuclein levels with clinical features of drug-naive patients with early Parkinson disease. *JAMA Neurology, 70*(10), 1277–1287. http://dx.doi.org/10.1001/jamaneurol.2013.3861.

Leverenz, J. B., Watson, G. S., Shofer, J., Zabetian, C. P., Zhang, J., & Montine, T. J. (2011). Cerebrospinal fluid biomarkers and cognitive performance in non-demented patients with Parkinson's disease. *Parkinsonism & Related Disorders, 17*(1), 61–64. http://dx.doi.org/10.1016/j.parkreldis.2010.10.003.

Lindqvist, D., Hall, S., Surova, Y., Nielsen, H. M., Janelidze, S., Brundin, L., & Hansson, O. (2013). Cerebrospinal fluid inflammatory markers in Parkinson's disease—Associations with depression, fatigue, and cognitive impairment. *Brain, Behavior, and Immunity, 33*, 183–189. http://dx.doi.org/10.1016/j.bbi.2013.07.007.

Litvan, I., Goldman, J. G., Troster, A. I., Schmand, B. A., Weintraub, D., Petersen, R. C., ... Emre, M. (2012). Diagnostic criteria for mild cognitive impairment in Parkinson's disease: Movement Disorder Society Task Force guidelines. *Movement Disorders, 27*(3), 349–356. http://dx.doi.org/10.1002/mds.24893.

Liu, C., Cholerton, B., Shi, M., Ginghina, C., Cain, K. C., Auinger, P., & Zhang, J. (2015). CSF tau and tau/Abeta42 predict cognitive decline in Parkinson's disease. *Parkinsonism & Related Disorders, 21*(3), 271–276. http://dx.doi.org/10.1016/j.parkreldis.2014.12.027.

Maetzler, W., Schmid, B., Synofzik, M., Schulte, C., Riester, K., Huber, H., ... Melms, A. (2010). The CST3 BB genotype and low cystatin C cerebrospinal fluid levels are associated with dementia in Lewy body disease. *Journal of Alzheimer's Disease, 19*(3), 937–942. http://dx.doi.org/10.3233/jad-2010-1289.

Maetzler, W., Stapf, A. K., Schulte, C., Hauser, A. K., Lerche, S., Wurster, I., ... Berg, D. (2011). Serum and cerebrospinal fluid uric acid levels in Lewy body disorders: Associations with disease occurrence and amyloid-beta pathway. *Journal of Alzheimer's Disease, 27*(1), 119–126. http://dx.doi.org/10.3233/jad-2011-110587.

Mathews, P. M., & Levy, E. (2016). Cystatin C in aging and in Alzheimer's disease. *Ageing Research Reviews, 32*, 38–50. http://dx.doi.org/10.1016/j.arr.2016.06.003.

McGeer, P. L., & McGeer, E. G. (2004). Inflammation and the degenerative diseases of aging. *The Annals of the New York Academy of Sciences, 1035*, 104–116. http://dx.doi.org/10.1196/annals.1332.007.

Mollenhauer, B., Parnetti, L., Rektorova, I., Kramberger, M. G., Pikkarainen, M., Schulz-Schaeffer, W. J., ... Schlossmacher, M. G. (2015). Biological confounders for the values of cerebrospinal fluid proteins in Parkinson's disease and related disorders. *Journal of Neurochemistry, 139*, 290–317. http://dx.doi.org/10.1111/jnc.13390.

Mollenhauer, B., Trenkwalder, C., von Ahsen, N., Bibl, M., Steinacker, P., Brechlin, P., ... Otto, M. (2006). Beta-amyloid 1-42 and tau-protein in cerebrospinal fluid of patients with Parkinson's disease dementia. *Dementia and Geriatric Cognitive Disorders, 22*(3), 200–208. http://dx.doi.org/10.1159/000094871.

Montine, T. J., Shi, M., Quinn, J. F., Peskind, E. R., Craft, S., Ginghina, C., ... Zhang, J. (2010). CSF Abeta(42) and tau in Parkinson's disease with cognitive impairment. *Movement Disorders, 25*(15), 2682–2685. http://dx.doi.org/10.1002/mds.23287.

Ohrfelt, A., Zetterberg, H., Andersson, K., Persson, R., Secic, D., Brinkmalm, G., ... Westman-Brinkmalm, A. (2011). Identification of novel alpha-synuclein isoforms in human brain tissue by using an online nanoLC-ESI-FTICR-MS method. *Neurochemical Research, 36*(11), 2029–2042. http://dx.doi.org/10.1007/s11064-011-0527-x.

Olsson, B., Lautner, R., Andreasson, U., Ohrfelt, A., Portelius, E., Bjerke, M., ... Zetterberg, H. (2016). CSF and blood biomarkers for the diagnosis of Alzheimer's disease: A systematic review and meta-analysis. *Lancet Neurology, 15*(7), 673–684. http://dx.doi.org/10.1016/s1474-4422(16)00070-3.

Otto, M., Esselmann, H., Schulz-Shaeffer, W., Neumann, M., Schroter, A., Ratzka, P., ... Wiltfang, J. (2000). Decreased beta-amyloid1-42 in cerebrospinal fluid of patients with Creutzfeldt-Jakob disease. *Neurology, 54*(5), 1099–1102.

Park, M. J., Cheon, S. M., Bae, H. R., Kim, S. H., & Kim, J. W. (2011). Elevated levels of alpha-synuclein oligomer in the cerebrospinal fluid of drug-naive patients with Parkinson's disease. *Journal of Clinical Neurology*, 7(4), 215–222. http://dx.doi.org/10.3988/jcn.2011.7.4.215.

Parnetti, L., Farotti, L., Eusebi, P., Chiasserini, D., De Carlo, C., Giannandrea, D., ... Calabresi, P. (2014). Differential role of CSF alpha-synuclein species, tau, and Abeta42 in Parkinson's disease. *Frontiers in Aging Neuroscience, 6*, 53. http://dx.doi.org/10.3389/fnagi.2014.00053.

Parnetti, L., Tiraboschi, P., Lanari, A., Peducci, M., Padiglioni, C., D'Amore, C., ... Calabresi, P. (2008). Cerebrospinal fluid biomarkers in Parkinson's disease with dementia and dementia with Lewy bodies. *Biological Psychiatry*, *64*(10), 850–855. http://dx.doi.org/10.1016/j.biopsych.2008.02.016.

Peskind, E., Nordberg, A., Darreh-Shori, T., & Soininen, H. (2009). Safety of lumbar puncture procedures in patients with Alzheimer's disease. *Current Alzheimer Research*, *6*(3), 290–292.

Peskind, E. R., Riekse, R., Quinn, J. F., Kaye, J., Clark, C. M., Farlow, M. R., … Galasko, D. (2005). Safety and acceptability of the research lumbar puncture. *Alzheimer Disease and Associated Disorders*, *19*(4), 220–225.

Pienaar, I. S., Burn, D., Morris, C., & Dexter, D. (2012). Synaptic protein alterations in Parkinson's disease. *Molecular Neurobiology*, *45*(1), 126–143. http://dx.doi.org/10.1007/s12035-011-8226-9.

Reiber, H. (2003). Proteins in cerebrospinal fluid and blood: Barriers, CSF flow rate and source-related dynamics. *Restorative Neurology and Neuroscience*, *21*(3–4), 79–96.

Schmid, A. W., Fauvet, B., Moniatte, M., & Lashuel, H. A. (2013). Alpha-synuclein post-translational modifications as potential biomarkers for Parkinson disease and other synucleinopathies. *Molecular & Cellular Proteomics*, *12*(12), 3543–3558. http://dx.doi.org/10.1074/mcp.R113.032730.

Schrag, A., Jahanshahi, M., & Quinn, N. (2000). What contributes to quality of life in patients with Parkinson's disease? *Journal of Neurology, Neurosurgery, and Psychiatry*, *69*(3), 308–312.

Schulz-Schaeffer, W. J. (2010). The synaptic pathology of alpha-synuclein aggregation in dementia with Lewy bodies, Parkinson's disease and Parkinson's disease dementia. *Acta Neuropathologica*, *120*(2), 131–143. http://dx.doi.org/10.1007/s00401-010-0711-0.

Siderowf, A., Xie, S. X., Hurtig, H., Weintraub, D., Duda, J., Chen-Plotkin, A., … Clark, C. (2010). CSF amyloid {beta} 1-42 predicts cognitive decline in Parkinson disease. *Neurology*, *75*(12), 1055–1061. http://dx.doi.org/10.1212/WNL.0b013e3181f39a78.

Simonsen, A. H., Kuiperij, B., El-Agnaf, O. M., Engelborghs, S., Herukka, S. K., Parnetti, L., … Mollenhauer, B. (2016). The utility of alpha-synuclein as biofluid marker in neurodegenerative diseases: A systematic review of the literature. *Biomarkers in Medicine*, *10*(1), 19–34. http://dx.doi.org/10.2217/bmm.14.105.

Skogseth, R. E., Bronnick, K., Pereira, J. B., Mollenhauer, B., Weintraub, D., Fladby, T., & Aarsland, D. (2015). Associations between cerebrospinal fluid biomarkers and cognition in early untreated Parkinson's disease. *Journal of Parkinson's Disease*, *5*(4), 783–792. http://dx.doi.org/10.3233/jpd-150682.

Stav, A. L., Aarsland, D., Johansen, K. K., Hessen, E., Auning, E., & Fladby, T. (2015). Amyloid-beta and alpha-synuclein cerebrospinal fluid biomarkers and cognition in early Parkinson's disease. *Parkinsonism & Related Disorders*, *21*(7), 758–764. http://dx.doi.org/10.1016/j.parkreldis.2015.04.027.

Stewart, T., Liu, C., Ginghina, C., Cain, K. C., Auinger, P., Cholerton, B., … Zhang, J. (2014). Cerebrospinal fluid alpha-synuclein predicts cognitive decline in Parkinson disease progression in the DATATOP cohort. *The American Journal of Pathology*, *184*(4), 966–975. http://dx.doi.org/10.1016/j.ajpath.2013.12.007.

Terrelonge, M., Jr., Marder, K. S., Weintraub, D., & Alcalay, R. N. (2016). CSF beta-amyloid 1-42 predicts progression to cognitive impairment in newly diagnosed Parkinson disease. *Journal of Molecular Neuroscience*, *58*(1), 88–92. http://dx.doi.org/10.1007/s12031-015-0647-x.

Tokuda, T., Qureshi, M. M., Ardah, M. T., Varghese, S., Shehab, S. A., Kasai, T., … El-Agnaf, O. M. (2010). Detection of elevated levels of alpha-synuclein oligomers in CSF from patients with Parkinson disease. *Neurology*, *75*(20), 1766–1772. http://dx.doi.org/10.1212/WNL.0b013e3181fd613b.

van de Beek, D., Drake, J. M., & Tunkel, A. R. (2010). Nosocomial bacterial meningitis. *New England Journal of Medicine*, *362*, 146–154. http://dx.doi/10.1056/NEJMra0804573.

Vidoni, E. D., Morris, J. K., Raider, K., & Burns, J. M. (2014). Reducing post-lumbar puncture headaches with small bore atraumatic needles. *Journal of Clinical Neuroscience*, *21*(3), 536–537. http://dx.doi.org/10.1016/j.jocn.2013.07.001.

Vranova, H. P., Henykova, E., Kaiserova, M., Mensikova, K., Vastik, M., Mares, J., ... Kanovsky, P. (2014). Tau protein, beta-amyloid(1)(-)(4)(2) and clusterin CSF levels in the differential diagnosis of Parkinsonian syndrome with dementia. *Journal of the Neurological Sciences*, *343*(1–2), 120–124. http://dx.doi.org/10.1016/j.jns.2014.05.052.

Whitfield, D. R., Vallortigara, J., Alghamdi, A., Howlett, D., Hortobagyi, T., Johnson, M., ... Francis, P. T. (2014). Assessment of ZnT3 and PSD95 protein levels in Lewy body dementias and Alzheimer's disease: Association with cognitive impairment. *Neurobiology of Aging*, *35*(12), 2836–2844. http://dx.doi.org/10.1016/j.neurobiolaging.2014.06.015.

Yarnall, A. J., Breen, D. P., Duncan, G. W., Khoo, T. K., Coleman, S. Y., Firbank, M. J., ... Burn, D. J. (2014). Characterizing mild cognitive impairment in incident Parkinson disease: The ICICLE-PD study. *Neurology*, *82*(4), 308–316. http://dx.doi.org/10.1212/wnl.0000000000000066.

Yu, S. Y., Zuo, L. J., Wang, F., Chen, Z. J., Hu, Y., Wang, Y. J., ... Zhang, W. (2014). Potential biomarkers relating pathological proteins, neuroinflammatory factors and free radicals in PD patients with cognitive impairment: A cross-sectional study. *BMC Neurology*, *14*, 113. http://dx.doi.org/10.1186/1471-2377-14-113.

Zetterberg, H., Tullhog, K., Hansson, O., Minthon, L., Londos, E., & Blennow, K. (2010). Low incidence of post-lumbar puncture headache in 1,089 consecutive memory clinic patients. *European Neurology*, *63*(6), 326–330. http://dx.doi.org/10.1159/000311703.

CHAPTER ELEVEN

Hallmarks of Treatment Aspects: Parkinson's Disease Throughout Centuries Including L-Dopa

Hee J. Kim*,†, Beom S. Jeon†,‡,1, Peter Jenner§
*Konkuk University School of Medicine, Seoul, South Korea
†Parkinson Disease Study Group, Seoul National University Hospital, Seoul, South Korea
‡Movement Disorder Center, Neuroscience Research Institute, College of Medicine, Seoul National University, Seoul, South Korea
§Institute of Pharmaceutical Science, King's College London, London, United Kingdom
[1]Corresponding author: e-mail address: brain@snu.ac.kr

Contents

International Review of Neurobiology, Volume 132
ISSN 0074-7742
http://dx.doi.org/10.1016/bs.irn.2017.01.006

Abstract

Deficit of striatal dopamine was first discovered in postmortem brain of patients with Parkinson's disease in 1960. This observation was the starting point for dopamine replacement therapy, and successful introduction of high dose L-dopa therapy in the 1969 revolutionized the treatment of Parkinson's disease. Since then, constant attempts have been made to enhance the efficacy of L-dopa and reduce motor complications by providing more continuous dopamine stimulation.

This chapter traces the hallmarks of medical treatments for Parkinson's disease throughout centuries including the first description of antiparkinsonian effects of anticholinergics, the birth of apomorphine in the 1900s, then discovery of L-dopa in the 1960s, and development of dopamine agonists since the 1970s.

1. INTRODUCTION

Parkinson's disease (PD) involves the progressive degeneration of the nigrostriatal neuron, and the resultant reduction of striatal dopamine is the neurochemical basis of PD. In 1960, the deficit of striatal dopamine in postmortem brain of PD patients was first discovered (Ehringer & Hornykiewicz, 1960), and this observation was the starting point for dopamine replacement therapy. After successful introduction of high dosage L-dopa therapy by Cotzias (Cotzias, Papavasiliou, & Gellene, 1969), L-dopa has been the mainstay of treatment for PD for about 50 years. In the meantime, a number of adjunctive therapies have been developed to enhance the efficacy of L-dopa including dopa decarboxylase inhibitors (DDI) (e.g., carbidopa, benserazide), monoamine oxidase (MAO)-B inhibitors (e.g., selegiline, rasagiline), catechol-*O*-methyltransferase (COMT) inhibitors (e.g., entacapone, tolcapone), and sustained release preparations (e.g., Madopar HBS (hydrodynamically balanced system), Sinemet CR (continuous release)). In addition to L-dopa, dopamine agonists (e.g., pramipexole, ropinirole), centrally acting antimuscarinic drugs (e.g., trihexyphenidyl, benztropine), and amantadine have been used in the treatment of PD.

This chapter traces the important steps in history of medical treatments for PD throughout centuries including the first description of antiparkinsonian effects of anticholinergics in 1868 by Ordenstein, the birth of apomorphine in the 1900s, then discovery of L-dopa in the 1960s, and start of development of dopamine agonists in the 1970s (Table 1).

Table 1 The Hallmarks of Medical Therapy for PD

1860s	Ordenstein introduced the use of belladonna extracts
	First synthesis of apomorphine
1910s	D,L-Dopa synthesized in laboratory Isoloation of L-dopa from *Vicia faba* (fava bean) seedlings
1920s	Chemical synthesis of L-dopa
1930s	Discovery of MAO as the mechanism for inactivating the monoamines L-Dopa decarboxylase enzyme identified
1940s	Introduction of synthetic anticholinergics
1950s	Report on antiparkinsonian effects of apomorphine
1960s	Coadministration of L-dopa and MAO inhibitor enhanced and prolonged L-dopa benefits First description of striatal dopamine deficiency in PD patients First clinical trial with intravenous L-dopa for parkinsonism Apomorphine noted to be structurally similar to dopamine Effectiveness of oral L-dopa demonstrated in patients with parkinsonism Coadministration of L-dopa and peripheral DDI shown beneficial First observation on antiparkinsonian effects of amantadine
1970s	Start of development of dopamine agonists Beneficial effects of apomorphine for PD patients rediscovered
	Sustained-release L-dopa formulation tried Discovery of L-deprenyl (selegiline) Continuous L-dopa administration tried for preventing motor complications L-dopa/benserazide (Madopar) and carbidopa/L-dopa (Sinemet) commercialized Introduction of domperidone, a peripheral dopamine receptor antagonist
1980s	Effectiveness of Lisuride, a soluble D2 receptor agonist, in patients with parkinsonism Pergolide, a potent D1- and D2-receptor agonist, shown effective as L-dopa adjunct in patients with long-term complications Dopamine agonists tested as monotherapy in early de novo PD Early administration of dopamine agonists with L-dopa tried for preventing motor fluctuations Two COMT inhibitor found to be orally active

Continued

Table 1 The Hallmarks of Medical Therapy for PD—cont'd

1990s	Cabergoline, a long-acting ergotic agonist, shown effective in de novo and fluctuating PD patients Part-time continuous L-dopa stimulation shown to improve severe "on–off" Introduction of nonergoline dopamine agonists Sustained-release carbidopa/L-dopa commercially available First clinical trial of enteral carbidopa/L-dopa infusion Description on antidyskinetic effect of amantadine Discovery of rasagiline First COMT inhibitor became commercially available (tolcapone; Tasmar)
2000s	Combination carbidopa/L-dopa/entacapone tablets (Stalevo) become commercially available Introduction of prolonged release dopamine agonists Introduction of dual-release formulation of L-dopa

COMT, catechol-*O*-methyltransferase; *DDI*, dopa decarboxylase inhibitor; *MAO*, monoamine oxidase; *PD*, Parkinson's disease.

Adapted from Hauser R. A. (2009). Levodopa: past, present, and future. *European Neurology, 62*, 1–8; Tolosa, E., Martí, M. J., Valldeoriola, F., & Molinuevo, J. L. (1998). History of levodopa and dopamine agonists in Parkinson's disease treatment. *Neurology, 50*, S2–S10.

2. ANTICHOLINERGICS

Anticholinergics are compounds originally derived from plants of the Solanaceae family (Adler, 2007). Anticholinergic agents are the oldest type of medication currently in use for the treatment of PD. They remained the only possible medical therapy for PD for almost a century prior to the introduction of amantadine and L-dopa in the late 1960s.

2.1 Treatment of PD With Natural Antimuscarinic Alkaloids

Antiparkinsonian effects of anticholinergics were first described by Ordenstein (1868), a student of Jean-Martin Charcot, who discovered the beneficial effect of the belladonna alkaloids (mainly containing atropine as active component) on tremor and other PD symptoms, when fortuitously administering tinctures of deadly nightshade (*Atropa belladonna*) and henbane (*Hyoscyamus niger*) to patients to control the excessive salivation and drooling (Lang & Blair, 1989). When Ordenstein wrote a thesis on PD and multiple sclerosis to obtain his medical degree, he mentions "Monsieur Charcot has begun to prescribe 2 or 3 granules of hyoscyamine daily, approximately 1 mg each. This medication was able to provide several hours of rest for some patients" (Fahn, 2015). At the end of the 19th century, subsequent investigators such as Erb, Mendel, and Gowers began using antimuscarinic substances, such as scopolamine (hyoscine), hyoscyamine (duboisine) and Indian hemp (containing *Cannabis sativa*) (Erb, 1887; Gowers, 1893; Mendel, 1893). Hyoscine was the preferred treatment for PD by the end of the 19th century (Oppenheim, 1905), and these natural antimuscarinic alkaloids were widely prescribed in the early 20th century (Fahn, 2015). In the early 1940s, stramonium, particularly the Bulgarian variety, was thought to be the most potent of the belladonna alkaloids and was often administered in the form of cigarettes, and in the form of wine extracts (Lang & Blair, 1989).

2.2 Introduction of Synthetic Anticholinergics and Antihistaminics

Then in the late 1940s and 1950s, several synthetic anticholinergic and antihistaminic agents were developed with more selective central actions than the naturally occurring alkaloids. In 1949, trihexiphenidyl (Artane) was found to be effective for PD in the several clinical trials (Corbin, 1949; Doshay & Constable, 1949; Schwab & Tillmann, 1949). The other commonly used synthetic anticholinergic agents have included benztropine mesylate (Congetin), procyclidine hydrochloride (Kemadrin), cycrimine hydrochloride (Pagitane), biperiden hydrochloride (Akineton), and ethopropazine hydrochloride (Parsitan, Parsidol) (Duvoisin, 1967). Antihistaminics such as diphenhydramine, orphenadrine hydrochloride (Disipal), and chlorphenoxene (Phenoxene) were also tested in PD patients (Duvoisin, 1965) and were recognized to have anticholinergic properties because of its similar effects to antimuscarinics. These antihistamines generally had milder benefit but less adverse effects than the antimuscarinics.

Although no studies compared the effects of one anticholinergic against another, it is generally felt that differences in potency are largely a matter of relative dose and no difference in the clinical effectiveness of various anticholinergic drugs exist (Yahr, Clough, & Bergmann, 1982). Beneficial effects of anticholinergics have been supported by contemporary reviews and investigations. The usefulness of anticholinergics, however, was limited by adverse effects from peripheral and central muscarinic blockage such as dry mouth and various psychological disturbances, especially in the elderly patients. Since the 1960s L-dopa and dopamine agonists have largely replaced anticholinergics as major antiparkinsonian agents.

2.3 The Mechanism of Action of the Anticholinergics

The precise action mechanism of the anticholinergics is still not clear. It is generally believed that they work (1) by restoration of the striatal dopamine–acetylcholine balance via a blockade of postsynaptic muscarinic receptors and (2) by blocking dopamine uptake in central dopaminergic neurons (some of the anticholinergic drugs such as benztropine). In the mid- to late 1920s, several studies reported that postencephalitic parkinsonism was exacerbated by administration of cholinergic agent, and exacerbation of parkinsonism by a cholinergic drug was reversed by an anticholinergic drug (Marinesco & Bourguignon, 1927; Zucker, 1925), supporting the role of the cholinergic system in parkinsonism. Later in 1941, Milhorat reported a marked exacerbation of parkinsonism in two patients with paralysis agitans after an injection of neostigmine and reversal by scopolamine or atropine (Milhorat, 1941). The mechanism of action of the anticholinergics, however, was believed to be due to peripheral muscarinic effects until Feldberg proposed a central effect for anticholinergic drugs (Feldberg, 1945). In 1945, Feldberg first discovered that acetylcholine was a central neurotransmitter that was abundant in the striatum at the synaptic vesicles of nerve terminals and that atropine had the opposite effect of acetylcholine in the central nervous system. In the 1960s, Duvoisin provided a rationale for the use of anticholinergics in PD and supported the notion that a state of striatal cholinergic preponderance exists in PD. He showed that physostigmine, centrally acting cholinesterase inhibitors, increased the severity of PD symptoms (Duvoisin, 1967). It has been postulated that dopamine depletion results in a state of cholinergic hypersensitivity which can be reversed by anticholinergics, such as benztropine. In 1969, Coyle and Snyder suggested that the mechanism of the therapeutic action of the anticholinergic drugs in PD is related to their ability to inhibit the neuronal reuptake of dopamine in striatal neurons, thus liberating more dopamine on striatal receptors (Coyle & Snyder, 1969).

3. AMANTADINE

Amantadine hydrochloride is a noncompetitive antagonist of *N*-methyl-D-aspartate receptor with rapid blocking and unblocking kinetics (Kornhuber et al., 1995). Amantadine was originally introduced in the 1960s as an antiviral agent effective against several strains of the influenza virus (Davies et al., 1964).

But soon afterward, it was noted to have antiparkinsonian effect in a single patient with PD (Schwab, England, Poskanzer, & Young, 1969).

3.1 Amantadine as an Antiviral Agent

Antiviral properties of amantadine were first reported in 1963 by Jackson and his colleagues at the University of Illinois Hospital in Chicago (Jackson, Muldoon, & Akers, 1963). Subsequent clinical trials demonstrated that the drug produced as much as a 70% reduction in clinical illness from influenza A (Maugh, 1979). Then, in October 1966, it was approved by the Food and Drug Administration (FDA) as a prophylactic agent specifically against Asian (H2N2) influenza and received approval for prophylactic use for influenza A infection in 1976 (Maugh, 1979). Currently, it is no longer a favored treatment for treatment or prophylaxis of influenza A due to the influenza virus' frequent mutations, and the advent of new drugs (Hubsher, Haider, & Okun, 2012).

3.2 Amantadine as a Treatment for PD

In the late 1960s, amantadine was fortuitously noted to be useful in relieving motor symptoms in a patient with PD (Schwab et al., 1969). In April 1968, a 58-year-old woman with advanced PD noted transient relief of rest tremor, rigidity, and akinesia while taking amantadine during the 6 weeks as prophylaxis against influenza A and then deterioration after stopping the medication. After this observation, the first clinical trial of amantadine for PD was performed in June 1968 by Schwab and colleagues of Massachusetts General Hospital in Boston. In an open-label study of 163 patients with PD, 107 (66%) reported an improvement of symptoms on amantadine with a maximum daily dosage of 200 mg (Schwab et al., 1969). In a subsequent report of 2 year experience with amantadine 200 mg/day for 60 days in 351 patients, they reported that maximum benefit occurred between 2 and 3 weeks with 64% improving at 60 days (Schwab, Poskanzer, England, & Young, 1972). In the early 1970s, numerous clinical trials established the beneficial effects of amantadine for PD as monotherapy (Butzer, Silver, & Sahs, 1975; Cox, Danta, Schnieden, & Yuill, 1973; Fahn & Isgreen, 1975; Mawdsley, Williams, Pullar, Davidson, & Kinloch, 1972; Parkes et al., 1971; Parkes, Baxter, Marsden, & Rees, 1974) and as an adjunctive therapy to L-dopa (Callagham, McIlroy, & O'Connor, 1974; Fehling, 1973; Millac, Hasan, Espir, & Slyfield, 1970) or anticholinergics

(Barbeau, Mars, Botez, & Joubert, 1971; Bauer & McHenry, 1974; Forssman, Kihlstrand, & Larsson, 1972; Rinne, Sonninen, & Siirtola, 1972; Silver & Sahs, 1971), although a decline in efficacy after several weeks or months has been noted in some studies (Dallos, Heathfield, Stone, & Allen, 1970; Hunter, Stern, Laurence, & Armitage, 1970; Schwab et al., 1969). In April 1973, the FDA approved the use of amantadine as a treatment for PD (Maugh, 1979).

3.3 Effect of Amantadine on L-Dopa-Induced Dyskinesia

Since the late 1970s, investigators' interest in amantadine waned. In the late 1990s, however, amantadine has received novel attention as a treatment of L-dopa-induced dyskinesia (LID). A small placebo-controlled crossover clinical trial by Metman et al. suggested its ability to alleviate LID (Metman et al., 1998). Amantadine reduced dyskinesia severity by 60% in the 14 patients completing this trial, compared with placebo, and its antidyskinetic effect was maintained in 13 out of 17 patients for 1 year (Metman et al., 1999). Since then, several randomized placebo-controlled trials have consistently shown antidyskinetic effects of amantadine in L-dopa-treated patients with advanced PD (Luginger, Wenning, Bösch, & Poewe, 2000; Sawada et al., 2010; Snow, Macdonald, Mcauley, & Wallis, 2000), although all of these had a relatively small sample size and were of short duration.

Meanwhile, there have been claims that antidyskinetic effects waned within a few months. Thomas et al. evaluated the duration of the antidyskinetic effect of amantadine over 12 months in 40 patients with advanced PD (Thomas et al., 2004). Although there was a reduction by 45% in the total dyskinesia scores after 15 days of amantadine treatment, the benefit was withdrawn in 3–8 months in their open-label series of 20 patients taking amantadine. However, several subjects experienced a rebound of dyskinesia severity after amantadine discontinuation (Thomas et al., 2004). Two recent randomized, controlled studies also reported that the withdrawal of amantadine worsens dyskinesias, even after years of treatment, suggesting relatively long-term antidyskinetic effects of amantadine (Ory-Magne et al., 2014; Wolf et al., 2010).

A few clinical trials recently suggested a beneficial effect of amantadine on freezing of gait (Giladi et al., 2001; Malkani et al., 2012) and pathologic gambling (Thomas, Bonanni, Gambi, Di Iorio, & Onofrj, 2010). However, trials with larger sample sizes are needed to confirm such efficacy because of the conflicting results (Kim et al., 2012; Lee, Kim, & Jeon, 2011; Lee et al., 2013; Macht et al., 2007).

4. APOMORPHINE

Dopamine agonists are the compounds which mimic the action of the natural neurotransmitter in stimulating striatal dopamine receptors. Apomorphine is a nonergoline dopamine agonist that interacts with dopamine D2, D3, and D4 receptors; adrenergic α1D, α2B, and α2C receptors; and to a lesser extent with D1 receptors and serotonin 5HT1A, 5HT2A, 5HT2B, and 5HT2C receptors (Gottwald & Aminoff, 2011). Because of extensive first-pass effect, orally administered apomorphine is not efficacious. With bolus injection, apomorphine has a rapid onset, usually within 10 min and a short duration of action, 45–90 min.

4.1 The Birth of Apomorphine and Its Use as an Antiparkinsonian Agent

Apomorphine was the first agonist used in PD. It was discovered in 1869 by Matthiessen and Wright (Matthiessen, 1868), and later synthesized by a procedure of morphine acidification at 100°C (Zurich, 1913). It had been initially used for many years due to its potent emetic properties. Then in 1884, its value in PD was recognized by Weil. He tried for the first time apomorphine in a patient with Sydenham's chorea, and suggested that it could be useful in the treatment of PD (Weil, 1884). Later in 1951, Schwab and colleagues confirmed his idea (Schwab, Amador, & Levine, 1951). They reported the favorable effects of apomorphine for all cardinal features of PD from a clinical trial on 20 patients with subcutaneous injection and 10 patients with an oral preparation. The effect of the subcutaneous apomorphine was shown to be more dramatic, but less sustained than oral preparation. Following this observation, Struppler and Von Uexkull reported antitremor effect of apomorphine in 1953 (Struppler & Von Uexkull, 1953). At that time, however, the dopaminergic properties of this drug were not known.

In subsequent years, several studies were conducted to determine the effect of apomorphine in the treatment of PD. Ernst outlined structural similarity of apomorphine to dopamine (Ernst, 1965) and its presumable action at the dopamine receptor (Ernst, 1967). In 1967, Andén and coworkers confirmed this hypothesis by reporting evidence of dopamine receptor stimulation by apomorphine in rats (Andén, Rubenson, Fuxe, & Hökfelt, 1967). Then in 1970, Cotzias and coworkers showed the efficiency of subcutaneous apomorphine in PD patients chronically treated with L-dopa in the first double-blind controlled trial (Cotzias, Papavasiliou, Fehling, Kaufman, & Mena, 1970). Braham et al. observed a regression in tremor within 5–10 min during 1–2 h following a 0.5–2-mg subcutaneous apomorphine injection in 11 out of 15 PD patients with a L-dopa-resistant tremor (Braham, Sarova-Pinhas, & Goldhammer, 1970). In 1972, Düby and coworkers initiated a first study of apomorphine action on motor fluctuations and demonstrated an improvement in "off" symptoms by apomorphine (Düby, Cotzias, Papavasiliou, & Lawrence, 1972). Use of apomorphine as an antiparkinsonian agent, however, was limited by its short half-life, multiple side effects, the necessity for high doses if given orally because of its extensive first-pass metabolism, and nephrotoxicity (Cotzias, Papavasiliou, Tolosa, Mendez, & Bell-Midura, 1976). These limitations coupled with the successful introduction of L-Dopa in the early 1970s, relegated apomorphine to a minor therapeutic option. Then in 1979, the introduction of domperidone, a peripheral dopamine receptor antagonist, made a breakthrough for the advancement of dopamine agonists therapy including apomorphine by reducing the side effects associated with administration of dopaminergic agonists (Agid, Bonnet, Pollak, Signoret, & Lhermitte, 1979; Corsini, Del Zompo, Gessa, & Mangoni, 1979).

4.2 Apomorphine as a Treatment for Motor Complications

In the 1980s, as limitation of L-dopa had become apparent, especially motor complications under long-term L-dopa therapy (Fahn, 1974; Lees, 1989; Marsden & Parkes, 1976), researchers' interest had returned to apomorphine as the treatment of motor fluctuation, with development of injector pens and continuous infusion pumps. In 1988, Stibe et al. reported the benefits of apomorphine administered subcutaneously (Stibe, Lees, Kempster, & Stern, 1988). In this trial, subcutaneous apomorphine was given by continuous infusion during the day or by repeated injections to 19 patients. In eight patients using apomorphine as a rescue medication, the total daily amount of "off" time was reduced by 55%. Continuous subcutaneous apomorphine infusion reduced the total daily amount of "off" time by 62% and the total L-dopa dose by approximately 20% in 11 patients. Subsequent clinical trials by a number of other groups replicated these results and confirmed apomorphine as a useful rescue drug in the treatment of PD (Dewey, Hutton, LeWitt, & Factor, 2001; Merello, Pikielny, Cammarota, & Leiguarda, 1997; Ostergaard et al., 1995; Poewe, Kleedorfer, Gerstenbrand, & Öertel, 1988; Pollak, Champay, Hommel, Perret, & Benabid, 1989; Stibe et al.,

1988; Van Laar et al., 1993). In 1993, apomorphine was first licensed in the United Kingdom for use in PD patients with disabling motor fluctuations (Chaudhuri, Critchley, Abbott, Pye, & Millac, 1988; Stibe et al., 1988). In the United States, it was approved as a rescue medication in PD, particularly to treat the "off" periods by subcutaneous injection in 2004 (Subramony, 2006).

4.3 Novel Formulations of Apomorphine

Although continuous subcutaneous apomorphine therapy has been shown to reduce L-dopa-induced motor fluctuations in advancing patients, its long-term use is limited due to skin complications, particularly nodule formation and focal panniculitis are seen in more than 50% of subjects (Koller & Stacy, 2004). Therefore, other routes of administration, including intranasal spray, sublingual film strip, and rectal suppository preparations (Hughes et al., 1991), have been examined.

Inhaled dry powder apomorphine (VR040) has been recently developed. Results from a double-blind clinic-based phase II study in 47 patients with fluctuating PD showed significantly greater improvement in Unified Parkinson's Disease Rating Scale motor score and rapid (mean, 10 min) reversal from the "off" state (Grosset, Malek, Morgan, & Grosset, 2013b). Similar results were observed in another trial with the same characteristics (Grosset, Malek, Morgan, & Grosset, 2013a).

A sublingually administered apomorphine film strip (APL-130277) has been recently developed for a recue treatment of "off" episodes, by rapidly delivering apomorphine from the oral cavity mucosa without inducing local skin or mucosal irritation or reactions. In a phase II, open-label, single-arm study, 40% turned fully "on" by 15 min, and the other 60% of responders turned fully "on" between 15 and 30 min. The most common adverse events were dizziness (36.8%), somnolence (31.6%), and nausea (21.1%) (Hauser et al., 2016; Titova & Chaudhuri, 2016).

5. L-DOPA

L-Dopa (L-3,4-dihydroxyphenylalanine), the precursor of dopamine, is the naturally occurring aromatic amino acid. Introduction of L-dopa in the 1960s revolutionized the treatment of PD. Since then, it, in fixed combination with a DDI, has been the standard and the most effective symptomatic therapy for motor symptoms in PD.

5.1 Discovery of Striatal Dopamine Deficiency in Patients With PD

In 1911, Funk, a Polish biochemist, chemically synthesized D,L-dopa (dihydroxyphenylalanine) (Funk, 1911), which was considered as a possible precursor of epinephrine at that time. Two years later, Guggenheim at the Hoffmann-LaRoche laboratories in Switzerland isolated L-dopa from the bean of *Vicia faba* (Guggenheim, 1913). He self-ingested 2.5 mg of L-dopa and discovered its emetic effect, which, however, was interpreted as unspecific irritation of the gastric mucosa. Then in 1921, L-dopa was chemically synthesized (Waser & Lewandowski, 1921) and in the late 1920s and early 1930s, it was found to be biologically active, causing hyperglycemia and hypotension in rabbits (Hornykiewicz, 2002). In 1956, Hornykiewicz showed that dopamine lowered blood pressure and that L-dopa had a similar effect (Hornykiewicz, 1958). In the late 1950s, dopamine was identified in many peripheral tissues such as adrenal medullar, heart, kidney, and sympathetic nerves, and the role of dopamine was discovered as an independent neurotransmitter in the central nervous system. The occurrence of dopamine in the mammalian brain including human was first demonstrated in August 1957 by Montagu (Montagu, 1957), soon followed by Weil-Malherbe and Bone (Weil-Malherbe & Bone, 1957). A month or so later, Holtz reported the central excitatory effect of L-dopa in rodents and suggested dopamine as the active L-dopa metabolite in the brain (Holtz, Balzer, Westermann, & Wezler, 1957). Following this observation, in November 1957, Carlsson (Carlsson, Lindqvist, & Magnusson, 1957) showed that L-dopa could reverse reserpine-induced akinesia in animals and postulated that dopamine appears to play a role in motor function. Three months later in February 1958, Carlsson and colleagues confirmed dopamine's occurrence in the brains of rabbits and found the depletion of dopamine by reserpine and restoration of depleted dopamine by L-dopa (Carlsson, Lindqvist, Magnusson, & Waldeck, 1958). Then, Bertler and Rosengren (Bertler & Rosengren, 1959) and Sano et al. (Sano et al., 1959) demonstrated high concentration of dopamine relatively localized to the striatum. This observation led Hornykiewicz to measure postmortem brain dopamine in patients with PD, postencephalitic parkinsonism and other extrapyramidal disorder as well as in control brain. While very high dopamine concentrations were found in the control basal ganglia, 90% loss of dopamine was found in the striatum of two patients with PD and four patients with postencephalitic parkinsonism. The results of this important observation were published in 1960 (Ehringer & Hornykiewicz, 1960,

1998), which changed understanding of pathophysiology of PD and provided a rational basis for the concept of "dopamine replacement therapy" with L-dopa. In the same year, Sano also reported depletion of dopamine in a single patient with PD (Sano, 2000). Two years later, Hornykiewicz found depletion of dopamine in the pars compacta of the substantia nigra in magnitude to the striatal dopamine loss and suggested that "the cell loss in the substantia nigra could well be the cause of the dopamine deficit in the striatum" (Hornykiewicz, 1963). Subsequently, the first convincing evidence that substantia nigra provided dopamine to the striatum was provided by fluorescence histochemical techniques (Andén et al., 1964).

5.2 Use of L-Dopa in Patients With Parkinsonism

Following the discoveries of dopamine deficit in the striatum, in July 1961, the first clinical trial with intravenous L-dopa was successfully carried out in 20 patients with PD or with postencephalitic parkinsonism by Birkmayer and Hornykiewicz (Birkmayer & Hornykiewicz, 1961). In this open-label trial, intravenous injection of 50–150 mg of L-dopa resulted in a complete abolition or substantial relief of akinesia transiently. The maximal effect of L-dopa reached within 2–3 h and lasted for up to 24 h. In 1962, Barbeau et al. independently observed transient improvement of rigidity with oral administration of 200 mg/day of L-dopa (Barbeau, Sourkes, & Murphy, 1962). In subsequent study by Birkmayer and Hornykiewicz, 200 patients with parkinsonism were treated with intravenous injections of L-dopa 25 mg once or twice weekly (together with a MAO inhibitor) (Birkmayer & Hornykiewicz, 1964). However, only 20% of the patients showed improvement of akinesia, 50% had some reduction in impaired speech or posture, and 30% had no improvement. Over the next several years, conflicting reports on the beneficial effects of L-dopa were published; several investigators (Pazzagli & Amaducci, 1966; Umbach & Baumann, 1964) found some benefit, while others (Fehling, 1966; McGeer & Zeldowicz, 1964; Rinaldi, Marghertia, & De Divitus, 1965) failed to find improvement with L-dopa or D,L-dopa.

Then 6 years after the initial studies in 1967, the major breakthrough occurred. George Cotzias in New York introduced a new approach of high-dose oral D,L-dopa regimen starting with a very low dose and then raising the dose gradually, which can avoid the gastrointestinal side effects (Cotzias, Van Woert, & Schiffer, 1967). Cotzias and colleagues treated 16 PD patients with oral D,L-dopa 3–16 g/day and reported remarkable improvement in akinesia, tremor, and rigidity. However, agranulocytopenia was seen in four patients. In 1969, Cotzias tried the pure L-dopa (up to 8 g/day) instead of the racemic D,L-dopa in 28 patients with parkinsonism, resulting in symptomatic improvement with less toxicity (Cotzias et al., 1969). During this study, a peripheral DDI, blocking peripheral conversion of L-dopa to dopamine was developed and became available for some participants. Coadministration of DDI with L-dopa reduced the dose of L-dopa required and eliminated anorexia and nausea in one case. Soon after that, in October 1969, Yahr in New York reported results of the first double-blind, placebo-controlled study to demonstrate dramatic effect of L-dopa in improving the symptoms of PD (Yahr, Duvoisin, Schear, Barrett, & Hoehn, 1969). Many subsequent open-label trials using slow titration strategy reported significant improvements, especially akinesia and rigidity. Tremor was reported to have a more variable response. Finally, L-dopa was approved as a treatment for PD by the FDA in 1970 and was introduced into the market (1970).

5.3 Complications of Long-Term L-Dopa Therapy and Strategies to Enhance the Effectiveness and Reduce the Adverse Effects of L-Dopa Therapy

Introduction of high dosage L-dopa therapy by Cotzias is a revolutionary treatment for PD. However, during their second study, dyskinesias became evident in half of them after exposure to L-dopa. Cotzias and colleagues proposed that the dyskinesias were dose dependent and that the presence of a nigrostriatal lesion had to be present for the dyskinesias. In the first review chapter on LIDs based on an analysis of L-dopa therapy in 116 patients with PD, Duvoisin found that 53% of patients had developed dyskinesias by 6 months of treatment and 81% by 12 months (Duvoisin, 1974). As motor fluctuations and dyskinesias were recognized as complications of high dose oral L-dopa therapy in the late 1960s, there have been attempts to overcome these complications with such techniques as addition of enzyme inhibitors, continuous L-dopa infusion, and long-acting L-dopa combinations.

5.3.1 DDI

In 1967, Bartholini et al. showed that small doses of Ro 4-4602 (benserazide), a selective inhibitor of the peripheral dopa decarboxylase, enhanced the concentration of cerebral catecholamines caused by L-dopa (Bartholini, Burkard, Pletscher, & Bates, 1967). These results were confirmed by Siegfried (Siegfried, 1969) and Tissot, Bartholini, and Pletscher (Tissot, Bartholini, & Pletscher, 1969). In 1969, Birkmayer et al. found that coadministration of L-dopa and Ro 4-4602 provided a clear potentiation and prolongation of the L-dopa's antiakinetic effect (Birkmayer, Linauer, & Mentasti, 1971). Meanwhile, Cotzias and colleagues began to use MK485 (carbidopa) with L-dopa in 1968 and found enhanced therapeutic benefits of L-dopa (Cotzias & Papavasiliou, 1971). Subsequently in the early 1970s, a number of studies showed the advantage of coadministration of L-dopa with a peripheral DDI compared to L-dopa alone (Barbeau, 1973; Calne et al., 1971; Lieberman, Goodgold, Jonas, & Leibowitz, 1975; Markham, Diamond, & Treciokas, 1974; Marsden, Barry, Parkes, & Zilkha, 1973; Martin et al., 1975; Papavasiliou et al., 1972; Sweet, McDowell, Wasterlain, & Stern, 1975; Yahr, Duvoisin, Mendoza, Schear, & Barrett, 1971). In 1972, Papavasiliou et al. reported that addition of a peripheral DDI to L-dopa showed several advantages such as much smaller doses of L-dopa needed for control of symptoms, more rapid induction of efficacy, better diurnal symptomatic control, and reduced gastrointestinal side effects (Papavasiliou et al., 1972). This publication established the combined use of L-dopa plus a peripheral DDI as the recommended standard manner for L-dopa therapy in PD, which is still in use today. The development of such peripheral DDIs made L-dopa more potent while reducing gastrointestinal adverse effects.

Consequentially, in 1975, the first combination of L-dopa plus carbidopa was commercialized by Merck, Sharp, and Dohme under the name of Sinemet (Tolosa, Martí, Valldeoriola, & Molinuevo, 1998). In same year, the combination of L-dopa plus benserazide was commercialized as Madopar by Hoffmann-La Roche. Sinemet (carbidopa/L-dopa) was initially sold in 1:10 ratios as 10/100 and 25/250 mg strength tablets. But because many patients require at least 50–75 mg/day of carbidopa to have adequate inhibition of peripheral dopa decarboxylase, a 25/100 mg tablet was later marketed and is probably the most common strength utilized today (Fahn, 2008).

5.3.2 COMT Inhibitor

The addition of COMT inhibitors is one of the many strategies used to prolong the "on" response. In 1957, inhibitor of COMT was found to inhibit the peripheral metabolism of L-dopa to 3-*O*-methyl-dopa, thereby increasing the bioavailability of L-dopa (Axelrod, 1957). Then in 1972, Cotzias proposed to block *O*-methyltransferase in peripheral tissues to further potentiate the potency of L-dopa, providing a prelude to the development of the COMT inhibitors now in use (Papavasiliou et al., 1972).

The first generation of COMT inhibitors, such as *N*-butyl gallate, pyrogallol, tropolone, and U-0521, was discarded because of nonspecific actions and significant clinical toxicity (Ericsson, 1971; Reches & Fahn, 1982). Then in the late 1980s, new, more selective COMT inhibitors, such as the pyridine derivatives (CGP 28014) or the nitrocatechol-type (entacapone, nitecapone, tolcapone), were developed (Backstrom et al., 1989; Borgulya, Bruderer, Bernauer, Zürcher, & Prada, 1989; Waldmeier et al., 1990). Two inhibitors of this enzyme, tolcapone (Ro 40-7592) and entacapone (OR-611), have been available since the mid-1990s. Entacapone acts mainly on extracerebral COMT and does not cross the blood–brain barrier. Tolcapone inhibits both extracerebral and cerebral COMT and thereby affects the synthesis and metabolism of dopamine in the brain (Bonifati & Meco, 1999). All are reversible inhibitors of the enzyme and inhibit COMT activity on erythrocytes in a dose-dependent fashion (Kaakkola, Gordin, & Männistö, 1994). Both of entacapone and tolcapone provided improvement in motor fluctuations when used as adjuncts to L-dopa in patients with PD (Davis, Roznoski, & Burns, 1995; Kaakkola, Teräväinen, Ahtila, Rita, & Gordin, 1994; Kurth et al., 1997; Limousin, Pollak, Gervason-Tournier, Hommel, & Perret, 1993; Merello, Lees, Webster, Bovingdon, & Gordin, 1994; Roberts et al., 1993; Ruottinen & Rinne, 1996). Tolcapone was approved in 1997 and entacapone in 1998 (2002a). In 1998, the first COMT inhibitor became commercially available (tolcapone; Tasmar). However, abnormalities in liver function tests were encountered in subjects participating in tolcapone clinical trials, and postmarketing surveillance revealed three cases of hepatocellular liver damage with death that were linked to the drug (Assal, Spahr, Hadengue, Rubbici-Brandt, & Burkhard, 1998; Olanow, 2000). Therefore, its use was suspended within the European Union (EU), and the labeling was changed in the United States. Specifically, FDA recommends serum ALT and AST to be determined at baseline, biweekly in the first year, every 4 weeks in the next 6 months, and every 8 weeks afterward (Olanow & Watkins, 2007). Tolcapone should be discontinued if either enzyme exceeds the upper limit of normal (Hauser, 2004). Entacapone has not been associated with hepatotoxicity, and liver monitoring is not required. Since 2003, combination carbidopa/L-dopa/entacapone tablets (Stalevo) became commercially available.

5.3.3 MAO-B Inhibitor

Another strategy to reduce dopamine degradation is inhibition of MAO-B because dopamine in the human brain is oxidized primarily by MAO-B.

MAO was discovered as the mechanism for inactivating the monoamines in 1937 (Blaschko, Richter, & Schlossmann, 1937). In 1959, Holzer and Hornykiewicz reported that the MAO inhibitors increased the dopamine content of rabbit brain (Holzer & Hornykiewicz, 1959). In the early 1960s, several researchers found that coadministration of MAO inhibitor and L-dopa enhanced and prolonged L-dopa benefits (Bernheimer, Birkmayer, & Hornykiewicz, 1962; Birkmayer & Hornykiewicz, 1962, 1998; Gerstenbrand, Pateisky, & Prosenz, 1963; McGeer, Boulding, Gibson, & Foulkes, 1961). Then, a MAO inhibitor was routinely used as an adjunct to L-dopa.

Two irreversible MAO-B inhibitors, selegiline and rasagiline, are commercially available. Both MAO-B inhibitors have been demonstrated to have antiparkinsonian effects particularly in reducing "off" time (Golbe et al., 1988; Parkinson Study Group, 2005; Rascol et al., 2005). The first MAO-B inhibitor studied was E-250 (Eldepryl, deprenyl, selegiline). The discovery of L-deprenyl (Knoll, Ecseri, Kelemen, Nievel, & Knoll, 1965; Knoll & Magyar, 1972; Knoll, Vizi, & Somogyi, 1968), a selective MAO-B inhibitor, devoid of the "cheese effect" (Knoll, 1976; Knoll & Magyar, 1972; Squires, 1972) has led to the application of this drug in combination with L-dopa for the management of PD since 1974 (Birkmayer et al., 1985; Birkmayer, Riederer, Youdim, & Linauer, 1975; Lieberman et al., 1984; Stern, Lees, Hardie, & Sandler, 1983). Rasagiline (Azilect, *N*-propargyl-*R*-aminoindan) mesylate is a second-generation MAO-B inhibitor. It was found by Youdim and coworkers in 1996 (Finberg, Lamensdorf, Commissiong, & Youdim, 1996) and was approved for the treatment of PD in the EU in February 2005 and by the FDA in May 2006.

Safinamide (Xadago) is a reversible MAO-B inhibitor, which also blocks Na^+/Ca^{2+} channels, and inhibits glutamate release (Caccia et al., 2006). A phase III, multicenter, double-blind, placebo-controlled, parallel-group study in 445 patients with fluctuating PD demonstrated that safinamide improved motor symptoms of parkinsonism without worsening LIDs (Borgohain et al., 2014a). Two years follow-up study in these patients showed no significant worsening of dyskinesia on safinamide compared with placebo. In moderate-to-severe dyskinetic patients, safinamide 100 mg/day vs placebo significantly improved dyskinesia (Borgohain et al., 2014b). In 2014, it was licensed by European Medicines Agency (EMA) for the treatment of PD as add-on therapy to a stable dose of L-dopa alone or in combination with other antiparkinsonian drugs in mid- to late-stage fluctuating patients.

5.3.4 Sustained Release Form of L-Dopa

Sustained release formulations of L-dopa were developed to prolong the plasma half-life of L-dopa and stabilize serum plasma levels, thus minimizing development of motor complications. These formulations produce a more constant rise in plasma L-dopa level owing to slower absorption but decreases bioavailability compared with immediate release (IR) formulations (Cedarbaum, Breck, Kutt, & McDowell, 1987; Crevoisier, Hoevels, Zürcher, & Da Prada, 1987; Jensen, Dupont, Hansen, Mikkelsen, & Mikkelsen, 1987; Malcolm et al., 1987; Nordera et al., 1987; Quinn, Marion, & Marsden, 1987; Wilding et al., 1991). Two such L-dopa formulations have become available in 1989. One is called carbidopa/L-dopa extended release (ER), with the brand name of Sinemet CR; another is Madopar HBS.

In several open-label and double-blind studies in patients with motor fluctuations, these preparations improved end of dose deterioration and prolonged "on" period (Cedarbaum et al., 1987; Cedarbaum, Hoey, Kutt, & McDowell, 1988; Chouza et al., 1990; Goetz, Tanner, Klawans, Shannon, & Carroll, 1987; Goetz et al., 1988; Juncos, Fabbrini, Mouradian, & Chase, 1987; Juncos, Fabbrini, Mouradian, Serrati, et al., 1987; Lees, 1987; Nutt, Woodward, & Carter, 1986; Pacchetti et al., 1990; Quinn et al., 1987; Rinne, 1987b; Rondot, Ziegler, Aymard, & Holzer, 1987; Sage & Mark, 1988; Siegfried, 1987). Others, however, have found a loss of clinical benefit mainly because of their relatively erratic absorption, tendency to be associated with low plasma levels, and the development or increase of peak dose or biphasic dyskinesias (Kleedorfer & Poewe, 1992; Pezzoli et al., 1988). The ER formulations of Madopar and Sinemet in comparison with their IR preparation failed to show significant advantage in postponing or reducing the long-term L-dopa complications (Block, Liss, Reines, Irr, & Nibbelink, 1997; Dupont et al., 1996; Koller, Hutton, Tolosa, Capilldeo, & The Carbidopa/Levodopa Study Group, 1999). Therefore, they are generally not suitable for control of motor complications.

5.3.5 Soluble Form of L-Dopa

Soluble L-dopa formulations dissolve and are absorbed quickly, and a clinical effect usually sets in very reliably around 20–30 min after ingestion, compared to 30–60 min with standard L-dopa (Tolosa, Marti, & Katzenschlager, 2015). They can be useful for the delayed early morning "on" or as a rescue therapy of bothersome or disabling "off" period, although chronic or very frequent use should be avoided in view of pulsatile dopaminergic stimulation (Tolosa et al., 2015). Such oral soluble forms of L-dopa include dispersible L-dopa preparations or L-dopa prodrugs with high water solubility. A dispersible formulation of L-dopa contains the same active ingredients as standard L-dopa/benserazide but with earlier release, more rapid absorption, and shorter time to peak and effective plasma concentration (Haglund & Hoogkamer, 1995). In open-label studies, this dispersible formulation was useful for treating early morning (Steiger, Stocchi, Bramante, Ruggieri, & Quinn, 1992; Ziégler, Ranoux, & de Recondo, 1994) and afternoon (Ziégler et al., 1994) "off" symptoms.

L-Dopa methyl ester (melevodopa hydrochloride), a L-dopa prodrug, is produced by esterification of the carboxylic moiety of the L-dopa molecule. It is about 250 times more soluble than L-dopa (Stocchi et al., 2007) and offers the potential for more rapid and consistent absorption that is not influenced by gastric pH (Rondelli, Acerbi, Mariotti, & Ventura, 1994; Sasahara, Nitanai, Habara, Morioka, & Nakajima, 1980; Vickers et al., 1978) and more rapid onset of action compared with standard oral L-dopa preparations (Stocchi, Barbato, Bramante, Bonamartini, & Ruggieri, 1994). In pilot studies, melevodopa in combination with carbidopa was demonstrated to lead a significantly more rapid reversal of morning and afternoon "off" period, compared with Sinemet or Madopar ensuring similar duration of action (Steiger et al., 1991, 1992; Stocchi et al., 1996; Stocchi, Quinn, et al., 1994; Stocchi, Ruggieri, Carta, Jenner, & Agnoli, 1989). Then, an effervescent tablet formulation containing melevodopa hydrochloride plus carbidopa (CHF 1512, Sirio) was developed. However, there had been conflicting results for the use of CHF 1512 in the treatment of motor fluctuations (Stocchi et al., 2007; Stocchi, Zappia, et al., 2010).

5.3.6 Duodenal Infusion

In 1975, continuous intravenous L-dopa infusion was tried, with success for preventing motor fluctuations (Shoulson, Glaubiger, & Chase, 1975). Then in the early 1980s, a series of clinical studies have reported that constant-rate intravenous infusion of L-dopa ameliorates motor fluctuations in patients with advanced PD (Hardie, Lees, & Stern, 1984; Hardie, Malcolm, Lees, Stern, & Allen, 1986; Marion, Stocchi, Quinn, Jenner, & Marsden, 1986; Nutt & Woodward, 1986; Nutt, Woodward, & Anderson, 1985; Nutt, Woodward, Hammerstad, Carter, & Anderson, 1984; Quinn, Marsden, & Parkes, 1982; Quinn, Parkes, & Marsden, 1984; Stocchi, Ruggieri, Brughitta, & Agnoli, 1986). However, it cannot be maintained in an individual patient for longer than several days because of the risk of thrombosis and lack of stability at room temperature (Pappert et al., 1996). In 1986, Kurlan et al. first reported a reduction in motor fluctuations after duodenal continuous infusion of L-dopa via a nasoduodenal tube in three advanced PD patients with resistant motor fluctuation, comparable with the effects of intravenous infusions (Kurlan et al., 1986). Since then, a number of studies have documented the efficacy of enteral L-dopa infusions not only to provide stable plasma L-dopa levels and reduce motor fluctuations but also to decrease preexisting dyskinesias (Cedarbaum, Silvestri, & Kutt, 1990; Kurth et al., 1993; Sage, Schuh, Heikkila, & Duvoisin, 1988; Sage, Trooskin, Sonsalla, & Heikkila, 1989; Syed, Murphy, Zimmerman, Mark, & Sage, 1998).

Earlier studies used percutaneous gastrostomy with a duodenal or jejunal tube linked to a portable pump and needed large volumes of liquid preparations for infusions due to the poor water solubility of L-dopa, which limited the practicality of infusion therapy. Then, Duodopa, a stable gel suspension with a uniform concentration of carbidopa/L-dopa (5/20 mg/mL in a carboxymethylcellulose mix) was developed and enabled controlled continuous delivery of the drug adjustable by small dosage increments (Nilsson, Nyholm, & Aquilonius, 2001; Nyholm et al., 2003). This therapy has proved to provide both reduced "off" time and less dyskinesia (Antonini et al., 2007, 2013; Fernandez et al., 2013; Nyholm, Klangemo, & Johansson, 2012; Nyholm et al., 2005, 2008; Olanow et al., 2014). The first country to approve the infusion therapy was Sweden in January 2004. Then it was approved in all EU in 2005, and in United States in 2015 (2015).

5.4 Novel Formulations of L-Dopa

5.4.1 Dual-Release Formulation

Another concept for achieving more constant L-dopa uptake has been a dual-release product. IPX066 (Rytary) is a novel, oral ER capsule that contains beads of carbidopa and L-dopa (carbidopa:L-dopa ratio, 1:4) that dissolves at various rate along their gastrointestinal passage. In a crossover comparison study of 27 patients with advanced PD, dual-release carbidopa/L-dopa produced plasma L-dopa profiles showing an onset of effect similar to that of carbidopa/L-dopa IR, but more sustained L-dopa plasma concentrations with less fluctuation compared with carbidopa/L-dopa IR (Hauser et al., 2011). The ADVANCE-PD (Hauser et al., 2013) and ASCEND-PD (Stocchi et al., 2014) studies in advanced PD reported that IPX066 significantly decreased "off" time and increased "on" time without troublesome dyskinesia. In ADVANCE-PD study, prevalence of adverse events was similar between the IPX066 and carbidopa/L-dopa IR groups. In January 2015, IPX066 received marketing authorization by the FDA for the treatment of patients with PD and parkinsonism from other causes. It is currently available only in the United States.

XP21279 is a novel L-dopa prodrug that is absorbed from the small and large intestine by high-capacity nutritional transporters throughout the gastrointestinal tract and then rapidly converted to L-dopa by carboxylesterases (LeWitt, Ellenbogen, et al., 2012). The capability for colonic absorption of XP21279 can extend the duration of maintaining therapeutic plasma concentrations of L-dopa (LeWitt et al., 2014). Relative bioavailability of XP21279 is approximately 88% of that of carbidopa/L-dopa IR (LeWitt, Ellenbogen, et al., 2012). In a phase II, randomized, double-blind, double-dummy, crossover study of carbidopa/XP21279 and carbidopa/L-dopa IR in 35 patients with PD with motor fluctuations, carbidopa/XP21279 significantly reduced variability in L-dopa concentrations compared with carbidopa/L-dopa IR, although carbidopa/XP21279 showed similar reduction in total daily "off" time to carbidopa/L-dopa IR (LeWitt et al., 2014).

Accordion pill is a novel gastric retention formulation of carbidopa/L-dopa consisting of a multilayer planar structure of biodegradable films that are folded in an accordion shape and then filled into standard-size capsules. A pilot phase II study of the accordion pill in 16 subjects reported significant reduction in total daily "off" time (mean of 2.4 vs 4.3 h; 44% reduction; $P < 0.0001$) and increase in percentage "on" time without troublesome dyskinesia, compared to optimized standard L-dopa therapy (LeWitt, Giladi, et al., 2012).

DM-1992 is a carbidopa/L-dopa bilayer tablet formulation combining IR and ER layers within a polymer-based gastroretentive drug delivery system. In an open-label, randomized crossover trial in 34 PD patients with fluctuating PD, DM-1992 significantly decreased the percentage of daily "off" time recorded in patient diaries from the baseline (Chaudhuri et al., 2016; Verhagen Metman, Stover, Chen, Cowles, & Sweeney, 2015).

5.4.2 Inhalation Powder Formulation

Pulmonary administration may offer an attractive alternative to oral administration, due to its immediate presentation of the drug to the absorption membrane, the large size of the absorption membrane and relatively low metabolic activity in the lung. CVT-301 is a novel self-administered, L-dopa inhalation powder formulated for pulmonary absorption and administered using a passive, breath-actuated delivery system (LeWitt et al., 2016). A phase IIa dose finding study performed by Acorda therapeutics showed that plasma L-dopa concentrations after pulmonary administration of L-dopa increased more rapidly and with less variability than was observed in the same patients after oral L-dopa dosing and that motor function improved significantly in an "off" period. In the phase IIb study, CVT-301 self-administered during "off" episodes provided rapid improvement of motor function, and daily "off" time was significantly reduced at the higher dose. Thus, pulmonary administration of L-dopa may be suitable for use as a rescue therapy during "off" periods (Luinstra et al., 2015). The most frequently reported adverse events in the CVT-301 group were dizziness, cough, and nausea, each in 7%.

5.4.3 Skin Patch

Transdermal administration of L-dopa may yield more continuous drug delivery (CDD). ND0611, a continuously delivered carbidopa solution administered subcutaneously by a patch, was developed. An adjunctive use of ND0611 to carbidopa/L-dopa IR was found to increase L-dopa half-life, area under the curve, and trough concentrations of L-dopa in preclinical studies and in a phase I study in healthy volunteers (Hauser, 2011).

ND0612 is a soluble carbidopa/L-dopa formulation for continuous subcutaneous delivery through a custom patch pump. The results of a phase I trial in healthy volunteers showed stable carbidopa/L-dopa plasma levels over 24-h infusion cycles, with peak concentrations of around 500 ng/mL at the highest infusion rate (Caraco, Oren, & LeWitt, 2013). In an early phase II study with fluctuating PD, patients on ND0612 showed reductions in "off" time and plasma L-dopa concentration fluctuations with complete abolition of the low trough levels compared with placebo (Giladi et al., 2015).

6. DOPAMINE AGONISTS

The use of dopamine agonists for the treatment of patients with PD started in the 1970s. Since the introduction of bromocriptine (2-bromo-α-ergocriptine) in the 1970s in an attempt to overcome the limitation of high-dose L-dopa therapy, several dopamine agonists have become available for the treatment of PD. Currently available dopamine receptor agonists fall into two major classes: (a) ergolines, which are derivatives of ergot alkaloids and include bromocriptine, pergolide, lisuride, α-dihydroergocryptine, and cabergoline and (b) nonergolines such as apomorphine, piribedil, ropinirole, pramipexole, and rotigotine.

Dopamine agonists were initially developed as an adjunctive therapy to L-dopa in advanced PD patients with motor complications (Calne et al., 1974; Hoehn & Elton, 1985; McDonald & Horowski, 1983). Later on, in the mid-1990s, some of researchers proposed that dopamine agonists should be used earlier in the course of disease, and even as first-line treatment, in order to delay or reduce the need for L-dopa, thereby reducing motor complications of long-term L-dopa therapy (Montastruc, Rascol, Senard, & Rascol, 1994). This strategy was generated from early observations that patients treated with bromocriptine monotherapy showed a notable lack of motor complication (Rascol, Guiraud, Montastruc, David, & Clanet, 1979; Rinne, 1985). Long-term follow-up studies of dopamine agonists such as bromocriptine, pergolide, ropinirole, pramipexole, or cabergoline have shown them to be effective in controlling motor symptoms of PD but with lesser frequency of dyskinesia than that occurring in patients treated with L-dopa (Bracco et al., 2004; Hauser et al., 2007; Hely et al., 1994; Holloway et al., 2004; Oertel et al., 2006; Ogawa et al., 1997; Parkinson Study Group CALM Cohort Investigators, 2009; Rascol et al., 1979, 2000; Rinne, 1985, 1987a; Rinne et al., 1998).

6.1 Ergot-Derived Dopamine Agonists

Bromocriptine is the first marketed dopamine receptor agonist. It was initially developed to reduce prolactin secretion and used to suppress lactation by dopaminergic production of prolactin inhibitory factor in the hypothalamus (Calne et al., 1974; Debono, Marsden, Asselman, & Parkes, 1976). In 1970, Fuxe and Hökfelt demonstrated ability of bromocriptine to reduce dopamine turnover in hypothalamic and nigrostriatal dopaminergic neurons (Fuxe & Hökfelt, 1970). Then in 1973, Corrodi et al. found effects of bromocriptine on motility in animal models of parkinsonism and suggested that bromocriptine appears to stimulate dopamine receptors (Corrodi, Fuxe, Hökfelt, Lidbrink, & Ungerstedt, 1973). Subsequently, Calne and colleagues conducted the first double-blind clinical trial with bromocriptine as an add-on therapy to L-dopa in 20 patients with PD (Calne et al., 1974), which showed that bromocriptine provided improvement of neurologic deficits by almost 20% in severely disabled patients and about 10% in mildly affected patients. Since then, others have reported various degrees of success with bromocriptine in the treatment of parkinsonism (Fahn, Cote, Snider, Barrett, & Isgreen, 1979; Kartzinel et al., 1976; Lieberman, Kupersmith, Estey, & Goldstein, 1976; Parkes, Debono, & Marsden, 1976).

A decade later in 1989, pergolide, an *N*-propylergoline derivative, was introduced on the market. In 1980, it was found to stimulate the D1 receptor as well as D2 receptor unlike bromocriptine which only stimulates D2 receptors (Goldstein et al., 1980). In an animal model of PD, pergolide induced rotatory behavior and relieved tremor, providing more potent and prolonged action than the other ergot alkaloids (Goldstein et al., 1980). Next year, Lieberman and colleagues tried the first small-scale, randomized, controlled trials of add-on therapy of pergolide to L-dopa in 13 patients with advanced PD with motor fluctuations and found a significant increase of the "on" time in 9 out of 13 who completed the study (Lieberman et al., 1981). In comparative studies of pergolide between the 1980s and 1990s, pergolide had similar (LeWitt et al., 1983; Mizuno, Kondo, & Narabayashi, 1995) or superior effect (Boas, Worm-Petersen, Dupont, Mikkelsen, & Wermuth, 1996; Pezzoli et al., 1994) on motor symptoms compared with bromocriptine. In a prospective, multicenter, double-blind, placebo-controlled, parallel-group study in 376 patients with motor fluctuations and dyskinesias, pergolide as an adjunctive therapy to L-dopa significantly improved activity of daily living (ADL) and Parkinson scores, and reduced "off" time and L-dopa daily dose, compared with placebo (Olanow et al., 1994).

Lisuride is a soluble alpha-amino-ergoline with D2 receptor agonist properties and also 5-HT2 activity, but has no apparent D1 receptor effects. It is a parenteral drug available in Europe. In 1981, Parkes et al. were the first to demonstrate antiparkinsonian effect of intravenous and oral lisuride in nine subjects with idiopathic, postencephalitic, or drug-induced parkinsonism (Parkes, Schachter, Marsden, Smith, & Wilson, 1981). Continuous subcutaneous infusions of lisuride in advanced PD patients provided significant reduction in both "off" time and dyskinesia in comparison to standard treatment (Stocchi, Ruggieri, Vacca, & Olanow, 2002).

Cabergoline, synthetic tetracyclic ergoline derivative, acts as a selective D2 receptor agonist with no substantial affinity for D1 receptors. It was the first that the antiparkinsonian activity of cabergoline was documented in an open, dose-ranging study by Jori et al. (Jori et al., 1990). One major characteristic of cabergoline is its long half-life of approximately 65 h with oral administration, thus allowing a once-daily dosing treatment regimen (2002b).

6.2 Adverse Effects of Ergot-Derived Dopamine Agonists

Common adverse effects of ergot-derived dopamine agonists are related to peripheral and central dopaminergic stimulation, which are shared with those of L-dopa or nonergoline dopamine agonists. These include nausea, vomiting, dizziness, orthostatic hypotension, bradycardia, other signs of autonomic peripheral stimulation, and psychiatric symptoms such as hallucinations, and delusions. Psychiatric adverse reactions are commonly seen with dopamine agonists rather than L-dopa (Factor, Molho, Podskalny, & Brown, 1995).

Some of the adverse effects are rare but seem to be related to their ergot structure, which are vasospasm, erythromelalgia, and pleuropulmonary or retroperitoneal fibrosis (Goetz & Diederich, 1992; Uitti & Ahlskog, 1996). Retroperitoneal, pleural, and pericardial fibrosis are well documented after bromocriptine therapy, and their prevalence has been reported to be 2%–5% over a 5-year period (McElvaney, Wilcox, Churg, & Fleetham, 1988). However, the occurrence of restrictive valvular heart disease during treatment with pergolide and cabergoline caused concern about the safety of dopamine agonists in PD. After Pritchett et al. reported three patients in 2002 (Pritchett et al., 2002), Van Camp et al. reported that restrictive valvular heart disease of any type was present in 33% of their 78 patients with PD treated with pergolide, 19% of whom had severe disease (Van Camp et al., 2004). The FDA issued a strong warning, and the pharmaceutical company discontinued manufacturing pergolide in 2007. The cardiac side effects are claimed to be potentially mediated by the 5-HT2B agonist activity on the serotoninergic receptors expressed on cardiac valvular fibroblasts (Antonini & Poewe, 2007). Other ergolinic dopamine agonists, such as lisuride, and nonergot dopamine agonists are devoid of 5-HT2B agonistic activity. Therefore, their use might not induce fibrotic changes in heart valves (Dewey, Reimold, & O'Suilleabhain, 2007). The extent to which fibrotic valvular changes are reversible after discontinuation and whether switching to a nonergot agonist prevents further progression are still unknown. Although the ergot-derived dopamine agonists have proved to be successful agents in the management of PD, these adverse effects limit their use only as a second-line alternative option.

6.3 Nonergot-Derived Dopamine Agonists

The newer nonergot-derived agents such as ropinirole, pramipexole, and piribedil are well known to provide clinical benefits both for advanced

PD patients as an add-on therapy to L-dopa and for early PD patients as a monotherapy (2002c; Fox et al., 2011). As the knowledge about the chemical configuration of dopamine receptors became sufficient by the end of the 1980s, nonergot dopamine agonists with the potential of achieving higher affinities, more specificity and longer duration of action were developed. Ropinirole was the first available nonergoline orally active dopamine agonist. It exhibits affinity specifically to D2-like receptors with a selectivity similar to that of dopamine (D3 > D2 > D4), but little or no interaction with other neurotransmitter receptors. Piribedil is a nonergot selective D2 and D3 agonist with α2 antagonist properties. It is marketed in a few European countries. Pramipexole, a synthetic amino-benzothiazole derivative, binds to D3 dopamine receptors with a sevenfold greater affinity than it does to D2 and D4 receptors. The receptor profile of pramipexole is similar to that of ropinirole (Watts, 1997). By the late 1990s, nonergot dopamine agonists, especially ropinirole and pramipexole, had largely replaced ergot dopamine agonists by due to fibrotic adverse events of ergot dopamine agonists such as restrictive valvular heart disease.

In the past decade, continuous delivery of dopamine agonists has been available by long-acting formulations of dopamine agonist such as prolonged release (PR) ropinirole, ER pramipexole, and rotigotine transdermal patch. Compared with the IR formulation, long-acting dopamine agonists not only provide more stable plasma concentrations over 24 h and possibly a more continuous dopamine stimulation (CDS) (Jenner, Könen-Bergmann, Schepers, & Haertter, 2009; Tompson & Vearer, 2007) but also improve patient's adherence to treatment (Grosset et al., 2009; Poewe et al., 2011; Schapira et al., 2011, 2013). However, Yun et al. showed that many patients preferred twice-daily combination of ropinirole PR over once-daily regimen in an open-label crossover study (Yun et al., 2013). Ropinirole PR is approved for the treatment of early and advanced PD (Pahwa et al., 2007; Stocchi, Hersh, Scott, Nausieda, & Giorgi, 2008). PREPARED study, comparison of ropinirole IR and PR in advanced PD, showed that ropinirole PR was more efficacious in maintaining a 20% or more reduction in "off" time compared with ropinirole IR (Stocchi, Giorgi, Hunter, & Schapira, 2011). Pramipexole ER is approved both as monotherapy in patients with early PD, and as adjunctive therapy with L-dopa in patients with advanced PD. In double-blind studies, short-term efficacy of pramipexole ER for motor symptoms and ADL was noninferior to that of pramipexole IR in patients with early PD as monotherapy (Hauser et al., 2010; Rascol et al., 2010;

Schapira et al., 2011) and similar to that of pramipexole IR in patients with advanced PD as adjunctive therapy to L-dopa (Schapira et al., 2011).

Rotigotine (SPM 962) is a novel, nonergolinic, lipid-soluble, selective dopamine D1, D2, and D3 receptor agonist formulated in a silicone-based transdermal system (Wood, Dubois, Scheller, & Gillard, 2015). Once-daily administration of a rotigotine provides stable plasma concentrations of rotigotine over 24 h (Elshoff, Braun, Andreas, Middle, & Cawello, 2012). Transdermal delivery is particularly useful in patients scheduled for surgery or in those with dysphagia (Wüllner et al., 2010) and also can prevent food interactions, variable absorption due to altered gastrointestinal motility, first-pass effects of the liver, and gastric emptying. Rotigotine was approved by the EMA in 2006 and for the treatment of patients with early stage PD by the FDA in May 2007. However, the marketing authorization of rotigotine was suspended by the FDA in March 2008 because of crystal formation at room temperature, therefore, possibly reducing its bioavailability and clinical efficacy (Chaudhuri, 2008). The crystals were composed of pure rotigotine and did not present any safety issues (Chaudhuri, 2008). Some batches of rotigotine transdermal patch were recalled following discussion with the EMA and the FDA. The EMA treatment restrictions between July 2008 and August 2009 limited prescribing to 1 month's supply and prevented new patients from being initiated on rotigotine. Later in 2012, with development of a room temperature stable patch, rotigotine was approved by both the FDA and the EMA and obtained additional indications for advanced stage PD in the United States (Elshoff et al., 2013). Rotigotine was confirmed to provide significant and sustained improvement in symptoms in patients with early or advanced stage PD in phase III randomized, placebo-controlled trials (Giladi et al., 2007; Jankovic, Watts, Martin, Boroojerdi, & The SP 512 Rotigotine Transdermal System Clinical Study Group, 2007; LeWitt, Lyons, Pahwa, & SP 650 Study Group, 2007; Nicholas et al., 2014; Poewe et al., 2007; Watts et al., 2007). A recent meta-analysis of six randomized controlled trials also showed that rotigotine improved motor symptoms and ADL, compared with placebo (Zhou et al., 2013).

6.4 Adverse Effects of nonergot-Derived Dopamine Agonists

Most of the adverse effects of nonergoline dopamine agonists are also related to dopaminergic hyperstimulation. Although gastrointestinal and cardiovascular adverse reactions occur at the beginning of therapy, tolerance can develop over time (Perez-Lloret & Rascol, 2010). Meanwhile, peripheral leg edema, which can be caused by both of ergot and nonergot dopamine agonists (Biglan, Holloway, McDermott, Richard, & The Parkinson Study Group CALM-PD Investigators, 2007), is not an early problem but tends to occur a few years of treatment. Sleep attacks in PD were initially reported to occur only with particular dopamine agonists, pramipexole and ropinirole (Frucht, Rogers, Greene, Gordon, & Fahn, 1999). It, however, can be associated with any dopaminergic medication. The prevalence of sleep attacks in PD has been reported variably ranging from 6% to 43% (Korner et al., 2004; Manni, Terzaghi, Sartori, Mancini, & Pacchetti, 2004; Montastruc et al., 2001; Paus et al., 2004; Videnovic & Golombek, 2013).

While nonergoline dopamine agonists do not seem to cause side effects specific to ergots such as skin inflammation, digital vasospasm, and paresthesias, pleural effusion, pulmonary infiltrates, or erythromelalgia, they can cause impulse control disorders (ICDs) and dopamine agonist withdrawal syndrome (DAWS). ICDs encompass a wide spectrum of abnormal behaviors including hypersexuality, pathological gambling, compulsive shopping, and binge eating (Weintraub & Nirenberg, 2013). ICD prevalence is significantly higher in PD patients who are on dopamine agonist therapy, although others are also considered as risk factors such as personal or familial history of alcoholism or gambling, impulsive or novelty seeking traits, younger age, male sex, early onset of PD, being unmarried, and past or current cigarette smoking (Weintraub, David, Evans, Grant, & Stacy, 2015). There, however, is no clear evidence for differential risk within the dopamine agonist class (Weintraub et al., 2015). In the DOMINION study of 3090 PD patients, dopamine agonist treatment in PD was associated with 2- to 3.5-fold increased odds of having an ICD, and ICD frequency was similar for pramipexole and ropinirole (17.7% and 15.5%, respectively) (Weintraub et al., 2010). In a recent multicenter transversal study, an ICD was detected by the Questionnaire for Impulsive–Compulsive Disorders in Parkinson's Disease-rating scale in 39% of the patients with PD chronically treated (>6 months) with a single nonergolinic dopamine agonist (Garcia-Ruiz et al., 2014).

The dose reduction or discontinuation of dopamine agonists can be complicated by DAWS. The symptoms of DAWS are similar to those of withdrawal from other psychostimulants and may include anxiety, panic, social phobia, agoraphobia, fatigue, irritability, dysphoria, depression, pain, nausea, vomiting, diaphoresis, orthostatic hypotension, drug cravings, and suicidal ideation (Pondal et al., 2013; Rabinak & Nirenberg, 2010).

Approximately one-third of patients with ICDs who attempt to taper dopamine agonists can develop DAWS, which makes weaning difficult or impossible (Bastiaens, Dorfman, Christos, & Nirenberg, 2013; Cunnington, White, & Hood, 2012; Pondal et al., 2013; Rabinak & Nirenberg, 2010). DAWS does not respond to substitution of L-dopa and other dopaminergic medications for the dopamine agonist, or to the addition of other medications and no known effective treatment exists (Samuel et al., 2015).

7. CDS STRATEGY AND THEN TRANSITION TO CDD STRATEGY

Dopaminergic replacement with repeated doses of short-acting drugs is associated with oscillating dopamine concentrations (Abercrombie, Bonatz, & Zigmond, 1990; de la Fuente-Fernández et al., 2004; Miller & Abercrombie, 1999) that are believed to induce maladaptive changes in basal ganglia motor circuits. The consequence of such nonphysiological, irregular, and pulsatile dopaminergic stimulation has been a central issue in attempts to explain mechanisms underlying motor complications such as dyskinesias and fluctuations in motor response. Therefore, it was proposed that achieving continuous stimulation of striatal dopamine receptors by using long-acting medicines such as dopamine agonists could delay or prevent the onset of motor complications. Actually, many of comparison studies of a dopamine agonist vs L-dopa as initial treatment in early PD showed that significantly decreased incidence of dyskinesia with dopamine agonist monotherapy (Holloway et al., 2004; Oertel et al., 2006; Parkinson Study Group, 2000; Rascol et al., 2000; Rinne et al., 1998). The effect of plasma half-life was thought to explain increased incidence of motor complications with L-dopa relative to dopamine agonists.

However, other such strategies to attempt to provide more CDS based on only half-life of the drugs have often failed to find evidence favoring these approaches over an intermittent therapy (Chaudhuri, Rizos, & Sethi, 2013), as following: carbidopa/L-dopa CR vs carbidopa/L-dopa IR in advanced PD (Pahwa et al., 2006); carbidopa/L-dopa/entacapone vs carbidopa/L-dopa (Stocchi, Rascol, et al., 2010); pramipexole ER vs pramipexole IR as an adjunct to L-dopa in advanced PD (Schapira et al., 2011); and transdermal rotigotine vs ropinirole IR as monotherapy in early PD (Giladi et al., 2007) or to pramipexole IR as an adjunct to L-dopa in advanced PD (Poewe et al., 2007). In contrast, the strategies to change the delivery method of the same agent even with short half-life such as the continuous infusion of

L-dopa (Nyholm & Aquilonius, 2004; Nyholm et al., 2005) or apomorphine (Manson et al., 2001; Pietz, Hagell, & Odin, 1998) have shown favorable outcomes in motor complications than intermittent therapy. In recent years, CDS has largely been displaced by the concept of CDD, which aims to minimize motor complications in PD by delivering the drug in as constant a manner as possible, regardless of serum half-life (Wright & Waters, 2013). To ensure more CDD, numerous efforts have been underway to develop various treatment strategies including transdermal very long-acting L-dopa preparations such as skin patch.

REFERENCES

(1970, 1970/06/15). PARKINSONISM: L-Dopa Goes Commercial. *Chemical & Engineering News Archive*. Retrieved 25, 48, from http://dx.doi.org/10.1021/cen-v048n025.p013.

(2002a). COMT inhibitors: Management of Parkinson's disease. *Movement Disorders, 17*-(Suppl. 4), S45–S51.

(2002b). DA agonists—Ergot derivatives: Cabergoline: Management of Parkinson's disease. *Movement Disorders, 17*(Suppl. 4), S68–S71.

(2002c). DA agonists—Non-ergot derivatives: Ropinirole: Management of Parkinson's disease. *Movement Disorders, 17*(Suppl. 4), S98–S102.

(2015). AbbVie announces U.S. FDA approval of DUOPA™ (carbidopa and levodopa) enteral suspension for the treatment of motor fluctuations in patients with advanced Parkinson's disease. Retrieved 12 Sep, 2016, from https://news.abbvie.com/news/abbvie-announces-us-fda-approval-duopa-carbidopa-and-levodopa-enteral-suspension-for-treatment-motor-fluctuations-in-patients-with-advanced-parkinsons-disease.htm.

Abercrombie, E. D., Bonatz, A. E., & Zigmond, M. J. (1990). Effects of L-DOPA on extracellular dopamine in striatum of normal and 6-hydroxydopamine-treated rats. *Brain Research, 525*, 36–44.

Adler, C. H. (2007). Amantaine and anticholinergics. In S. Factor & W. Weiner (Eds.), *Parkinson's disease: Diagnosis & clinical management* (2nd ed., pp. 491–497). New York, NY: Demos Medical Publishing.

Agid, Y., Bonnet, A. M., Pollak, P., Signoret, J. L., & Lhermitte, F. (1979). Bromocriptine associated with a peripheral dopamine blocking agent in treatment of Parkinson's disease. *The Lancet, 1*, 570–572.

Andén, N. E., Carlsson, A., Dahlström, A., Fuxe, K., Hillarp, N. Å., & Larsson, K. (1964). Demonstration and mapping out of nigro-neostriatal dopamine neurons. *Life Sciences, 3*, 523–530.

Andén, N. E., Rubenson, A., Fuxe, K., & Hökfelt, T. (1967). Evidence for dopamine receptor stimulation by apomorphine. *Journal of Pharmacy and Pharmacology, 19*, 627–629.

Antonini, A., Isaias, I. U., Canesi, M., Zibetti, M., Mancini, F., Manfredi, L., et al. (2007). Duodenal levodopa infusion for advanced Parkinson's disease: 12-month treatment outcome. *Movement Disorders, 22*, 1145–1149.

Antonini, A., Odin, P., Opiano, L., Tomantschger, V., Pacchetti, C., Pickut, B., et al. (2013). Effect and safety of duodenal levodopa infusion in advanced Parkinson's disease: A retrospective multicenter outcome assessment in patient routine care. *Journal of Neural Transmission, 120*, 1553–1558.

Antonini, A., & Poewe, W. (2007). Fibrotic heart-valve reactions to dopamine-agonist treatment in Parkinson's disease. *The Lancet. Neurology, 6*, 826–829.

Assal, F., Spahr, L., Hadengue, A., Rubbici-Brandt, L., & Burkhard, P. R. (1998). Tolcapone and fulminant hepatitis. *The Lancet, 352*, 958.

Axelrod, J. (1957). O-methylation of epinephrine and other catechols in vitro and in vivo. *Science, 126*, 400–401.

Backstrom, R., Honkanen, E., Pippuri, A., Kairisalo, P., Pystynen, J., Heinola, K., et al. (1989). Synthesis of some novel potent and selective catechol O-methyltransferase inhibitors. *Journal of Medicinal Chemistry, 32*, 841–846.

Barbeau, A. (1973). Treatment of Parkinson's disease with L-DOPA and Ro 4-4602: Review and present status. In M. Yahr (Ed.), *Treatment of parkinsonism: The role of dopa decarboxylase inhibitors* (pp. 173–198). New York: Raven Press.

Barbeau, A., Mars, H., Botez, M. I., & Joubert, M. (1971). Amantadine-HCl (Symmetrel) in the management of Parkinson's disease: A double-blind cross-over study. *Canadian Medical Association Journal, 105*, 42–47.

Barbeau, A., Sourkes, T. L., & Murphy, G. F. (1962). Les catecholamines dans la maladie de Parkinson. In J. de Ajuriaguerra (Ed.), *Monoamines et Systeme Nerveaux Central* (pp. 925–927). Paris: Masson.

Bartholini, G., Burkard, W. P., Pletscher, A., & Bates, H. M. (1967). Increase of cerebral catecholamines caused by 3,4-dihydroxyphenylalanine after inhibition of peripheral decarboxylase. *Nature, 215*, 852–853.

Bastiaens, J., Dorfman, B. J., Christos, P. J., & Nirenberg, M. J. (2013). Prospective cohort study of impulse control disorders in Parkinson's disease. *Movement Disorders, 28*, 327–333.

Bauer, R. B., & McHenry, J. T. (1974). Comparison of amantadine, placebo, and levodopa in Parkinson's disease. *Neurology, 24*, 715–720.

Bernheimer, H., Birkmayer, W., & Hornykiewicz, O. (1962). Verhalten der monoaminoxydase im gehirn des menschen nach therapie mit monoaminoxydase-hemmern. Behavior of monoamine oxidase in the brain of man after therapy with monoamine oxidase inhibitors *Wiener Klinische Wochenschrift, 74*, 558–559.

Bertler, Å., & Rosengren, E. (1959). Occurrence and distribution of dopamine in brain and other tissues. *Experientia, 15*, 10–11.

Biglan, K. M., Holloway, R. G., McDermott, M. P., Richard, I. H., & The Parkinson Study Group CALM-PD Investigators. (2007). Risk factors for somnolence, edema, and hallucinations in early Parkinson disease. *Neurology, 69*, 187–195.

Birkmayer, W., & Hornykiewicz, O. (1961). The L-3,4-dioxyphenylalanine (DOPA)-effect in Parkinson-akinesia. *Wiener Klinische Wochenschrift, 73*, 787–788.

Birkmayer, W., & Hornykiewicz, O. (1962). Der L-Dioxyphenylalanin (L-DOPA)-Effekt beim Parkinson-Syndrom des Menschen: Zur Pathogenese und Behandlung der Parkinson-Akinese. The L-dihydroxyphenylalanine (L-DOPA) effect in Parkinson's syndrome in man: On the pathogenesis and treatment of Parkinson akinesis *Archiv für Psychiatrie und Nervenkrankheiten, vereinigt mit Zeitschrift für die gesamte Neurologie und Psychiatrie, 203*, 560–574.

Birkmayer, W., & Hornykiewicz, O. (1964). Weitere experimentelle Untersuchungen über L-DOPA beim Parkinson-Syndrom und Reserpin-Parkinsonismus. Additional experimental studies on L-dopa in Parkinson's syndrome and reserpine Parkinsonism *Archiv für Psychiatrie und Nervenkrankheiten, 206*, 367–381.

Birkmayer, W., & Hornykiewicz, O. (1998). The effect of L-3,4-dihydroxyphenylalanine (=DOPA) on akinesia in parkinsonism. *Parkinsonism & Related Disorders, 4*, 59–60.

Birkmayer, W., Knoll, J., Riederer, P., Youdim, M. B. H., Hars, V., & Marton, J. (1985). Increased life expectancy resulting from addition of L-deprenyl to Madopar® treatment in Parkinson's disease: A longterm study. *Journal of Neural Transmission, 64*, 113–127.

Birkmayer, W., Linauer, W., & Mentasti, M. (1971). Traitement à la L-dopa combinée avec un inhibiteur de la décarboxylase (RO4-4602). *Monoamines noyaux gris centraux et syndrome de Parkinson* (pp. 435–441). Geneva: Georg.

Birkmayer, W., Riederer, P., Youdim, M. B. H., & Linauer, W. (1975). The potentiation of the anti akinetic effect after L-Dopa treatment by an inhibitor of MAO-B, deprenil. *Journal of Neural Transmission, 36*, 303–326.

Blaschko, H., Richter, D., & Schlossmann, H. (1937). The inactivation of adrenaline. *The Journal of Physiology, 90*, 1–17.

Block, G., Liss, C., Reines, S., Irr, J., & Nibbelink, D. (1997). Comparison of immediate-release and controlled release carbidopa/levodopa in Parkinson's disease. A multicenter 5-year study. The CR first study group. *European Neurology, 37*, 23–27.

Boas, J., Worm-Petersen, J., Dupont, E., Mikkelsen, B., & Wermuth, L. (1996). The levodopa dose-sparing capacity of pergolide compared with that of bromocriptine in an open-label, crossover study. *European Journal of Neurology, 3*, 44–49.

Bonifati, V., & Meco, G. (1999). New, selective catechol-O-methyltransferase inhibitors as therapeutic agents in Parkinson's disease. *Pharmacology & Therapeutics, 81*, 1–36.

Borgohain, R., Szasz, J., Stanzione, P., Meshram, C., Bhatt, M., Chirilineau, D., et al. (2014a). Randomized trial of safinamide add-on to levodopa in Parkinson's disease with motor fluctuations. *Movement Disorders, 29*, 229–237.

Borgohain, R., Szasz, J., Stanzione, P., Meshram, C., Bhatt, M., Chirilineau, D., et al. (2014b). Two-year, randomized, controlled study of safinamide as add-on to levodopa in mid to late Parkinson's disease. *Movement Disorders, 29*, 1273–1280.

Borgulya, J., Bruderer, H., Bernauer, K., Zürcher, G., & Prada, M. D. (1989). Catechol-O-methyltransferase-inhibiting pyrocatechol derivatives: Synthesis and structure-activity studies. *Helvetica Chimica Acta, 72*, 952–968.

Bracco, F., Battaglia, A., Chouza, C., Dupont, E., Gershanik, O., Masso, J. F. M., et al. (2004). The long-acting dopamine receptor agonist cabergoline in early Parkinson's disease: Final results of a 5-year, double-blind, levodopa-controlled study. *CNS Drugs, 18*, 733–746.

Braham, J., Sarova-Pinhas, I., & Goldhammer, Y. (1970). Apomorphine in Parkinsonian tremor. *British Medical Journal, 3*, 768.

Butzer, J. F., Silver, D. E., & Sahs, A. L. (1975). Amantadine in Parkinson's disease. A double-blind, placebo-controlled, crossover study with long-term follow-up. *Neurology, 25*, 603–606.

Caccia, C., Maj, R., Calabresi, M., Maestroni, S., Faravelli, L., Curatolo, L., et al. (2006). Safinamide: From molecular targets to a new anti-Parkinson drug. *Neurology, 67*, S18–S23.

Callagham, N., Mcllroy, M., & O'Connor, M. (1974). Treatment of Parkinson's disease with levodopa and amantadine used as single drugs and in combined therapy. *Irish Journal of Medical Science, 143*, 67–78.

Calne, D. B., Reid, J. L., Vakil, S. D., Rao, S., Petrie, A., Pallis, C. A., et al. (1971). Idiopathic Parkinsonism treated with an extracerebral decarboxylase inhibitor in combination with levodopa. *British Medical Journal, 3*, 729–732.

Calne, D. B., Teychenne, P. F., Claveria, L. E., Eastman, R., Greenacre, J. K., & Petrie, A. (1974). Bromocriptine in Parkinsonism. *British Medical Journal, 4*, 442–444.

Caraco, Y., Oren, S., & LeWitt, P. (2013). Constant therapeutic levodopa (LD) plasma concentrations maintained by continuous subcutaneous (SC) administration of ND-0612, a novel formulation of LD/carbidopa (CD). *Movement Disorders, 28*, S162.

Carlsson, A., Lindqvist, M., & Magnusson, T. (1957). 3,4-Dihydroxyphenylalanine and 5-hydroxytryptophan as reserpine antagonists. *Nature, 180*, 1200.

Carlsson, A., Lindqvist, M., Magnusson, T., & Waldeck, B. (1958). On the presence of 3-hydroxytyramine in brain. *Science, 127*, 471.

Cedarbaum, J. M., Breck, L., Kutt, H., & McDowell, F. H. (1987). Controlled-release levodopa/carbidopa: I. Sinemet CR3 treatment of response fluctuations in Parkinson's disease. *Neurology, 37*, 233–241.

Cedarbaum, J. M., Hoey, M., Kutt, H., & McDowell, F. H. (1988). Controlled-release levodopa/carbidopa III: Sinemet CR5 treatment of response fluctuations in Parkinson's disease. *Clinical Neuropharmacology, 11*, 168–173.

Cedarbaum, J. M., Silvestri, M., & Kutt, H. (1990). Sustained enteral administration of levodopa increases and interrupted infusion decreases levodopa dose requirement. *Neurology, 40*, 995–997.

Chaudhuri, K. R. (2008). Crystallisation within transdermal rotigotine patch: Is there cause for concern? *Expert Opinion on Drug Delivery, 5*, 1169–1171.

Chaudhuri, K. R., Critchley, P., Abbott, R. J., Pye, I. F., & Millac, P. A. (1988). Subcutaneous apomorphine for on-off oscillations in Parkinson's disease. *Lancet, 2*(8622), 1260.

Chaudhuri, K. R., Qamar, M. A., Rajah, T., Loehrer, P., Sauerbier, A., Odin, P., et al. (2016). Non-oral dopaminergic therapies for Parkinson's disease: Current treatments and the future. *NPJ Parkinson's Disease, 2*, 16023.

Chaudhuri, K. R., Rizos, A., & Sethi, K. D. (2013). Motor and nonmotor complications in Parkinson's disease: An argument for continuous drug delivery? *Journal of Neural Transmission, 120*, 1305–1320.

Chouza, C., Aljanati, R., Caamaño, J. L., De Medina, O., Scaramelli, A., Buzó, R., et al. (1990). Long-term treatment with Madopar HBS in parkinsonians with fluctuations. *Advances in Neurology, 53*, 519–526.

Corbin, K. B. (1949). Trihexyphenidyl: Evaluation of the new agent in the treatment of parkinsonism. *Journal of the American Medical Association, 141*, 377–382.

Corrodi, H., Fuxe, K., Hökfelt, T., Lidbrink, P., & Ungerstedt, U. (1973). Effect of ergot drugs on central catecholamine neurons: Evidence for a stimulation of central dopamine neurons. *Journal of Pharmacy and Pharmacology, 25*, 409–412.

Corsini, G. U., Del Zompo, M., Gessa, G. L., & Mangoni, A. (1979). Therapeutic efficacy of apomorphine combined with an extracerebral inhibitor of dopamine receptors in Parkinson's disease. *The Lancet, 1*, 954–956.

Cotzias, G. C., & Papavasiliou, P. S. (1971). Blocking the negative effects of pyridoxine on patients receiving levodopa. *JAMA, 215*, 1504–1505.

Cotzias, G. C., Papavasiliou, P. S., Fehling, C., Kaufman, B., & Mena, I. (1970). Similarities between neurologic effects of L-dopa and of apomorphine. *The New England Journal of Medicine, 282*, 31–33.

Cotzias, G. C., Papavasiliou, P. S., & Gellene, R. (1969). Modification of Parkinsonism—Chronic treatment with L-dopa. *The New England Journal of Medicine, 280*, 337–345.

Cotzias, G. C., Papavasiliou, P. S., Tolosa, E. S., Mendez, J. S., & Bell-Midura, M. (1976). Treatment of Parkinson's disease with aporphines. *The New England Journal of Medicine, 294*, 567–572.

Cotzias, G. C., Van Woert, M. H., & Schiffer, L. M. (1967). Aromatic amino acids and modification of Parkinsonism. *The New England Journal of Medicine, 276*, 374–379.

Cox, B., Danta, G., Schnieden, H., & Yuill, G. M. (1973). Interactions of L-dopa and amantadine in patients with Parkinsonism. *Journal of Neurology, Neurosurgery, and Psychiatry, 36*, 354–361.

Coyle, J. T., & Snyder, S. H. (1969). Antiparkinsonian drugs: Inhibition of dopamine uptake in the corpus striatum as a possible mechanism of action. *Science, 166*, 899–901.

Crevoisier, C., Hoevels, B., Zürcher, G., & Da Prada, M. (1987). Bioavailability of L-dopa after Madopar HBS administration in healthy volunteers. *European Neurology, 27*(Suppl. 1), 36–46.

Cunnington, A. L., White, L., & Hood, K. (2012). Identification of possible risk factors for the development of dopamine agonist withdrawal syndrome in Parkinson's disease. *Parkinsonism & Related Disorders, 18*, 1051–1052.

Dallos, V., Heathfield, K., Stone, P., & Allen, F. A. D. (1970). Use of amantadine in Parkinson's disease. Results of a double-blind trial. *British Medical Journal, 4*, 24–26.

Davies, W. L., Grunert, R. R., Haff, R. F., Mcgahen, J. W., Neumayer, E. M., Paulshock, M., et al. (1964). Antiviral acitivity of 1-adamantanamine (amantadine). *Science, 144*, 862–863.
Davis, T. L., Roznoski, M., & Burns, R. S. (1995). Effects of tolcapone in Parkinson's patients taking L-dihydroxyphenylalanine/carbidopa and selegiline. *Movement Disorders, 10*, 349–351.
de la Fuente-Fernández, R., Sossi, V., Huang, Z., Furtado, S., Lu, J.-Q., Calne, D. B., et al. (2004). Levodopa-induced changes in synaptic dopamine levels increase with progression of Parkinson's disease: Implications for dyskinesias. *Brain, 127*, 2747–2754.
Debono, A. G., Marsden, C. D., Asselman, P., & Parkes, J. D. (1976). Bromocriptine and dopamine receptor stimulation. *British Journal of Clinical Pharmacology, 3*, 977–982.
Dewey, R. B., Hutton, J., LeWitt, P. A., & Factor, S. A. (2001). A randomized, double-blind, placebo-controlled trial of subcutaneously injected apomorphine for parkinsonian off-state events. *Archives of Neurology, 58*, 1385–1392.
Dewey, R. B., Reimold, S. C., & O'Suilleabhain, P. E. (2007). Cardiac valve regurgitation with pergolide compared with nonergot agonists in Parkinson disease. *Archives of Neurology, 64*, 377–380.
Doshay, L. J., & Constable, K. (1949). Artane® therapy for parkinsonism: A preliminary study of results in one hundred and seventeen cases. *Journal of the American Medical Association, 140*, 1317–1322.
Düby, S. E., Cotzias, G. C., Papavasiliou, P. S., & Lawrence, W. H. (1972). Injected apomorphine and orally administered levodopa in parkinsonism. *Archives of Neurology, 27*, 474–480.
Dupont, E., Andersen, A., Boas, J., Boisen, E., Borgmann, R., Helgetveit, A. C., et al. (1996). Sustained-release Madopar HBS® compared with standard Madopar® in the long-term treatment of de novo parkinsonian patients. *Acta Neurologica Scandinavica, 93*, 14–20.
Duvoisin, R. C. (1965). A review of drug therapy in parkinsonism. *Bulletin of the New York Academy of Medicine, 41*, 898–910.
Duvoisin, R. C. (1967). Cholinergic-anticholinergic antagonism in parkinsonism. *Archives of Neurology, 17*, 124–136.
Duvoisin, R. C. (1974). Hyperkinetic reactions with L-DOPA. In M. D. Yahr (Ed.), *Current concepts in the treatment of Parkinsonism* (pp. 203–210). New York: Raven Press.
Ehringer, H., & Hornykiewicz, O. (1960). Distribution of noradrenaline and dopamine (3-hydroxytyramine) in the human brain and their behavior in diseases of the extrapyramidal system. *Klinische Wochenschrift, 38*, 1236–1239.
Ehringer, H., & Hornykiewicz, O. (1998). Distribution of noradrenaline and dopamine (3-hydroxytyramine) in the human brain and their behavior in diseases of the extrapyramidal system1. *Parkinsonism & Related Disorders, 4*, 53–57.
Elshoff, J.-P., Braun, M., Andreas, J.-O., Middle, M., & Cawello, W. (2012). Steady-state plasma concentration profile of transdermal rotigotine: An integrated analysis of three, open-Label, randomized, phase I multiple dose studies. *Clinical Therapeutics, 34*, 966–978.
Elshoff, J.-P., Timmermann, L., Schmid, M., Arth, C., Komenda, M., Brunnert, M., et al. (2013). Comparison of the bioavailability and adhesiveness of different rotigotine transdermal patch formulations. *Current Medical Research and Opinion, 29*, 1657–1662.
Erb, W. H. (1887). Uber Hyoscin. About hyoscine *Therapeutische Monatshefte, 1*, 252–254.
Ericsson, A. D. (1971). Potentiation of the L-dopa effect in man by the use of catechol-O-methyltransferase inhibitors. *Journal of the Neurological Sciences, 14*, 193–197.
Ernst, A. M. (1965). Relation between the action of dopamine and apomorphine and their O-methylated derivatives upon the CNS. *Psychopharmacologia, 7*, 391–399.
Ernst, A. M. (1967). Mode of action of apomorphine and dexamphetamine on gnawing compulsion in rats. *Psychopharmacologia, 10*, 316–323.

Factor, S. A., Molho, E. S., Podskalny, G. D., & Brown, D. (1995). Parkinson's disease: Drug-induced psychiatric states. *Advances in Neurology, 65*, 115–138.

Fahn, S. (1974). "On-off" phenomenon with levodopa therapy in parkinsonism: Clinical and pharmacologic correlations and the effect of intramuscular pyridoxine. *Neurology, 24*, 431–441.

Fahn, S. (2008). The history of dopamine and levodopa in the treatment of Parkinson's disease. *Movement Disorders, 23*, S497–S508.

Fahn, S. (2015). The medical treatment of Parkinson disease from James Parkinson to George Cotzias. *Movement Disorders, 30*, 4–18.

Fahn, S., Cote, L. J., Snider, S. R., Barrett, R. E., & Isgreen, W. P. (1979). The role of bromocriptine in the treatment of parkinsonism. *Neurology, 29*, 1077–1083.

Fahn, S., & Isgreen, W. P. (1975). Long-term evaluation of amantadine and levodopa combination in parkinsonism by double-blind corssover analyses. *Neurology, 25*, 695–700.

Fehling, C. (1966). Treatment of Parkinson's syndrome with L-dopa. A double blind study. *Acta Neurologica Scandinavica, 42*, 367–372.

Fehling, C. (1973). The effect of adding amantadine to optimum L-dopa dosage in Parkinson's syndrome. *Acta Neurologica Scandinavica, 49*, 245–251.

Feldberg, W. (1945). Present views on the mode of action of acetylcholine in the central nervous system. *Physiological Reviews, 25*, 596–642.

Fernandez, H. H., Vanagunas, A., Odin, P., Espay, A. J., Hauser, R. A., Standaert, D. G., et al. (2013). Levodopa–carbidopa intestinal gel in advanced Parkinson's disease open-label study: Interim results. *Parkinsonism & Related Disorders, 19*, 339–345.

Finberg, J. P. M., Lamensdorf, I., Commissiong, J. W., & Youdim, M. B. H. (1996). Pharmacology and neuroprotective properties of rasagiline. In W. Kuhn, P. Kraus, & H. Przuntek (Eds.), *Deprenyl—Past and future: Journal of Neural Transmission Supplement 48* (pp. 95–101). Vienna: Springer Vienna.

Forssman, B., Kihlstrand, S., & Larsson, L. E. (1972). Amantadine therapy in parkinsonism. *Acta Neurologica Scandinavica, 48*, 1–18.

Fox, S. H., Katzenschlager, R., Lim, S.-Y., Ravina, B., Seppi, K., Coelho, M., et al. (2011). The movement disorder society evidence-based medicine review update: Treatments for the motor symptoms of Parkinson's disease. *Movement Disorders, 26*, S2–S41.

Frucht, S., Rogers, J. D., Greene, P. E., Gordon, M. F., & Fahn, S. (1999). Falling asleep at the wheel: Motor vehicle mishaps in persons taking pramipexole and ropinirole. *Neurology, 52*, 1908–1910.

Funk, C. (1911). LXV.—Synthesis of dl–3: 4-dihydroxyphenylalanine. *Journal of the Chemical Society, Transactions, 99*, 554–557.

Fuxe, K., & Hökfelt, T. (1970). Central monoaminergic systems and hypothalamic function. In T. L. Martini, M. Motta, & F. Fraschini (Eds.), *The hypothalamus* (pp. 123–138). New York: Academic Press.

Garcia-Ruiz, P. J., Martinez Castrillo, J. C., Alonso-Canovas, A., Herranz Barcenas, A., Vela, L., Sanchez Alonso, P., et al. (2014). Impulse control disorder in patients with Parkinson's disease under dopamine agonist therapy: A multicentre study. *Journal of Neurology, Neurosurgery & Psychiatry, 85*, 840–844.

Gerstenbrand, F., Pateisky, K., & Prosenz, P. (1963). Erfahrungen mit L-dopa in der therapie des parkinsonismus. Experiences with L-dopa in the therapy of parkinsonism *Psychiatria et Neurologia, 146*, 246–261.

Giladi, N., Boroojerdi, B., Korczyn, A. D., Burn, D. J., Clarke, C. E., & Schapira, A. H. V. (2007). Rotigotine transdermal patch in early Parkinson's disease: A randomized, double-blind, controlled study versus placebo and ropinirole. *Movement Disorders, 22*, 2398–2404.

Giladi, N., Caraco, Y., Gureritch, T., Djaldetti, R., Cohen, Y., Yacobi-Zeevi, O., et al. (2015). Pharmacokinetics and safety of ND0612L (levodopa/carbidopa for subcutaneous infusion): Results from a phase II study in moderate to severe Parkinson's disease. *Neurology*, *84*, P1.187.

Giladi, N., Treves, A. T., Simon, S. E., Shabtai, H., Orlov, Y., Kandinov, B., et al. (2001). Freezing of gait in patients with advanced Parkinson's disease. *Journal of Neural Transmission*, *108*, 53–61.

Goetz, C. G., & Diederich, N. J. (1992). Dopaminergic agonists in the treatment of Parkinson's disease. *Neurologic Clinics*, *10*, 527–540.

Goetz, C. G., Tanner, C. M., Klawans, H. L., Shannon, K. M., & Carroll, V. S. (1987). Parkinson's disease and motor fluctuations: Long-acting carbidopa/levodopa (CR-4-Sinemet). *Neurology*, *37*, 875–878.

Goetz, C. G., Tanner, C. M., Shannon, K. M., Carroll, V. S., Klawans, H. L., Carvey, P. M., et al. (1988). Controlled-release carbidopa/levodopa (CR4-Sinemet) in Parkinson's disease patients with and without motor fluctuations. *Neurology*, *38*, 1143–1146.

Golbe, L. I., Lieberman, A. N., Muenter, M. D., Ahlskog, J. E., Gopinathan, G., Neophytides, A. N., et al. (1988). Deprenyl in the treatment of symptom fluctuations in advanced Parkinson's disease. *Clinical Neuropharmacology*, *11*, 45–55.

Goldstein, M., Lieberman, A., Lew, J. Y., Asano, T., Rosenfeld, M. R., & Makman, M. H. (1980). Interaction of pergolide with central dopaminergic receptors. *Proceedings of the National Academy of Sciences of the United States of America*, *77*, 3725–3728.

Gottwald, M. D., & Aminoff, M. J. (2011). Therapies for dopaminergic-induced dyskinesias in Parkinson disease. *Annals of Neurology*, *69*, 919–927.

Gowers, W. R. (1893). *A manual of diseases of the nervous system: Vol. II* (2nd ed.). Philadelphia, PA: Blakiston.

Grosset, D., Antonini, A., Canesi, M., Pezzoli, G., Lees, A., Shaw, K., et al. (2009). Adherence to antiparkinson medication in a multicenter European study. *Movement Disorders*, *24*, 826–832.

Grosset, K. A., Malek, N., Morgan, F., & Grosset, D. G. (2013a). Inhaled apomorphine in patients with 'on-off' fluctuations: A randomized, double-blind, placebo-controlled, clinic and home based, parallel-group study. *Journal of Parkinson's Disease*, *3*, 31–37.

Grosset, K. A., Malek, N., Morgan, F., & Grosset, D. G. (2013b). Inhaled dry powder apomorphine (VR040) for 'off' periods in Parkinson's disease: An in-clinic double-blind dose ranging study. *Acta Neurologica Scandinavica*, *128*, 166–171.

Guggenheim, M. (1913). Dioxyphenylalanin, eine neue Aminosäure aus Vicia faba. *Hoppe-Seyler's Zeitschrift für physiologische Chemie*, *88*, 276–284.

Haglund, L., & Hoogkamer, J. F. W. (1995). Madopar® dispensible: Pharmacokinetics and bioavailability in healthy volunteers. *Journal of Neurology*, *242*, S140.

Hardie, R. J., Lees, A. J., & Stern, G. M. (1984). On-off fluctuations in Parkinson's disease. A clinical and neuropharmacological study. *Brain*, *107*, 487–506.

Hardie, R. J., Malcolm, S. L., Lees, A. J., Stern, G. M., & Allen, J. G. (1986). The pharmacokinetics of intravenous and oral levodopa in patients with Parkinson's disease who exhibit on-off fluctuations. *British Journal of Clinical Pharmacology*, *22*, 429–436.

Hauser, R. A. (2004). Levodopa/carbidopa/entacapone (Stalevo). *Neurology*, *62*, S64–S71.

Hauser, R. A. (2011). Future treatments for Parkinson's disease: Surfing the PD pipeline. *International Journal of Neuroscience*, *121*, 53–62.

Hauser, R. A., Ellenbogen, A. L., Metman, L. V., Hsu, A., O'Connell, M. J., Modi, N. B., et al. (2011). Crossover comparison of IPX066 and a standard levodopa formulation in advanced Parkinson's disease. *Movement Disorders*, *26*, 2246–2252.

Hauser, R. A., Hsu, A., Kell, S., Espay, A. J., Sethi, K., Stacy, M., et al. (2013). Extended-release carbidopa-levodopa (IPX066) compared with immediate-release carbidopa-levodopa in patients with Parkinson's disease and motor fluctuations: A phase 3 randomised, double-blind trial. *The Lancet. Neurology*, *12*, 346–356.

Hauser, R. A., Olanow, C. W., Dzyngel, B., Bilbault, T., Shill, H., Isaacson, S., et al. (2016). Sublingual apomorphine (APL-130277) for the acute conversion of OFF to ON in Parkinson's disease. *Movement Disorders*, *31*, 1366–1372.
Hauser, R. A., Rascol, O., Korczyn, A. D., Jon Stoessl, A., Watts, R. L., Poewe, W., et al. (2007). Ten-year follow-up of Parkinson's disease patients randomized to initial therapy with ropinirole or levodopa. *Movement Disorders*, *22*, 2409–2417.
Hauser, R. A., Schapira, A. H. V., Rascol, O., Barone, P., Mizuno, Y., Salin, L., et al. (2010). Randomized, double-blind, multicenter evaluation of pramipexole extended release once daily in early Parkinson's disease. *Movement Disorders*, *25*, 2542–2549.
Hely, M. A., Morris, J. G., Reid, W. G., O'Sullivan, D. J., Williamson, P. M., Rail, D., et al. (1994). The Sydney Multicentre Study of Parkinson's disease: A randomised, prospective five year study comparing low dose bromocriptine with low dose levodopa-carbidopa. *Journal of Neurology, Neurosurgery & Psychiatry*, *57*, 903–910.
Hoehn, M. M., & Elton, R. L. (1985). Low dosages of bromocriptine added to levodopa in Parkinson's disease. *Neurology*, *35*, 199–206.
Holloway, R. G., Shoulson, I., Fahn, S., Kieburtz, K., Lang, A., Marek, K., et al. (2004). Pramipexole vs levodopa as initial treatment for Parkinson disease: A 4-year randomized controlled trial. *Archives of Neurology*, *61*, 1044–1053.
Holtz, P., Balzer, H., Westermann, E., & Wezler, E. (1957). Beeinflussung der Evipannarkose durch Reserpin, Iproniazid und biogene Amine. *Naunyn-Schmiedeberg's Archives of Pharmacology*, *231*, 333–348.
Holzer, G., & Hornykiewicz, O. (1959). On dopamine (hydroxytyramine) metabolism in the rat brain. *Naunyn-Schmiedebergs Archiv für Experimentelle Pathologie und Pharmakologie*, *237*, 27–33.
Hornykiewicz, O. (1958). The action of dopamine on the arterial blood pressure of the guinea-pig. *British Journal of Pharmacology and Chemotherapy*, *13*, 91–94.
Hornykiewicz, O. (1963). The tropical localization and content of noradrenalin and dopamine (3-hydroxytyramine) in the substantia nigra of normal persons and patients with Parkinson's disease. *Wiener Klinische Wochenschrift*, *75*, 309–312.
Hornykiewicz, O. (2002). L-DOPA: From a biologically inactive amino acid to a successful therapeutic agent. *Amino Acids*, *23*, 65–70.
Hubsher, G., Haider, M., & Okun, M. S. (2012). Amantadine: The journey from fighting flu to treating Parkinson disease. *Neurology*, *78*, 1096–1099.
Hughes, A. J., Bishop, S., Lees, A. J., Stern, G. M., Webster, R., & Bovingdon, M. (1991). Rectal apomorphine in Parkinson's disease. *The Lancet*, *337*, 118.
Hunter, K. R., Stern, G. M., Laurence, D. R., & Armitage, P. (1970). Amantadine in parkinsonism. *The Lancet*, *1*, 1127–1129.
Jackson, G. G., Muldoon, R. L., & Akers, L. W. (1963). Serological evidence for prevention of influenzal infection in volunteers by an anti-influenzal drug adamantanamine hydrochloride. *Antimicrobial Agents and Chemotherapy*, *161*, 703–707.
Jankovic, J., Watts, R. L., Martin, W., Boroojerdi, B., & The SP 512 Rotigotine Transdermal System Clinical Study Group. (2007). Transdermal rotigotine: Double-blind, placebo-controlled trial in Parkinson disease. *Archives of Neurology*, *64*, 676–682.
Jenner, P., Könen-Bergmann, M., Schepers, C., & Haertter, S. (2009). Pharmacokinetics of a once-daily extended-release formulation of pramipexole in healthy male volunteers: Three studies. *Clinical Therapeutics*, *31*, 2698–2711.
Jensen, N. O., Dupont, E., Hansen, E., Mikkelsen, B., & Mikkelsen, B. O. (1987). Madopar HBS: Slow-release levodopa and benserazide in Parkinsonian patients presenting marked fluctuations in symptoms on standard L-dopa treatment. *European Neurology*, *27*(Suppl. 1), 68–72.

Jori, M. C., Franceschi, M., Giusti, M. C., Canal, N., Piolti, R., Frattola, L., et al. (1990). Clinical experience with cabergoline, a new ergoline derivative, in the treatment of Parkinson's disease. *Advances in Neurology*, *53*, 539–543.

Juncos, J. L., Fabbrini, G. G., Mouradian, M. M., & Chase, T. N. (1987a). Controlled release levodopa-carbidopa (CR-5) in the management of parkinsonian motor fluctuations. *Archives of Neurology*, *44*, 1010–1012.

Juncos, J. L., Fabbrini, G., Mouradian, M. M., Serrati, C., Kask, A. M., & Chase, T. N. (1987b). Controlled release levodopa treatment of motor fluctuations in Parkinson's disease. *Journal of Neurology, Neurosurgery & Psychiatry*, *50*, 194–198.

Kaakkola, S., Gordin, A., & Männistö, P. T. (1994). General properties and clinical possibilities of new selective inhibitors of catechol O-methyltransferase. *General Pharmacology: The Vascular System*, *25*, 813–824.

Kaakkola, S., Teräväinen, H., Ahtila, S., Rita, H., & Gordin, A. (1994). Effect of entacapone, a COMT inhibitor, on clinical disability and levodopa metabolism in parkinsonian patients. *Neurology*, *44*, 77–80.

Kartzinel, R., Teychenne, P., Gillespie, M. M., Perlow, M., Gielen, A. C., Sadowsky, D. A., et al. (1976). Bromocriptine and levodopa (with or without carbidopa) in parkinsonism. *The Lancet*, *308*, 272–275.

Kim, Y. E., Yun, J. Y., Yang, H. J., Kim, H. J., Gu, N., Yoon, S. H., et al. (2012). Intravenous amantadine for freezing of gait resistant to dopaminergic therapy: A randomized, double-blind, placebo-controlled, cross-over clinical trial. *PloS One*, *7*, e48890.

Kleedorfer, B., & Poewe, W. (1992). Comparative efficacy of two oral sustained-release preparations of L-dopa in fluctuating Parkinson's disease. Preliminary findings in 20 patients. *Journal of Neural Transmission. Parkinson's Disease and Dementia Section*, *4*, 173–178.

Knoll, J. (1976). Analysis of the pharmacological effects of selective monoamine oxidase inhibitors. In M. L. C. Bernheim (Ed.), *Ciba Foundation Symposium 39—Monoamine oxidase and its inhibition* (pp. 135–161). Chichester, UK: John Wiley & Sons, Ltd.

Knoll, J., Ecseri, Z., Kelemen, K., Nievel, J., & Knoll, B. (1965). Phenylisopropylmethylpropinylamine (E-250), a new spectrum psychic energizer. *Archives Internationales de Pharmacodynamie et de Thérapie*, *155*, 154–164.

Knoll, J., & Magyar, K. (1972). Some puzzling pharmacological effects of monoamine oxidase inhibitors. *Advances in Biochemical Psychopharmacology*, *5*, 393–408.

Knoll, J., Vizi, E. S., & Somogyi, G. (1968). Phenylisopropylmethylpropynylamine (E-250), a monoamine oxidase inhibitor antagonising the effects of tyramine. *Arzneimittel-Forschung*, *18*, 109–112.

Koller, W., Hutton, J. T., Tolosa, E., Capilldeo, R., & The Carbidopa/Levodopa Study Group. (1999). Immediate-release and controlled-release carbidopa/levodopa in PD: A 5-year randomized multicenter study. *Neurology*, *53*, 1012–1019.

Koller, W., & Stacy, M. (2004). Other formulations and future considerations for apomorphine for subcutaneous injection therapy. *Neurology*, *62*, S22–S26.

Korner, Y., Meindorfner, C., Moller, J. C., Stiasny-Kolster, K., Haja, D., Cassel, W., et al. (2004). Predictors of sudden onset of sleep in Parkinson's disease. *Movement Disorders*, *19*, 1298–1305.

Kornhuber, J., Quack, G., Danysz, W., Jellinger, K., Danielczyk, W., Gsell, W., et al. (1995). Therapeutic brain concentration of the NMDA receptor antagonist amantadine. *Neuropharmacology*, *34*, 3–21.

Kurlan, R., Rubin, A., Miller, C., Rivera-Calimlim, L., Clarke, A., & Shoulson, I. (1986). Duodenal delivery of levodopa for on-off fluctuations in parkinsonism: Preliminary observations. *Annals of Neurology*, *20*, 262–265.

Kurth, M. C., Adler, C. H., St. Hilaire, M., Singer, C., Waters, C., LeWitt, P., et al. (1997). Tolcapone improves motor function and reduces levodopa requirement in patients with Parkinson's disease experiencing motor fluctuations: A multicenter, double-blind, randomized, placebo-controlled trial. Tolcapone fluctuator study group I. *Neurology*, *48*, 81–87.

Kurth, M. C., Tetrud, J. W., Tanner, C. M., Irwin, I., Stebbins, G. T., Goetz, C. G., et al. (1993). Double-blind, placebo-controlled, crossover study of duodenal infusion of levodopa/carbidopa in Parkinson's disease patients with 'on-off' fluctuations. *Neurology*, *43*, 1698–1703.

Lang, A. E., & Blair, R. D. G. (1989). Anitcholinergic drugs and amantadine in the treatment of Parkinson´s disease. In D. Calne (Ed.), *Handbook of experimental pharmacology: 88.* (pp. 307–323). Berlin Heidelberg: Springer-Verlag.

Lee, J. Y., Kim, H. J., & Jeon, B. S. (2011). Is pathological gambling in Parkinson's disease reduced by amantadine? *Annals of Neurology*, *69*, 213–214; author reply 214–215.

Lee, J. Y., Oh, S., Kim, J. M., Kim, J. S., Oh, E., Kim, H. T., et al. (2013). Intravenous amantadine on freezing of gait in Parkinson's disease: A randomized controlled trial. *Journal of Neurology, Neurosurgery & Psychiatry*, *260*, 3030–3038.

Lees, A. J. (1987). A sustained-release formulation of L-dopa (Madopar HBS) in the treatment of nocturnal and early-morning disabilities in Parkinson's disease. *European Neurology*, *27*(Suppl. 1), 126–134.

Lees, A. J. (1989). The on-off phenomenon. *Journal of Neurology, Neurosurgery & Psychiatry*, *52*, 29–37.

LeWitt, P. A., Ellenbogen, A., Chen, D., Lal, R., McGuire, K., Zomorodi, K., et al. (2012). Actively transported levodopa prodrug XP21279: A study in patients with Parkinson disease who experience motor fluctuations. *Clinical Neuropharmacology*, *35*, 103–110.

LeWitt, P. A., Giladi, N., Gurevich, T., Shabtai, H., Djaldetti, R., Roizen, N., et al. (2012). Accordion pill carbidopa/levodopa (AP CD/LD) for treatment of advanced PD. *Movement Disorders*, *27*, S248.

LeWitt, P. A., Hauser, R. A., Grosset, D. G., Stocchi, F., Saint-Hilaire, M.-H., Ellenbogen, A., et al. (2016). A randomized trial of inhaled levodopa (CVT-301) for motor fluctuations in Parkinson's disease. *Movement Disorders*, *31*, 1356–1365.

LeWitt, P. A., Huff, F. J., Hauser, R. A., Chen, D., Lissin, D., Zomorodi, K., et al. (2014). Double-blind study of the actively transported levodopa prodrug XP21279 in Parkinson's disease. *Movement Disorders*, *29*, 75–82.

LeWitt, P. A., Lyons, K. E., Pahwa, R., & SP 650 Study Group. (2007). Advanced Parkinson disease treated with rotigotine transdermal system: PREFER Study. *Neurology*, *68*, 1262–1267.

LeWitt, P. A., Ward, C. D., Larsen, T. A., Raphaelson, M. I., Newman, R. P., Foster, N., et al. (1983). Comparison of pergolide and bromocriptine therapy in parkinsonism. *Neurology*, *33*, 1009–1014.

Lieberman, A., Goldstein, M., Leibowitz, M., Neophytides, A., Kupersmith, M., Pact, V., et al. (1981). Treatment of advanced Parkinson disease with pergolide. *Neurology*, *31*, 675–682.

Lieberman, A., Goodgold, A., Jonas, S., & Leibowitz, M. (1975). Comparison of dopa decarboxylase inhibitor (carbidopa) combined with levodopa and levodopa alone in Parkinson's disease. *Neurology*, *25*, 911.

Lieberman, A. N., Gopinathan, G., Neophytides, A., Hiesiger, E., Nelson, J., Walker, R., et al. (1984). Deprenyl in the treatment of Parkinson's disease. A specific type B monoamine oxidase inhibitor. *The New York State Journal of Medicine*, *84*, 13–16.

Lieberman, A., Kupersmith, M., Estey, E., & Goldstein, M. (1976). Treatment of Parkinson's disease with bromocriptine. *The New England Journal of Medicine*, *295*, 1400–1404.

Limousin, P., Pollak, P., Gervason-Tournier, C. L., Hommel, M., & Perret, J. (1993). Ro 40-7592, a COMT inhibitor, plus levodopa in Parkinson's disease. *The Lancet*, *341*, 1605.

Luginger, E., Wenning, G. K., Bösch, S., & Poewe, W. (2000). Beneficial effects of amantadine on L-dopa-induced dyskinesias in Parkinson's disease. *Movement Disorders, 15*, 873–878.

Luinstra, M., Rutgers, A. W. F., Dijkstra, H., Grasmeijer, F., Hagedoorn, P., Vogelzang, J. M. J., et al. (2015). Can patients with Parkinson's disease use dry powder inhalers during Off periods? *PloS One, 10*, e0132714

Macht, M., Kaussner, Y., Möller, J. C., Stiasny-Kolster, K., Eggert, K. M., Krüger, H.-P., et al. (2007). Predictors of freezing in Parkinson's disease: A survey of 6,620 patients. *Movement Disorders, 22*, 953–956.

Malcolm, S. L., Allen, J. G., Bird, H., Quinn, N. P., Marion, M. H., Marsden, C. D., et al. (1987). Single-dose pharmacokinetics of Madopar HBS in patients and effect of food and antacid on the absorption of Madopar HBS in volunteers. *European Neurology, 27*(Suppl. 1), 28–35.

Malkani, R., Zadikoff, C., Melen, O., Videnovic, A., Borushko, E., & Simuni, T. (2012). Amantadine for freezing of gait in patients with Parkinson disease. *Clinical Neuropharmacology, 35*, 266–268.

Manni, R., Terzaghi, M., Sartori, I., Mancini, F., & Pacchetti, C. (2004). Dopamine agonists and sleepiness in PD: Review of the literature and personal findings. *Sleep Medicine, 5*, 189–193.

Manson, A. J., Hanagasi, H., Turner, K., Patsalos, P. N., Carey, P., Ratnaraj, N., et al. (2001). Intravenous apomorphine therapy in Parkinson's disease. *Brain, 124*, 331–340.

Marinesco, G., & Bourguignon, G. (1927). Variations de la chronaxie et de l'attitude des membres sous l'influence de la scopolamine et de l'ésérine etc. *Comptes Rendus des Seances de la Societe de Biologie et de Ses Filiales, 97*, 207.

Marion, M. H., Stocchi, F., Quinn, N. P., Jenner, P., & Marsden, C. D. (1986). Repeated levodopa infusions in fluctuating Parkinson's disease: Clinical and pharmacokinetic data. *Clinical Neuropharmacology, 9*, 165–181.

Markham, C. H., Diamond, S. G., & Treciokas, L. J. (1974). Carbidopa in Parkinson disease and in nausea and vomiting of levodopa. *Archives of Neurology, 31*, 128–133.

Marsden, C. D., Barry, P. E., Parkes, J. D., & Zilkha, K. J. (1973). Treatment of Parkinson's disease with levodopa combined with L-alpha-methyldopahydrazine, an inhibitor of extracerebral DOPA decarboxylase. *Journal of Neurology, Neurosurgery & Psychiatry, 36*, 10–14.

Marsden, C. D., & Parkes, J. D. (1976). "On-off" effects in patients with Parkinson's disease on chronic levodopa therapy. *The Lancet, 1*, 292–296.

Martin, W. E., Tolosa, E. S., Loewenson, R. B., Lee, M. C., Resch, J. A., & Baker, A. B. (1975). The effects of combining carbidopa with levodopa for Parkinson's disease. *Geriatrics, 30*, 39–44.

Matthiessen, A. (1868). Researches into the chemical constitution of the opium bases. Part I. On the action of hydrochloric acid on morphia. *Proceedings of the Royal Society of London, 17*, 455–460.

Maugh, T. H. (1979). Panel urges wide use of antiviral drug. *Science, 206*, 1058–1060.

Mawdsley, C., Williams, I. R., Pullar, I. A., Davidson, D. L., & Kinloch, N. E. (1972). Treatment of parkinsonism by amantadine and levodopa. *Clinical Pharmacology & Therapeutics, 13*, 575–583.

McDonald, R. J., & Horowski, R. (1983). Lisuride in the treatment of Parkinsonism. *European Neurology, 22*, 240–255.

McElvaney, N. G., Wilcox, P. G., Churg, A. A., & Fleetham, J. A. (1988). Pleuropulmonary disease during bromocriptine treatment of Parkinson's disease. *Archives of Internal Medicine, 148*, 2231–2236.

McGeer, P. L., Boulding, J. E., Gibson, W. C., & Foulkes, R. G. (1961). Drug-induced extrapyramidal reactions: Treatment with diphenhydramine hydrochloride and dihydroxyphenylalanine. *JAMA, 177*, 665–670.

McGeer, P. L., & Zeldowicz, L. R. (1964). Administration of dihydroxyphenylalanine to Parkinsonian patients. *Canadian Medical Association Journal, 90*, 463–466.

Mendel, E. (1893). Uber Duboisin. About duboisine *Neurologisches Centralblatt, 12*, 89–93.

Merello, M., Lees, A. J., Webster, R., Bovingdon, M., & Gordin, A. (1994). Effect of entacapone, a peripherally acting catechol-O-methyltransferase inhibitor, on the motor response to acute treatment with levodopa in patients with Parkinson's disease. *Journal of Neurology, Neurosurgery & Psychiatry, 57*, 186–189.

Merello, M., Pikielny, R., Cammarota, A., & Leiguarda, R. (1997). Comparison of subcutaneous apomorphine versus dispersible madopar latency and effect duration in Parkinson's disease patients: A double-blind single-dose study. *Clinical Neuropharmacology, 20*, 165–167.

Metman, L. V., Del Dotto, P., LePoole, K., Konitsiotis, S., Fang, J., & Chase, T. N. (1999). Amantadine for levodopa-induced dyskinesias: A 1-year follow-up study. *Archives of Neurology, 56*, 1383–1386.

Metman, L. V., Del Dotto, P., van den Munckhof, P., Fang, J., Mouradian, M. M., & Chase, T. N. (1998). Amantadine as treatment for dyskinesias and motor fluctuations in Parkinson's disease. *Neurology, 50*, 1323–1326.

Milhorat, A. T. (1941). Studies in diseases of muscle: IX. Effect of quinine and prostigmine methyl sulfate on muscular rigidity in paralysis agitans. *Archives of Neurology & Psychiatry, 45*, 74–85.

Millac, P., Hasan, I., Espir, M. L., & Slyfield, D. G. (1970). Treatment of Parkinsonism with L-dopa and amantadine. *The Lancet, 2*, 720.

Miller, D. W., & Abercrombie, E. D. (1999). Role of high-affinity dopamine uptake and impulse activity in the appearance of extracellular dopamine in striatum after administration of exogenous L-DOPA: Studies in intact and 6-hydroxydopamine-treated rats. *Journal of Neurochemistry, 72*, 1516–1522.

Mizuno, Y., Kondo, T., & Narabayashi, H. (1995). Pergolide in the treatment of Parkinson's disease. *Neurology, 45*, S13–S21.

Montagu, K. A. (1957). Catechol compounds in rat tissues and in brains of different animals. *Nature, 180*, 244–245.

Montastruc, J. L., Brefel-Courbon, C., Senard, J. M., Bagheri, H., Ferreira, J., Rascol, O., et al. (2001). Sleep attacks and antiparkinsonian drugs: A pilot prospective pharmacoepidemiologic study. *Clinical Neuropharmacology, 24*, 181–183.

Montastruc, J. L., Rascol, O., Senard, J. M., & Rascol, A. (1994). A randomised controlled study comparing bromocriptine to which levodopa was later added, with levodopa alone in previously untreated patients with Parkinson's disease: A five year follow up. *Journal of Neurology, Neurosurgery, and Psychiatry, 57*, 1034–1038.

Nicholas, A. P., Borgohain, R., Chaná, P., Surmann, E., Thompson, E. L., Bauer, L., et al. (2014). A randomized study of rotigotine dose response on 'off' time in advanced Parkinson's disease. *Journal of Parkinson's Disease, 4*, 361–373.

Nilsson, D., Nyholm, D., & Aquilonius, S. M. (2001). Duodenal levodopa infusion in Parkinson's disease—Long-term experience. *Acta Neurologica Scandinavica, 104*, 343–348.

Nordera, G. P., Lorizio, A., Lion, P., Durisotti, C., D'Andrea, G., & Ferro-Milone, F. (1987). Treatment of parkinsonian conditions with a controlled-release form of levodopa—Preliminary study. *European Neurology, 27*(Suppl. 1), 76–80.

Nutt, J. G., & Woodward, W. R. (1986). Levodopa pharmacokinetics and pharmacodynamics in fluctuating parkinsonian patients. *Neurology, 36*, 739–744.

Nutt, J. G., Woodward, W. R., & Anderson, J. L. (1985). The effect of carbidopa on the pharmacokinetics of intravenously administered levodopa: The mechanism of action in the treatment of parkinsonism. *Annals of Neurology, 18*, 537–543.

Nutt, J. G., Woodward, W. R., & Carter, J. H. (1986). Clinical and biochemical studies with controlled-release levodopa/carbidopa. *Neurology*, *36*, 1206–1211.

Nutt, J. G., Woodward, W. R., Hammerstad, J. P., Carter, J. H., & Anderson, J. L. (1984). The on–off phenomenon in Parkinson's disease: Relation to levodopa absorption and transport. *The New England Journal of Medicine*, *310*, 483–488.

Nyholm, D., & Aquilonius, S. M. (2004). Levodopa infusion therapy in Parkinson disease: State of the art in 2004. *Clinical Neuropharmacology*, *27*, 245–256.

Nyholm, D., Askmark, H., Gomes-Trolin, C., Knutson, T., Lennernäs, H., Nyström, C., et al. (2003). Optimizing levodopa pharmacokinetics: Intestinal infusion versus oral sustained-release tablets. *Clinical Neuropharmacology*, *26*, 156–163.

Nyholm, D., Klangemo, K., & Johansson, A. (2012). Levodopa/carbidopa intestinal gel infusion long-term therapy in advanced Parkinson's disease. *European Journal of Neurology*, *19*, 1079–1085.

Nyholm, D., Lewander, T., Johansson, A., LeWitt, P. A., Lundqvist, C., & Aquilonius, S. M. (2008). Enteral levodopa/carbidopa infusion in advanced Parkinson disease: Long-term exposure. *Clinical Neuropharmacology*, *31*, 63–73.

Nyholm, D., Nilsson Remahl, A. I., Dizdar, N., Constantinescu, R., Holmberg, B., Jansson, R., et al. (2005). Duodenal levodopa infusion monotherapy vs oral polypharmacy in advanced Parkinson disease. *Neurology*, *64*, 216–223.

Oertel, W. H., Wolters, E., Sampaio, C., Gimenez-Roldan, S., Bergamasco, B., Dujardin, M., et al. (2006). Pergolide versus levodopa monotherapy in early Parkinson's disease patients: The PELMOPET study. *Movement Disorders*, *21*, 343–353.

Ogawa, N., Kanazawa, I., Kowa, H., Kuno, S., Mizuno, Y., Tashiro, K., et al. (1997). Nationwide multicenter prospective study on the long-term effects of bromocriptine for Parkinson's disease. *European Neurology*, *38*, 37–49.

Olanow, C. W. (2000). Tolcapone and hepatotoxic effects. Tasmar advisory panel. *Archives of Neurology*, *57*, 263–267.

Olanow, C. W., Fahn, S., Muenter, M., Klawans, H., Hurtig, H., Stern, M., et al. (1994). A multicenter double-blind placebo-controlled trial of pergolide as an adjunct to sinemet® in Parkinson's disease. *Movement Disorders*, *9*, 40–47.

Olanow, C. W., Kieburtz, K., Odin, P., Espay, A. J., Standaert, D. G., Fernandez, H. H., et al. (2014). Continuous intrajejunal infusion of levodopa-carbidopa intestinal gel for patients with advanced Parkinson's disease: A randomised, controlled, double-blind, double-dummy study. *The Lancet. Neurology*, *13*, 141–149.

Olanow, C. W., & Watkins, P. B. (2007). Tolcapone: An efficacy and safety review (2007). *Clinical Neuropharmacology*, *30*, 287–294.

Oppenheim, H. (1905). Zur Diagnose, Prognose und Therapie der Paralysis agitans. Toward the diagnosis, prognosis and treatment of paralysis agitans *DMW-Deutsche Medizinische Wochenschrift*, *31*, 1705–1710.

Ordenstein, L. (1868). *Sur la paralysie agitante et la sclérose en plaques généralisée.* On paralysis agitans and multiple sclerosis Paris: Delahaye.

Ory-Magne, F., Corvol, J. C., Azulay, J. P., Bonnet, A. M., Brefel-Courbon, C., Damier, P., et al. (2014). Withdrawing amantadine in dyskinetic patients with Parkinson disease: The AMANDYSK trial. *Neurology*, *82*, 300–307.

Ostergaard, L., Werdelin, L., Odin, P., Lindvall, O., Dupont, E., Christensen, P. B., et al. (1995). Pen injected apomorphine against off phenomena in late Parkinson's disease: A double blind, placebo controlled study. *Journal of Neurology, Neurosurgery & Psychiatry*, *58*, 681–687.

Pacchetti, C., Martignoni, E., Sibilla, L., Bruggi, P., Turla, M., & Nappi, G. (1990). Effectiveness of Madopar HBS plus Madopar standard in patients with fluctuating Parkinson's disease: Two years of follow-up. *European Neurology*, *30*, 319–323.

Pahwa, R., Factor, S. A., Lyons, K. E., Ondo, W. G., Gronseth, G., Bronte-Stewart, H., et al. (2006). Practice parameter: Treatment of Parkinson disease with motor fluctuations and dyskinesia (an evidence-based review) report of the Quality Standards Subcommittee of the American Academy of neurology. *Neurology, 66*, 983–995.

Pahwa, R., Stacy, M. A., Factor, S. A., Lyons, K. E., Stocchi, F., Hersh, B. P., et al. (2007). Ropinirole 24-hour prolonged release: Randomized, controlled study in advanced Parkinson disease. *Neurology, 68*, 1108–1115.

Papavasiliou, P. S., Cotzias, G. C., Düby, S. E., Stec, A. J., Fehling, C., & Bell, M. A. (1972). Levodopa in Parkinsonism: Potentiation of central effects with a peripheral inhibitor. *The New England Journal of Medicine, 286*, 8–14.

Pappert, E. J., Buhrfiend, C., Lipton, J. W., Carvey, P. M., Stebbins, G. T., & Goetz, C. G. (1996). Levodopa stability in solution: Time course, environmental effects, and practical recommendations for clinical use. *Movement Disorders, 11*, 24–26.

Parkes, J. D., Baxter, R. C., Curzon, G., Knill-Jones, R. P., Knott, P. J., Marsden, C. D., et al. (1971). Treatment of Parkinson's disease with amantadine and levodopa. A one-year study. *The Lancet, 1*, 1083–1086.

Parkes, J. D., Baxter, R. C., Marsden, C. D., & Rees, J. E. (1974). Comparative trial of benzhexol, amantadine, and levodopa in the treatment of Parkinson's disease. *Journal of Neurology, Neurosurgery, and Psychiatry, 37*, 422–426.

Parkes, J. D., Debono, A. G., & Marsden, C. D. (1976). Bromocriptine in Parkinsonism: Long-term treatment, dose response, and comparison with levodopa. *Journal of Neurology, Neurosurgery, and Psychiatry, 39*, 1101–1108.

Parkes, J. D., Schachter, M., Marsden, C. D., Smith, B., & Wilson, A. (1981). Lisuride in parkinsonism. *Annals of Neurology, 9*, 48–52.

Parkinson Study Group. (2000). Pramipexole vs levodopa as initial treatment for Parkinson disease: A randomized controlled trial. *JAMA, 284*, 1931–1938.

Parkinson Study Group. (2005). A randomized placebo-controlled trial of rasagiline in levodopa-treated patients with Parkinson disease and motor fluctuations: The presto study. *Archives of Neurology, 62*, 241–248.

Parkinson Study Group CALM Cohort Investigators. (2009). Long-term effect of initiating pramipexole vs levodopa in early Parkinson disease. *Archives of Neurology, 66*, 563–570.

Paus, S., Seeger, G., Brecht, H. M., Koster, J., El-Faddagh, M., Nothen, M. M., et al. (2004). Association study of dopamine D2, D3, D4 receptor and serotonin transporter gene polymorphisms with sleep attacks in Parkinson's disease. *Movement Disorders, 19*, 705–707.

Pazzagli, A., & Amaducci, L. (1966). La Sperimentazione clinica del Dopa nelle sindromi parkinsoniane. *Rivista di Neurobiologia, 12*, 138–145.

Perez-Lloret, S., & Rascol, O. (2010). Dopamine receptor agonists for the treatment of early or advanced Parkinson's disease. *CNS Drugs, 24*, 941–968.

Pezzoli, G., Martignoni, E., Pacchetti, C., Angeleri, V. A., Lamberti, P., Muratorio, A., et al. (1994). Pergolide compared with bromocriptine in Parkinson's disease: A multicenter, crossover, controlled study. *Movement Disorders, 9*, 431–436.

Pezzoli, G., Tesei, S., Ferrante, C., Cossutta, E., Zecchinelli, A., & Scarlato, G. (1988). Madopar HBS in fluctuating parkinsonian patients: Two-year treatment. *Movement Disorders, 3*, 37–45.

Pietz, K., Hagell, P., & Odin, P. (1998). Subcutaneous apomorphine in late stage Parkinson's disease: A long term follow up. *Journal of Neurology, Neurosurgery & Psychiatry, 65*, 709–716.

Poewe, W., Kleedorfer, B., Gerstenbrand, F., & Öertel, W. (1988). Subcutaneous apomorphine in Parkinson's disease. *The Lancet, 331*, 943.

Poewe, W., Rascol, O., Barone, P., Hauser, R. A., Mizuno, Y., Haaksma, M., et al. (2011). Extended-release pramipexole in early Parkinson disease: A 33-week randomized controlled trial. *Neurology, 77*, 759–766.

Poewe, W. H., Rascol, O., Quinn, N., Tolosa, E., Oertel, W. H., Martignoni, E., et al. (2007). Efficacy of pramipexole and transdermal rotigotine in advanced Parkinson's disease: A double-blind, double-dummy, randomised controlled trial. *The Lancet. Neurology, 6*, 513–520.

Pollak, P., Champay, A. S., Hommel, M., Perret, J. E., & Benabid, A. L. (1989). Subcutaneous apomorphine in Parkinson's disease. *Journal of Neurology, Neurosurgery, and Psychiatry, 52*, 544.

Pondal, M., Marras, C., Miyasaki, J., Moro, E., Armstrong, M. J., Strafella, A. P., et al. (2013). Clinical features of dopamine agonist withdrawal syndrome in a movement disorders clinic. *Journal of Neurology, Neurosurgery & Psychiatry, 84*, 130–135.

Pritchett, A. M., Morrison, J. F., Edwards, W. D., Schaff, H. V., Connolly, H. M., & Espinosa, R. E. (2002). Valvular heart disease in patients taking pergolide. *Mayo Clinic Proceedings, 77*, 1280–1286.

Quinn, N. P., Marion, M. H., & Marsden, C. D. (1987). Open study of Madopar HBS, a new formulation of levodopa with benserazide, in 13 patients with Parkinson's disease and 'on-off' fluctuations. *European Neurology, 27*(Suppl. 1), 105–113.

Quinn, N., Marsden, C. D., & Parkes, J. D. (1982). Complicated response fluctuations in Parkinson's disease: Response to intravenous infusion of levodopa. *The Lancet, 320*, 412–415.

Quinn, N., Parkes, J. D., & Marsden, C. D. (1984). Control of on/off phenomenon by continuous intravenous infusion of levodopa. *Neurology, 34*, 1131–1136.

Rabinak, C. A., & Nirenberg, M. J. (2010). Dopamine agonist withdrawal syndrome in Parkinson disease. *Archives of Neurology, 67*, 58–63.

Rascol, O., Barone, P., Hauser, R. A., Mizuno, Y., Poewe, W., Schapira, A. H. V., et al. (2010). Efficacy, safety, and tolerability of overnight switching from immediate- to once daily extended-release pramipexole in early Parkinson's disease. *Movement Disorders, 25*, 2326–2332.

Rascol, O., Brooks, D. J., Korczyn, A. D., De Deyn, P. P., Clarke, C. E., & Lang, A. E. (2000). A five-year study of the incidence of dyskinesia in patients with early Parkinson's disease who were treated with ropinirole or levodopa. *The New England Journal of Medicine, 342*, 1484–1491.

Rascol, O., Brooks, D. J., Melamed, E., Oertel, W., Poewe, W., Stocchi, F., et al. (2005). Rasagiline as an adjunct to levodopa in patients with Parkinson's disease and motor fluctuations (LARGO, lasting effect in adjunct therapy with rasagiline given once daily, study): A randomised, double-blind, parallel-group trial. *The Lancet, 365*, 947–954.

Rascol, A., Guiraud, B., Montastruc, J., David, J., & Clanet, M. (1979). Long-term treatment of Parkinson's disease with bromocriptine. *Journal of Neurology, Neurosurgery, and Psychiatry, 42*, 143–150.

Reches, A., & Fahn, S. (1982). 3-O- methyldopa blocks dopa metabolism in rat corpus striatum. *Annals of Neurology, 12*, 267–271.

Rinaldi, F., Marghertia, G., & De Divitus, E. (1965). Effetti della somministrazione de DOPA a pazienti parkinsoniani pretrattati con inhibitore delle monoaminossidasi. *Annali di Freniatria e Scienze Affini, 78*, 105–113.

Rinne, U. K. (1985). Combined bromocriptine-levodopa therapy early in Parkinson's disease. *Neurology, 35*, 1196–1198.

Rinne, U. K. (1987a). Early combination of bromocriptine and levodopa in the treatment of Parkinson's disease: A 5-year follow-up. *Neurology, 37*, 826–828.

Rinne, U. K. (1987b). Madopar HBS in the long-term treatment of Parkinsonian patients with fluctuations in disability. *European Neurology, 27*(Suppl. 1), 120–125.

Rinne, U. K., Bracco, F., Chouza, C., Dupont, E., Gershanik, O., Marti Masso, J. F., et al. (1998). Early treatment of Parkinson's disease with cabergoline delays the onset of motor complications. *Drugs*, *55*, 23–30.

Rinne, U. K., Sonninen, V., & Siirtola, T. (1972). Treatment of Parkinson's disease with amantadine and L-Dopa. *European Neurology*, 7, 228–240.

Roberts, J. W., Cora-Locatelli, G., Bravi, D., Amantea, M. A., Mouradian, M. M., & Chase, T. N. (1993). Catechol-O-methyltransferase inhibitor tolcapone prolongs levodopa/carbidopa action in parkinsonian patients. *Neurology*, *43*, 2685.

Rondelli, I., Acerbi, D., Mariotti, F., & Ventura, P. (1994). Simultaneous determination of levodopa methyl ester, levodopa, 3-O-methyldopa and dopamine in plasma by high-performance liquid chromatography with electrochemical detection. *Journal of Chromatography B: Biomedical Sciences and Applications*, *653*, 17–23.

Rondot, P., Ziegler, M., Aymard, N., & Holzer, J. (1987). Clinical trial of Madopar HBS in Parkinsonian patients with fluctuating drug response after long-term levodopa therapy. *European Neurology*, *27*(Suppl. 1), 114–119.

Ruottinen, H. M., & Rinne, U. K. (1996). Entacapone prolongs levodopa response in a one month double blind study in parkinsonian patients with levodopa related fluctuations. *Journal of Neurology, Neurosurgery & Psychiatry*, *60*, 36–40.

Sage, J. I., & Mark, M. H. (1988). Comparison of controlled-release Sinemet (CR4) and standard Sinemet (25 mg/100 mg) in advanced Parkinson's disease: A double-blind, crossover study. *Clinical Neuropharmacology*, *11*, 174–179.

Sage, J. I., Schuh, L., Heikkila, R. E., & Duvoisin, R. C. (1988). Continuous duodenal infusions of levodopa: Plasma concentrations and motor fluctuations in Parkinson's disease. *Clinical Neuropharmacology*, *11*, 36–44.

Sage, J. I., Trooskin, S., Sonsalla, P. K., & Heikkila, R. E. (1989). Experience with continuous enteral levodopa infusions in the treatment of 9 patients with advanced Parkinson's disease. *Neurology*, *39*, 60–63.

Samuel, M., Rodriguez-Oroz, M., Antonini, A., Brotchie, J. M., Chaudhuri, K. R., Brown, R. G., et al. (2015). Management of impulse control disorders in Parkinson's disease: Controversies and future approaches. *Movement Disorders*, *30*, 150–159.

Sano, H. (2000). Biochemistry of the extrapyramidal system: Shinkei Kennkyu No Shinpo, Advances in Neurological Sciences. (ISSN 0001-8724) Tokyo, October 1960;5:42–48. *Parkinsonism & Related Disorders*, *6*, 3–6.

Sano, I., Gamo, T., Kakimoto, Y., Taniguchi, K., Takesada, M., & Nishinuma, K. (1959). Distribution of catechol compounds in human brain. *Biochimica et Biophysica Acta*, *32*, 586–587.

Sasahara, K., Nitanai, T., Habara, T., Morioka, T., & Nakajima, E. (1980). Dosage form design for improvement of bioavailability of levodopa III: Influence of dose on pharmacokinetic behavior of levodopa in dogs and parkinsonian patients. *Journal of Pharmaceutical Sciences*, *69*, 1374–1378.

Sawada, H., Oeda, T., Kuno, S., Nomoto, M., Yamamoto, K., Yamamoto, M., et al. (2010). Amantadine for dyskinesias in Parkinson's disease: A randomized controlled trial. *PloS One*, *5*, e15298

Schapira, A. H. V., Barone, P., Hauser, R. A., Mizuno, Y., Rascol, O., Busse, M., et al. (2011). Extended-release pramipexole in advanced Parkinson disease: A randomized controlled trial. *Neurology*, 77, 767–774.

Schapira, A. H. V., Barone, P., Hauser, R. A., Mizuno, Y., Rascol, O., Busse, M., et al. (2013). Patient-reported convenience of once-daily versus three-times-daily dosing during long-term studies of pramipexole in early and advanced Parkinson's disease. *European Journal of Neurology*, *20*, 50–56.

Schwab, R. S., Amador, L. V., & Levine, J. Y. (1951). Apomorphine in Parkinson's disease. *Transactions of the American Neurological Association*, *56*, 251–253.

Schwab, R. S., England, A. C., Poskanzer, D. C., & Young, R. R. (1969). Amantadine in the treatment of Parkinson's disease. *JAMA*, *208*, 1168–1170.

Schwab, R. S., Poskanzer, D. C., England, A. C., & Young, R. R. (1972). Amantadine in Parkinson's disease: Review of more than two years' experience. *JAMA*, *222*, 792–795.

Schwab, R. S., & Tillmann, W. R. (1949). Artane in the treatment of Parkinson's disease. *The New England Journal of Medicine*, *241*, 483–485.

Shoulson, I., Glaubiger, G. A., & Chase, T. N. (1975). On-off response: Clinical and biochemical correlations during oral and intravenous levodopa administration in parkinsonian patients. *Neurology*, *25*, 1144–1148.

Siegfried, J. (1969). Traitement du Parkinsonisme avec la L-DOPA associée à un inhibiteur de la decarboxylase. *Médecine et Hygiène*, *27*, 543–545.

Siegfried, J. (1987). Therapeutic value of Madopar HBS: Judgment after 2 years experience. *European Neurology*, *27*, 98–104.

Silver, D. E., & Sahs, A. L. (1971). Double blind study using amantadine hydrochloride in the therapy of Parkinson's disease. *Transactions of the American Neurological Association*, *96*, 307–308.

Snow, B. J., Macdonald, L., Mcauley, D., & Wallis, W. (2000). The effect of amantadine on levodopa-induced dyskinesias in Parkinson's disease: A double-blind, placebo-controlled study. *Clinical Neuropharmacology*, *23*, 82–85.

Squires, R. F. (1972). Multiple forms of monoamine oxidase in intact mitochondria as characterized by selective inhibitors and thermal stability: A comparison of eight mammalian species. *Advances in Biochemical Psychopharmacology*, *5*, 355.

Steiger, M. J., Stocchi, F., Bramante, L., Ruggieri, S., & Quinn, N. P. (1992). The clinical efficacy of single morning doses of levodopa methyl ester: Dispersible Madopar and Sinemet plus in Parkinson disease. *Clinical Neuropharmacology*, *15*, 501–504.

Steiger, M. J., Stocchi, F., Carta, A., Ruggieri, S., Agnoli, A., Quinn, N. P., et al. (1991). The clinical efficacy of oral levodopa methyl ester solution in reversing afternoon "off" periods in Parkinson's disease. *Clinical Neuropharmacology*, *14*, 241–244.

Stern, G. M., Lees, A. J., Hardie, R. J., & Sandler, M. (1983). Clinical and pharmacological problems of deprenyl (selegiline) treatment in Parkinson's disease. *Acta Neurologica Scandinavica. Supplementum*, *95*, 113–116.

Stibe, C. M., Lees, A. J., Kempster, P. A., & Stern, G. M. (1988). Subcutaneous apomorphine in parkinsonian on-off oscillations. *The Lancet*, *331*, 403–406.

Stocchi, F., Barbato, L., Bramante, L., Bonamartini, A., & Ruggieri, S. (1994). The clinical efficacy of a single afternoon dose of levodopa methyl ester: A double-blind cross-over study versus placebo. *Functional Neurology*, *9*, 259–264.

Stocchi, F., Barbato, L., Bramante, L., Nordera, G., Vacca, L., & Ruggieri, S. (1996). Fluctuating parkinsonism: A pilot study of single afternoon dose of levodopa methyl ester. *Journal of Neurology*, *243*, 377–380.

Stocchi, F., Fabbri, L., Vecsei, L., Krygowska-Wajs, A., Monici Preti, P. A., & Ruggieri, S. A. (2007). Clinical efficacy of a single afternoon dose of effervescent levodopa-carbidopa preparation (CHF 1512) in fluctuating Parkinson disease. *Clinical Neuropharmacology*, *30*, 18–24.

Stocchi, F., Giorgi, L., Hunter, B., & Schapira, A. H. V. (2011). PREPARED: Comparison of prolonged and immediate release ropinirole in advanced Parkinson's disease. *Movement Disorders*, *26*, 1259–1265.

Stocchi, F., Hersh, B. P., Scott, B. L., Nausieda, P. A., & Giorgi, L. (2008). Ropinirole 24-hour prolonged release and ropinirole immediate release in early Parkinson's disease: A randomized, double-blind, non-inferiority crossover study. *Current Medical Research and Opinion*, *24*, 2883–2895.

Stocchi, F., Hsu, A., Khanna, S., Ellenbogen, A., Mahler, A., Liang, G., et al. (2014). Comparison of IPX066 with carbidopa–levodopa plus entacapone in advanced PD patients. *Parkinsonism & Related Disorders*, *20*, 1335–1340.

Stocchi, F., Quinn, N. P., Barbato, L., Patsalos, P. N., O'Connel, M. T., Ruggieri, S., et al. (1994). Comparison between a fast and a slow release preparation of levodopa and a combination of the two: A clinical and pharmacokinetic study. *Clinical Neuropharmacology*, *17*, 38–44.
Stocchi, F., Rascol, O., Kieburtz, K., Poewe, W., Jankovic, J., Tolosa, E., et al. (2010). Initiating levodopa/carbidopa therapy with and without entacapone in early Parkinson disease: The STRIDE-PD study. *Annals of Neurology*, *68*, 18–27.
Stocchi, F., Ruggieri, S., Brughitta, G., & Agnoli, A. (1986). Problems in daily motor performances in Parkinson's disease: The continuous dopaminergic stimulation. *Journal of Neural Transmission. Supplementum*, *22*, 209–218.
Stocchi, F., Ruggieri, S., Carta, A., Jenner, P., & Agnoli, A. (1989). Different therapeutic approaches to complicated Parkinson's disease. Clinical, pharmacological and physiological aspects. In N. P. Quinn & P. G. Jenner (Eds.), *Disorders of movement* (pp. 137–146). London, UK: Academic Press.
Stocchi, F., Ruggieri, S., Vacca, L., & Olanow, C. W. (2002). Prospective randomized trial of lisuride infusion versus oral levodopa in patients with Parkinson's disease. *Brain*, *125*, 2058–2066.
Stocchi, F., Zappia, M., Dall'Armi, V., Kulisevsky, J., Lamberti, P., & Obeso, J. A. (2010). Melevodopa/carbidopa effervescent formulation in the treatment of motor fluctuations in advanced Parkinson's disease. *Movement Disorders*, *25*, 1881–1887.
Struppler, A., & Von Uexkull, T. (1953). Studies of mechanism of action of apormorphine on Parkinson's tremor. *Zeitschrift für Klinische Medizin*, *152*, 46–57.
Subramony, J. A. (2006). Apomorphine in dopaminergic therapy. *Molecular Pharmaceutics*, *3*, 380–385.
Sweet, R. D., McDowell, F. H., Wasterlain, C. G., & Stern, P. H. (1975). Treatment of "on-off effect" with a dopa decarboxylase inhibitor. *Archives of Neurology*, *32*, 560–563.
Syed, N., Murphy, J., Zimmerman, T., Mark, M. H., & Sage, J. I. (1998). Ten years' experience with enteral levodopa infusions for motor fluctuations in Parkinson's disease. *Movement Disorders*, *13*, 336–338.
Thomas, A., Bonanni, L., Gambi, F., Di Iorio, A., & Onofrj, M. (2010). Pathological gambling in Parkinson disease is reduced by amantadine. *Annals of Neurology*, *68*, 400–404.
Thomas, A., Iacono, D., Luciano, A. L., Armellino, K., Di Iorio, A., & Onofrj, M. (2004). Duration of amantadine benefit on dyskinesia of severe Parkinson's disease. *Journal of Neurology, Neurosurgery & Psychiatry*, *75*, 141–143.
Tissot, R. R., Bartholini, G. G., & Pletscher, A. A. (1969). Drug-induced changes of extracerebral dopa metabolism in man. *Archives of Neurology*, *20*, 187–190.
Titova, N., & Chaudhuri, K. R. (2016). Apomorphine therapy in Parkinson's and future directions. *Parkinsonism & Related Disorders*, *33*(Suppl. 1), S56–S60. http://www.prd-journal.com/article/S1353-8020(16)30458-8/fulltext.
Tolosa, E., Marti, M. J., & Katzenschlager, R. (2015). Pharmacologic management of Parkinson's disease. In J. Jankovic & E. Tolosa (Eds.), *Parkinson's disease and movement disorders* (6th ed., pp. 86–111). Philadelphia, Baltimore, New York, London, Buenos Aires, Hong Kong, Sydney, Tokyo: Wolters Kluwer.
Tolosa, E., Martí, M. J., Valldeoriola, F., & Molinuevo, J. L. (1998). History of levodopa and dopamine agonists in Parkinson's disease treatment. *Neurology*, *50*, S2–S10.
Tompson, D. J., & Vearer, D. (2007). Steady-state pharmacokinetic properties of a 24-hour prolonged-release formulation of ropinirole: Results of two randomized studies in patients with Parkinson's disease. *Clinical Therapeutics*, *29*, 2654–2666.
Uitti, R. J., & Ahlskog, J. E. (1996). Comparative review of dopamine receptor agonists in Parkinson's disease. *CNS Drugs*, *5*, 369–388.
Umbach, W., & Baumann, D. (1964). Die Wirksamkeit von L-dopa bei Parkinson: Patienten mit und ohne stereotaktischem Hirneingriff. The efficacy of L-dopa in Parkinson patients with and without stereotactic brain sugery *Archiv für Psychiatrie und Nervenkrankheiten*, *205*, 281–292.

Van Camp, G., Flamez, A., Cosyns, B., Weytjens, C., Muyldermans, L., Van Zandijcke, M., et al. (2004). Treatment of Parkinson's disease with pergolide and relation to restrictive valvular heart disease. *The Lancet, 363*, 1179–1183.

Van Laar, T., Jansen, E. N. H., Essink, A. W. G., Neef, C., Oosterloo, S., & Roos, R. A. C. (1993). A double-blind study of the efficacy of apomorphine and its assessment in 'off'-periods in Parkinson's disease. *Clinical Neurology and Neurosurgery, 95*, 231–235.

Verhagen Metman, L., Stover, N., Chen, C., Cowles, V. E., & Sweeney, M. (2015). Gastroretentive carbidopa/levodopa, DM-1992, for the treatment of advanced Parkinson's disease. *Movement Disorders, 30*, 1222–1228.

Vickers, S., Duncan, C. A., White, S. D., Breault, G. O., Royds, R. B., de Schepper, P. J., et al. (1978). Evaluation of succinimidoethyl and pivaloyloxyethyl esters as progenitors of methyldopa in man, rhesus monkey, dog, and rat. *Drug Metabolism and Disposition, 6*, 640–646.

Videnovic, A., & Golombek, D. (2013). Circadian and sleep disorders in Parkinson's disease. *Experimental Neurology, 243*, 45–56.

Waldmeier, P. C., Baumann, P. A., Feldtrauer, J. J., Hauser, K., Bittiger, H., Bischoff, S., et al. (1990). CGP 28014, a new inhibitor of cerebral catechol-O-methylation with a non-catechol structure. *Naunyn-Schmiedeberg's Archives of Pharmacology, 342*, 305–311.

Waser, E., & Lewandowski, M. (1921). Untersuchungen in der Phenylalanin-Reihe I. Synthese des L-3,4-Dioxy-phenylalanins. Studies on the phenylalanine series. I. Synthesis of L-3,4-dihydroxyphenylala-nine *Helvetica Chimica Acta, 4*, 657–666.

Watts, R. L. (1997). The role of dopamine agonists in early Parkinson's disease. *Neurology, 49*, S34–S48.

Watts, R. L., Jankovic, J., Waters, C., Rajput, A., Boroojerdi, B., & Rao, J. (2007). Randomized, blind, controlled trial of transdermal rotigotine in early Parkinson disease. *Neurology, 68*, 272–276.

Weil, E. (1884). De l'apomorphine dans certain troubles nerveux. *Lyon Médical, 48*, 411–419.

Weil-Malherbe, H., & Bone, A. D. (1957). Intracellular distribution of catecholamines in the brain. *Nature, 180*, 1050–1051.

Weintraub, D., David, A. S., Evans, A. H., Grant, J. E., & Stacy, M. (2015). Clinical spectrum of impulse control disorders in Parkinson's disease. *Movement Disorders, 30*, 121–127.

Weintraub, D., Koester, J., Potenza, M. N., Siderowf, A. D., Stacy, M., Voon, V., et al. (2010). Impulse control disorders in Parkinson disease: A cross-sectional study of 3090 patients. *Archives of Neurology, 67*, 589–595.

Weintraub, D., & Nirenberg, M. J. (2013). Impulse control and related disorders in Parkinson's disease. *Neurodegenerative Diseases, 11*, 63–71.

Wilding, I. R., Hardy, J. G., Davis, S. S., Melia, C. D., Evans, D. F., Short, A. H., et al. (1991). Characterisation of the in vivo behaviour of a controlled-release formulation of levodopa (Sinemet CR). *Clinical Neuropharmacology, 14*, 305–321.

Wolf, E., Seppi, K., Katzenschlager, R., Hochschorner, G., Ransmayr, G., Schwingenschuh, P., et al. (2010). Long-term antidyskinetic efficacy of amantadine in Parkinson's disease. *Movement Disorders, 25*, 1357–1363.

Wood, M., Dubois, V., Scheller, D., & Gillard, M. (2015). Rotigotine is a potent agonist at dopamine D1 receptors as well as at dopamine D2 and D3 receptors. *British Journal of Pharmacology, 172*, 1124–1135.

Wright, B. A., & Waters, C. H. (2013). Continuous dopaminergic delivery to minimize motor complications in Parkinson's disease. *Expert Review of Neurotherapeutics, 13*, 719–729.

Wüllner, U., Kassubek, J., Odin, P., Schwarz, M., Naumann, M., Häck, H.-J., et al. (2010). Transdermal rotigotine for the perioperative management of Parkinson's disease. *Journal of Neural Transmission, 117*, 855–859.

Yahr, M. D., Clough, C. G., & Bergmann, K. J. (1982). Cholinergic and dopaminergic mechanisms in Parkinson's disease after long term levodopa administration. *The Lancet, 320*, 709–710.

Yahr, M. D., Duvoisin, R. C., Mendoza, M. R., Schear, M. J., & Barrett, R. E. (1971). Modification of L-dopa therapy of Parkinsonism by alpha-methyldopa hydrazine (MK-486). *Transactions of the American Neurological Association, 96*, 55–58.

Yahr, M. D., Duvoisin, R. C., Schear, M. J., Barrett, R. E., & Hoehn, M. M. (1969). Treatment of parkinsonism with levodopa. *Archives of Neurology, 21*, 343–354.

Yun, J. Y., Kim, H.-J., Lee, J.-Y., Kim, Y. E., Kim, J. S., Kim, J.-M., et al. (2013). Comparison of once-daily versus twice-daily combination of Ropinirole prolonged release in Parkinson's disease. *BMC Neurology, 13*, 113.

Zhou, C. Q., Li, S. S., Chen, Z. M., Li, F. Q., Lei, P., & Peng, G. G. (2013). Rotigotine transdermal patch in Parkinson's disease: A systematic review and meta-analysis. *PloS One, 8*, e69738

Ziégler, M., Ranoux, D., & de Recondo, J. (1994). Clinical efficacy of a liquid formulation of levodopa (Madopar Dispersible) in reversing afternoon "Off" periods in Parkinson's disease. *Clinical Neuropharmacology, 17*, S21–S25.

Zucker, D. (1925). Über die Wirkung des Physostigmins bei Erkrankungen des extrapyramidalen Systems. *European Neurology, 58*, 11–30.

Zurich, F. M. (1913). Apomorphine. The formation of Apomorphine on heating and preserving morphine solutions. *Hoppe-Seyler's Zeitschrift für Physiologische Chemie, 84*, 363–378.

CHAPTER TWELVE

Treatment Strategies in Early Parkinson's Disease

Luca Marsili*,†, Roberto Marconi†, Carlo Colosimo‡,1
*Sapienza University of Rome, Rome, Italy
†Misericordia Hospital, Grosseto, Italy
‡Santa Maria University Hospital, Terni, Italy
[1]Corresponding author: e-mail addresses: carlo.colosimo@uniroma1.it; c.colosimo@aospterni.it

Contents

Abstract

The clinicians' approach to the treatment of early Parkinson's disease (PD) should take into account numerous aspects, including how to inform a patient upon diagnosis and the critical decision of what therapy to adopt and when to start it. The treatment of the motor disorder associated with early PD needs to consider several crucial factors, such as age at onset, comorbidities, and the patient's functional requirements, and cannot be summarized in a simple formula. In younger patients (i.e., before the age of 70) and in those without high functional requirements, treatment is usually initiated with dopamine agonists and/or monoamine oxidase-B enzyme inhibitors (MAO-B I). By contrast, in older patients, or in those with high functional requirements, low doses of levodopa are generally used when treatment is started. In younger patients, levodopa should be added to dopamine agonists and/or MAO-B I, as required by disease progression, whereas in older patients, when response to levodopa alone is not satisfactory, dopamine agonists or catechol-*O*-methyltransferase inhibitors may subsequently be added.

International Review of Neurobiology, Volume 132
ISSN 0074-7742
http://dx.doi.org/10.1016/bs.irn.2017.01.002

1. INTRODUCTION

The appropriate choice of pharmacological therapy for early Parkinson's disease (PD) depends on many factors, including the patient's age at onset, employment-related features, lifestyle, phenomenology and severity of motor symptoms, presence of nonmotor features such as cognitive or behavioral abnormalities, and comorbidities. However, even when all these variables have been considered, the question of when pharmacological therapy should be initiated remains controversial. There are two different approaches: one is the classical "watch-and-wait" strategy (Aminoff, 2006), which implies delaying treatment until the patient's clinical condition is such that pharmacological therapy is indispensable, and the other is based on the initiation of treatment as soon as the diagnosis is made (Aminoff, 2006; Löhle et al., 2014; Rascol, Goetz, Koller, et al., 2002; Schapira & Obeso, 2006). Early initiation of therapy in PD allows the motor symptoms of the disease to be controlled more effectively and the quality of life to be improved (Grosset, Taurah, Burn, et al., 2007; Horstink, Tolosa, Bonuccelli, et al., 2006) and is consequently likely to be cost effective by maintaining the productivity of patients. Although it has been claimed that early pharmacotherapy may rebalance altered neurotransmitter levels in the basal ganglia (Schapira & Obeso, 2006) and lead to disease-modifying effects, no studies have unequivocally shown that early PD therapy slows down the clinical progression of PD (Rascol et al., 2016). Delayed initiation of PD treatment instead has other advantages, which include reduced adverse effects of anti-PD medication and lower costs for health services (Miyasaki, Martin, Suchowersky, et al., 2002). Unfortunately, delayed initiation of therapy is also associated with a greater disability and a higher likelihood of loss of productivity, which have consequences for both patients and society in the long term (Fox, Katzenschlager, Lim, et al., 2011, 2016). There is thus a widespread consensus among neurologists that delayed initiation of therapy cannot be considered a successful strategy because the primary goal of treatment should be the improvement in patients' function and quality of life (Pahwa & Lyons, 2014).

In this chapter, we will review the main drugs used in early PD stages, including levodopa, dopamine agonists (DAs), monoamine oxidase-B enzyme inhibitors (MAO-B I), catechol-O-methyltransferase (COMT) enzyme inhibitors (even though this class of drugs is only recommended for patients who already manifest some form of symptom fluctuation),

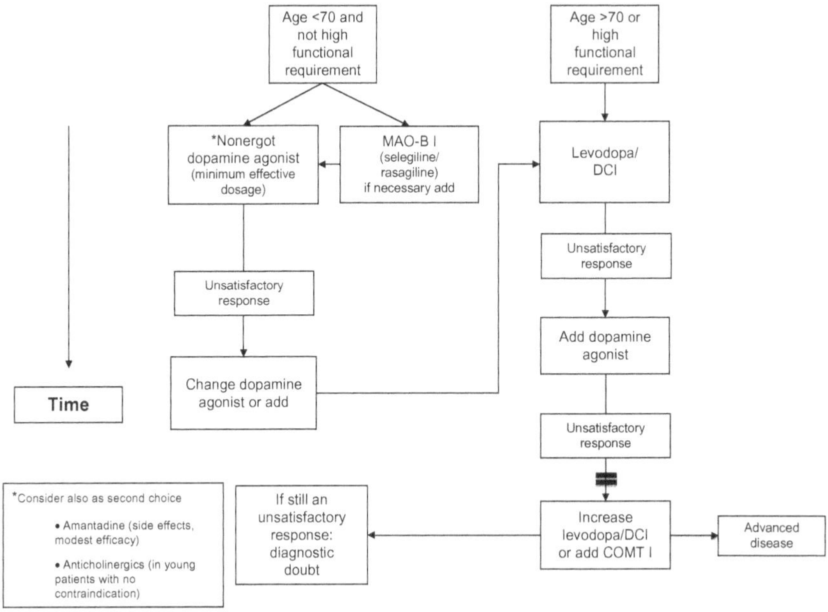

Fig. 1 Management of early Parkinson's disease. *COMT I*, catechol-*O*-methyltransferase inhibitors; *DCI*, dopa decarboxylase inhibitors; *MAO-B I*, monoamine oxidase-B inhibitors.

amantadine, anticholinergics, and possible disease-modifying strategies. Last, we will consider the nonpharmacological therapies recommended in early PD. Our ultimate aim is to provide clinicians with a practical guide to effectively manage PD from the very outset (Fig. 1).

2. PHARMACOLOGICAL THERAPY

Current treatment options for early PD include levodopa/carbidopa, DAs (particularly immediate and extended release [ER] formulations of pramipexole and ropinirole, and transdermal rotigotine), and MAO-B I (rasagiline, selegiline, and, more recently, safinamide). COMT enzyme inhibitors are used above all when motor fluctuations appear, typically during middle-stage PD. Amantadine is a wide action mechanism drug that acts on various PD symptoms and is thus used for both initial and advanced PD stages. Despite having been abandoned by many specialists, anticholinergics may be used in younger patients because of their efficacy on tremor, though their use is somewhat limited owing to the risk of adverse events, including cognitive impairment. The antiparkinsonian drugs most commonly used in clinical practice to treat early PD are summarized in Table 1.

2.1 Levodopa

Levodopa remains the drug with the best therapeutic index for symptomatic antiparkinsonian medication in all PD stages. This compound, which is the natural precursor of dopamine, is activated through its decarboxylation by the cytosolic aromatic amino acid decarboxylase (AADC). In commercial preparations, levodopa is combined with the AADC peripheral inhibitors carbidopa or benserazide, thus allowing the administration of levodopa at doses that are four times lower than those of levodopa administered on its own and reducing its potential peripheral side effects. Levodopa is combined in a single tablet with carbidopa at a 1:10 or 1:5 ratio, or with benserazide at a 1:4 ratio. Generally, the initial dosage of levodopa is from 50 to 100 mg b.i.d. to t.i.d.; this dose can progressively be titrated up to the individual's optimal dosage (100–250 t.i.d. or q.i.d.). Although levodopa is a very effective drug, its long-term use is associated with motor complications: fluctuations and dyskinesia. The development of these complications increases at an estimated rate of 10% per year. Standard levodopa has a very short half-life (~90 min), whereas controlled-release formulations of levodopa/carbidopa have been studied to produce delayed enteric absorption (~3- to 4-h half-life) and may reduce long-term complications, though their effect is, unfortunately, scarce and unpredictable. Controlled-release formulations of levodopa are not routinely recommended in early PD, whereas they may be considered in patients with motor fluctuations or in those with nocturnal problems. Dispersible levodopa preparations, which are designed to have symptomatic effects more promptly, are also available, though they too are indicated in advanced PD patients. In early 2015, the Food and Drug Administration and the European Medicines Agency (EMA) approved a novel levodopa–carbidopa oral formulation, called IPX066, that combines immediate release and ER levodopa–carbidopa at a 4:1 ratio. This compound, which is already available in the United States, is usually administered t.i.d. and is designed to dissolve at different rates so as to ensure the release and absorption of levodopa over a longer time frame than that provided by standard levodopa. IPX066 has been tested in both early (levodopa naïve) (Pahwa et al., 2014; Waters, Nausieda, Dzyak, et al., 2015) and advanced (Hauser, Hsu, Kell, et al., 2013; Nausieda, Hsu, Elmer, et al., 2015; Stocchi, Hsu, Khanna, et al., 2014; Waters et al., 2015) PD stages,

Table 1 Synoptic Table of Antiparkinsonian Drugs Used in Early Parkinson's Disease

Name	Dosage Unit	Daily Dose (mg)	Mechanism of Action
Selegiline	5–10 mg	5–10	MAO-B I
Rasagiline	1 mg	1	MAO-B I
Safinamide[a]	50–100 mg	50–100	MAO-B I and antiglutamatergic
Trihexyphenidyl	2 mg	6–8	Anticholinergic
Biperidene	2 mg; 4 mg CR; 5 mg/1 mL ampules	1–12	Anticholinergic
Amantadine	100 mg	200–300	Mixed (dopamine release, anticholinergic, NMDA antagonist)
Levodopa/carbidopa	100/10 mg; 100/25 mg; 200/50 mg; 250/25 mg 200/50 mg CR; 100/25 mg CR	200/50–2000/250	DA precursor/dopa decarboxylase inhibitor
Levodopa/ benserazide	100/25 mg; 200/50 mg 100/25 mg CR 100/25 mg dispersible	200/50–2000/250	DA precursor/dopa decarboxylase inhibitor
Bromocriptine	2.5; 5; 10 mg	7.5–40	DA agonist
Cabergoline[b]	0.5; 1; 2 mg	2–10	DA agonist
Pergolide[b]	0.05; 0.25; 1 mg	1.5–6	DA agonist
Dihydroergocryptine	20 mg	20–120	DA agonist
Ropinirole Ropinirole ER	0.25; 0.5; 1; 2; 5 mg 2; 4; 8 mg	4–24	DA agonist
Pramipexole Pramipexole ER	0.18; 0.7 mg 0.26; 0.52; 1.0 mg	3–4.5	DA agonist DA agonist

Continued

Table 1 Synoptic Table of Antiparkinsonian Drugs Used in Early Parkinson's Disease—cont'd

Name	Dosage Unit	Daily Dose (mg)	Mechanism of Action
Piribedil	20 mg; 50 mg CR	20–100	DA agonist
Rotigotine (transdermal)	Patch (2; 4; 6; 8 mg)	4–8	DA agonist

[a]Safinamide is currently licensed only as an adjunct therapy to levodopa.
[b]Note that cabergoline and pergolide are second-choice drugs owing to their possible toxicity.
CR, sustained release; *DA*, dopamine; *ER*, extended release; *MAO-B I*, monoamine oxidase-B enzyme inhibitors; *mg*, milligrams; *NMDA*, *N*-methyl-D-aspartate.

yielding beneficial results. In summary, IPX066 has proved to effectively reduce daily OFF time and to improve motor function and quality of life in both early and advanced PD (Waters et al., 2015). Its long-term benefits over standard levodopa, particularly on dyskinesia, is not yet known.

Ongoing trials are also evaluating newer levodopa formulations currently being designed to achieve better drug delivery and absorption; worthy of mention are DM-1992 (Verhagen Metman, Stover, Chen, Cowles, & Sweeney, 2015) and the "accordion pill" (AP09004) (LeWitt, Friedman, & Giladi, 2012), which are both ER levodopa–carbidopa formulations with gastroretentive properties designed to improve the pharmacokinetics of levodopa. XP21279, which is an ester conjugate of levodopa, designed to improve absorption of the active drug and to reduce motor fluctuations (LeWitt, Huff, Hauser, et al., 2014). ND0612 is a liquid subcutaneous formulation of levodopa–carbidopa administered via a patch-pump device (Giladi, Caraco, Gurevitch, et al., 2015), while CVT-301 is an inhalation powder of levodopa that acts rapidly; both these formulations are currently being tested in studies on advanced PD (LeWitt, Saint-Hilaire, Grosset, et al., 2015).

Possible side effects of levodopa include gastrointestinal adverse reactions (nausea, vomiting, constipation). These adverse events tend to be dose dependent and to decrease over time. When severe, they may be treated by adding the peripheral dopamine receptor blocker domperidone 10–20 mg t.i.d. An electrocardiogram that calculates the QT/QTc interval is mandatory before domperidone is started because of this drug's cardiac side effects. Orthostatic hypotension, hallucinations, and mental confusion may also be observed during levodopa therapy. Dopaminergic drug-induced hallucinations are typically visual, though they may also occasionally present under other sensory forms. These psychotic phenomena frequently herald the onset of cognitive impairment in PD patients.

2.2 Dopamine Agonists

DAs are synthetic drugs that act directly on striatal postsynaptic dopamine receptors. They have a better pharmacokinetic profile than levodopa and are divided into two classes: ergot derived and nonergot derived. The older ergot-derived drugs, such as bromocriptine, cabergoline, lisuride, dihydroergocryptine, and pergolide, are all second-line drugs because of their severe side effects, which include retroperitoneal, pleuropulmonar, and valvular heart fibrosis (Zanettini et al., 2007). Nonergot-derived DAs, such as pramipexole (D2, D3 agonist), ropinirole (D2, D3, D4 agonist), piribedil (D2, D3 agonist and α2 antagonist), and rotigotine (D1, D2, D3 agonist), are used in monotherapy or as adjunctive therapy to levodopa in early-to-moderate PD stages. Apomorphine, which is the oldest drug in this class, has attracted renewed interest in recent years on account of its potential use in advanced PD stages. This compound, which acts on both D1 and D2 dopamine receptors, displays the most complete pharmacological profile of all clinically available DAs. However, since its half-life is short and its oral bioavailability is poor, it is unsuitable for use in early PD cases (Colosimo, Merello, & Albanese, 1994).

In order to find the optimum dose and avoid side effects, all agonists must be progressively titrated. Classical formulations are usually given t.i.d., though more practical ER formulations taken once daily are now available for ropinirole and pramipexole (oral preparations) as well as for rotigotine (marketed as transdermal formulations). DA monotherapy induces fewer long-term motor complications, such as dyskinesia or wearing-off, than levodopa monotherapy. The motor benefit (i.e., reduction in the Movement Disorder Society-sponsored revision of the Unified PD Rating Scale—MDS UPDRS score, part III) when DAs are used alone is less marked than that achieved by using levodopa, a difference that increases as the disease progresses (Chaudhuri & Schapira, 2009; PD Med Collaborative Group, 2014). Accordingly, the majority of patients require add-on levodopa after a few years. The adverse effects of DAs include nausea, daytime somnolence, confusion, hallucinations, leg edema, orthostatic hypotension, and erythromelalgia (particularly ergot derivatives). The advantages and disadvantages of the various DAs should be compared in clinical practice.

All available DAs, with the exception of apomorphine, share the same efficacy profile. However, the level of evidence available for the different drugs tends to vary because the effects of some older DAs have never been thoroughly assessed. The best levels of evidence are, consequently, associated with newer nonergot derivatives, despite a lack of empirical evidence showing that older agonists are less effective than more recent ones. Safety is a critical aspect and, since fibrotic reactions appear to be much more frequent with ergot than with nonergot derivatives, ergot DAs are a second-line therapy (Horstink et al., 2006).

Impulse control disorders (ICDs), defined as a failure to resist an impulse or temptation that is harmful to one or others, may develop in PD as a consequence of dopamine replacement therapy. The most commonly reported ICDs are pathological gambling, hypersexuality, compulsive shopping, and compulsive eating, while their overall prevalence in some studies is as high as 14%. Treatment with DAs is the main risk factor for ICDs. Although levodopa has also been reported to induce ICDs, it does so to a far lesser extent than DAs.

2.3 Monoamine Oxidase-B Enzyme Inhibitors

These drugs are strong, irreversible, selective MAO-B I that reduce the catabolism of dopamine, thereby increasing the availability of this neurotransmitter at the synaptic level. The two classical compounds available on the market are selegiline and rasagiline. In 2015, a new MAO-B I, safinamide, was introduced in Europe as an adjunct therapy to levodopa. This compound actually has a double mechanism of action: a dopaminergic action as a reversible, selective MAO-B I, and a nondopaminergic action as an antiglutamatergic drug that acts on the voltage-gated sodium channel (Borgohain et al., 2014; Stocchi, Borgohain, Onofrj, et al., 2012). Selegiline and rasagiline exert a moderate benefit on PD motor symptoms, as well as on fatigue and mood, when used in early PD. They also play a marginal role, as an adjunct therapy to levodopa, in advanced PD. Their possible neuroprotective, or disease modifying, role on dopaminergic cell loss is as yet unclear (Rascol et al., 2016). Rasagiline is given at a dose of 1 mg once daily and selegiline at 5–10 mg once daily; titration is not required. Uncommon side effects are insomnia, nausea, dizziness, and orthostatic hypotension. There are no direct comparative trials between selegiline and rasagiline. Drug interactions leading to a serotonine syndrome type may occur on rare occasions when MAO-B I are combined with some serotonine reuptake inhibitors or with meperidine. Safinamide has been approved by the EMA only as add-on therapy to levodopa in moderate-advanced stages of PD at dosages of 50–100 mg once daily; safinamide provides an alternative strategy to merely increasing the DA dose, thereby reducing the theoretical risk of DA-related side effects (Stocchi et al., 2012).

2.4 COMT Enzyme Inhibitors

Add-on COMT inhibiting drugs may be used to extend the effects of levodopa and reduce motor fluctuations, particularly in patients with advanced disease (Fig. 1). These compounds, which are named tolcapone and entacapone and are always administrated with levodopa, delay the enzymatic degradation of levodopa and dopamine. Tolcapone enhances the release of dopamine in the central nervous system and is more powerful and longer acting than entacapone. The side effects of tolcapone include diarrhea and, in rare cases, serious hepatotoxicity; liver function tests must be performed periodically. Entacapone, which exerts its effects exclusively at the peripheral level, has a milder effect than tolcapone but is safer (side effects include increased dyskinesia, urine discoloration, diarrhea). The dosage given with each dose of levodopa (t.i.d. or more frequently) is 200 mg. A recent study suggested that entacapone should not be combined with levodopa therapy in early PD, but should be limited to patients who are already experiencing fluctuations (Stocchi, Rascol, Kieburtz, et al., 2010). It should, however, be borne in mind that the reported inefficacy of entacapone as adjunct therapy in stable PD patients may be incorrect because of biases in the design of the aforementioned study. With regard to the moderate efficacy of entacapone and the suboptimal safety profile of tolcapone, a potent third-generation COMT inhibitor with a good safety and efficacy profile, named opicapone, has recently been proposed for PD at a dosage of 50 mg once daily (Ferreira et al., 2016). Opicapone is already marketed in Germany and United Kingdom, though further studies are needed to better validate the efficacy and long-term risk–benefit ratio of this new drug.

2.5 Amantadine

Amantadine is an old antiviral compound (Schwab & England, 1969) that can be used to reduce tremor and rigidity at any stage of the disease (also as initial symptomatic PD therapy); in addition, amantadine reduces dyskinesia in about half of the PD patients in the advanced stages (Ory-Magne,

Corvol, Azulay, et al., 2014). Although its mechanisms of action have yet to be fully understood, they are known to include not only a dopaminergic action but also antiglutamatergic and anticholinergic properties. The usual dosage is 100 mg two or three times a day. Side effects include sleep disorders, confusion, constipation, xerostomia, hallucinations, erythromelalgia, and livedo reticularis. In a recent clinical trial based on PD patients with troublesome dyskinesia, a once-daily ER formulation of amantadine led to a considerable reduction in dyskinesia, as measured by means of the Unified Dyskinesia Rating Scale score, and an increased ON time (Pahwa, Tanner, Hauser, et al., 2015). Although ER formulations of amantadine have not yet been marketed, they might represent a valid and simple option for dyskinetic PD patients in the future.

2.6 Anticholinergics

Anticholinergics (antimuscarinics) are old drugs used as a second/third choice to reduce tremor in young patients with early PD. Owing to their common neuropsychiatric (memory loss, confusion) and autonomic (constipation, urinary retention, dry mouth) side effects and their limited clinical efficacy, these drugs are not usually recommended in patients over 65 years. The main compounds of anticholinergics are trihexyphenidyl and biperidene (2 mg t.i.d.).

2.7 Studies on Possible Neuroprotective Agents

Neuroprotection refers to a treatment that modifies the natural history of PD by reducing dopaminergic cell loss and disease progression and represents one of the main unmet needs in PD therapy. Despite a number of interesting data on experimental models of PD, there is not as yet sufficient evidence to unequivocally demonstrate that substances such as neurotrophic agents, antioxidants (e.g., iron chelators, glutathione, inosine), vitamins, omega-3 fatty acids, coenzyme Q10, creatine, peroxisome proliferator-activated receptor gamma inhibitors (e.g., pioglitazione, rosiglitazione), DAs, and MAO-B I exert a true neuroprotective effect in PD (Rascol et al., 2016). Several difficulties seriously hamper the possibility of identifying particular molecules to be used for neuroprotective drug purposes. Major limitations in the development of neuroprotective agents include a lack of understanding of the mechanisms underlying neurodegeneration in PD, the lack of a reliable animal model (i.e., one that accurately reflects the progressive nature of PD) to be used to test possible molecules, and the difficulty in discriminating between an early symptomatic effect and a true neuroprotective effect when a hypothetical disease-modifying drug is being tested. Last but not least, there are difficulties involved in correctly selecting idiopathic PD patients for clinical trials, given that there is a higher likelihood of an incorrect diagnosis and of a subject dropping out in early disease stages when these patients eventually need symptomatic treatment (Stocchi, 2014).

A growing body of evidence has linked alpha-synuclein (α-SYN) aggregation to the pathogenesis of PD, with α-SYN oligomers appearing to be toxic to neuronal cells and Lewy bodies providing a compensatory-like response. A number of strategies may be used to reduce α-SYN toxicity: antioxidants act by inhibiting oligomer accumulation, whereas immunotherapy acts by impeding it (Kalia, Kalia, & Lang, 2015). Several molecules designed to induce active or passive immunization against α-SYN are currently being studied (Games et al., 2014), and the first results from randomized clinical trials on immunotherapy in PD will hopefully be presented in the coming years. In particular, promising preliminary data (unpublished) have emerged from one randomized controlled phase I study (NCT02267434) that is investigating the safety and tolerability of the vaccine AFFITOPE® PD03A, which targets α-SYN in early PD.

3. NONPHARMACOLOGICAL THERAPIES

Nonpharmacological therapies include surgical therapy and physical therapy. Surgical therapy (deep brain stimulation—DBS) is not usually recommended in early-stage PD; however, recent pilot studies, (Camalier, Konrad, Gill, et al., 2014; Charles, Konrad, Neimat, et al., 2014; Goetz, Poewe, Rascol, et al., 2005) designed to test bilateral subthalamic (STN) DBS in PD patients with Hoehn and Yahr stage II (measured in OFF condition) and a mean disease duration not exceeding 2 years, have suggested that DBS is safe in early PD stages, at least in patients with a young age at disease onset. Further studies on larger and more representative samples of PD patients are needed to better assess the efficacy of DBS in early PD and reconsider the timing of surgery. Physical therapy should instead be considered as an adjunctive therapy in all PD stages, even when patients present premature postural or gait abnormalities in the early PD stages; this is particularly important if we consider the widely acknowledged poor effect of pharmacological therapy on gait disturbances and postural instability (Table 2). Most studies that have assessed physical therapy, speech therapy,

Table 2 Parkinson's Disease Symptoms That Respond Poorly to Dopaminergic Drugs

Postural instability
Freezing
Dysarthria
Cognitive impairment
REM sleep behavior disorder
Orthostatic hypotension
Constipation
Bladder hyperreflexia
Sweating abnormalities
Sensory phenomena

and rehabilitation programs in PD have reported an improvement in at least one outcome measure (Bloem, de Vries, & Ebersbach, 2015). However, it is difficult to unravel the importance of these clinical improvements, particularly of their long-term cost effectiveness. The use of alternative motor strategies which can be easily taught to patients (e.g., military step-like walking, marching on the spot before walking, making oscillatory trunk movements) or the addition of auditory or visual stimuli (walking in time to a metronome, following the lines of the paving stones, attempting to reach a target placed on the floor) may prove useful for the often disabling gait disturbances.

4. SUMMARY OF THE GUIDELINES AVAILABLE

The treatment of the motor disorder in early PD needs to take into account several crucial factors and cannot be summarized in a simple recipe (Pahwa & Lyons, 2014). The question of when and how pharmacological therapy should be initiated remains controversial, with no general consensus being reached in international guidelines on the definition of patients according to their age at the onset of motor symptoms (Horstink et al., 2006; Miyasaki et al., 2002). As a practical suggestion, we recommend that treatment in younger patients (i.e., younger than 70) or in those without high functional requirements be started with DAs and/or MAO-B I

(Colosimo & Marsili, 2015). By contrast, treatment in older patients or in those with high functional requirements should start directly with low doses of levodopa. In younger patients, levodopa may be added to DAs and/or MAO-B I according to disease progression. In older patients, when response to levodopa alone is not satisfactory (or to avoid adverse events related to high dosages of levodopa, such as dyskinesia), DAs or COMT enzyme inhibitors may be added. As disease progresses and these therapeutic strategies often become inadequate, increasingly complex pharmacological therapies, or other approaches, such as DBS, warrant consideration. Fig. 1 shows a flowchart with basic recommendations on how to treat early (untreated) PD.

Practical and widely accepted recommendations for patients on levodopa include chewing the tablets instead of swallowing them and taking medication on an empty stomach, to achieve a quicker onset of action of each dose (although drug-naïve PD patients may be advised to start by taking levodopa after meals to avoid adverse gastrointestinal effects). Carefully administered dietary protein restriction has been shown to yield a stable response to levodopa therapy. It is important to refer patients to nutritional therapists to prevent obesity or malnutrition even in the early stages of the disease. Reduced gastric motility and constipation, which are frequent symptoms in PD, are often aggravated by antiparkinsonian medications and may reduce drug absorption (Stirpe, Hoffman, Badiali, & Colosimo, 2016). General measures need to be adopted to avoid constipation, such as a correct diet (with plenty of liquids and high-fiber foods), taking smaller doses of, or even cutting out, some antiparkinsonian drugs (particularly anticholinergics) and taking laxatives (macrogol) may be necessary. IPX066, a new ER levodopa formulation (Hauser et al., 2013; Nausieda et al., 2015; Pahwa et al., 2014; Stocchi et al., 2014; Waters et al., 2015), which is designed to maintain stable plasmatic concentrations of the drug, has recently been marketed for advanced as well as early PD to increase compliance and avoid some of the complications associated with long-term treatment. Since levodopa remains the most effective medication for all PD symptoms, trials with new ER (LeWitt et al., 2012, 2014; Verhagen Metman et al., 2015), subcutaneous (Giladi et al., 2015), and inhaled (LeWitt et al., 2015) levodopa formulations are currently being undertaken to find ways of improving the bioavailability of levodopa, extending its duration and maximizing its effect.

REFERENCES

Aminoff, M. J. (2006). Treatment should not be initiated too soon in Parkinson's disease. *Annals of Neurology*, *59*(3), 562–564.

Bloem, B. R., de Vries, N. M., & Ebersbach, G. (2015). Nonpharmacological treatments for patients with Parkinson's disease. *Movement Disorders*, *30*(11), 1504–1520.

Borgohain, R., Szasz, J., Stanzione, P., Meshram, C., Bhatt, M. H., Chirilineau, D., et al. (2014). Two-year, randomized, controlled study of safinamide as add-on to levodopa in mid to late Parkinson's disease. *Movement Disorders*, *29*(10), 1273–1280.

Camalier, C. R., Konrad, P. E., Gill, C. E., et al. (2014). Methods for surgical targeting of the STN in early-stage Parkinson's disease. *Frontiers in Neurology*, *5*, 1–6.

Charles, D., Konrad, P. E., Neimat, J. S., et al. (2014). Subthalamic nucleus deep brain stimulation in early stage Parkinson's disease. *Parkinsonism & Related Disorders*, *20*, 731–737.

Chaudhuri, K. R., & Schapira, A. H. (2009). Non-motor symptoms of Parkinson's disease: Dopaminergic pathophysiology and treatment. *Lancet Neurology*, *8*, 464–474.

Colosimo, C., & Marsili, L. (2015). Treatment of Parkinson's disease. In C. Colosimo, A. Gil-Nagel, N. E. Gilhus, A. Rapoport, & O. Williams (Eds.), *Handbook of neurological therapy* (pp. 293–306). USA: Oxford University Press.

Colosimo, C., Merello, M., & Albanese, A. (1994). Clinical usefulness of apomorphine in movement disorders. *Clinical Neuropharmacology*, *17*(3), 243–259.

Ferreira, J. J., Lees, A., Rocha, J. F., Poewe, W., Rascol, O., Soares da Silva, P., et al. (2016). Opicapone as an adjunct to levodopa in patients with Parkinson's disease and end-of-dose motor fluctuations: A randomised, double-blind, placebo-controlled and active-controlled parallel-group trial. *Lancet Neurology*, *15*(2), 154–165.

Fox, S. H., Katzenschlager, R., Lim, S. Y., et al. (2011). The movement disorder society evidence-based medicine review update: Treatments for the motor symptoms of Parkinson's disease. *Movement Disorders*, *26*(3), S2–S41.

Fox, S. H., Katzenschlager, R., Lim, S. Y., et al. (2016). Evidence based medicine publications. In *International Parkinson and movement disorder society*. www.movementdisorders.org/MDS/Resources/Publications-Reviews/EBM-Reviews1.htm. Accessed June 17.

Games, D., Valera, E., Spencer, B., Rockenstein, E., Mante, M., Adame, A., et al. (2014). Reducing C-terminal-truncated alpha-synuclein by immunotherapy attenuates neurodegeneration and propagation in Parkinson's disease-like models. *The Journal of Neuroscience*, *34*(28), 9441–9954.

Giladi, N., Caraco, Y., Gurevitch, T., et al. (2015). Pharmacokinetics and safety of ND0612L (levodopa/carbidopa for subcutaneous infusion): Results from a phase II study in moderate to severe Parkinson's disease. *Neurology*, *84*, P1.187.

Goetz, C. G., Poewe, W., Rascol, O., et al. (2005). Evidence-based medical review update: Pharmacological and surgical treatments of Parkinson's disease: 2001 to 2004. *Movement Disorders*, *20*, 523–539.

Grosset, D., Taurah, L., Burn, D. J., et al. (2007). A multicentre longitudinal observational study of changes in self-reported health status in people with Parkinson's disease left untreated at diagnosis. *Journal of Neurology, Neurosurgery, and Psychiatry*, *78*, 465–469.

Hauser, R. A., Hsu, A., Kell, S., et al. (2013). Extended-release carbidopa-levodopa (IPX066) compared with immediate-release carbidopa-levodopa in patients with Parkinson's disease and motor fluctuations: A phase 3 randomised, double-blind trial. *Lancet Neurology*, *12*, 346–356.

Horstink, M., Tolosa, E., Bonuccelli, U., European Federation of Neurological Societies, Movement Disorder Society-European Section, et al. (2006). Review of the therapeutic management of Parkinson's disease. Report of a joint task force of the European Federation of Neurological Societies and the Movement Disorder Society-European Section.

Part I: Early (uncomplicated) Parkinson's disease. *European Journal of Neurology, 13*, 1170–1185.
Kalia, L. V., Kalia, S. K., & Lang, A. E. (2015). Disease-modifying strategies for Parkinson's disease. *Movement Disorders, 30*, 1442–1450.
LeWitt, P. A., Friedman, H., & Giladi, N. (2012). Accordion pill carbidopa/levodopa for improved treatment of advanced Parkinson's disease symptoms [abstract]. *Movement Disorders, 27*(1), S408.
LeWitt, P. A., Huff, F. J., Hauser, R., et al. (2014). Double-blind study of an actively-transported levodopa prodrug, XP21279, in Parkinson disease. *Movement Disorders, 29*, 75e82.
LeWitt, P. A., Saint-Hilaire, M. H., Grosset, D. G., et al. (2015). Inhaled levodopa (CVT-301) provides rapid motor improvements after administration to Parkinson's disease patients when OFF [abstract]. *Movement Disorders, 30*, 260.
Löhle, M., Ramberg, C. J., Reichmann, H., & Schapira, A. H. V. (2014). Early versus delayed initiation of pharmacotherapy in Parkinson's disease. *Drugs, 74*, 645–657.
Miyasaki, J. M., Martin, W., Suchowersky, O., et al. (2002). Practice parameter: Initiation of treatment for Parkinson's disease: An evidence-based review: Report of the Quality Standards Subcommittee of the American Academy of Neurology. *Neurology, 58*, 11–17.
Nausieda, P. A., Hsu, A., Elmer, L., et al. (2015). Conversion to IPX066 from standard levodopa formulations in advanced Parkinson's disease: Experience in clinical trials. *Journal of Parkinson's Disease, 5*, 837–845.
Ory-Magne, F., Corvol, J. C., Azulay, J. P., et al. (2014). Withdrawing amantadine in dyskinetic patients with Parkinson disease: The AMANDYSK trial. *Neurology, 82*(4), 300–307.
Pahwa, R., & Lyons, K. E. (2014). Treatment of early Parkinson's disease. *Current Opinion in Neurology, 27*(4), 442–449.
Pahwa, R., Lyons, K. E., Hauser, R. A., Fahn, S., Jankovic, J., Pourcher, E., et al. (2014). Randomized trial of IPX066, carbidopa/levodopa extended release, in early Parkinson's disease. *Parkinsonism & Related Disorders, 20*, 142–148.
Pahwa, R., Tanner, C. M., Hauser, R. A., et al. (2015). Amantadine extended release for levodopa-induced dyskinesia in Parkinson's disease (EASED Study). *Movement Disorders, 30*, 788–795.
PD Med Collaborative Group, Gray, R., Ives, N., Rick, C., et al. (2014). Long-term effectiveness of dopamine agonists and monoamine oxidase B inhibitors compared with levodopa as initial treatment for Parkinson's disease (PD MED): A large, open-label, pragmatic randomised trial. *Lancet, 384*(9949), 1196–1205.
Rascol, O., Goetz, C., Koller, W., et al. (2002). Treatment interventions for Parkinson's disease: An evidence based assessment. *Lancet, 359*, 1589–1598.
Rascol, O., Hauser, R. A., Stocchi, F., Fitzer-Attas, C. J., Sidi, Y., Abler, V., et al. (2016). Long-term effects of rasagiline and the natural history of treated Parkinson's disease. *Movement Disorders, 31*, 1489–1496. http://dx.doi.org/10.1002/mds.26724.
Schapira, A. H., & Obeso, J. (2006). Timing of treatment initiation in Parkinson's disease: A need for reappraisal? *Annals of Neurology, 59*(3), 559–562.
Schwab, R. S., & England, A. C., Jr. (1969). Amantadine HCL (Symmetrel) and its relation to levo-dopa in the treatment of Parkinson's disease. *Transactions of the American Neurological Association, 94*, 85–90.
Stirpe, P., Hoffman, M., Badiali, D., & Colosimo, C. (2016). Constipation: An emerging risk factor for Parkinson's disease? *European Journal of Neurology, 23*(11), 1606–1613.
Stocchi, F. (2014). Therapy for Parkinson's disease: What is in the pipeline? *Neurotherapeutics, 11*, 24–33.

Stocchi, F., Borgohain, R., Onofrj, M., et al. (2012). A randomized, double-blind, placebo-controlled trial of safinamide as add-on therapy in early Parkinson's disease patients. *Movement Disorders*, *27*(1), 106–112.

Stocchi, F., Hsu, A., Khanna, S., et al. (2014). Comparison of IPX066 with carbidopa-levodopa plus entacapone in advanced PD patients. *Parkinsonism & Related Disorders*, *20*, 1335–1340.

Stocchi, F., Rascol, O., Kieburtz, K., et al. (2010). Initiating levodopa/carbidopa therapy with and without entacapone in early Parkinson disease: The STRIDE-PD study. *Annals of Neurology*, *68*(1), 18–27.

Verhagen Metman, L., Stover, N., Chen, C., Cowles, V. E., & Sweeney, M. (2015). Gastro-retentive carbidopa/levodopa, DM-1992, for the treatment of advanced Parkinson's disease. *Movement Disorders*, *30*, 1222–1228. http://dx.doi.org/10.1002/mds.26219.

Waters, C. H., Nausieda, P., Dzyak, L., et al. (2015). Long-term treatment with extended-release carbidopa-levodopa (IPX066) in early and advanced Parkinson's disease: A 9-month open-label extension trial. *CNS Drugs*, *29*, 341–350.

Zanettini, R., Antonini, A., Gatto, G., Gentile, R., Tesei, S., & Pezzoli, G. (2007). Valvular heart disease and the use of dopamine agonists for Parkinson's disease. *The New England Journal of Medicine*, *356*(1), 39–46.

CHAPTER THIRTEEN

Treatment of Nonmotor Symptoms in Parkinson's Disease

Anna Sauerbier*,[1], Ilaria Cova[†], Miguel Rosa-Grilo*, Raquel N. Taddei*, Laurie K. Mischley[‡,§,¶], K. Ray Chaudhuri[||,#,**]

*King's College London and King's College Hospital, London, United Kingdom
[†]Center for Research and Treatment on Cognitive Dysfunctions, Institute of Clinical Neurology, Luigi Sacco' Hospital, University of Milan, Milan, Italy
[‡]Bastyr University Research Institute, Kenmore, WA, United States
[§]UW Graduate Program in Nutritional Sciences, Seattle, WA, United States
[¶]University of Washington (UW), Seattle, WA, United States
[||]National Parkinson Foundation International Centre of Excellence, Kings College and Kings College Hospital, London, United Kingdom
[#]Maurice Wohl Clinical Neuroscience Institute, Kings College, London, United Kingdom
**National Institute for Health Research (NIHR) Mental Health Biomedical Research Centre (BRC) and Dementia Unit at South London and Maudsley NHS Foundation Trust, London, United Kingdom
[1]Corresponding author: e-mail address: annasauerbier@nhs.net

Contents

Abstract

Nonmotor symptoms (NMS) are integral to Parkinson's disease (PD) and the management can often be challenging. In spite of the growing evidence that NMS have a key impact on the quality of life of patients and caregivers, most clinical trials still focus on motor symptoms as primary outcomes. As a consequence strong evidence-based treatment recommendations for NMS occurring in PD are spare. In this chapter, the current data addressing the treatment of major NMS such as sleep, cognitive and autonomic dysfunction, and depression and anxiety are described.

International Review of Neurobiology, Volume 132
ISSN 0074-7742
http://dx.doi.org/10.1016/bs.irn.2017.03.002

1. INTRODUCTION

Nonmotor symptoms (NMS) are integral to the course of Parkinson's disease (PD) (Sauerbier & Ray Chaudhuri, 2014), and being one of the key factors for the quality of life of both patients and caregivers, NMS play a major role in the management of this neurodegenerative condition (Martinez-Martin, 2014). Since 2006, objective measurements of NMS with validated tools (questionnaires and scales) have been developed, which are now in widespread use in standard clinical care and clinical trials. The two main NMS tools are the patient-completed NMS Questionnaire (NMS Quest) and health-professional-completed NMS Scale (NMSS) (Chaudhuri, Healy, & Schapira, 2006; Chaudhuri et al., 2007; Chaudhuri, Martinez-Martin, et al., 2006). In addition, NMS can also be measured, although in a limited fashion, by the NMS section of the Movement Disorders Society-Unified Parkinson's Disease Rating Scale (MDS-UPDRS) (Goetz et al., 2008). Fig. 1 summarizes a proposed pathway that might help to assess and manage NMS in clinical practice.

In this chapter, the published clinical trials addressing the treatment of NMS in PD will be reviewed with a particular focus on trials using the NMS Quest and NMSS, which have the most widely published clinometric data. Major NMS, including sleep, cognitive and autonomic dysfunction, as well as depression and anxiety, will be described in detail.

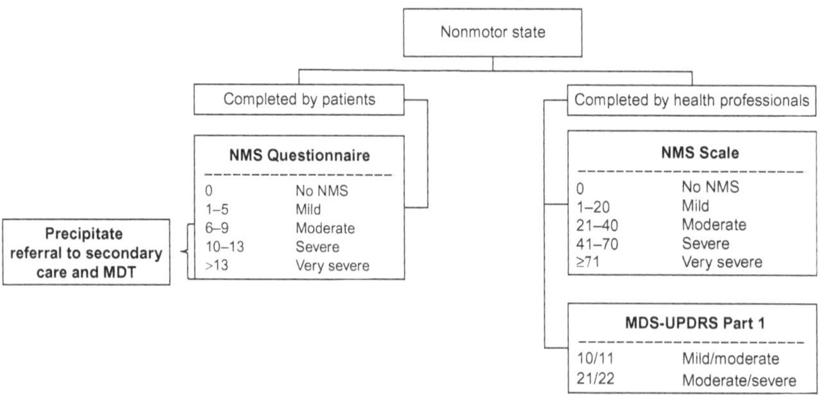

Fig. 1 Proposed pathway to assess NMS in a holistic manner in clinic and consider further management. *MDT*, multidisciplinary team; *MDS-UPDRS*, Movement Disorders Society-Unified Parkinson's Disease Rating Scale; *NMS*, nonmotor symptoms. *Adapted from Sauerbier, A., Qamar, M. A., Rajah, T., & Chaudhuri, K.R. (2016). New concepts in the pathogenesis and presentation of Parkinson's disease.* Clinical Medicine (London, England), 16, *365–370.*

2. SLEEP DISTURBANCES

Sleep disturbances are common in PD and consist mainly of nighttime sleep difficulties such as insomnia, rapid eye movement (REM) sleep behavior disorder (RBD), restless legs syndrome (RLS), periodic limb movement (PLM), and sleep-disordered breathing, but also of excessive daytime sleepiness (EDS) and early morning "off" (Chahine, Amara, & Videnovic, 2016). In clinical practice, apart from the NMS Quest and NMSS, more specific tools, such as the Parkinson's disease Sleep Scale version 1 and 2 (PDSS-1 and PDSS-2) (Chaudhuri et al., 2007; Trenkwalder, Kohnen, et al., 2011) and the Epworth Sleepiness Scale (ESS) (Hagell & Broman, 2007; Johns, 1991), are available to investigate sleep disturbances in the bedside.

Despite the overwhelming importance, only few randomized controlled trials and high-quality open-label studies have approached the management of sleep disturbance in PD (Chahine et al., 2016; Rodrigues, Caldas, & Ferreira, 2016; Schrag, Sauerbier, & Chaudhuri, 2015).

As first-line interventions, general sleep hygiene recommendations cannot be overemphasized, and the potential effects of dopaminergic therapy on sleep investigated. It has been recognized that some sleep symptoms can be improved while others can be worsened by dopaminergic therapy. EDS can worsen with the initiation of dopamine agonists for example, possibly due to the action of dopamine D3 agonists, as has been suggested in the proposed Park Sleep subtype (Sauerbier, Qamar, Rajah, & Chaudhuri, 2016).

On the other hand, sleep fragmentation can be partly explained by nighttime motor fluctuations and RLS. Continuous drug delivery, as well as controlled-release formulations of levodopa or dopamine agonists, transdermal delivery of rotigotine, and addition of inhibitors of catechol-O-methyltransferase or monoamine oxidase-B might be effective improving nocturnal motor disability, fluctuation, as well as early morning "off." Aforesaid observations have been previously reported with cabergoline (Marco, Appiah-Kubi, & Chaudhuri, 2002; Romigi et al., 2006). A recent open-label, multicenter study has shown a positive effect of the monoamine oxidase-B inhibitor rasagiline as mono- or add-on therapy on sleep disturbances as assessed by PDSS (Panisset et al., 2016). Additionally, rotigotine transdermal patches have shown to ameliorate sleep dysfunction in PD in randomized trials. The multicenter, randomized, double-blind, placebo-controlled "RECOVER" trial investigated the effect of the rotigotine transdermal patch on sleep dysfunction and showed a significant improvement in nocturnal sleep disturbances as assessed by PDSS-2 and NMSS (Trenkwalder, Kies, et al., 2011). These results are in line with findings of open-label studies and a randomized trial using subjective clinical scales and objective recordings, including polysomnography (Calandra-Buonaura et al., 2016; Pagonabarraga et al., 2015; Pierantozzi et al., 2016). Furthermore, the "RECOVER" study reported a low incidence of EDS as an adverse event (Trenkwalder, Kies, et al., 2011). It has been hypothesized that this might be at least partly explained by the fact that rotigotine does not share the high-affinity D3 receptor profile of other dopamine agonists as discussed above (Chaudhuri & Sauerbier, 2016; Sauerbier et al., 2016).

Beneficial effects have been observed with PD advanced therapies in open-label studies as well. Results from a surveillance-based study on apomorphine showed a significant improvement in the domain of sleep/fatigue of NMSS at follow-up, of particular importance in individual items assessing fatigue, sleep-onset insomnia, and RLS (Martinez-Martin et al., 2011). The open-label, prospective, observational, multicenter "Euroinf" study compared patients on apomorphine infusion to patients on intrajejunal levodopa infusion (IJLI) which demonstrated a significantly higher improvement in NMSS sleep domain for those on IJLI (Martinez-Martin et al., 2015). Zibetti et al. also noted improvement in subjective sleep quality and EDS as assessed by PDSS-2 and ESS in patients treated with IJLI (Zibetti et al., 2013).

Significant improvement has been described after bilateral subthalamic stimulation measured by the sleep domain on the NMSS and PDSS (Dafsari et al., 2016). Furthermore, similar results have been achieved after microsubthalamotomy in a small sample of 15 patients (Merlino et al., 2014). However, a recent systematic review on deep brain stimulation (DBS) and sleep–wake functions in PD has summarized that the current literature is conflicting and more work is needed in this field (Eugster, Bargiotas, Bassetti, & Michael Schuepbach, 2016).

When further pharmacological intervention is warranted to treat insomnia, antidepressants (including tricyclics, trazodone, agomelatine), nonbenzodiazepine hypnotics (including eszopiclone), as well as melatonin have been tried (Dowling et al., 2005; Rios Romenets et al., 2013; Seppi et al., 2011). In a pilot study doxepin, a tricyclic antidepressant (TCA) with selective histaminergic antagonistic action, has been reported to be effective at low dosages (Rios Romenets et al., 2013).

Additionally, it is important to consider the sleep environment and ensure that RBD sleep-related injury is prevented (Chahine et al., 2016).

Melatonin and clonazepam are prescribed routinely to control RBD, with the former showing a more favorable adverse event profile in patients with concomitant sleep-disordered breathing (Aurora et al., 2010). A randomized, double-blind, placebo-controlled trial investigated the effects of rivastigmine transdermal patch (4.6 mg/day) in a small sample of PD patients with severe RBD (>5 episodes/week) refractory to clonazepam (2 mg/day) and melatonin (5 mg/day). Rivastigmine was found to significantly decrease the number of RBD episodes at 3-week follow-up (Di Giacopo et al., 2012).

RLS in PD is currently not yet fully understood, and there are currently no randomized controlled trials addressing the different therapies to improve RLS specifically occurring in PD. Generally, iron deficiency should be excluded as a cause of RLS in PD. Studies investigating the effect of DBS have reported conflicting findings (Chahine et al., 2016).

EDS should be primarily addressed by reducing potentially causative medications. Combined analysis of three randomized, double-blind, placebo-controlled trials supports the evidence that modafinil (100–200 mg/day) taken in the morning improves EDS in PD patients (Rodrigues et al., 2016). Other stimulants such as caffeine and methylphenidate have been investigated as well; however, these therapies remain investigational (Chahine et al., 2016; Postuma et al., 2012). Sodium oxybate at nighttime has also been suggested for the treatment of EDS (with caution because of addictive potential), and further studies are currently investigating this effect (Ondo et al., 2008). One study has shown that when continuous positive airway pressure is used to treat sleep apnea, it has an additional positive effect on EDS as well (Neikrug et al., 2014).

Apart from pharmacological therapies, some nonpharmacological interventions have reported interesting positive results, such as a multidisciplinary intensive rehabilitation treatment (Frazzitta et al., 2015) and bright light therapy (Rutten et al., 2012). However, such treatments are not readily available worldwide.

In conclusion, management of sleep dysfunction is complex and needs accurate diagnosis of the specific type of disturbance, which can be achieved with clinical tools such as the PDSS. Therapy should then be tailored according to specific issues such as early morning "off," nocturnal motor symptoms, sleep fragmentation, RLS, and RBD. Apart from the few but increasing number of studies addressing sleep disturbances in PD, strong recommendations cannot be made at this point.

3. COGNITIVE IMPAIRMENT

Cognitive impairment is a common NMS in PD (Broeders et al., 2013). Initial deficits presenting as mild cognitive impairment (MCI) can be detected in 15% of patients at the time of diagnosis (Aarsland & Kramberger, 2015). Those may remain stable or progress to PD dementia (PDD) over time. Only a few systematic studies are currently available which addressed the treatment of cognitive impairment specifically in PD. In a recent systematic review, physical activity was shown to positively impact cognition in PD (Cusso, Donald, & Khoo, 2016). The effect of drug therapy on MCI is currently controversial (Strohle et al., 2015). A recent study highlighted that application of anodal transcranial direct current stimulation could improve cognitive abilities in MCI PD in particular in combination with physical therapy (Manenti et al., 2016).

Treatment of PDD in clinical practice can involve the use of cholinergic agents. Rivastigmine has been shown to be efficacious in large, randomized placebo-controlled trials (Seppi et al., 2011). Furthermore, open-label and randomized controlled studies also suggested that donepezil can improve cognition in PD, but the results are inconclusive and as such no general recommendations could be made (Cooney & Stacy, 2016). Galantamine has only been evaluated for PDD in open-label studies and evidence is currently insufficient for the recommendation in PDD treatment (Seppi et al., 2011). A recent systematic meta-analysis suggested that memantine, a low-affinity antagonist to glutamate NMDA receptors, possibly shows a slight improvement in global impression of cognitive dysfunctions in PD (Wang et al., 2015).

Moreover, a small, open-label, pilot study of atomoxetine, a norepinephrine reuptake inhibitor, for cognitive impairment found an improvement in executive functions measures (Marsh, Biglan, Gerstenhaber, & Williams, 2009).

In conclusion, cognitive dysfunction may occur in PD even at early stages, now recognized as Park Cognitive subtype (Sauerbier et al., 2016). Cognitive dysfunction is one of the key problems in advanced PD and reasonable evidence base exists with cholinergic agents in PD. However, further research needs to be conducted.

4. DEPRESSIVE SYMPTOMS AND ANXIETY

The prevalence of depression and anxiety disorders in PD varies considerably across different settings and the screening tools used. Recently published systematic reviews estimate a prevalence for both major and minor depression and any anxiety disorder to be around 30% (Broen, Narayen, Kuijf, Dissanayaka, & Leentjens, 2016; Goodarzi et al., 2016).

Behavioral and psychosocial interventions in PD patients have been shown to have a beneficial effect particularly during the acute management of episodes with depression and anxiety, while longer-term effects are still unclear (Yang, Sajatovic, & Walter, 2012). In this context, cognitive behavioral therapy (CBT), with some studies looking at telephone-administered CBT, has shown promising results (Armento et al., 2012; Bomasang-Layno, Fadlon, Murray, & Himelhoch, 2015). Bright light therapy has been suggested as beneficial for depressive symptoms in PD, possibly through restoring the circadian rhythm which may be involved in the development of depressive symptoms (Rutten et al., 2012). A recent systematic review has highlighted the potential positive impact of physical activity on NMS such as depression; however, further studies are needed to confirm this (Cusso et al., 2016). The first treatment with electroconvulsive therapy (ECT) for psychiatric and neurological disorders goes back to 1947 (Moellentine et al., 1998; Narang, Glowacki, & Lippman, 2015). ECT has been performed in the past, however the role of ECT in clinical practice is disputed and further robust clinical trial data is needed before ECT is recommended for refractory depression (Borisovskaya, Bryson, Buchholz, Samii, & Borson, 2016).

Regarding pharmacological interventions, it is important to establish if depressive symptoms and anxiety are related to nonmotor fluctuations in which case adjustment of dopaminergic medication should be considered (Storch et al., 2013).

There is now also good evidence that several dopaminergic drugs are useful to treat depressive symptoms in PD. Pramipexole, a dopamine agonist, has been shown to be efficacious for the treatment of depressive symptoms in PD (Barone et al., 2010). The "RECOVER" study showed an improvement in depressive symptoms assessed by the Beck Depression Inventory (BDI-II) and NMSS with rotigotine (Trenkwalder, Kies, et al., 2011). Furthermore, a prospective open-label multicenter study investigating the effect of ropinirole over 6 months showed a significant improvement in depressive symptoms and anxiety measured by the Hamilton Anxiety Scale (HAM-A) and Montgomery–Asberg Depression Rating Scale in patients with motor fluctuations (Rektorova et al., 2008). Other studies have demonstrated similar results, describing considerable improvements in depressive symptoms with ropinirole (Buchwald, Angersbach, & Jost, 2007). Published data of the effect of rasagiline on depressive symptoms in PD patients are controversial. A post hoc analysis of the data from the ADAGIO study in drug-naïve PD patients showed that the add-on therapy with rasagiline (1 or 2 mg per day) had a beneficial effect on depression in PD patients on antidepressive medication (Smith, Eyal, & Weintraub, 2015). However, other studies do not confirm this positive finding (Barone et al., 2015). A multicenter, open-label, prospective, observational 6-month study comparing the effect of apomorphine to IJLI on NMS, motor symptoms, and quality of life indicated that both advanced therapies improve the NMSS domain mood/apathy with a superiority observed with apomorphine (Martinez-Martin et al., 2015).

Furthermore, serotonin–norepinephrine reuptake inhibitors such as mirtazapine and venlafaxine as well as serotonin selective reuptake inhibitors (SSRIs) such as fluoxetine, sertraline, citalopram, and paroxetine are among the commonly used treatments for depressive symptoms and anxiety in PD. Moreover, TCAs including amitriptyline and nortriptyline are commonly used in clinical practice. Many would regard SSRIs as first choice, even though published literature is conflicting (Pena et al., 2016).

In addition, omega-3 fatty-acid supplementation has been reported to be useful for depressive symptoms in PD (Da Silva et al., 2008).

DBS with subthalamic nucleus (STN) or internal globus pallidus stimulation showed a short-term improvement in depression (mainly class I and II data) and anxiety (class I data) with a waning in effect over the longer term (Couto, Monteiro, Oliveira, Lunet, & Massano, 2014). Differences between both targets could not be elucidated.

In conclusion, depression and anxiety is integral to PD and can occur as part of the disease process or nonmotor fluctuations. Management therefore needs to address the underlying cause; however, robust evidence based for good antidepressants and antianxiolytics including NSRIs, SSRIs TCA, dopamine agonists, and other agents is still lacking. At this moment in time, current data do not indicate toward one specific class of antidepressants when compared with a placebo.

5. ORTHOSTATIC HYPOTENSION

Orthostatic hypotension (OH) is a clinical sign defined by a drop of systolic blood pressure (SBP) of at least 20 mmHg or diastolic blood pressure of at least 10 mmHg within 3 min after assuming a standing position. It may be asymptomatic or accompanied with orthostatic symptoms such as dizziness, lightheadedness, or syncope (Freeman et al., 2011). Prevalence of OH in PD is estimated to be around 30%–40% (Velseboer, De Haan, Wieling, Goldstein, & De Bie, 2011). OH prevalence increases with disease duration (Rocchi et al., 2015) and might be worsened by dopaminergic therapy in which case a dose reduction in symptomatic and refractory cases should be considered (Park & Stacy, 2011).

The management of neurogenic OH (nOH) in PD is complex and requires patient education to optimally control symptoms that have functional impact on activities of daily living. Recommended practical values are a standing SBP $\geq$90 mmHg and a supine SBP $\leq$180 mmHg (Low & Tomalia, 2015).

Nonpharmacological therapies are first-line interventions. Increased salt intake, increased water intake, and compression stockings ameliorate orthostatic symptoms (Wu & Hohler, 2015). Furthermore, drinking caffeine-rich beverages, practice regular exercise, and avoiding hot baths might provide benefit for some patients (Figueroa, Basford, & Low, 2010; Sánchez-Ferro, Benito-León, & Gómez-Esteban, 2013).

Several pharmacological therapies are available, and these are often administered in conjunction with nonpharmacologic interventions. Fludrocortisone, midodrine, droxidopa, domperidone, pyridostigmine, and yohimbine have been used with different profiles of efficacy, mechanisms of action, and side effects (Wu & Hohler, 2015). Domperidone might help OH; however, owing to cardiovascular risks this cannot be routinely recommended. Furthermore, drug therapies vary between countries.

Droxidopa (L-*threo*-dihydroxyphenylserine) is a synthetic catechol-amino acid that is converted to norepinephrine by the enzyme DOPA decarboxylase. Droxidopa has been approved by the Food and Drug Administration (FDA) in the United States for use in nOH in PD since 2014, partly based on results from several studies including multicenter, double-blind, randomized placebo-controlled studies (Biaggioni et al., 2015; Hauser, Isaacson, Lisk, Hewitt, & Rowse, 2015; Kaufmann et al., 2014). However, not all studies confirmed the beneficial effect of droxidopa and further investigations are needed (Schrag et al., 2015).

Only a few studies assessed the effect of DBS on autonomous symptoms including OH problems in PD patients. In a small study involving 14 PD patients, an improvement in autonomic regulation in PD patients was observed (Stemper et al., 2006), and this positive effect on OH has been confirmed by other groups (Kurtis, Rajah, Delgado, & Dafsari, 2017).

In contrast, other studies could not find major effects of DBS on cardiovascular autonomic nervous system functions (Erola, Haapaniemi, Heikkinen, Huikuri, & Myllya, 2006; Lipp et al., 2005; Ludwig et al., 2007). Whether this potential positive effect is secondary to the reduction of oral medication after surgery or is a direct result of stimulating central pathways remains to be clarified and needs further investigation.

In summary, OH occurs more commonly in PD than initially thought. Newer promising pharmacological treatments such as droxidopa are adding to the currently widely available therapies including midodrine or fludrocortisone. While conventional and supportive therapies are effective, large-scale control studies with new investigational products are required.

6. URINARY DYSFUNCTION

Lower urinary tract symptoms (LUTS) and dysfunction are commonly reported to play a key role in the quality of life of PD patients; however, randomized clinical trials addressing urinary dysfunction are currently sparse. LUTS are composed of two major categories: storage symptoms (e.g., urgency, frequency, nocturia, and incontinence) and voiding symptoms (e.g., hesitancy, interrupted or poor stream, and double voiding), and both are reported to occur in PD (Sakakibara et al., 2014). Storage symptoms are thought to be related to detrusor overactivity, and voiding symptoms may result from bladder hypoactivity or an obstruction in the lower urinary tract. Nocturia is one of the most reported symptoms followed by frequency (Mcdonald, Winge, & Burn, 2017).

When addressing urinary dysfunction, it is important to establish if the symptoms are related to fluctuations in which case adjustment of dopaminergic medication can be considered. However, the role of dopaminergic medication in the management of LUTS is unclear, with most studies using urodynamic studies to date showing conflicting results (Mcdonald et al., 2017; Sakakibara, Panicker, Finazzi-Agro, Iacovelli, & Bruschini, 2016). Even though bladder dysfunction might be related to PD itself, it is important to check for common bladder diseases as recently summarized by Sakakibara et al. (2016). Male and female patients over 50 years old should be investigated for benign prostatic enlargement and stress-induced urinary incontinence, respectively (Sakakibara et al., 2016).

Antimuscarinics are used routinely in clinical practice to treat overactive bladder, with oxybutynin being the most investigated one.

Solifenacin, darifenacin, and trospium were approved by the FDA in 2004 for their use in overactive bladder (Hesch, 2007). A recent study by the Parkinson Study Group with a randomized, placebo-controlled three-site setting (measuring the mean number of micturitions per 24 h as a primary outcome) showed no significant improvement among the treated group with Solifenacin, but showed a significant reduction in the number of incontinence and nocturia episodes (Zesiewicz et al., 2015). Propiverine and tolterodine have also been investigated in people with detrusor overactivity and have shown beneficial results, however, well designed studies in PD are currently lacking (Sakakibara et al., 2016).

Intravesical botulinum toxin injections have been reported to be successful in treating hyperactive bladder dysfunction (Giannantoni et al., 2011; Kulaksizoglu & Parman, 2010).

Newer treatment options currently being investigated for bladder dysfunction include: a beta-3 adrenergic agonist such as mirabegron, DBS, as well as posterior tibial nerve stimulation (Sakakibara et al., 2016; Schrag et al., 2015).

In conclusion, urinary dysfunction may complicate PD from an early stage and might even be a prodromal sign. Management of urinary dysfunction remains a key unmet need, although recent clinical trials with solifenacin seem promising. Newer drugs such as mirabegron might provide an important pharmacological alternative to anticholinergics in patients with cognitive impairment.

7. GASTROINTESTINAL DYSFUNCTION

Gastrointestinal dysfunction plays a key role in PD, with constipation being the most common symptom (Rossi, Merello, & Perez-Lloret, 2015). In the literature, constipation is characterized as less than three bowel movements a week or having to strain to pass a stool (Chaudhuri, Martinez-Martin, et al., 2006; Poirier et al., 2016; Postuma, Romenets, & Rakheja, 2012). Limited data are published on the management of constipation in PD patients. In the literature, constipation in PD is sometimes divided into two types: constipation due to slow colonic transit and constipation due to defecatory dysfunction, which is often related to pelvic floor dyssynergia (Rossi et al., 2015).

In relation to the first type of constipation, after exclusion of secondary causes, lifestyle changes are among the first-line recommendation as they can have a significant positive impact. These include an increase in the amount of fiber and water intake as well as physical activity (Barboza, Okun, & Moshiree, 2015; Rossi et al., 2015). In case these nonpharmacological strategies are not sufficiently successful, bulk-forming laxatives such as ispaghula husk and hyperosmotic laxatives including polyethylene glycol (PEG, macrogol) have been shown to be useful to treat constipation in PD. Additionally, the FDA-approved chloride channel activator called lubiprostone has been shown to be useful to treat constipation. Also, the serotonin 5-HT4 receptor agonist prucalopride has been studied (Barboza et al., 2015; Shin et al., 2014).

Stimulant laxatives such as bisacodyl are effective but long-term use is not recommended due to potential side effects.

On the other hand, levodopa or apomorphine injection, botulinum toxin injections into the puborectalis muscle, and nonpharmacological interventions like biofeedback therapy or functional magnetic stimulation have been reported to improve the defecatory dysfunction-related constipation (Rossi et al., 2015).

Another development has addressed the effect of ghrelin receptor agonist (HM01) in rats, in vitro as well as in vivo, and found promising results; however, these need further investigation (Karasawa et al., 2014).

In conclusion, gastrointestinal dysfunction is a common nonmotor feature in PD, with constipation being the most frequent one. Exclusion of secondary causes is important, and nonpharmacological treatment strategies can often offer a considerable improvement. Several pharmacological treatments such as laxatives are routinely used in clinical practice, while new drugs are currently under development.

8. NUTRITION AND PARKINSON'S DISEASE

While historically relegated to the symptomatic management of dysphagia, constipation, and interactions between dietary protein and levodopa, it is now evident that the topic of nutrition in PD is more complex than once thought. Epidemiological studies suggest coffee, tea, dark berries, a plant-based diet, and dairy avoidance decrease PD incidence (Gao, Cassidy, Schwarzschild, Rimm, & Ascherio, 2012; Gao et al., 2007; Jiang, Ju, Jiang, & Zhang, 2014; Qi & Li, 2014), and studies are underway to evaluate whether these variables are associated with PD progression (Mischley, 2015). Early involvement of the gastrointestinal tract is supported by the finding that constipation and α-synuclein aggregation are observed in the salivary glands and intestinal mucosa over a decade prior to the onset of PD motor symptoms (Adams-Carr et al., 2016; Mukherjee, Biswas, & Das, 2016). Recently, alterations in the intestinal microbiome have been described (Scheperjans, 2016), and a dietary *Lactobacillus* supplement was shown to improve bowel health (Cassani et al., 2011). Beyond diet, perturbations in essential metabolites have also been demonstrated in PD; patients are more likely to be deficient in glutathione (Zeevalk, Razmpour, & Bernard, 2008), coenzyme Q10 (Mischley, Allen, & Bradley, 2012), lithium (Mischley, 2013), and folic acid, the latter attributable to a levodopa side effect (Paul & Borah, 2016). Not all drug–nutrient interactions are negative, as several studies suggest cytidine diphosphate choline has a levodopa-sparing effect (Cubells & Hernando, 1988). It is unclear whether a subset of PD symptoms are manifestations of nutritional deficiency symptoms or whether depletion of nutrients is associated with disease progression (Mischley, 2014). To date, no guidelines exist for the screening, evaluation, and management of nutrition in PD.

9. CONCLUSION: NONMOTOR SUBTYPE-SPECIFIC TREATMENT IN PARKINSON'S DISEASE?

NMS in PD remain a major clinical and research challenge. Fifty years since the discovery of Levodopa dramatically reversed the motor syndrome of PD, research and clinical care in PD has focused on motor PD. NMS have remained underresearched, underfunded, and underexplored. Treatment also remains a key unmet need. In this chapter, some recent advances in the management of NMS in PD are highlighted. However, this is just a drop in the ocean, and much needs to be done in the coming years. The recognition of specific NMS subtypes is likely to generate trials focused on subtype-specific medicine and more individualized treatment in future (Marras & Chaudhuri, 2016; Sauerbier et al., 2016). Such strategy will enhance the quality of life of many PD patients with the high nonmotor burden in future.

REFERENCES

Aarsland, D., & Kramberger, M. G. (2015). Neuropsychiatric symptoms in Parkinson's disease. *Journal of Parkinson's Disease*, *5*, 659–667.

Adams-Carr, K. L., Bestwick, J. P., Shribman, S., Lees, A., Schrag, A., & Noyce, A. J. (2016). Constipation preceding Parkinson's disease: A systematic review and meta-analysis. *Journal of Neurology, Neurosurgery & Psychiatry*, *87*, 710–716.

Armento, M. E., Stanley, M. A., Marsh, L., Kunik, M. E., York, M. K., Bush, A. L., et al. (2012). Cognitive behavioral therapy for depression and anxiety in Parkinson's disease: A clinical review. *Journal of Parkinson's Disease*, *2*, 135–151.

Aurora, R. N., Zak, R. S., Maganti, R. K., Auerbach, S. H., Casey, K. R., Chowdhuri, S., et al. (2010). Best practice guide for the treatment of REM sleep behavior disorder (RBD). *Journal of Clinical Sleep Medicine*, *6*, 85–95.

Barboza, J. L., Okun, M. S., & Moshiree, B. (2015). The treatment of gastroparesis, constipation and small intestinal bacterial overgrowth syndrome in patients with Parkinson's disease. *Expert Opinion on Pharmacotherapy*, *16*, 2449–2464.

Barone, P., Poewe, W., Albrecht, S., Debieuvre, C., Massey, D., Rascol, O., et al. (2010). Pramipexole for the treatment of depressive symptoms in patients with Parkinson's disease: A randomised, double-blind, placebo-controlled trial. *Lancet Neurology*, *9*, 573–580.

Barone, P., Santangelo, G., Morgante, L., Onofrj, M., Meco, G., Abbruzzese, G., et al. (2015). A randomized clinical trial to evaluate the effects of rasagiline on depressive symptoms in non-demented Parkinson's disease patients. *European Journal of Neurology*, *22*, 1184–1191.

Biaggioni, I., Freeman, R., Mathias, C. J., Low, P., Hewitt, L. A., & Kaufmann, H. (2015). Randomized withdrawal study of patients with symptomatic neurogenic orthostatic hypotension responsive to droxidopa. *Hypertension*, *65*, 101–107.

Bomasang-Layno, E., Fadlon, I., Murray, A. N., & Himelhoch, S. (2015). Antidepressive treatments for Parkinson's disease: A systematic review and meta-analysis. *Parkinsonism & Related Disorders*, *21*, 833–842. discussion 833.

Borisovskaya, A., Bryson, W. C., Buchholz, J., Samii, A., & Borson, S. (2016). Electroconvulsive therapy for depression in Parkinson's disease: Systematic review of evidence and recommendations. *Neurodegenerative Disease Management*, *6*, 161–176.

Broeders, M., De Bie, R. M., Velseboer, D. C., Speelman, J. D., Muslimovic, D., & Schmand, B. (2013). Evolution of mild cognitive impairment in Parkinson disease. *Neurology*, *81*, 346–352.

Broen, M. P., Narayen, N. E., Kuijf, M. L., Dissanayaka, N. N., & Leentjens, A. F. (2016). Prevalence of anxiety in Parkinson's disease: A systematic review and meta-analysis. *Movement Disorders*, *31*, 1125–1133.

Buchwald, B., Angersbach, D., & Jost, W. H. (2007). Improvements in motor and nonmotor symptoms in parkinson patients under ropinirole therapy. *Fortschritte der Neurologie-Psychiatrie*, *75*, 236–241.

Calandra-Buonaura, G., Guaraldi, P., Doria, A., Zanigni, S., Nassetti, S., Favoni, V., et al. (2016). Rotigotine objectively improves sleep in Parkinson's disease: An open-label pilot study with actigraphic recording. *Parkinson's Disease*, *2016*, 3724148.

Cassani, E., Privitera, G., Pezzoli, G., Pusani, C., Madio, C., Iorio, L., et al. (2011). Use of probiotics for the treatment of constipation in Parkinson's disease patients. *Minerva Gastroenterologica e Dietologica*, *57*, 117–121.

Chahine, L. M., Amara, A. W., & Videnovic, A. (2016). A systematic review of the literature on disorders of sleep and wakefulness in Parkinson's disease from 2005 to 2015. *Sleep Medicine Review*. pii: S1087-0792(16)30075-2. http://dx.doi.org/10.1016/j.smrv.2016.08.001.

Chaudhuri, K. R., Healy, D. G., & Schapira, A. H. (2006). Non-motor symptoms of Parkinson's disease: Diagnosis and management. *Lancet Neurology*, *5*, 235–245.

Chaudhuri, K. R., Martinez-Martin, P., Brown, R. G., Sethi, K., Stocchi, F., Odin, P., et al. (2007). The metric properties of a novel non-motor symptoms scale for Parkinson's disease: Results from an international pilot study. *Movement Disorders*, *22*, 1901–1911.

Chaudhuri, K. R., Martinez-Martin, P., Schapira, A. H., Stocchi, F., Sethi, K., Odin, P., et al. (2006). International multicenter pilot study of the first comprehensive self-completed nonmotor symptoms questionnaire for Parkinson's disease: The NMSQuest study. *Movement Disorders*, *21*, 916–923.

Chaudhuri, K. R., & Sauerbier, A. (2016). Parkinson disease. Unravelling the nonmotor mysteries of Parkinson disease. *Nature Reviews. Neurology*, *12*, 10–11.

Cooney, J. W., & Stacy, M. (2016). Neuropsychiatric issues in Parkinson's disease. *Current Neurology and Neuroscience Reports*, *16*, 49.

Couto, M. I., Monteiro, A., Oliveira, A., Lunet, N., & Massano, J. (2014). Depression and anxiety following deep brain stimulation in Parkinson's disease: Systematic review and meta-analysis. *Acta Médica Portuguesa, 27*, 372–382.

Cubells, J. M., & Hernando, C. (1988). Clinical trial on the use of cytidine diphosphate choline in Parkinson's disease. *Clinical Therapeutics, 10*, 664–671.

Cusso, M. E., Donald, K. J., & Khoo, T. K. (2016). The impact of physical activity on non-motor symptoms in Parkinson's disease: A systematic review. *Frontiers in Medicine (Lausanne), 3*, 35.

Dafsari, H. S., Reddy, P., Herchenbach, C., Wawro, S., Petry-Schmelzer, J. N., Visser-Vandewalle, V., et al. (2016). Beneficial effects of bilateral subthalamic stimulation on non-motor symptoms in Parkinson's disease. *Brain Stimulation, 9*, 78–85.

Da Silva, T. M., Munhoz, R. P., Alvarez, C., Naliwaiko, K., Kiss, A., Andreatini, R., et al. (2008). Depression in Parkinson's disease: A double-blind, randomized, placebo-controlled pilot study of omega-3 fatty-acid supplementation. *Journal of Affective Disorders, 111*, 351–359.

Di Giacopo, R., Fasano, A., Quaranta, D., Della Marca, G., Bove, F., & Bentivoglio, A. R. (2012). Rivastigmine as alternative treatment for refractory REM behavior disorder in Parkinson's disease. *Movement Disorders, 27*, 559–561.

Dowling, G. A., Mastick, J., Colling, E., Carter, J. H., Singer, C. M., & Aminoff, M. J. (2005). Melatonin for sleep disturbances in Parkinson's disease. *Sleep Medicine, 6*, 459–466.

Erola, T., Haapaniemi, T., Heikkinen, E., Huikuri, H., & Myllya, V. (2006). Subthalamic nucleus deep brain stimulation does not alter long-term heart rate variability in Parkinson's disease. *Clinical Autonomic Research, 16*, 286–288.

Eugster, L., Bargiotas, P., Bassetti, C. L., & Michael Schuepbach, W. M. (2016). Deep brain stimulation and sleep-wake functions in Parkinson's disease: A systematic review. *Parkinsonism & Related Disorders, 32*, 12–19.

Figueroa, J. J., Basford, F. R., & Low, P. A. (2010). Preventing and treating orthostatic hypotension: As easy as A, B, C. *Cleveland Clinic Journal of Medicine, 77*, 298–306.

Frazzitta, G., Maestri, R., Ferrazzoli, D., Riboldazzi, G., Bera, R., Fontanesi, C., et al. (2015). Multidisciplinary intensive rehabilitation treatment improves sleep quality in Parkinson's disease. *Journal of Clinical Movement Disorders, 2*, 11.

Freeman, R., Wieling, W., Axelrod, F. B., Benditt, D. G., Benarroch, E., Biaggioni, I., et al. (2011). Consensus statement on the definition of orthostatic hypotension, neurally mediated syncope and the postural tachycardia syndrome. *Clinical Autonomic Research, 21*, 69–72.

Gao, X., Cassidy, A., Schwarzschild, M. A., Rimm, E. B., & Ascherio, A. (2012). Habitual intake of dietary flavonoids and risk of Parkinson disease. *Neurology, 78*, 1138–1145.

Gao, X., Chen, H., Fung, T. T., Logroscino, G., Schwarzschild, M. A., Hu, F. B., et al. (2007). Prospective study of dietary pattern and risk of Parkinson disease. *American Journal of Clinical Nutrition, 86*, 1486–1494.

Giannantoni, A., Conte, A., Proietti, S., Giovannozzi, S., Rossi, A., Fabbrini, G., et al. (2011). Botulinum toxin type A in patients with Parkinson's disease and refractory overactive bladder. *Journal of Urology, 186*, 960–964.

Goetz, C. G., Tilley, B. C., Shaftman, S. R., Stebbins, G. T., Fahn, S., Martinez-Martin, P., et al. (2008). Movement disorder society-sponsored revision of the unified Parkinson's Disease Rating Scale (MDS-UPDRS): Scale presentation and clinimetric testing results. *Movement Disorders, 23*, 2129–2170.

Goodarzi, Z., Mrklas, K. J., Roberts, D. J., Jette, N., Pringsheim, T., & Holroyd-Leduc, J. (2016). Detecting depression in Parkinson disease: A systematic review and meta-analysis. *Neurology, 87*, 426–437.

Hagell, P., & Broman, J. E. (2007). Measurement properties and hierarchical item structure of the Epworth sleepiness scale in Parkinson's disease. *Journal of Sleep Research, 16*, 102–109.

Hauser, R. A., Isaacson, S., Lisk, J. P., Hewitt, L. A., & Rowse, G. (2015). Droxidopa for the short-term treatment of symptomatic neurogenic orthostatic hypotension in Parkinson's disease (nOH306B). *Movement Disorders, 30*, 646–654.

Hesch, K. (2007). Agents for treatment of overactive bladder: A therapeutic class review. *Proceedings (Baylor University Medical Center), 20*, 307–314.

Jiang, W., Ju, C., Jiang, H., & Zhang, D. (2014). Dairy foods intake and risk of Parkinson's disease: A dose-response meta-analysis of prospective cohort studies. *European Journal of Epidemiology, 29*, 613–619.

Johns, M. W. (1991). A new method for measuring daytime sleepiness: The Epworth sleepiness scale. *Sleep, 14*, 540–545.

Karasawa, H., Pietra, C., Giuliano, C., Garcia-Rubio, S., Xu, X., Yakabi, S., et al. (2014). New ghrelin agonist, HM01 alleviates constipation and L-dopa-delayed gastric emptying in 6-hydroxydopamine rat model of Parkinson's disease. *Neurogastroenterology and Motility, 26*, 1771–1782.

Kaufmann, H., Freeman, R., Biaggioni, I., Low, P., Pedder, S., Hewitt, L. A., et al. (2014). Droxidopa for neurogenic orthostatic hypotension: A randomized, placebo-controlled, phase 3 trial. *Neurology, 83*, 328–335.

Kulaksizoglu, H., & Parman, Y. (2010). Use of botulinum toxin-A for the treatment of overactive bladder symptoms in patients with Parkinson's disease. *Parkinsonism & Related Disorders, 16*, 531–534.

Kurtis, M. M., Rajah, T., Delgado, L. F., & Dafsari, H. S. (2017). The effect of deep brain stimulation on the non-motor symptoms of Parkinson's disease: A critical review of the current evidence. *npj Parkinson's Disease, 3*, 16024.

Lipp, A., Tank, J., Trottenberg, T., Kupsch, A., Arnold, G., & Jordan, J. (2005). Sympathetic activation due to deep brain stimulation in the region of the STN. *Neurology, 65*, 774–775.

Low, P. A., & Tomalia, V. A. (2015). Orthostatic hypotension: Mechanisms, causes, management. *Journal of Clinical Neurology, 11*, 220–226.

Ludwig, J., Remien, P., Guballa, C., Binder, A., Binder, S., Schattschneider, J., et al. (2007). Effects of subthalamic nucleus stimulation and levodopa on the autonomic nervous system in Parkinson's disease. *Journal of Neurology, Neurosurgery & Psychiatry, 78*, 742–745.

Manenti, R., Brambilla, M., Benussi, A., Rosini, S., Cobelli, C., Ferrari, C., et al. (2016). Mild cognitive impairment in Parkinson's disease is improved by transcranial direct current stimulation combined with physical therapy. *Movement Disorders, 31*, 715–724.

Marco, A. D., Appiah-Kubi, L. S., & Chaudhuri, K. R. (2002). Use of the dopamine agonist cabergoline in the treatment of movement disorders. *Expert Opinion on Pharmacotherapy, 3*, 1481–1487.

Marras, C., & Chaudhuri, K. R. (2016). Nonmotor features of Parkinson's disease subtypes. *Movement Disorders, 31*, 1095–1102.

Marsh, L., Biglan, K., Gerstenhaber, M., & Williams, J. R. (2009). Atomoxetine for the treatment of executive dysfunction in Parkinson's disease: A pilot open-label study. *Movement Disorders, 24*, 277–282.

Martinez-Martin, P. (2014). Nonmotor symptoms and health-related quality of life in early Parkinson's disease. *Movement Disorders, 29*, 166–168.

Martinez-Martin, P., Reddy, P., Antonini, A., Henriksen, T., Katzenschlager, R., Odin, P., et al. (2011). Chronic subcutaneous infusion therapy with apomorphine in advanced Parkinson's disease compared to conventional therapy: A real life study of non motor effect. *Journal of Parkinson's Disease, 1*, 197–203.

Martinez-Martin, P., Reddy, P., Katzenschlager, R., Antonini, A., Todorova, A., Odin, P., et al. (2015). EuroInf: A multicenter comparative observational study of apomorphine and levodopa infusion in Parkinson's disease. *Movement Disorders*, *30*, 510–516.

Mcdonald, C., Winge, K., & Burn, D. J. (2017). Lower urinary tract symptoms in Parkinson's disease: Prevalence, aetiology and management. *Parkinsonism & Related Disorders*, *35*, 8–16.

Merlino, G., Lettieri, C., Mondani, M., Belgrado, E., Devigili, G., Mucchiut, M., et al. (2014). Microsubthalamotomy improves sleep in patients affected by advanced Parkinson's disease. *Sleep Medicine*, *15*, 637–641.

Mischley, L. K. (2013). *Lithium deficiency in Parkinson's disease*. Master of Public Health, University of Washington.

Mischley, L. K. (2014). Conditionally essential nutrients: The state of the science. *Journal of Food and Nutrition*, *1*, 1–4.

Mischley, L. K. (2015). *Complementary & alternative medicine in Parkinson's disease (CAM care in PD)*. ClinicalTrials.gov. U.S. National Institutes of Health.

Mischley, L. K., Allen, J., & Bradley, R. (2012). Coenzyme Q10 deficiency in patients with Parkinson's disease. *Journal of Neurological Sciences*, *318*, 72–75.

Moellentine, C., Rummans, T., Ahlskog, J. E., Harmsen, W. S., Suman, V. J., O'Connor, M. K., et al. (1998). Effectiveness of ECT in patients with parkinsonism. *Journal of Neuropsychiatry and Clinical Neurosciences*, *10*, 187–193.

Mukherjee, A., Biswas, A., & Das, S. K. (2016). Gut dysfunction in Parkinson's disease. *World Journal of Gastroenterology*, *22*, 5742–5752.

Narang, P., Glowacki, A., & Lippman, S. (2015). Electroconvulsive therapy intervention for Parkinson's disease. *Innovations in Clinical Neuroscience*, *12*, 25–28.

Neikrug, A. B., Liu, L., Avanzino, J. A., Maglione, J. E., Natarajan, L., Bradley, L., et al. (2014). Continuous positive airway pressure improves sleep and daytime sleepiness in patients with Parkinson disease and sleep apnea. *Sleep*, *37*, 177–185.

Ondo, W. G., Perkins, T., Swick, T., Hull, K. L., Jr., Jimenez, J. E., Garris, T. S., et al. (2008). Sodium oxybate for excessive daytime sleepiness in Parkinson disease: An open-label polysomnographic study. *Archives of Neurology*, *65*, 1337–1340.

Pagonabarraga, J., Pinol, G., Cardozo, A., Sanz, P., Puente, V., Otermin, P., et al. (2015). Transdermal rotigotine improves sleep fragmentation in Parkinson's disease: Results of the multicenter, prospective SLEEP-FRAM study. *Parkinson's Disease*, *2015*, 131508.

Panisset, M., Stril, J. L., Belanger, M., Lehoux, G., Coffin, D., & Chouinard, S. (2016). Open-label study of sleep disturbances in patients with Parkinson's disease treated with rasagiline. *Canadian Journal of Neurological Sciences*, *43*, 809–814.

Park, A., & Stacy, M. (2011). Dopamine-induced nonmotor symptoms of Parkinson's disease. *Parkinson's Disease*, *2011*, 485063.

Paul, R., & Borah, A. (2016). L-DOPA-induced hyperhomocysteinemia in Parkinson's disease: Elephant in the room. *Biochimica et Biophysica Acta*, *1860*, 1989–1997.

Pena, E., Mata, M., Lopez-Manzanares, L., Kurtis, M., Eimil, M., Martinez-Castrillo, J. C., et al. (2016). Antidepressants in Parkinson's disease. Recommendations by the movement disorder study group of the Neurological Association of Madrid. *Neurologia*. pii: S0213-4853(16)00055-4. http://dx.doi.org/10.1016/j.nrl.2016.02.002.

Pierantozzi, M., Placidi, F., Liguori, C., Albanese, M., Imbriani, P., Marciani, M. G., et al. (2016). Rotigotine may improve sleep architecture in Parkinson's disease: A double-blind, randomized, placebo-controlled polysomnographic study. *Sleep Medicine*, *21*, 140–144.

Poirier, A., Aubé, B., Côté, M., Morin, N., Di Paolo, T., & Soulet, D. (2016). Gastrointestinal dysfunctions in Parkinson's disease: Symptoms and treatments. *Parkinson's Disease*, *2016*, 6762528.

Postuma, R. B., Lang, A. E., Munhoz, R. P., Charland, K., Pelletier, A., Moscovich, M., et al. (2012). Caffeine for treatment of Parkinson disease: A randomized controlled trial. *Neurology, 79*, 651–658.

Postuma, R., Romenets, S. R., & Rakheja, R. (2012). *Physician guide: Non-motor symptoms of Parkinson's disease*. Montreal, Canada: McGill University Health Centre.

Qi, H., & Li, S. (2014). Dose-response meta-analysis on coffee, tea and caffeine consumption with risk of Parkinson's disease. *Geriatrics & Gerontology International, 14*, 430–439.

Rektorova, I., Balaz, M., Svatova, J., Zarubova, K., Honig, I., Dostal, V., et al. (2008). Effects of ropinirole on nonmotor symptoms of Parkinson disease: A prospective multicenter study. *Clinical Neuropharmacology, 31*, 261–266.

Rios Romenets, S., Creti, L., Fichten, C., Bailes, S., Libman, E., Pelletier, A., et al. (2013). Doxepin and cognitive behavioural therapy for insomnia in patients with Parkinson's disease—A randomized study. *Parkinsonism & Related Disorders, 19*, 670–675.

Rocchi, C., Pierantozzi, M., Galati, S., Chiaravalloti, A., Pisani, V., Prosperetti, C., et al. (2015). Autonomic function tests and MIBG in Parkinson's disease: Correlation to disease duration and motor symptoms. *CNS Neuroscience & Therapeutics, 21*, 727–732.

Rodrigues, T. M., Caldas, A. C., & Ferreira, J. J. (2016). Pharmacological interventions for daytime sleepiness and sleep disorders in Parkinson's disease: Systematic review and meta-analysis. *Parkinsonism & Related Disorders, 27*, 25–34.

Romigi, A., Stanzione, P., Marciani, M. G., Izzi, F., Placidi, F., Cervellino, A., et al. (2006). Effect of cabergoline added to levodopa treatment on sleep-wake cycle in idiopathic Parkinson's disease: An open label 24-hour polysomnographic study. *Journal of Neural Transmission (Vienna, Austria), 113*, 1909–1913.

Rossi, M., Merello, M., & Perez-Lloret, S. (2015). Management of constipation in Parkinson's disease. *Expert Opinion on Pharmacotherapy, 16*, 547–557.

Rutten, S., Vriend, C., Van Den Heuvel, O. A., Smit, J. H., Berendse, H. W., & Van Der Werf, Y. D. (2012). Bright light therapy in Parkinson's disease: An overview of the background and evidence. *Parkinson's Disease, 2012*, 767105.

Sakakibara, R., Panicker, J., Finazzi-Agro, E., Iacovelli, V., & Bruschini, H. (2016). A guideline for the management of bladder dysfunction in Parkinson's disease and other gait disorders. *Neurourology and Urodynamics, 35*, 551–563.

Sakakibara, R., Tateno, F., Nagao, T., Yamamoto, T., Uchiyama, T., Yamanishi, T., et al. (2014). Bladder function of patients with Parkinson's disease. *International Journal of Urology, 21*, 638–646.

Sánchez-Ferro, A., Benito-León, J., & Gómez-Esteban, J. C. (2013). The management of orthostatic hypotension in Parkinson's disease. *Frontiers in Neurology, 4*, 64.

Sauerbier, A., Jenner, P., Todorova, A., & Chaudhuri, K. (2016). Non motor subtypes and Parkinson's disease. *Parkinsonism & Related Disorders, 22*, S41–S46.

Sauerbier, A., & Ray Chaudhuri, K. (2014). Non-motor symptoms: The core of multi-morbid Parkinson's disease. *British Journal of Hospital Medicine (London, England), 75*, 18–24.

Sauerbier, A., Qamar, M. A., Rajah, T., & Chaudhuri, K. R. (2016). New concepts in the pathogenesis and presentation of Parkinson's disease. *Clinical Medicine (London, England), 16*, 365–370.

Scheperjans, F. (2016). Gut microbiota, 1013 new pieces in the Parkinson's disease puzzle. *Current Opinion in Neurology, 29*, 773–780.

Schrag, A., Sauerbier, A., & Chaudhuri, K. R. (2015). New clinical trials for nonmotor manifestations of Parkinson's disease. *Movement Disorders, 30*, 1490–1504.

Seppi, K., Weintraub, D., Coelho, M., Perez-Lloret, S., Fox, S. H., Katzenschlager, R., et al. (2011). The movement disorder society evidence-based medicine review update: Treatments for the non-motor symptoms of Parkinson's disease. *Movement Disorders, 26*(Suppl. 3), S42–S80.

Shin, A., Camilleri, M., Kolar, G., Erwin, P., West, C. P., & Murad, M. H. (2014). Systematic review with meta-analysis: Highly selective 5-HT4 agonists (prucalopride, velusetrag or naronapride) in chronic constipation. *Alimentary Pharmacology & Therapeutics*, *39*, 239–253.
Smith, K. M., Eyal, E., & Weintraub, D. (2015). Combined rasagiline and antidepressant use in Parkinson disease in the ADAGIO study: Effects on nonmotor symptoms and tolerability. *JAMA Neurology*, *72*, 88–95.
Stemper, B., Beric, A., Welsch, G., Haendl, T., Sterio, D., & Hilz, M. J. (2006). Deep brain stimulation improves orthostatic regulation of patients with Parkinson disease. *Neurology*, *67*, 1781–1785.
Storch, A., Schneider, C. B., Wolz, M., Stürwald, Y., Nebe, A., Odin, P., et al. (2013). Nonmotor fluctuations in Parkinson disease: Severity and correlation with motor complications. *Neurology*, *80*, 800–809.
Strohle, A., Schmidt, D. K., Schultz, F., Fricke, N., Staden, T., Hellweg, R., et al. (2015). Drug and exercise treatment of Alzheimer disease and mild cognitive impairment: A systematic review and meta-analysis of effects on cognition in randomized controlled trials. *The American Journal of Geriatric Psychiatry*, *23*, 1234–1249.
Trenkwalder, C., Kies, B., Rudzinska, M., Fine, J., Nikl, J., Honczarenko, K., et al. (2011). Rotigotine effects on early morning motor function and sleep in Parkinson's disease: A double-blind, randomized, placebo-controlled study (RECOVER). *Movement Disorders*, *26*, 90–99.
Trenkwalder, C., Kohnen, R., Hogl, B., Metta, V., Sixel-Doring, F., Frauscher, B., et al. (2011). Parkinson's disease sleep scale—Validation of the revised version PDSS-2. *Movement Disorders*, *26*, 644–652.
Velseboer, D. C., De Haan, R. J., Wieling, W., Goldstein, D. S., & De Bie, R. M. (2011). Prevalence of orthostatic hypotension in Parkinson's disease: A systematic review and meta-analysis. *Parkinsonism & Related Disorders*, *17*, 724–729.
Wang, H. F., Yu, J. T., Tang, S. W., Jiang, T., Tan, C. C., Meng, X. F., et al. (2015). Efficacy and safety of cholinesterase inhibitors and memantine in cognitive impairment in Parkinson's disease, Parkinson's disease dementia, and dementia with Lewy bodies: Systematic review with meta-analysis and trial sequential analysis. *Journal of Neurology, Neurosurgery, and Psychiatry*, *86*, 135–143.
Wu, C. K., & Hohler, A. D. (2015). Management of orthostatic hypotension in patients with Parkinson's disease. *Practical Neurology*, *15*, 100–104.
Yang, S., Sajatovic, M., & Walter, B. L. (2012). Psychosocial interventions for depression and anxiety in Parkinson's disease. *Journal of Geriatric Psychiatry and Neurology*, *25*, 113–121.
Zeevalk, G. D., Razmpour, R., & Bernard, L. P. (2008). Glutathione and Parkinson's disease: Is this the elephant in the room? *Biomedicine & Pharmacotherapy*, *62*, 236–249.
Zesiewicz, T. A., Evatt, M., Vaughan, C. P., Jahan, I., Singer, C., Ordorica, R., et al. (2015). Randomized, controlled pilot trial of solifenacin succinate for overactive bladder in Parkinson's disease. *Parkinsonism & Related Disorders*, *21*, 514–520.
Zibetti, M., Rizzone, M., Merola, A., Angrisano, S., Rizzi, L., Montanaro, E., et al. (2013). Sleep improvement with levodopa/carbidopa intestinal gel infusion in Parkinson disease. *Acta Neurologica Scandinavica*, *127*, e28–e32.

CHAPTER FOURTEEN

Treatment of Older Parkinson's Disease

Abhishek Lenka*, Chandrasekharapillai Padmakumar†, Pramod K. Pal*,[1]

*National Institute of Mental Health & Neurosciences, Bangalore, Karnataka, India
†Parkinson's Disease Service for the Older Person, Rankin Park Centre, John Hunter Hospital, Newcastle, NSW, Australia
[1]Corresponding author: e-mail address: pal.pramod@rediffmail.com

Contents

Abstract

Parkinson's disease (PD) is the second most common neurodegenerative disorder after Alzheimer's disease. The prevalence of PD increases with age. The spectrum of clinical features, the rate of progression of the disease, the burden of nonmotor symptoms, and the response to medications are different in older patients with PD from the relatively younger patients. Management of symptoms of PD in older patients is challenging because of possible existence of several age-related systemic illness. While dealing with older patients, it is crucial not to attribute all the physical symptoms to PD. Thorough evaluation for existence of diseases such as normal pressure hydrocephalus and vascular parkinsonism which partially mimic the symptoms of PD carries immense importance. Medical management of parkinsonian symptoms should be preferred with levodopa monotherapy. However, in patients with significant motor fluctuations, dopaminergic agents may be added with caution, as they are notorious for several adverse reactions. Nonmotor symptoms must be provided high importance as they substantially worsen the quality of life. In addition to parkinsonian symptoms, older patients with PD may need to undergo surgery for several conditions. Meticulous perioperative management is crucial as older patients with PD may face several surgery-related complications compared to the younger patients. Compliance to treatment is an important issue in old age. Hence multidisciplinary approach to management of PD in older patients should be emphasized.

International Review of Neurobiology, Volume 132
ISSN 0074-7742
http://dx.doi.org/10.1016/bs.irn.2017.01.005

1. INTRODUCTION

Parkinson's disease (PD) is a chronic progressive neurologic disorder. It is the second most common neurodegenerative disorder after Alzheimer's disease. In industrialized countries, the prevalence of PD in entire population has been estimated to be approximately 0.3%, whereas in population older than 60 years of age, the prevalence raises approximately to 1% (de Lau & Breteler, 2006). With each decade, the prevalence of PD becomes higher as a recent meta-analysis has estimated the prevalence of PD to be 1087 per 100,000 in individuals aged 70–79 years and 1903 per 100,000 in individuals over age 80 years (Pringsheim, Jette, Frolkis, & Steeves, 2014).

Loss of dopaminergic neurons in the substantia nigra and presence of Lewy bodies are the major pathological findings of PD (Braak et al., 2003). Motor symptoms such as tremor at rest, bradykinesia, rigidity, and postural instability are the hallmark motor symptoms of PD (Jankovic, 2008). As per the UK Parkinson's Disease Society Brain Bank clinical diagnostic criteria, bradykinesia must be present along with any of the other three aforementioned motor symptoms for the diagnosis of clinically probable PD (Hughes, Daniel, Kilford, & Lees, 1992). In addition to motor symptoms, patients with PD may also develop several nonmotor symptoms (NMSs) such as depression, psychosis, cognitive impairment, sleep disturbances, autonomic dysfunction, constipation, and hyposmia, which significantly worsen the health-related quality of life of the patients (Chaudhuri, Healy, & Schapira, 2006; Martinez-Martin, Rodriguez-Blazquez, Kurtis, Chaudhuri, & NMSS Validation Group, 2011). Certain NMSs such as sleep disturbance, autonomic dysfunction, hallucinations, and cognitive dysfunction are observed more frequently in older patients with PD (Szewczyk-Krolikowski et al., 2014; Zhou et al., 2013) (a list of possible NMSs is provided in Table 1). The motor symptoms and NMSs may have a differential response to antiparkinsonian medications. While improvement in motor symptoms secondary to dopaminergic therapy is one of the hallmark features of PD, treatment with dopaminergic agents alone may not be sufficient enough to ameliorate many of the NMS. Response to antiparkinsonian medications may also depend on several factors such as age of the patients, phenotype of PD, and stage of PD.

The term *older PD* may include patients with onset of PD at old age as well as those having young or middle-age onset of PD with long duration of illness. In either of the cases, management of the older PD patients poses

Table 1 Nonmotor Symptoms in Parkinson's Disease

Domains	Symptoms
Cardiovascular	[a]Light headedness, fainting
Sleep/fatigue	[a]Excessive daytime sleep, [a]difficulty in falling asleep, restless legs, fatigue
Mood/ cognition	Loss of interest in surroundings, lack of motivation, feel nervous, seem sad, flat mood, difficulty in experiencing pleasure
Perceptual problems	[a]Hallucinations, delusions, double vision
Attention/ memory	Concentration, [a]forget things or events, [a]forget to do things
Gastrointestinal	[a]Increased saliva/drooling, swallowing problems, constipation
Urinary	[a]Urgency, frequency, nocturia
Sexual dysfunction	[a]Loss of interest in sex, [a]problems in having sex
Miscellaneous	Unexplainable pain, change in weight, excessive sweating, reduced taste, or smell sensation

[a]NMS commonly observed in older patients with PD.
Chaudhuri, K. R., et al. (2007). The metric properties of a novel nonmotor symptoms scale for Parkinson's disease: Results from an international pilot study. *Movement Disorders: Official Journal of the Movement Disorder Society, 22*, 1901–1911.

different challenges compared to the management of the relatively younger patients. The major issue that makes the management of older PD patients difficult is the presence of other neurological and nonneurological comorbidities. In addition, the clinical characteristics, the response to medications, and the profile of adverse drug reactions are not as favorable as in patients with PD in young age or in middle age. Patients with old-age onset of PD have greater motor impairment and accelerated course of disease compared to those with onset of PD in middle-age onset having similar duration illness (Diederich, Moore, Leurgans, Chmura, & Goetz, 2003; Halliday & McCann, 2010). Not just the greater severity of motor dysfunction, older patients with PD have been reported to have a more intense NMS burden as well (Pagano, Ferrara, Brooks, & Pavese, 2016). Arevalo et al. in a study comparing the response to levodopa challenge in patients with early-onset PD and late-onset PD have reported significant age-related differences (Gomez Arevalo, Jorge, Garcia, Scipioni, & Gershanik, 1997). Some of the adverse effects of dopaminergic medications such as hallucinations and sleep disturbances are more common in older PD patients compared to the younger ones. In addition to symptoms related to PD, the older patients may also have other comorbidities, which may lead to requirement of polypharmacy. Hence the treatment of older PD patients is of immense importance and it underscores the importance of judicious use of the dopaminergic medications and meticulous monitoring of their adverse effects. Along with the careful approach toward management of physical symptoms, psychosocial support needs to be addressed, both to the patient and to the caregiver.

2. TREATMENT STRATEGIES FOR OLDER PD PATIENTS

2.1 Management of Motor Symptoms

Pharmacotherapy for the management of older PD patients must be individualized based on stage of the disease, presence and severity of motor fluctuations, spectrum of NMS, and adverse drug reactions. One of the important things that need to be considered is that all the physical symptoms present in older PD patients may not be attributed only to PD. "Missed diagnosis" and "misdiagnosis" are not uncommon in older patients with PD. For example, gait problems and slowness in an older patient with PD may also be secondary to osteoarthritis. Similarly, older patients must also be evaluated for other neurological illnesses such as normal pressure hydrocephalus (NPH) and vascular parkinsonism, which can mimic PD. Fig. 1 summarizes possible physical symptoms observed in older patients with PD.

2.1.1 Levodopa and Other Dopaminergic Agents

Irrespective of the age of the patients, levodopa unequivocally offers the greatest symptomatic benefit for PD (Connolly & Lang, 2014; Ferreira et al., 2013). Considering a better adverse effect profile compared to the dopamine receptor agonists such as pramipexole and ropinirole, levodopa is preferred as the initial drug of choice in patients with PD older than 60 years of age. Several adverse effects associated with dopamine agonists such as hallucinations and sleep disturbances are more common in older patients (Knie, Mitra, Logishetty, & Chaudhuri, 2011; Poewe, 2003). Pramipexole, a commonly used D_2 receptor agonist, has been reported to be associated with higher risk of heart failure in elderly PD patients compared to non-PD controls (Mokhles et al., 2012). Elderly patients, especially those with preexisting cognitive dysfunction, are at higher risk of developing psychiatric adverse effects during the course of illness. The only factor in

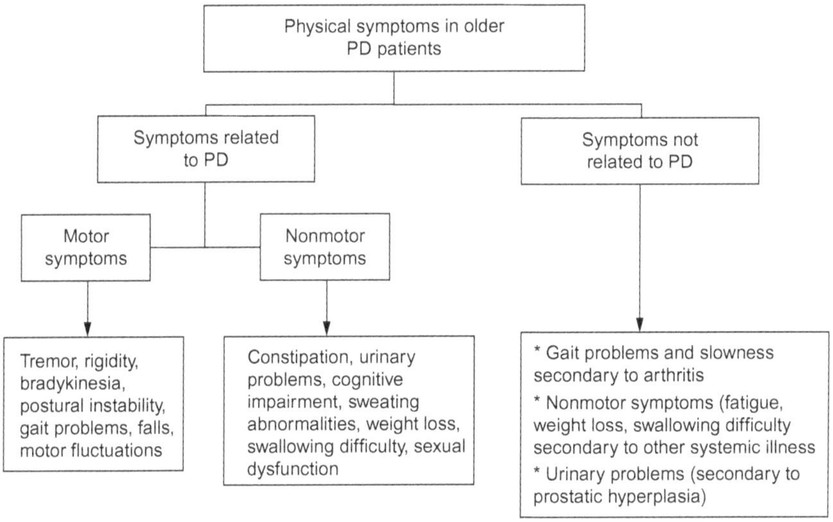

Fig. 1 A summary of possible physical symptoms observed in older patients with Parkinson's disease.

favoring treatment with dopamine receptor agonists is to delay the drug-induced dyskinesia. Thus, to summarize, in older patients, the risk to benefit ratio favors levodopa compared to dopamine agonists and alternative therapies. The safest method to initiate treatment in an elderly patient with PD is to begin with half a tablet of combination of levodopa (100 mg) and carbidopa (25 mg) three times a day. The dose should be slowly titrated upward based on clinical response and adverse effects. Sometimes patients may develop nausea and vomiting after taking levodopa tablets, which may be tackled by advising peripheral selective dopamine receptor antagonist such as domperidone. However, considering its cardiac side effects especially QT_c prolongation, which may be more common in elderly population, domperidone should be used only as a short-term measure (Johannes, Varas-Lorenzo, McQuay, Midkiff, & Fife, 2010).

Although motor fluctuations, especially dyskinesia, are more common in patients with young onset PD and with longer duration of symptoms, it is not uncommon for older patients with PD to develop dyskinesia. In such cases leading to troublesome dyskinesia in older patients, dopamine receptor agonists need to be started with lot of precautions, as the adverse effect profile is not very favorable. Pramipexole may be started at the dose of 0.375 mg/day in three divided doses, and the dose can be slowly titrated upward by 0.375 mg every week up to a maximum of 4.5 mg/day in three divided doses. Ropinirole is the alternative to pramipexole, and it can be started at the dose of 0.75 mg in three divided doses, and based on the response and side effects, the dose may be increased up to 24 mg/day in three divided doses. The dilemma for a movement disorder neurologist is compounded when the patient develops both dyskinesia and neuropsychiatric symptoms. In such scenarios, reducing the dose of levodopa in order to combat dyskinesia expectedly worsens the motor symptoms and adding or escalating the dose of dopamine agonists may worsen the neuropsychiatric complications. Amantadine (*N*-methyl-D-aspartate blocker) has been regarded as an antidyskinetic agent (Sawada et al., 2010). It also increases the striatal dopamine release and has neuroprotective properties. However, the use of amantadine may be limited in elderly patients considering its propensity to develop several adverse effects such as hallucinations, pedal edema, and livedo reticularis (Hayes, Cook-Norris, Miller, Rodriguez, & Zic, 2006; Postma & Van Tilburg, 1975). Hence the drug combinations need to be individualized in such cases after analyzing the presence and severity of other symptoms.

In addition to dyskinesia, chronic therapy with levodopa/carbidopa may be associated with the "wearing-off" phenomenon. Patients having wearing-off phenomenon report a loss of response to a dose of levodopa/carbidopa before taking the next dose (Stocchi, 2006). Entacapone, which is a catechol-*O*-methyltransferase, has been reported to be beneficial for ameliorating the wearing-off symptoms by increasing the ON duration (Schrag, 2005). Pellicano et al. (2009) have studied the efficacy, safety, and tolerability of entacapone in elderly PD patients (>70 years) and have reported significant improvement in the frequency and severity of OFF periods without any significant adverse effects. However, if prescribed to patients with preexisting dyskinesias, entacapone has the propensity to worsen dyskinesia (Schrag, 2005). Hence entacapone may be useful for wearing-off symptoms in elderly PD patients not having dyskinesias. If prescribed, patients must also be counseled regarding the common adverse effects (orange discoloration of urine, nausea, and giddiness), and the rare incidences of hepatic injury related to entacapone (Fisher, Croft-Baker, Davis, Purcell, & McLean, 2002; Myllylä et al., 2001). Monoamine oxidase (MAO-B) inhibitors such as rasagiline and selegiline may significantly improve the motor symptoms in PD and have been used commonly for monotherapy in early stages of PD or as an adjuvant to levodopa/carbidopa. As studies have reported no statistical relationship between adverse effects of rasagiline and age (Goetz, Schwid, Eberly, Oakes, & Shoulson, 2006), rasagiline (up to 1 mg/day) may be prescribed to older patients. The use of selegiline may be limited because of relatively unfavorable adverse effect profile (anorexia, postural hypotension, dry mouth) compared to rasagiline (Volz & Gleiter, 1998).

As discussed earlier, causes of reduced mobility other than PD itself in elderly patients should be vigorously searched for as these may significantly affect the quality of life. Joint pains secondary to osteoarthritis, back pain secondary to prolapse, or degenerative disc changes are common in old age, and they may also affect the mobility of elderly patients with PD. Referrals to appropriate specialists are of paramount importance in patients with aforementioned comorbidities. Similarly, both physiotherapy and occupational therapy may prove invaluable. Walking aids as well as modifications of home environment can not only improve mobility but also reduce the risk of falls. As older patients with PD have higher risk of falls compared to healthy individuals (Kalilani, Asgharnejad, Palokangas, & Durgin, 2016), both patients and caregivers must be counseled regarding measures to prevent falls. Older age and longer duration of disease have been reported to be associated with higher risk of falls (Hiorth, Larsen, Lode, & Pedersen, 2014; Kalilani et al., 2016; Wood, Bilclough, Bowron, & Walker, 2002). Patients with onset of PD at the age >70 years may experience falls much earlier in the disease course compared to younger patients (Contreras & Grandas, 2012). Hence modifications in home environment such as avoidance of slippery floors, use of walkers, and use of grab bars in bathrooms may be useful in preventing falls and fall-related injuries. In addition, gait and balance training after consultation with physiotherapists also helps in reducing the risk of falls (Conradsson et al., 2015; Shen & Mak, 2014). A phase-2 study of a recently conducted clinical trial (ReSPonD trial) has reported significant improvement in gait stability and reduction in the frequency of falls in patients taking rivastigmine; however, the findings remain to be confirmed in phase-3 trials (Henderson et al., 2016).

In addition to falls, the other comorbidity, which substantiates the risk of fractures, is osteoporosis. It should also be recognized that both PD and osteoporosis may affect a substantial portion of the elderly population, and they have a significant socioeconomic impact (Invernizzi, Carda, Viscontini, & Cisari, 2009). Osteoporosis represents a significant comorbidity in elderly population and, considering the greater risk of fracture secondary to falls, should be actively screened for and treated prospectively. The use of simple measures, such as hip pads, can also be an effective method for reducing fracture, which would necessitate a lengthy admission and commonly triggers transition into institutional care.

2.1.2 Continuous Drug Delivery Systems and Deep Brain Stimulation

Motor fluctuations may often necessitate the use of continuous drug delivery systems such as duodenal infusion pump (duodopa) and subcutaneous apomorphine. Both duodopa and apomorphine have been effective for reducing motor fluctuations in patients with PD. Duodopa not only reduces the burden of motor and NMSs but also improves the quality of life in patients with advanced PD (Nyholm, 2012). Although there is no clear age cutoff for patients undergoing continuous delivery of duodopa by infusion pump, adverse effects secondary to infusion system or surgical procedure may be bothersome for elderly patients who may already have some comorbidities (Nyholm, 2012). Apomorphine, which is a D_1 and D_2 receptor agonist, has been reported to be effective as a rescue medication for unpredictable and predictable OFF episodes. In addition to the management of unpredictable OFF periods, apomorphine indirectly helps in ameliorating the NMSs associated with OFF state (Trenkwalder et al., 2015). It may also be considered in older persons with advanced PD having wearing-off symptoms. However, the neurologist should be aware about the common adverse effects such as nausea, which may be bothersome for most of the patients. Rotigotine, a dopamine receptor agonist, is an attractive option for older patients having motor fluctuations. With single daily application, transdermal patches provide stable plasma concentration of rotigotine for 24 h. Because of the nature of application, the side effects of rotigotine are not as severe as that of other dopaminergic agents. However, several side effects such as application site reaction, somnolence, nausea, dizziness, and falls have been reported in patients using rotigotine transdermal patches (Giladi, Boroojerdi, & Surmann, 2013). Studies exploring age-related safety and tolerability of rotigotine have observed higher frequency of dizziness and falls in older patients compared to the younger ones (Oertel et al., 2013). Hence, the use of rotigotine patches may be considered in older patients with motor fluctuations because of the favorable side effect profile and high compliance rate (Schnitzler, Leffers, & Häck, 2010).

Deep brain stimulation (DBS) has been a revolutionary modality of treatment for patients with advanced PD having motor fluctuations. DBS may be of immense help in elderly patients with motor fluctuations but again the issue, which may limit its use in this population, is the presence of neuropsychiatric symptoms and other comorbidities. Although DBS unequivocally improves motor fluctuation, apprehension regarding higher postoperative morbidities in older patients often brings dilemma while selecting older patients for DBS. The literature on safety and efficacy of DBS in elderly population is limited in number, and their results have been nonuniform. Large longitudinal studies have reported significant improvement in motor fluctuations after DBS in older patients, which is comparable to the younger ones (Derost et al., 2007; Russmann et al., 2004). However, these studies have also reported a relative worsening of axial symptoms (gait problems and postural instability) in older patients after DBS. Previous trials with DBS have also reported worsening of cognitive functions after bilateral subthalamic stimulation in elderly PD patients compared to the younger ones (Bouwyn et al., 2016). A recent study by Cozac et al. has reported a higher prevalence of psychiatric complications in older patients compared to the younger PD patients undergoing bilateral subthalamic nucleus stimulation (Cozac et al., 2016). Although postoperative morbidities like hematoma, pneumonia, wound infections, and embolisms are expected to be more in elderly population, large retrospective studies have reported no difference in the rate of complications between old (>75 years) and young patients with PD after DBS (DeLong et al., 2014). This not only indicates the existing controversy regarding the safety and efficacy of DBS in older patients but also underscores the fact that selection of older patients with PD should be based on the cost–benefit ratio and should be individualized.

2.2 Management of NMSs in Old Patients

2.2.1 Cognitive Impairment

Cognitive impairment is a common NMS of PD and its prevalence increases with age of the patients, duration, severity, and stage of PD (Giladi et al., 2000; Xu, Yang, & Shang, 2016). The spectrum of cognitive impairment in PD may range from mild cognitive impairment (PD-MCI) to dementia (PDD). Cognitive impairment should be dealt with utmost importance in old patients with PD because old age itself is a risk factor for emergence of cognitive impairment, and it has been reported that cognitive impairment is significantly associated with poor quality of life and higher caregiver distress in patients with PD (Lawson et al., 2014; Leroi, McDonald, Pantula, & Harbishettar, 2012; Martinez-Martin et al., 2015). In addition to the risk factors described earlier, certain medications such as trihexyphenidyl hydrochloride and benzhexol can also lead to cognitive dysfunction. Other possible factors, which may lead to cognitive impairment in older PD patients, should be vigorously screened. As poor balance and tendency to fall are common in older PD patients, subdural hematoma should always be kept as a differential diagnosis in case of subacute onset of memory disturbance. Although common in PD, other comorbidities, which may also lead to cognitive impairment, should not be missed. Hence evaluation for hypothyroidism, vitamin B12 deficiency, dyselectrolytemia, NPH, systemic infections, and intracranial tumors carries paramount importance. Depression is one of the commonly observed NMSs in older PD patients. Since severe depression may also present as dementia (pseudodementia), referral to a psychiatrist for management of depression may also be considered.

Several clinical trials have been conducted for drugs to treat PD-MCI and PDD (Broadstock, Ballard, & Corbett, 2014). Cholinesterase inhibitors such as rivastigmine and donepezil have been reported to be effective in treating cognitive dysfunction in PD and thus have been widely used in demented PD patients. Results of several large clinical trials have strongly favored the use of rivastigmine in patients with PDD (Emre et al., 2004; Schmitt, Farlow, Meng, Tekin, & Olin, 2010). Recent studies have also reported efficacy of rivastigmine in reducing psychotic symptoms in patients with PD (Reading, Luce, & McKeith, 2001). As there is a strong association between psychosis and cognitive impairment in patients with PD (Lenka, Hegde, Jhunjhunwala, & Pal, 2016), rivastigmine can be an attractive option for patients having both the symptoms. As described earlier, rivastigmine may also improve the stability of gait resulting in reduction in the frequency of falls (Henderson et al., 2016). However, the physicians must be aware of the adverse effects of rivastigmine as it may result in nausea and vomiting, and though uncommon, it may worsen the parkinsonian tremor in some patients (Emre et al., 2004). In addition to pharmacological management, cognitive training may also be considered in older PD patients with cognitive impairment (Leung et al., 2015).

2.2.2 Psychosis in Older Patients With PD

Old age is one of the well-known risk factors for emergence of psychosis in PD (Fénelon & Alves, 2010). The spectrum of psychosis in PD may range from the minor hallucinations such as presence and passage hallucinations to formed complex visual hallucinations. Delusions, illusions, and hallucinations of modalities other than vision are relatively rare and usually coexist with visual hallucinations (Bountouni, Zis, Chaudhuri, & Schrag, 2015). The healthcare providers must also be aware of the comorbidities, which may precipitate acute or subacute onset psychosis in older PD patients. Systemic infections, dehydration, sleep deprivation, psychosocial stress, and metabolic derangements are the common causes of acute and subacute onset psychosis, and their presence must be thoroughly explored. Abnormalities in vision are one of the factors, which may predispose to symptoms mimicking the minor hallucinations. Hence patients complaining of minor hallucinations should undergo detailed evaluations to rule out conditions such as cataract and macular degeneration that are common in elderly population. Addressing the comorbid conditions leading to psychosis and withholding the medications (dopaminergic agents, anticholinergics), which may cause psychosis are the cornerstones of management of florid psychosis in old patients with PD. Parkinsonian symptoms should be preferably managed with monotherapy with the lowest possible dose of levodopa in older patients with PD having psychosis because other antiparkinsonian medications such as dopamine receptor agonists, amantadine, and MAO-B inhibitors have propensity to cause psychosis.

Failure of the above-described steps to reduce the symptoms of psychosis may necessitate the administration of antipsychotic medications. Clozapine has been used as the first-line drug and is the most potent atypical antipsychotic against psychosis in PD. However, considering the adverse effect profile of clozapine and the necessity to monitor hematological parameters regularly, it may become a difficult choice to treat psychotic symptoms in elderly patients with PD (Pollak et al., 2004). Among atypical psychotics, quetiapine has been one of the off-label drugs of choice because of its favorable adverse effect profile (Bloomfield, Macdonald, Finucane, Snow, & Roxburgh, 2012; Friedman & Factor, 2000). Other atypical antipsychotics such as olanzapine and aripiprazole, though effective, should be avoided in older PD patients considering their adverse effects. Recently the FDA has approved pimavanserin (selective 5-HT2A inverse agonist) for the treatment of psychosis in PD. As a clinical trial has reported significant improvement in psychotic symptoms by pimavanserin, which was well tolerated by the patients (Cummings et al., 2014), it may be an attractive option in future. Cognitive impairment is a well-established risk factor for emergence of psychosis, and this fact necessitates the evaluation for cognitive dysfunction in PD patients with psychosis (Fénelon et al., 2000). In case of coexistence of cognitive impairment and psychosis, rivastigmine can be an excellent choice as it has been reported to be effective in both PDD and visual hallucinations in PD (Bullock & Cameron, 2002; Reading et al., 2001).

2.2.3 Affective Disorders

Affective disorders such as depression, apathy, and anxiety are extremely common in PD, and they often remain undiagnosed because the major attention goes to management of motor symptoms. Depression is one of the common psychiatric manifestations in patients with PD. Nonpharmacological approaches such as counseling and cognitive behavior therapy should be preferred for mild symptoms (Dobkin et al., 2011). Apathy is also commonly observed in PD patients, and it is difficult to differentiate apathy and depression as often they coexist (Pluck & Brown, 2002). Currently there are no clear therapeutic guidelines to manage apathy in PD. However, cholinesterase inhibitors have emerged as an option to treat apathy in PD as rivastigmine was reported to be beneficial in one of the recent clinical trials involving nondemented euthymic PD patients (Devos et al., 2014). Patients with apathy may be referred to a psychiatrist as a thorough evaluation for the presence of underlying depression becomes important in such scenarios. Large clinical trials have reported significant improvement of symptoms of depression by nortriptyline compared to paroxetine, a selective serotonin reuptake inhibitor (SSRI) (Menza et al., 2009). In case of adverse effects secondary to nortriptyline (nausea, vomiting, urinary problems, vision problems), SSRIs such as paroxetine and escitalopram may be considered for depression in PD. Antidepressants may be individualized based on the presence of other NMSs. For example, in patients with no cognitive impairment and who suffer from pain, insomnia and hypersalivation, nortriptyline, or in those with poor appetite and insomnia, mirtazapine may be useful (Djamshidian & Friedman, 2014).

2.2.4 Bladder and Bowel Problems

Urological problems are very common in older patients in PD, and a wide range of prevalence has been reported (24%–96%) (Jost, 2013). Increased urgency, increased frequency, urge incontinence, and nocturia are common urological problems in PD, and their severity as well as frequency correlates positively with age, disease duration, and severity of motor symptoms. Although the exact pathophysiology of these problems is not clearly understood, the final common pathway is believed to be the result of instability of the detrusor muscle in bladder. However, before attributing the urological problems to PD, possibility of benign prostatic hyperplasia, which is extremely common in elderly population, must be considered. Hence detailed urological evaluation must be considered in older PD patients to rule out the primary urological problems. The treating neurologists should also be aware of the medications, which may cause urinary problems. Tricyclic antidepressants and anticholinergic agents especially trihexyphenidyl, which may be prescribed to patients with tremor dominant PD and those with depression, are commonly associated with urinary disturbance. Antimuscarinic agents such as tolterodine, darifenacin, and solifenacin are effective for symptoms related to detrusor overactivity and have been commonly used in patients with PD. However, these agents should be judiciously used in older PD patients as these antimuscarinic agents have high propensity to cause several behavioral (confusion, agitation, disorientation), visual (blurring of vision, double vision, worsening of glaucoma), cardiovascular (arrhythmias, orthostatic hypotension), and gastrointestinal (dry mouth, constipation) adverse effects. Nocturia, which is a common urological symptom in older PD patients, may improve with intranasal desmopressin (Yeo, Singh, Gundeti, Barua, & Masood, 2012). However, neurologists should be aware of the desmopressin-related side effects such as hyponatremia and confusional states in older PD patients (Fowler, 2007).

Constipation is a common gastroenterological problem. It may be present in 30% of the general population with higher prevalence in the elderly population (De Giorgio et al., 2015). It is one of the commonest NMSs of PD, and it may be present much before the onset of motor symptoms (Kaye, Gage, Kimber, Storey, & Trend, 2006). Constipation may occur secondary to involvement of both central and peripheral nervous system. Slow colonic transit and defecatory dysfunctions possibly result in constipation in PD. Modification in the lifestyle to increase the intake of fibrous food and fluids should be the first step to treat constipation. If the results are not satisfactory with lifestyle modification, sequential introduction and combination of bulking agents, softeners and lubricants, osmotics, and stimulants should be tried and titrated against the needs of the individual patient (Rossi, Merello, & Perez-Lloret, 2015).

2.2.5 Bulbar, Autonomic, and Sleep Disturbances

Difficulty in speaking and swallowing is common in older patients as well as in patients with long-standing PD and is very troublesome for both patients and the caregivers (Tjaden, 2008). Hence speech therapy early in the course of the illness should be strongly encouraged, as it has proven to have a beneficial effect on both of these symptoms (Claassen et al., 2010). Lee Silverman vocal treatment (LSVT) has become popular because of its beneficial effects on the speech quality in patients with PD (Sapir, Ramig, & Fox, 2011; Sapir, Spielman, Ramig, Story, & Fox, 2007). Hence it may be tried in older patients with the help of the speech pathologists. The early involvement of a speech pathologist may also help in the assessment of swallowing, with advice on dietary preparation to reduce aspiration. In a small number of cases, enteral feeding via a percutaneous endoscopic gastrostomy tube may be considered. In those patients with troubling sialorrhea, promoting deglutition with chewing gum or by sucking sweets is often less troublesome than trying to harness the benefits of pharmacological approaches such as anticholinergics (e.g., hyoscine skin patch, atropine eye drops applied topically, TCAs) or injectable agents (e.g., botulinum toxin, glycopyrrolate). As described many times earlier, other neurological comorbidities, which may result in speech and swallowing disturbances, should be carefully scrutinized.

Postural hypotension is a commonly observed symptom, which occurs secondary to autonomic dysfunction in patients with PD. Symptomatic orthostatic hypotension occurs in 15%–20% of PD patients (Senard et al., 1997). It is crucial to delineate the causes of postural hypotension in older PD patients as it increases the risk of falls, which may have devastating consequences in patients with older age group. Although postural hypotension may occur as a part of autonomic dysfunction in PD, a thorough review of the medication chart should be considered as several antiparkinsonian medications may cause postural hypotension. In such scenario, discontinuation of the offending drugs must be considered. Nonpharmacological measures such as increasing fluid intake, adding extra salt in the diet, and using elastic stockings may be effective in reducing the symptoms of orthostatic hypotension (Mathias & Kimber, 1999). If postural hypotension persists even after trying the aforementioned measures, pharmacological therapy may be considered. Fludrocortisone, midodrine, pyridostigmine, and domperidone have been reported to be effective in managing postural hypotension (Sánchez-Ferro, Benito-León, & Gómez-Esteban, 2013). Fludrocortisone primarily acts by restricting the salt loss and expanding the blood volume, and it has been the mainstay of pharmacotherapy for orthostatic hypotension. However, the physicians should also be aware of the fludrocortisone-related side effects such as hypokalemia, supine hypertension, and headache, which may be troublesome in older PD patients. If patients remain symptomatic even with nonpharmacological management as well as with fludrocortisone, midodrine (an alpha agonist) may be considered. The major contraindications for the use of midodrine are coronary heart disease, cardiac failure, urinary retention, and acute renal failure (Gupta & Lipsitz, 2007). Pyridostigmine acts principally by augmenting ganglionic cholinergic transmissions by inhibiting cholinesterase. It favors normal physiologic responses upon standing, without worsening supine hypertension. The adverse effects include diarrhea, nausea, and other cholinergic symptoms (Sánchez-Ferro et al., 2013).

Sleep disturbances are extremely common in patients with PD, and the prevalence is higher in the elderly population. Insomnia, excessive daytime sleepiness, rapid eye movement (REM) sleep behavior disorder (RBD), restless leg syndrome, periodic limb movement, and obstructive sleep apnea are commonly observed in PD (French & Muthusamy, 2016). The exact cause of higher prevalence of excessive daytime sleepiness is not clear, but it may occur as adverse reaction of dopamine receptor agonists (pramipexole and ropinirole) (Gjerstad, Alves, Wentzel-Larsen, Aarsland, & Larsen, 2006). Hence proper titration of antiparkinsonian medications is of immense importance as excessive daytime sleepiness may substantially hamper the quality of life. It is prudent to rule out obstructive sleep apnea as it is one of the major causes of excessive daytime sleepiness (Pagel, 2009). Increasing sleep fragmentation with difficulties entering into and remaining in the deeper stages of REM and non-REM sleep is also associated with normal aging, and these features are further exacerbated in PD. RBD may be present in more than half of the patients with PD, and its onset may even precede the onset of motor symptoms of PD (RBD, 2010). As RBD is characterized by the presence of dream enactment behaviors, the patient as well as their bed partners is prone to injuries. Hence proper counseling must be done to reduce the risk of injuries. Clonazepam is effective in reducing the severity and frequency of RBD episodes. However, the older patients taking clonazepam should be thoroughly evaluated for the presence of any side effects and as far as possible, clonazepam should be avoided in older patients. Oral melatonin may also be considered for managing symptoms of RBD in elderly population (McGrane, Leung, St. Louis, & Boeve, 2015). Medications such as zolpidem and zopiclone may be beneficial for patients with sleep onset insomnia.

2.2.6 Adherence to Treatment: A Big Issue in Elderly Patients

One of the critical issues that need to be considered while treating older patients with PD is adherence to treatment. Several factors such as comorbidities, cognitive impairment, psychosocial issues, financial condition, adverse drug effects, and communication with the physicians may affect the adherence to treatment in older PD patients (Schlenk, Dunbar-Jacob, & Engberg, 2004). Adverse effects of drugs and higher expenses related to multiple medications may prompt the older patients with PD either to discontinue the medications or to reduce the dose. Active communication with the health care provider is of immense importance in such scenarios. The physicians must also look for other causes of nonadherence to treatment especially the nonadherence secondary to comorbidities. For example, patients with disturbance of memory may find it difficult to remember the exact schedule of medications. A study by Schlenk et al. has revealed that forgetting to take medicines is the most commonly reported reason for nonadherence (Schlenk et al., 2004). Similarly, presence of depression has also been described as a risk factor for nonadherence to treatments in patients with PD. DiMatteo and colleagues have reported poor adherence to medication is three times more likely in patients with depression compared to those without depression (DiMatteo, Lepper, & Croghan, 2000). Hence such comorbidities affecting adherence should be properly addressed in elderly PD patients. Adequate counseling and collaborative approach including the participation of nurse practitioners, social workers, pharmacists may help in improving the adherence to treatment. Use of several adherence aids such as weekly pillboxes, and hour-by-hour organizational charts may improve the treatment adherence in elderly PD patients (Park, Morrell, Frieske, & Kincaid, 1992).

2.3 Emergencies, Hospital Admissions, and Perioperative Issues in Older Patients With PD

Emergencies in patients with PD are common in older patients. The major causes of emergency hospitalization include (i) age-related systemic illnesses, (ii) adverse effect of certain medications, and (iii) complications of advanced disease (motor fluctuations, falls, psychiatric complications) (Factor & Molho, 2000; Woodford & Walker, 2005). Treatment of older patients with PD in emergency department is challenging because of the multiple age-related systemic illnesses such as infections (pneumonia, urinary tract infection), cardiovascular diseases (angina, myocardial infarction, transient ischemic attack, stroke, deep vein thrombosis, arrhythmia), and urinary retention. PD patients are nearly twice as likely to be admitted for complications of disease and its treatment rather than for management of primary motor deficit and 30% of hospital admission caused by complications of advanced PD and its treatment may be prevented by early intervention (Temlett & Thompson, 2006). Hence older patients with PD must be routinely evaluated for age-related systemic illnesses, which may prevent hospitalizations.

Many older patients with PD may require surgery for several comorbidities, which are common in old age. The common indications for surgery in old age include urological (benign prostatic hyperplasia), ophthalmological (cataract), orthopedic (joint replacement for arthritis, fractures), neurosurgical (head injuries secondary to fall), cardiac (ischemic heart disease), and gastrointestinal (intestinal obstruction) problems. In addition, patients may be selected for surgeries specific for PD such as DBS, thalamotomy, and pallidotomy. The overall management may be challenging because of several postoperative issues such as effect of anesthesia, withdrawal of anti-PD medications, swallowing difficulties, pain, tightness of bandages, immobility, and metabolic alterations (Gálvez-Jiménez & Lang, 2004). Emergencies related to pulmonary dysfunctions are common in older patients during postoperative state. Pneumonia, upper airway obstruction, and laryngospasm are the commonly encountered pulmonary dysfunctions in the intraoperative and postoperative state. Underlying subclinical pulmonary dysfunctions, abrupt withdrawal of dopaminergic agents, and adverse effects of anesthetic and neuroleptic medications may precipitate pulmonary dysfunctions. This underscores the importance of preoperative pulmonary function tests, judicious use of anesthetic agents, and preoperative and postoperative breathing exercise in older patients. Delirium, agitation, psychosis, and sleep disturbances are common in the postoperative period, and emergence of these symptoms necessitates gradual withdrawal of several anti-PD medications such as anticholinergics, amantadine, MAO-B inhibitors, dopamine agonists, and COMT inhibitors. In such scenarios, it is ideal to maintain the lowest possible dose of levodopa. Atypical antipsychotics such as clozapine and quetiapine may be preferred in severe cases. If the patients cannot take oral formulations of levodopa, administration through nasogastric tube may be preferred. However, if postoperative periods need restriction of food by mouth or nasogastric tube, subcutaneous apomorphine may be considered. In an open-label trial (Wüllner et al., 2010), the use of transdermal rotigotine patch during perioperative period was considered feasible and acceptable for patients as well as the neurologists and anesthesiologists. In the same study, rotigotine patches resulted in good control of PD symptoms and swift switching/reswitching of the oral antiparkinsonian medications in the same study. Hence rotigotine patches may be considered in older PD patients in the perioperative period. One of the serious postoperative issues in PD is parkinsonism hyperpyrexia syndrome (PHS), which usually occurs due to abrupt withdrawal of anti-PD medications prior to surgery (Newman, Grosset, & Kennedy, 2009). Metabolic alterations such as hypernatremia may also result in PHS. The initial symptoms of PHS include severe rigidity, tremor, and respiratory distress, which are followed by fever, altered sensorium, autonomic dysfunction, leukocytosis, and raised creatine kinase levels (Newman et al., 2009). Correction of the metabolic parameters and reinstitution of dopaminergic medications are the cornerstone of the management of PHS. In severe cases dantrolene may be preferred. As older age is a poor prognostic indicator of PHS (Takubo et al., 2003), prompt actions should be taken to prevent and manage this condition.

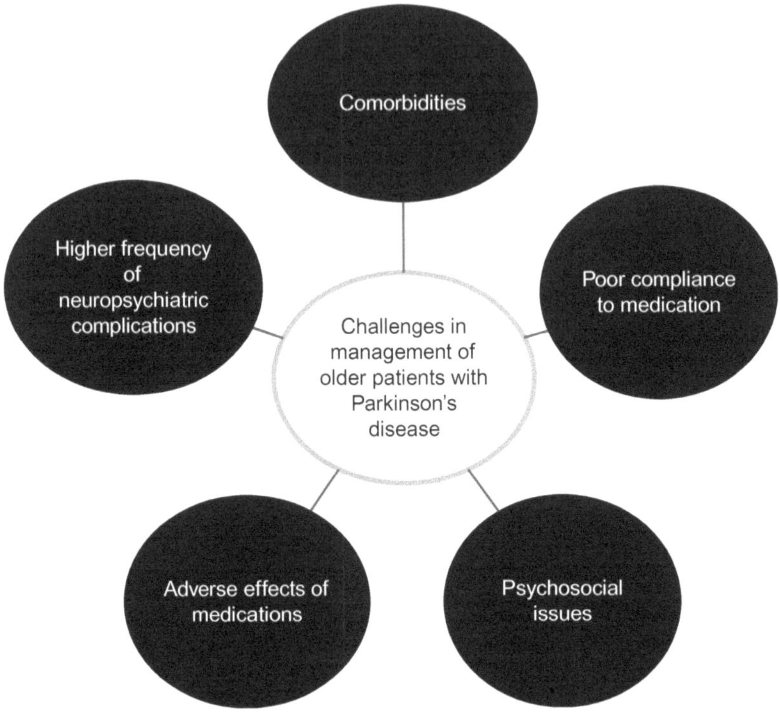

Fig. 2 A summary of challenges associated with management of older patients with Parkinson's disease.

To summarize, perioperative issues in older PD patients may be challenging to manage. Hence meticulous preoperative assessments carry immense importance in preventing or minimizing some of the serious postoperative issues. In addition, proper cardiopulmonary assessments, preoperative breathing exercises, judicial use of anesthetic agents, early administration of dopaminergic agents, and early mobilization hold the key to an uneventful postoperative outcome of the surgeries in old age.

Fig. 2 highlights the challenges associated with management of older patients with PD, and Table 2 lists the important take-home messages.

3. CONCLUSION

Managing the older patients with PD is challenging mainly because of the overlap of some of symptoms related to PD and the comorbidities commonly observed in old age. As described earlier, the key is not to ascribe

Table 2 Take-Home Messages

• Management of older patients with idiopathic Parkinson's disease has to be individualized taking into account the specific care needs of the patients
• As with every other geriatric syndrome, management should be tailor made to address the impact that the disease has made on the life of the older patients, both medical and nonmedical, including psychosocial elements
• Measuring the nonmotor symptom burden and introducing measures to address them will have a tremendous impact on improving the health-related quality of life of both patients and the caregivers
• Because of the increased prevalence of multiple comorbidities, management of PD in an older person, especially with significant comorbidities, should be preferably limited to L-dopa monotherapy
• In the context of worsening cognition in an older person with PDD, the clinical question that needs to be addressed should be not which drug to start but which drug to withdraw/avoid
• Dopamine agonists are not well tolerated in older PD Patients with cognitive impairment
• Clozapine has the most evidence base to be used as treatment for PD psychosis; however, the side-effect profile restricts its use in older persons with PD. Quetiapine is a reasonable alternative in those cases
• Autonomic impairment producing postural hypotension is a very important clinical problem in the older person restricting in many occasions the use of L-dopa in high doses
• A comprehensive geriatric assessment emphasizing the impact of PD in an older person complemented by a patient centered multidisciplinary team led case management is the corner stone of management of Parkinson's disease

every physical or mental discomfort to PD. Thorough exploration of the comorbid conditions, which mimic symptoms of PD, is crucial. The neurologists should be careful regarding the pharmacological therapy as the drug-related adverse events are more common in elderly patients, and presence neuropsychiatric symptoms requires strict vigilance on the drug chart. Levodopa remains the mainstay of pharmacological management, as its adverse effect profile is more favorable compared to the dopamine receptor agonists. The care of older patients with PD warrants involvement of multiple specialists based on requirement. In addition, creation of a better psychosocial environment remains another key as what really important is a perfect balance between the psychological and physiological state.

Financial Disclosure/Conflict of Interest: None of the authors have any financial disclosure to make or have any conflict of interest.

Source of funding: Nil.

REFERENCES

Bloomfield, K., Macdonald, L., Finucane, G., Snow, B., & Roxburgh, R. (2012). Use of antipsychotic medications in patients with Parkinson's disease at Auckland City Hospital. *Internal Medicine Journal, 42*(7), e151–e156.

Bountouni, I., Zis, P., Chaudhuri, K. R., & Schrag, A. (2015). Psychosis in Parkinson's disease. In *Neuropsychiatric symptoms of movement disorders, Springer Series: Neuropsychiatric Symptoms in Neurological Diseases* (pp. 113–140). http://dx.doi.org/10.1007/978-3-319-09537-0_6.

Bouwyn, J.-P., Derrey, S., Lefaucheur, R., Fetter, D., Rouille, A., Le Goff, F., et al. (2016). Age limits for deep brain stimulation of subthalamic nuclei in Parkinson's disease. *Journal of Parkinson's Disease, 6*(2), 393–400.

Braak, H., Del Tredici, K., Rüb, U., De Vos, R. A. I., Jansen Steur, E. N. H., & Braak, E. (2003). Staging of brain pathology related to sporadic Parkinson's disease. *Neurobiology of Aging, 24*(2), 197–211.

Broadstock, M., Ballard, C., & Corbett, A. (2014). Latest treatment options for Alzheimer's disease, Parkinson's disease dementia and dementia with Lewy bodies. *Expert Opinion on Pharmacotherapy, 15*, 1797–1810.

Bullock, R., & Cameron, A. (2002). Rivastigmine for the treatment of dementia and visual hallucinations associated with Parkinson's disease: A case series. *Current Medical Research and Opinion, 18*(5), 258–264.

Chaudhuri, K. R., Healy, D. G., & Schapira, A. H. (2006). Non-motor symptoms of Parkinson's disease: Diagnosis and management. *Lancet Neurology, 5*(3), 235–245.

Claassen, D. O., Josephs, K. A., Ahlskog, J. E., Silber, M. H., Tippmann-Peikert, M., & Boeve, B. F. (2010). REM sleep behavior disorder preceding other aspects of synucleinopathies by up to half a century. *Neurology, 75*(6), 494–499.

Connolly, B. S., & Lang, A. E. (2014). Pharmacological treatment of Parkinson disease: A review. *JAMA, 311*(16), 1670–1683.

Conradsson, D., Löfgren, N., Nero, H., Hagströmer, M., Ståhle, A., Lökk, J., et al. (2015). The effects of highly challenging balance training in elderly with Parkinson's disease: A randomized controlled trial. *Neurorehabilitation and Neural Repair, 29*(9), 827–836.

Contreras, A., & Grandas, F. (2012). Risk of falls in Parkinson's disease: A cross-sectional study of 160 patients. *Parkinson's Disease 2012*, http://dx.doi.org/10.1155/2012/362572

Cozac, V. V., Ehrensperger, M. M., Gschwandtner, U., Hatz, F., Meyer, A., Monsch, A. U., et al. (2016). Older candidates for subthalamic deep brain stimulation in Parkinson's disease have a higher incidence of psychiatric serious adverse events. *Frontiers in Aging Neuroscience, 8*(13), 132.

Cummings, J., Isaacson, S., Mills, R., Williams, H., Chi-Burris, K., Corbett, A., et al. (2014). Pimavanserin for patients with Parkinson's disease psychosis: A randomised, placebo-controlled phase 3 trial. *Lancet, 383*, 533–540.

De Giorgio, R., Ruggeri, E., Stanghellini, V., Eusebi, L. H., Bazzoli, F., & Chiarioni, G. (2015). Chronic constipation in the elderly: A primer for the gastroenterologist. *BMC Gastroenterology, 15*(1), 130.

de Lau, L. M. L., & Breteler, M. M. B. (2006). Epidemiology of Parkinson's disease. *Lancet Neurology, 5*(6), 525–535.

DeLong, M. R., Huang, K. T., Gallis, J., Lokhnygina, Y., Parente, B., Hickey, P., et al. (2014). Effect of advancing age on outcomes of deep brain stimulation for Parkinson disease. *JAMA Neurology, 71*(10), 1290–1295.

Derost, P.-P., Ouchchane, L., Morand, D., Ulla, M., Llorca, P.-M., Barget, M., et al. (2007). Is DBS-STN appropriate to treat severe Parkinson disease in an elderly population? *Neurology*, *68*(17), 1345–1355.

Devos, D., Moreau, C., Maltête, D., Lefaucheur, R., Kreisler, A., Eusebio, A., et al. (2014). Rivastigmine in apathetic but dementia and depression-free patients with Parkinson's disease: A double-blind, placebo-controlled, randomised clinical trial. *Journal of Neurology, Neurosurgery, and Psychiatry*, *85*(6), 668–674.

Diederich, N. J., Moore, C. G., Leurgans, S. E., Chmura, T. A., & Goetz, C. G. (2003). Parkinson disease with old-age onset: A comparative study with subjects with middle-age onset. *Archives of Neurology*, *60*(4), 529–533.

DiMatteo, M. R., Lepper, H. S., & Croghan, T. W. (2000). Depression is a risk factor for noncompliance with medical treatment. *Archives of Internal Medicine*, *160*(14), 2101.

Djamshidian, A., & Friedman, J. H. (2014). Anxiety and depression in Parkinson's disease. *Current Treatment Options in Neurology*, *16*(4), 285.

Dobkin, R. D., Menza, M., Allen, L. A., Gara, M. A., Mark, M. H., Tiu, J., et al. (2011). Cognitive-behavioral therapy for depression in Parkinson's disease: A randomized, controlled trial. *The American Journal of Psychiatry*, *168*(10), 1066–1074.

Emre, M., Aarsland, D., Albanese, A., Byrne, E. J., Deuschl, G., De Deyn, P. P., et al. (2004). Rivastigmine for dementia associated with Parkinson's disease. *The New England Journal of Medicine*, *351*, 2509–2518.

Factor, S. A., & Molho, E. S. (2000). Emergency department presentations of patients with Parkinson's disease. *The American Journal of Emergency Medicine*, *18*(2), 209–215.

Fénelon, G., & Alves, G. (2010). Epidemiology of psychosis in Parkinson's disease. *Journal of the Neurological Sciences*, *289*(1–2), 12–17.

Fénelon, G., Mahieux, F., Huon, R., & Ziégler, M. (2000). Hallucinations in Parkinson's disease: Prevalence, phenomenology and risk factors. *Brain*, *123*(Pt. 4), 733–745.

Ferreira, J. J., Katzenschlager, R., Bloem, B. R., Bonuccelli, U., Burn, D., Deuschl, G., et al. (2013). Summary of the recommendations of the EFNS/MDS-ES review on therapeutic management of Parkinson's disease. *European Journal of Neurology*, *20*(1), 5–15.

Fisher, A., Croft-Baker, J., Davis, M., Purcell, P., & McLean, A. J. (2002). Entacapone-induced hepatotoxicity and hepatic dysfunction. *Movement Disorders*, *17*(6), 1362–1365.

Fowler, C. J. (2007). Update on the neurology of Parkinson's disease. *Neurourology and Urodynamics*, *26*, 103–109.

French, I. T., & Muthusamy, K. A. (2016). A review of sleep and its disorders in patients with Parkinson's disease in relation to various brain structures. *Frontiers in Aging Neuroscience*, *8*(6), 114.

Friedman, J. H., & Factor, S. A. (2000). Atypical antipsychotics in the treatment of drug-induced psychosis in Parkinson's disease. *Movement Disorders*, *15*, 201–211.

Gálvez-Jiménez, N., & Lang, A. E. (2004). The perioperative management of Parkinson's disease revisited. *Neurologic Clinics*, *22*, 367–377.

Giladi, N., Boroojerdi, B., & Surmann, E. (2013). The safety and tolerability of rotigotine transdermal system over a 6-year period in patients with early-stage Parkinson's disease. *Journal of Neural Transmission*, *120*(9), 1321–1329.

Giladi, N., Treves, T. A., Paleacu, D., Shabtai, H., Orlov, Y., Kandinov, B., et al. (2000). Risk factors for dementia, depression and psychosis in long-standing Parkinson's disease. *Journal of Neural Transmission*, *107*(1), 59–71.

Gjerstad, M. D., Alves, G., Wentzel-Larsen, T., Aarsland, D., & Larsen, J. P. (2006). Excessive daytime sleepiness in Parkinson disease: Is it the drugs or the disease? *Neurology*, *67*(5), 853–858.

Goetz, C. G., Schwid, S. R., Eberly, S. W., Oakes, D., & Shoulson, I. (2006). Safety of rasagiline in elderly patients with Parkinson disease. *Neurology, 66*(9), 1427–1429.
Gomez Arevalo, G., Jorge, R., Garcia, S., Scipioni, O., & Gershanik, O. (1997). Clinical and pharmacological differences in early- versus late-onset Parkinson's disease. *Movement Disorders, 12*(3), 277–284.
Gupta, V., & Lipsitz, L. A. (2007). Orthostatic hypotension in the elderly: Diagnosis and treatment. *The American Journal of Medicine, 120*(10), 841–847.
Halliday, G. M., & McCann, H. (2010). The progression of pathology in Parkinson's disease. *Annals of the New York Academy of Sciences, 1184,* 188–195.
Hayes, B. B., Cook-Norris, R. H., Miller, J. L., Rodriguez, A., & Zic, J. A. (2006). Amantadine-induced livedo reticularis: A report of two cases. *Journal of Drugs in Dermatology, 5,* 288–289.
Henderson, E. J., Lord, S. R., Brodie, M. A., Gaunt, D. M., Lawrence, A. D., Close, J. C. T., et al. (2016). Rivastigmine for gait stability in patients with Parkinson's disease (ReSPonD): A randomised, double-blind, placebo-controlled, phase 2 trial. *Lancet Neurology, 15*(3), 249–258.
Hiorth, Y. H., Larsen, J. P., Lode, K., & Pedersen, K. F. (2014). Natural history of falls in a population-based cohort of patients with Parkinson's disease: An 8-year prospective study. *Parkinsonism & Related Disorders, 20*(10), 1059–1064.
Hughes, A. J., Daniel, S. E., Kilford, L., & Lees, A. J. (1992). Accuracy of clinical diagnosis of idiopathic Parkinson's disease: A clinico-pathological study of 100 cases. *Journal of Neurology, Neurosurgery, and Psychiatry, 55*(3), 181–184.
Invernizzi, M., Carda, S., Viscontini, G. S., & Cisari, C. (2009). Osteoporosis in Parkinson's disease. *Parkinsonism & Related Disorders, 15,* 339–346.
Jankovic, J. (2008). Parkinson's disease: Clinical features and diagnosis. *Journal of Neurology, Neurosurgery, and Psychiatry, 79*(4), 368–376.
Johannes, C. B., Varas-Lorenzo, C., McQuay, L. J., Midkiff, K. D., & Fife, D. (2010). Risk of serious ventricular arrhythmia and sudden cardiac death in a cohort of users of domperidone: A nested case-control study. *Pharmacoepidemiology and Drug Safety, 19*(9), 881–888.
Jost, W. H. (2013). Urological problems in Parkinson's disease: Clinical aspects. *Journal of Neural Transmission, 120*(4), 587–591.
Kalilani, L., Asgharnejad, M., Palokangas, T., & Durgin, T. (2016). Comparing the incidence of falls/fractures in Parkinson's disease patients in the US population. *PLoS One, 11*(9),e0161689
Kaye, J., Gage, H., Kimber, A., Storey, L., & Trend, P. (2006). Excess burden of constipation in Parkinson's disease: A pilot study. *Movement Disorders, 21*(8), 1270–1273.
Knie, B., Mitra, M. T., Logishetty, K., & Chaudhuri, K. R. (2011). Excessive daytime sleepiness in patients with Parkinson's disease. *CNS Drugs, 25,* 203–212.
Lawson, R. A., Yarnall, A. J., Duncan, G. W., Khoo, T. K., Breen, D. P., Barker, R. A., et al. (2014). Severity of mild cognitive impairment in early Parkinson's disease contributes to poorer quality of life. *Parkinsonism & Related Disorders, 20*(10), 1071–1075.
Lenka, A., Hegde, S., Jhunjhunwala, K. R., & Pal, P. K. (2016). Interactions of visual hallucinations, rapid eye movement sleep behavior disorder and cognitive impairment in Parkinson's disease: A review. *Parkinsonism & Related Disorders, 22,* 1–8.
Leroi, I., McDonald, K., Pantula, H., & Harbishettar, V. (2012). Cognitive impairment in Parkinson disease: Impact on quality of life, disability, and caregiver burden. *Journal of Geriatric Psychiatry and Neurology, 25*(4), 208–214.
Leung, I., Walton, C., Hallock, H., Lewis, S., Valenzuela, M., & Lampit, A. (2015). Cognitive training in Parkinson disease: A systematic review and meta-analysis. *Neurology, 85*(21), 1843–1851.
Martinez-Martin, P., Rodriguez-Blazquez, C., Forjaz, M. J., Frades-Payo, B., Agüera-Ortiz, L., Weintraub, D., et al. (2015). Neuropsychiatric symptoms and caregiver's burden in Parkinson's disease. *Parkinsonism & Related Disorders, 21*(6), 629–634.

Martinez-Martin, P., Rodriguez-Blazquez, C., Kurtis, M. M., Chaudhuri, K. R., & NMSS Validation Group. (2011). The impact of non-motor symptoms on health-related quality of life of patients with Parkinson's disease. *Movement Disorders, 26*(3), 399–406.

Mathias, C. J., & Kimber, J. R. (1999). Postural hypotension: Causes, clinical features, investigation, and management. *Annual Review of Medicine, 50*, 317–336.

McGrane, I. R., Leung, J. G., St. Louis, E. K., & Boeve, B. F. (2015). Melatonin therapy for REM sleep behavior disorder: A critical review of evidence. *Sleep Medicine, 16*, 19–26.

Menza, M., Dobkin, R. D., Marin, H., Mark, M. H., Gara, M., Buyske, S., et al. (2009). A controlled trial of antidepressants in patients with Parkinson disease and depression. *Neurology, 72*(10), 886–892.

Mokhles, M. M., Trifirò, G., Dieleman, J. P., Haag, M. D., van Soest, E. M., Verhamme, K. M. C., et al. (2012). The risk of new onset heart failure associated with dopamine agonist use in Parkinson's disease. *Pharmacological Research, 65*(3), 358–364.

Myllylä, V. V., Kultalahti, E. R., Haapaniemi, H., Leinonen, M., Aho, K., Alhainen, K., et al. (2001). Twelve-month safety of entacapone in patients with Parkinson's disease. *European Journal of Neurology, 8*(1), 53–60.

Newman, E. J., Grosset, D. G., & Kennedy, P. G. E. (2009). The parkinsonism-hyperpyrexia syndrome. *Neurocritical Care, 10*, 136–140.

Nyholm, D. (2012). Duodopa® treatment for advanced Parkinson's disease: A review of efficacy and safety. *Parkinsonism & Related Disorders, 18*(8), 916–929.

Oertel, W., LeWitt, P., Giladi, N., Ghys, L., Grieger, F., & Boroojerdi, B. (2013). Treatment of patients with early and advanced Parkinson's disease with rotigotine transdermal system: Age-relationship to safety and tolerability. *Parkinsonism & Related Disorders, 19*(1), 37–42.

Pagano, G., Ferrara, N., Brooks, D. J., & Pavese, N. (2016). Age at onset and Parkinson disease phenotype. *Neurology, 86*(15), 1400–1407.

Pagel, J. F. (2009). Excessive daytime sleepiness. *American Family Physician, 79*, 391–396.

Park, D. C., Morrell, R. W., Frieske, D., & Kincaid, D. (1992). Medication adherence behaviors in older adults: Effects of external cognitive supports. *Psychology and Aging, 7*(2), 252–256.

Pellicano, C., Benincasa, D., Giovannelli, M., Buttarelli, F. R., Ruggieri, S., & Pontieri, F. E. (2009). Entacapone in elderly parkinsonian patients experiencing levodopa-related wearing-off: A pilot study. *Neurological Research, 31*(1), 74–76.

Pluck, G. C., & Brown, R. G. (2002). Apathy in Parkinson's disease. *Journal of Neurology, Neurosurgery, and Psychiatry, 73*(6), 636–642.

Poewe, W. (2003). Psychosis in Parkinson's disease. *Movement Disorders, 18*(Suppl. 6), S80–S87.

Pollak, P., Tison, F., Rascol, O., Destée, A., Péré, J. J., Senard, J. M., et al. (2004). Clozapine in drug induced psychosis in Parkinson's disease: A randomised, placebo controlled study with open follow up. *Journal of Neurology, Neurosurgery, and Psychiatry, 75*(5), 689–695.

Postma, J. U., & Van Tilburg, W. (1975). Visual hallucinations and delirium during treatment with amantadine (Symmetrel). *Journal of the American Geriatrics Society, 23*(5), 212–215.

Pringsheim, T., Jette, N., Frolkis, A., & Steeves, T. D. L. (2014). The prevalence of Parkinson's disease: A systematic review and meta-analysis. *Movement Disorders, 29*, 1583–1590.

RBD, C. C. (2010). *Movement Disorders, 25*, S596–S597.

Reading, P. J., Luce, A. K., & McKeith, I. G. (2001). Rivastigmine in the treatment of parkinsonian psychosis and cognitive impairment: Preliminary findings from an open trial. *Movement Disorders, 16*(6), 1171–1174.

Rossi, M., Merello, M., & Perez-Lloret, S. (2015). Management of constipation in Parkinson's disease. *Expert Opinion on Pharmacotherapy, 16*(4), 547–557.

Russmann, H., Ghika, J., Villemure, J. G., Robert, B., Bogousslavsky, J., Burkhard, P. R., et al. (2004). Subthalamic nucleus deep brain stimulation in Parkinson disease patients over age 70 years. *Neurology*, *63*(10), 1952–1954.

Sánchez-Ferro, A., Benito-León, J., & Gómez-Esteban, J. C. (2013). The management of orthostatic hypotension in Parkinson's disease. *Frontiers in Neurology*, *4*, 64.

Sapir, S., Ramig, L. O., & Fox, C. M. (2011). Intensive voice treatment in Parkinson's disease: Lee Silverman Voice Treatment. *Expert Review of Neurotherapeutics*, *11*(6), 815–830.

Sapir, S., Spielman, J. L., Ramig, L. O., Story, B. H., & Fox, C. (2007). Effects of intensive voice treatment (the Lee Silverman Voice Treatment [LSVT]) on vowel articulation in dysarthric individuals with idiopathic Parkinson disease: Acoustic and perceptual findings. *Journal of Speech, Language, and Hearing Research*, *50*(4), 899–912.

Sawada, H., Oeda, T., Kuno, S., Nomoto, M., Yamamoto, K., Yamamoto, M., et al. (2010). Amantadine for dyskinesias in Parkinson's disease: A randomized controlled trial. *PLoS One*, *5*(12), 1–7.

Schlenk, E. A., Dunbar-Jacob, J., & Engberg, S. (2004). Medication non-adherence among older adults: A review of strategies and interventions for improvement. *Journal of Gerontological Nursing*, *30*(7), 33–43.

Schmitt, F. A., Farlow, M. R., Meng, X., Tekin, S., & Olin, J. T. (2010). Efficacy of rivastigmine on executive function in patients with Parkinson's disease dementia. *CNS Neuroscience & Therapeutics*, *16*, 330–336.

Schnitzler, A., Leffers, K. W., & Häck, H. J. (2010). High compliance with rotigotine transdermal patch in the treatment of idiopathic Parkinson's disease. *Parkinsonism & Related Disorders*, *16*(8), 513–516.

Schrag, A. (2005). Entacapone in the treatment of Parkinson's disease. *Lancet Neurology*, *4*, 366–370.

Senard, J. M., Raï, S., Lapeyre-Mestre, M., Brefel, C., Rascol, O., Rascol, A., et al. (1997). Prevalence of orthostatic hypotension in Parkinson's disease. *Journal of Neurology, Neurosurgery, and Psychiatry*, *63*(5), 584–589.

Shen, X., & Mak, M. K. Y. (2014). Technology-assisted balance and gait training reduces falls in patients with Parkinson's disease: A randomized controlled trial with 12-month follow-up. *Neurorehabilitation and Neural Repair*, *29*(2), 103–111.

Stocchi, F. (2006). The levodopa wearing-off phenomenon in Parkinson's disease: Pharmacokinetic considerations. *Expert Opinion on Pharmacotherapy*, 7(10), 1399–1407.

Szewczyk-Krolikowski, K., Tomlinson, P., Nithi, K., Wade-Martins, R., Talbot, K., Ben-Shlomo, Y., et al. (2014). The influence of age and gender on motor and non-motor features of early Parkinson's disease: Initial findings from the Oxford Parkinson Disease Center (OPDC) discovery cohort. *Parkinsonism & Related Disorders*, *20*(1), 99–105.

Takubo, H., Harada, T., Hashimoto, T., Inaba, Y., Kanazawa, I., Kuno, S., et al. (2003). A collaborative study on the malignant syndrome in Parkinson's disease and related disorders. *Parkinsonism & Related Disorders*, *9*(Suppl. 1), S31–S41.

Temlett, J. A., & Thompson, P. D. (2006). Reasons for admission to hospital for Parkinson's disease. *Internal Medicine Journal*, *36*, 524–526.

Tjaden, K. (2008). Speech and swallowing in Parkinson's disease. *Topics in Geriatric Rehabilitation*, *24*(2), 115–126.

Trenkwalder, C., Chaudhuri, K. R., García Ruiz, P. J., LeWitt, P., Katzenschlager, R., Sixel-Döring, F., et al. (2015). Expert Consensus Group report on the use of apomorphine in the treatment of Parkinson's disease—Clinical practice recommendations. *Parkinsonism & Related Disorders*, *21*(9), 1023–1030.

Volz, H. P., & Gleiter, C. H. (1998). Monoamine oxidase inhibitors. A perspective on their use in the elderly. *Drugs & Aging*, *13*(5), 341–355.

Wood, B. H., Bilclough, J., Bowron, A., & Walker, R. W. (2002). Incidence and prediction of falls in Parkinson's disease: A prospective multidisciplinary study. *Journal of Neurology, Neurosurgery, and Psychiatry*, *72*(6), 721–725.

Woodford, H., & Walker, R. (2005). Emergency hospital admissions in idiopathic Parkinson's disease. *Movement Disorders*, *20*(9), 1104–1108.

Wüllner, U., Kassubek, J., Odin, P., Schwarz, M., Naumann, M., Häck, H. J., et al. (2010). Transdermal rotigotine for the perioperative management of Parkinson's disease. *Journal of Neural Transmission*, *117*(7), 855–859.

Xu, Y., Yang, J., & Shang, H. (2016). Meta-analysis of risk factors for Parkinson's disease dementia. *Translational Neurodegeneration*, *5*(5), 11.

Yeo, L., Singh, R., Gundeti, M., Barua, J. M., & Masood, J. (2012). Urinary tract dysfunction in Parkinson's disease: A review. *International Urology and Nephrology*, *44*, 415–424.

Zhou, M.-Z., Gan, J., Wei, Y.-R., Ren, X.-Y., Chen, W., & Liu, Z.-G. (2013). The association between non-motor symptoms in Parkinson's disease and age at onset. *Clinical Neurology and Neurosurgery*, *115*(10), 2103–2107.

CHAPTER FIFTEEN

New Symptomatic Treatments for the Management of Motor and Nonmotor Symptoms of Parkinson's Disease

Raquel N. Taddei*[,1], **Federica Spinnato**[†], **Peter Jenner**[‡]
*King's College London and King's College Hospital, London, United Kingdom
[†]University of Palermo, Faculty of Medicine, Palermo, Italy
[‡]Institute of Pharmaceutical Science, King's College London, London, United Kingdom
[1]Corresponding author: e-mail address: raqueltaddei@hotmail.com

Contents

Abstract

Motor symptoms are core features of Parkinson's disease, while nonmotor symptoms are present from the prodromal stage. Management strategies for the motor symptoms of Parkinson's disease have been widely researched and there have been many advances. Therapy has evolved from oral therapy to once a day to nonoral strategies, both for rescue and for infusion therapy. Treatment for nonmotor symptoms, however, has remained a key unmet need, although of late evidence base for management of

International Review of Neurobiology, Volume 132
ISSN 0074-7742
http://dx.doi.org/10.1016/bs.irn.2017.03.004

some nonmotor symptoms such as pain, dementia, aspects of sleep dysfunction, and constipation has emerged. However, management of many nonmotor symptoms such as anxiety, apathy, fatigue, and insomnia remains uncharted. In this review, we address these management strategies and discuss the evidence base of available therapies.

1. INTRODUCTION

The discovery of dopaminergic cell loss in substantia nigra and the ensuing striatal dopamine deficiency identified the major pathological and biochemical hallmarks of Parkinson's disease (PD) and led to the introduction of dopamine replacement therapy in the form of L-dopa and dopamine agonist drugs (Hornykiewicz, 2010). In recent times, the management of the motor symptoms of PD has undergone immense development with the discovery and use of novel classes of dopamine agonists and enzyme inhibitors to prevent L-dopa and dopamine degradation and nonoral and continuous drug delivery systems. Significant progress has also been made in the treatment of common motor complications and motor fluctuations associated with the therapy of PD, most notably dyskinesia and "wearing off" through the use of dopaminergic and nondopaminergic medications.

Recently, there has been an acceptance that not only is the pathology of PD widespread in both brain and the periphery but that the multiple neuronal and neurotransmitter systems affected contribute to a broad spectrum of nonmotor symptoms (NMSs) of PD that can occur before, at the same time, or after the onset of motor signs. However, the NMSs of PD have proved a challenge in terms of their recognition and management even though they represent a key determinant of quality of life in PD. The level of understanding of the pathophysiological basis of NMSs is low, and there has been too little development of appropriate animal models for their study and even more limited pharmacological investigation into new potential drug treatments. Consequently, there are limited treatment options currently available. However, NMSs and their preclinical and clinical investigation offer an opportunity for a step change in the treatment of PD in the foreseeable future.

2. NEW DOPAMINERGIC APPROACHES TO THE TREATMENT OF MOTOR SYMPTOMS IN PD

The treatment of the motor symptoms of PD is almost entirely centered on dopamine replacement in one form or another using L-dopa or dopamine agonist drugs, such as ropinirole, pramipexole, and apomorphine. This strategy has revolutionized therapy and novel approaches aimed at further improving dopaminergic therapy continue. New formulations of L-dopa are under investigation along with novel delivery routes for both L-dopa and dopamine agonist drugs. This is particularly evident for L-dopa where its erratic absorption, short plasma half-life, and propensity to induce motor complications and motor fluctuations have proved difficult to overcome using standard formulation techniques.

2.1 New Formulations and Delivery Systems for L-Dopa

The use of immediate-release formulations of L-dopa came associated with an erratic drug response and with a high incidence of "wearing off" and dyskinesia associated with the short plasma half-life of the drug and its pulsatile mode of action. Attempts to make controlled or sustained release formulations of L-dopa have been largely unsuccessful, and until recently, finding an alternative route of administration to oral therapies has also proved difficult.

2.1.1 Duodopa-Percutaneous Delivery

Currently, an observational clinical trial on Duodopa (DUOGLOBE) is under way, assessing long-term outcome of percutaneous treatment with Duodopa/Duopa in advanced PD patients, who will be assessed at baseline and in regular follow-ups to an expected timeline of 3 years. Effectiveness of treatment by means of changes in "off" time will be assessed as a primary outcome, along with various motor, nonmotor, and quality of life-related features as secondary measures. Study completion is expected by December 2020.

2.1.2 IPX-066/Rytary-Oral Extended Release L-Dopa/Carbidopa

IPX-066 or Rytary is an oral extended-release therapy of L-dopa/carbidopa microbeads, which dissolves at different rates, thus allowing a stable plasma level. A phase 2 study performed by Hauser et al. (2011) showed a rapid absorption and sustained plasma L-dopa (LD) concentrations with less fluctuation compared to immediate-release carbidopa/L-dopa (IR-CD/LD). Further phase 3 studies including the ADVANCE-PD (Hauser et al., 2013) and the ASCEND-PD (Stocchi et al., 2014) could show a significant reduction in "off" time without an increase in dyskinesia in advanced PD patients treated with Rytary when compared to L-dopa/carbidopa plus entacapone as seen in Fig. 1, where L-dopa/carbidopa/entacapone was

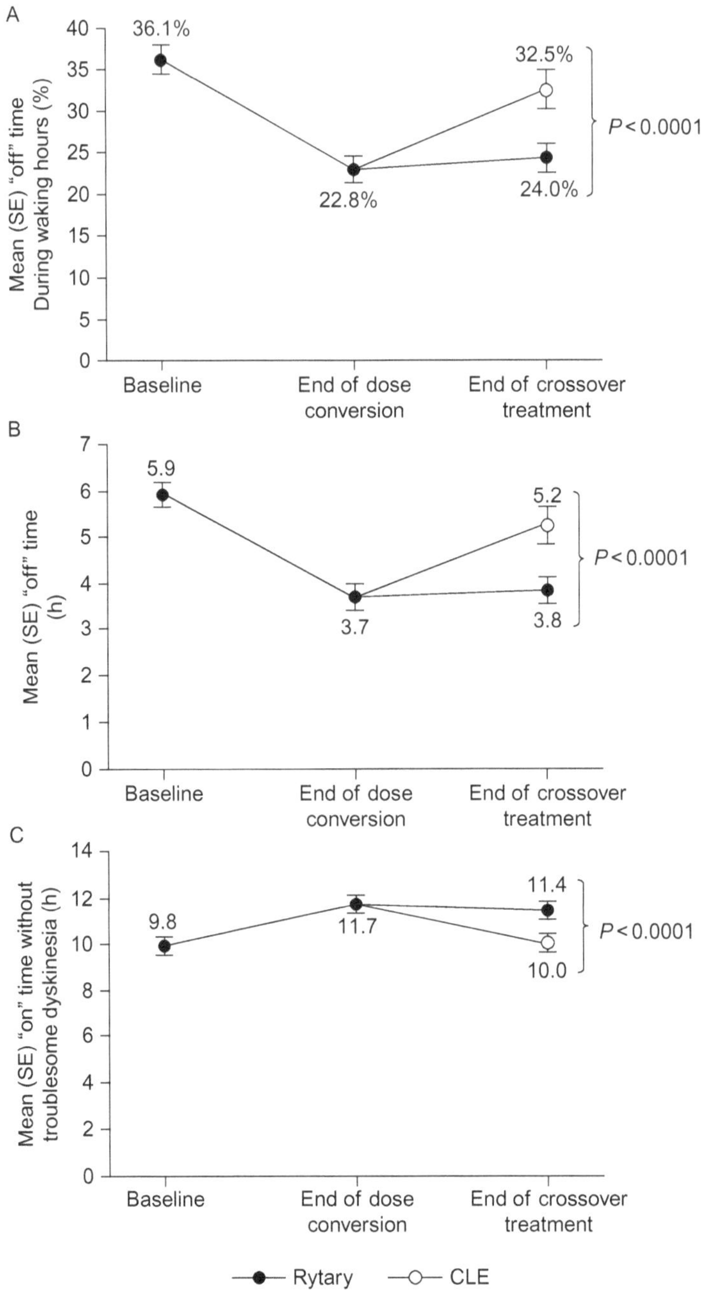

Fig. 1 Mean "off" time and mean "on" time with troublesome dyskinesia under Rytary or under L-dopa/carbidopa plus entacapone therapy. *CLE*, carbidopa–levodopa plus entacapone; *SE*, standard error. *From Hinson, V. K., et al. (2009). Reducing dosing frequency of carbidopa/levodopa: Double-blind crossover study comparing twice-daily bilayer formulation of carbidopa/levodopa (IPX054) versus 4 daily doses of standard carbidopa/levodopa in stable Parkinson disease patients.* Clinical Neuropharmacology, 32, *189–192.*

compared with Rytary (Nausieda et al., 2015; Stocchi et al., 2014). The use of Rytary was approved by the FDA in January 2015.

2.1.3 ND0612—Liquid L-Dopa/Carbidopa

Currently, two clinical trials led by the pharmaceutical company Neuroderm are under way on ND0612, a novel liquid formulation of L-dopa/carbidopa administered subcutaneously through a mini-pump with the aim of achieving steady L-dopa concentrations over a 24-h period. The first of the studies is a randomized, parallel study on 36 advanced PD patients treated with more than four doses of L-dopa per day and having at least 2.5 h of "off" time a day, which will be randomized to two doses of ND0612, with the primary outcome measure being the changes in daytime "off" time. The second clinical trial on ND0612 is a phase 2 open-label clinical study on 120 advanced PD patients treated with more than four doses of L-dopa per day and having at least 2.5 h of "off" time per day, who will be followed up over 12 months in order to assess the long-term efficacy and safety profile of this novel formulation. Completion of the study is expected by February 2018.

2.1.4 Oral L-Dopa-Ongoing Trials

An observational cross-sectional trial on classical oral L-dopa is currently ongoing to assess its effect on postural motor learning in PD patients, being the primary outcome measure the change in movement of the center of mass after postural perturbation between "on" and "off" state under L-dopa treatment. As a secondary outcome, transcranial magnetic stimulation will be performed in order to capture cortical excitability and its correlation with postural motor learning, being the hypothesis of this study, that dopamine has a negative effect on postural motor learning.

A further study on oral L-dopa/carbidopa has recently been completed on IPX054, a bilayered tablet of extended-release L-dopa/carbidopa, comparing this compound with standard L-dopa/carbidopa. The results showed a similar maintenance of efficacy of IPX054 twice a day and classic L-dopa/carbidopa four times a day, thus being IPX054 of benefit in its twice-daily regime, potentially enhancing compliance (Hinson et al., 2009).

2.2 Enzyme Inhibitors

The pharmacokinetic profile and the efficacy of L-dopa have been enhanced by its combination with a range of enzyme inhibitors. The peripheral decarboxylase inhibitors, either carbidopa or benserazide, are routinely used to prevent the breakdown of L-dopa outside of the brain. Inhibitors of catechol-O-methyl transferase (COMT), entacapone and tolcapone, are used to inhibit the other major pathway of peripheral L-dopa metabolism, and these also serve to increase the bioavailability of L-dopa and extend its plasma half-life. Finally, inhibitors of monoamine-oxidase B, selegiline and rasagiline, are used to prevent the degradation of dopamine in the striatum that is either remaining endogenous dopamine or dopamine formed from L-dopa. But while current enzyme inhibitors improve the actions of L-dopa, a new generation of drugs has been recently introduced to further enhance their utility.

2.2.1 Opicapone (Ongentys)

Opicapone (OPC) is a novel third-generation COMT inhibitor, which has been approved by the European Commission in 2016 as an adjunctive therapy to preparations of L-dopa/dopa-decarboxylase inhibitors (DDCIs) in adult PD patients with end-of-dose motor fluctuations. OPC has a high COMT inhibitory potency and a slow complex dissociation rate constant that can be translated in a long duration of action in vivo (Kiss et al., 2010; Palma & Soares-da-Silva, 2013). Several studies proved a longer and safer efficacy in prolonging L-dopa action than the commonly used COMT inhibitors, tolcapone and entacapone (Bonifacio et al., 2015). The first study on men (healthy male volunteers) showed a good tolerance after single doses of OPC ranging from 10 to 1200 mg. The adverse events did not differ from placebo. Despite the short half-life (0.8–3.2 h) the inhibitory effect was dose dependent (from 34.5% with 10 mg to 100% with 1200 mg) and long-lasting (from 25.1% with 10 mg to 76.5% with 1200 mg after 24 h postdose) (Almeida, Falcao, et al., 2013; Rocha et al., 2015). Different dosages were tested, showing a dose-dependent effect and a high efficacy in inhibiting COMT, enhancing L-dopa action and reducing "off" periods, thus improving motor abilities. A three-center, double-blind, randomized, placebo-controlled crossover study undertaken in Portugal, Romania, and Ukraine tested 10 patients who were randomized to 1 of 4 different study treatments (25, 50, and 100 mg of OPC and placebo) (Rocha et al., 2015). The main aim was to test the effectiveness of OPC in inhibiting COMT activity (AUEC, area under the effect–time curve), increasing L-dopa-concentration–time profiles (AUC, area under the concentration–time curve), improving motor performance (UPDRS, unified PD rating scale), and the risk of dyskinesias (abnormal involuntary movement scale). Results showed a marked dose-dependent efficacy of OPC as well as an increase in dyskinesias with the administration of 100 mg OPC (Fig. 2).

A more recent phase 3, randomized, double-blind, placebo-controlled trial tested oral treatment with OPC (5, 25, or 50 mg once daily), placebo, or entacapone (200 mg with every levodopa intake) for 14–15 weeks among 537 patients (112 in the placebo group, 104 in the entacapone group, 110 in the OPC 5 mg group, 105 in the OPC 25 mg group, and 106 in the OPC 50 mg group) (Ferreira et al., 2015). The primary endpoint was the change from baseline to end of study treatment in absolute time in the "off" state, assessed by daily patients' diaries. The mean change in time in the "off" state with OPC 50 mg was significantly superior to placebo and noninferior to entacapone. The most common adverse events were dyskinesias, reported in all groups, but higher among the patients taking 50 mg OPC. In summary, OPC is an acceptable adjunctive therapy for PD patients under dopamine replacement therapy, as a single daily dose of 50 mg taken at bedtime at least 1 h before or after levodopa combinations. Evidence of relevant adverse effect, apart from "on" state dyskinesias, has so far not been reported and are being assessed in a currently ongoing clinical trial among Europe and the United States, aiming at including 550 PD patients (Pintor et al., 2012).

2.2.2 Xadago/Safinamide

Safinamide is a reversible MAO-B inhibitor such as the already available compound rasagiline, thought to work on dopaminergic as well as on non-dopaminergic pathways by increasing dopamine within the brain on one hand and modulating the release of glutamate through voltage-gated sodium channel modulation on the other hand (http://www.mims.co.uk; Schapira, 2010). A phase 3 double-blind, placebo-controlled study on 568 patients, comparing two dosages (50 and 100 mg) of safinamide as an add-on therapy to L-dopa and other dopaminergic treatments in PD patients with motor fluctuations (Borgohain et al., 2014), showed an improvement in "off" time as well as no significant increase in dyskinesias while increasing "on" time, in contrast to rasagiline, where an increase in dyskinesias alongside improvement in "on" time was seen in the PRESTO study (Starkstein, Brockman, & Hayhow, 2012). Safinamide has already been approved and is available in the United Kingdom since May 2016.

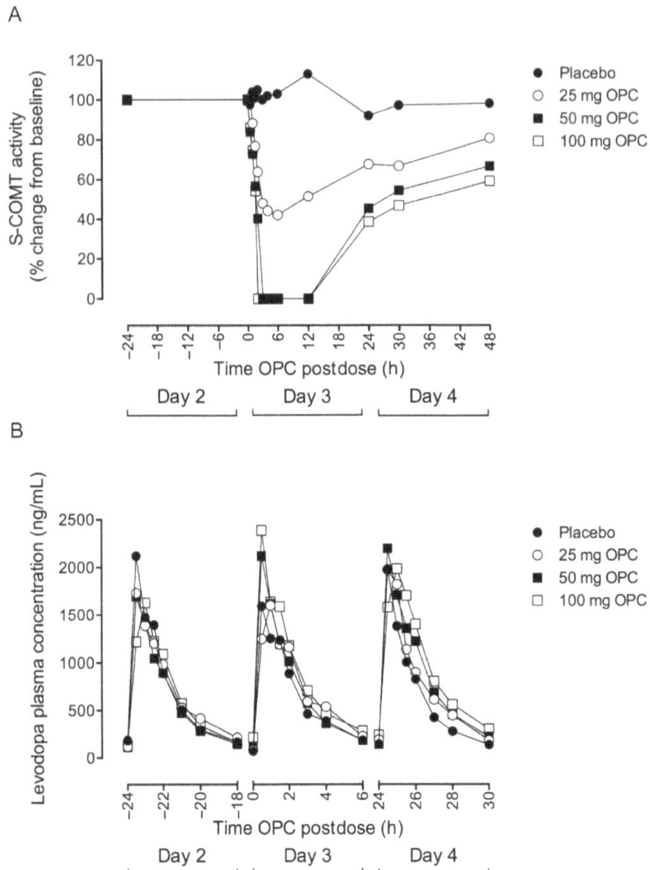

Fig. 2 (A) Mean S-COMT activity (% of baseline, day 2) vs time following oral administration of levodopa/carbidopa or levodopa/benserazide concomitantly with placebo, 25, 50, and 100 mg OPC on day 3 and day 4. (B) Mean plasma levodopa concentration–time profile following oral administration of levodopa/carbidopa or levodopa/benserazide alone on days 2 and 4 and concomitantly with placebo, 25, 50, and 100 mg OPC on day 3. *OPC*, opicapone; *S-COMT*, soluble-catechol-*O*-methyltransferase. *From Rocha, J. F., et al. (2015). Effect of single-dose regimens of opicapone on levodopa pharmacokinetics, catechol-O-methyltransferase activity and motor response in patients with Parkinson disease.* Clinical Pharmacology in Drug Development, 5, *232–240.*

2.3 Dopamine Agonists

The lack of potency, erratic absorption, and short half-life of L-dopa led to the introduction of more potent, longer acting synthetic dopamine agonist drugs. Initially piribedil and the ergot derivatives, bromocriptine, pergolide, and cabergoline, were developed, but because of unfavorable short- and long-term side-effect profiles, these were superseded by the nonergots, ropinirole and pramipexole. These longer acting oral agonists produced less dyskinesia than L-dopa on prolonged use but also had less efficacy and new unwanted effects in the form of impulse control disorders (ICDs) and sudden onset of sleep. Despite having longer plasma half-lives than L-dopa, ropinirole and pramipexole were administered three times daily, and for convenience, extended-release versions were introduced to improve their effectiveness. At this time, there has been little interest in the development of further oral dopamine agonist compounds. One exception has been in attempts to target the D1 dopamine receptor as current oral agonists are relatively selective for D2-like dopamine receptors, while dopamine derived from L-dopa acts on both D1 and D2 receptors.

2.3.1 D1-Agonists: Dihydrexidine, A-68930, A77636, Rotigotine, CVT-301

Studies on full dopamine D1-agonists, such as dihydrexidine, have so far shown little benefit with regard to motor symptoms, having a broad variety of side effects including flushing, hypotension, and tachycardia, thus limiting their use (Blanchet et al., 1998). Preliminary studies on other D1-agonist compounds, including A-68930 and A77636 on animals, have shown a greater than 20-h duration of contralateral turning, but no response on the second day of treatment (Blanchet et al., 1998). As to the compound A77636, increases in locomotor activity and decreases in Parkinson-like symptoms in MPTP-treated marmosets and monkeys with no substantial increase in dyskinesia were observed, but its effect was already reduced on the second day of application (Antonini et al., 2016; Voon & Fox, 2007). Further studies are awaited.

Perhaps surprisingly, the most interest has been in dopamine agonists that have poor oral bioavailability due to extensive first-pass metabolism. Rotigotine, which is a broad-spectrum dopamine agonist, has been developed into a transdermal patch providing continual drug delivery over a 24-h period based on its optimal physicochemical properties. There has also been interest in developing depot microsphere rotigotine preparations for long-term effect. These were first studied in 6-OHDA-lesioned rats, where nonetheless no therapeutic benefit between rotigotine-loaded microspheres and pulsatile L-dopa administration and no significant reduction of dyskinesias comparing both could be found (Wang et al., 2012). A recently published study on in vitro evaluation of rotigotine-loaded implants by the same group (Wang et al., 2016) could show a sustained drug release for a period of time of 40 days, thus posing a potential drug to overcome fluctuations in advanced PD patients. In a clinical trial on Cynomolgus monkeys, with intramuscular administration of rotigotine-loaded microspheres, finding an absent treatment-related overall toxicity with a potentially safe long-term benefit could open up potential studies in humans soon (Tian et al., 2013).

However, the most interest has been centered on the mixed D1/D2 agonist apomorphine, which is the only dopamine agonist with efficacy approaching that of L-dopa. Not only does it have poor bioavailability, but it also has a short plasma half-life. However, its utility as a rescue therapy by subcutaneous injection and as a treatment for "wearing off" by subcutaneous infusion has led to a number of attempts to deliver the drug by alternative routes, both acutely and over the longer term.

2.3.2 CVT-301

CVT-301 is currently being developed as a self-administered, inhaled levodopa (L-dopa)-based powder for the "rescue" treatment of "off" periods in PD, and is being studied to provide delivery of a precise dose of L-dopa through the lungs to gain a rapid return to the "on" state. The device used for the administration of this inhaled L-dopa compound is a passive, breath-actuated system, clinically tested several times for the delivery of big inhaled molecules, such as proteins (GH, insulin) (DeLong et al., 2005). A phase 2a dose-finding study (Freed, Batycky, DeFeo-Fraulini, & CVT-301-002 Study Investigators, 2014) was done enrolling 24 PD patients that received a single in-clinic dose of standard oral L-dopa and each of 3 inhaled double-blind treatments: placebo, CVT-301 as 25 mg fine-particle dose (FPD), and CVT-301 as 50 mg FPD. Plasma L-dopa concentrations were found to increase more rapidly and with less variability with the inhalation of CVT-301 than after oral L-dopa. UPDRS part III score improved after few minutes (5–15 min) and persisted until the 90-min assessment. The phase 2b study (a randomized, double-blind, placebo-controlled, multicenter, parallel-group dose-escalation trial) enrolled 89 PD patients, 75 of which completed the entire trial (LeWitt et al., 2016). They were divided into two groups, one taking inhaled CVT-301 and the other taking placebo (maximum three capsules/day, on-needed basis in order to treat "off" episodes, without stopping the standard treatment plan) for 4 weeks. Unified Parkinson Disease Rating Scale (UPDRS) part III score was used on baseline and at the end of weeks 1, 2, and 4 (predose "off" state, 10, 20, 30, and 60 min postdose). The results showed a marked difference between the two groups, with a statistically significant improvement after drug inhalation. No severe adverse effects were noticed, despite the known dopaminergic ones (nausea and dizziness), and no increase in "on" state with dyskinesia was reported. A phase 3 study is currently underway (Fig. 3).

2.3.3 *Apomorphine-Based Therapies*

2.3.3.1 Sublingual Apomorphine: APL-130277

APL-130277 is a sublingually administered apomorphine film strip, developed by Cynapsus Therapeutics Inc. (Toronto, Canada). Apomorphine is actually commercialized just as an injectable solution (intermittent "rescue" injection with a pen and continuous diurnal subcutaneous infusion with a pump). It is a short-acting nonergoline dopamine agonist with a 10 times stronger affinity for D1 and D2 receptors than dopamine (Goetz, Koller, Poewe, et al., 2002; Playfer & Hindle, 2010). Its major indication is the treatment of sudden motor fluctuations and early morning "off" episodes in patients with advanced PD, which cannot be tackled with the

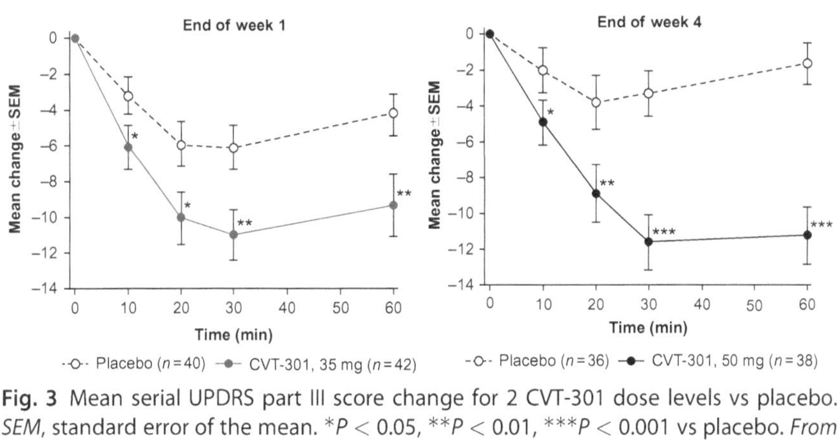

Fig. 3 Mean serial UPDRS part III score change for 2 CVT-301 dose levels vs placebo. *SEM*, standard error of the mean. $^{*}P < 0.05$, $^{**}P < 0.01$, $^{***}P < 0.001$ vs placebo. *From LeWitt, P. A., et al. (2016). A randomized trial of inhaled levodopa (CVT-301) for motor fluctuations in Parkinson's disease.* Movement Disorders, 31, *1356–1365.*

standard dopamine replacement therapies. The oral route is not currently available since apomorphine undergoes an extensive inactivation during its hepatic first-pass metabolism. This led to the sublingual route of administration and its study over the last years, where the latency before the onset of symptomatic relief was shown to be double compared with the subcutaneous route and the dose required was quite high even being the degree of the motor response between both ways of administration equivalent (Durif et al., 1991).

APL-130277 as a sublingual way of administration is a bilayered film with an optimal disintegration and a compatibility with buccal tissue. The first layer is the drug composed one and the second layer is designed to rapidly neutralize the acid generation following drug absorption to enhance drug permeability. The latter avoids the risk of inducing local skin or mucosal irritation or reactions that have been seen with the administration of apomorphine sublingual tablets. A recent open-label study tested this new formulation of sublingual apomorphine on humans and enrolled a total of 20 patients with Idiopathic PD (Hauser et al., 2016). A 10 mg dose of APL-130277 (that could have been dosed up to 15 mg, two times per day) was administered in the morning, while patients were in "off" state as they were asked to skip their levodopa morning dose. They were tested with UPDRS part III scores at predose and at 15, 30, 45, 60, and 90 min after each administration. Just 19 patients were dosed, and 15 of them reached the full "on" response within 30 min from the administration. The four nonresponders seemed to have swallowed the film, not allowing it to be absorbed properly. The UPDRS part III score improved by 30% at each assessment, reaching a maximum of a 51.3% improvement in the responder population. The most common adverse events were the dopaminergic ones, including nausea and dizziness. No evidence of local oral mucosal irritation was reported. A phase 3 study (CTH-300, a placebo-controlled, double-blind, parallel-design trial) is currently in progress to further evaluate the safety and efficacy of this new formulation of apomorphine.

2.3.3.2 Inhaled Apomorphine: VR040

VR040 is a dry powder formulation of apomorphine contained within a unit-dose blister administered using an inhaler. The first study (Grosset, Malek, Morgan, & Grosset, 2013a) on it tested its safety, tolerability, and pharmacokinetic properties administering three escalating doses of VR040 (0.2, 0.5, and 0.8 mg FPD) to 24 PD patients in a defined "off" state. Inhaled apomorphine was rapidly absorbed, giving peak concentrations (C_{max}) at 1–3 min, which compares favorably to subcutaneous apomorphine. The effect lasted for approximately 20–40 min for the doses used in the study and no significant improvement was registered in converting patients to a complete "on" state and in decreasing "off" time. A second study on 47 PD patients assessed the tolerability of VR040 with higher doses (1.5, 2.3, 3.0, and 4.0 mg) until the achievement of an "on" state while they were in a defined "off" (Grosset, Malek, Morgan, & Grosset, 2013b). A mean of 10 min was needed to reverse completely the "off" state and the UPDRS part III score improved significantly more in patients taking VR040 than in the ones taking placebo. No clinically significant changes in electrocardiogram or lung function were reported. These results have been confirmed by another trial (Grosset, Malek, Morgan, & Grosset, 2013c). Supposedly, higher doses were needed and the results seem promising as this route of administration did not show any local adverse events apart from the known dopaminergic side effects.

2.3.3.3 ND0701 (Neuroderm, Israel)

ND0701 is a novel apomorphine-based formulation for continuous delivery through a patch-pump technology that, differently from the readily available commercial apomorphine hydrochloride, induces less local skin reactions in the sense of skin nodules and an equivalent pharmacokinetic profile, even being concentrated up to fivefold (Shaltiel-Karyo et al., 2016). This new formulation provides a safer and more convenient alternative to the actual commercial preparations.

2.3.3.4 Lipophilic Prodrugs of Apomorphine: DLA, DPA, FKK01PD

Dilauroyl apomorphine (DLA) and dipalmitoyl apomorphine (DPA) are two lipophilic diesters of apomorphine that can be made resistant to hydrolysis by gastrointestinal enzymes by adding self-emulsifying drug delivery system (SEDDS) (Borkar et al., 2015). These two diesters have been recently orally administered to rats and have been studied comparing their absorption to the one of apomorphine, administered as an emulsion or an aqueous solution (Borkar, Holm, Yang, Mullertz, & Mu, 2016). Concentration and relative bioavailability of apomorphine seemed to be higher after DLA-SEDDS administration, indicating an improvement in absorption through the addition of triglycerides and surfactants.

FKK01PD is an orally active D1 and D2 agonist in development by Fabre-Kramer Pharmaceuticals (Houston, USA). It has a similar action to the one of apomorphine, but with a longer half-life and less toxicity issues. It has been tested on rats as an enteric-coated capsule, and its dopaminergic effect has been showed to last for up to 10 h. In MPTP-lesioned L-dopa-treated marmosets, the administration of this prodrug produced an antiparkinsonian effect that lasted for 33 h (http://www.fabrekramer.com/?page_id=78).

2.3.3.5 L-Dopa Prodrug: XP21279

This is a new compound that is actively absorbed through the small and large intestine and is then converted to L-dopa rapidly (Lewitt et al., 2012). In a double-blind, randomized study with patients receiving either immediate-release L-dopa/carbidopa or XP21279, no statistically significant difference in reduction in "off" time could be found (LeWitt et al., 2014). Nonetheless, but less fluctuation in L-dopa concentrations could be seen, being this of potential benefit with further studies with bigger sample sizes needed (Table 1).

3. NEW NONDOPAMINERGIC APPROACHES TO THE TREATMENT OF MOTOR SYMPTOMS IN PD

The loss of dopamine in the basal ganglia in PD causes adaptive change in many neuronal input and output pathways that affect multiple neurotransmitter systems, such as gamma-aminobutyric acid (GABA), acetylcholine, glutamate, noradrenaline, 5-hydroxytryptamin (5-HT), histamine, adenosine, opiate, and cannabinoid receptors. Many of these will contribute to the motor deficits that characterize PD and as such offer potential targets for pharmacological intervention. These have been exploited to a limited degree through the use of anticholinergic drugs and the weak *N*-methyl-D-aspartic acid (NMDA) glutamate antagonist, amantadine. This compound, initially used as an antiviral drug, has shown to be effective in noncontrolled clinical trials, but has failed to prove significant efficacy measures in the treatment of PD so far (Crosby, Deane, & Clarke, 2003). The side-effect profile of muscarinic antagonists has limited their use in PD, but there is now interest in pursuing subtype selective M4 antagonists as a means of affecting the basal ganglia without causing cognitive impairment, blurred vision, dry mouth, or urinary retention. The use of amantadine has also been limited by its side-effect profile, but a new controlled release version of the drug is under development to avoid those adverse effects occurring at peak plasma concentrations.

Table 1 Summary of L-Dopa-Based Approaches in Development

	Drug	Mechanism	Trial Status
Novel LD formulation	IPX O66	LD-ER	Phase 3, completed
	XP21279	ER LD prodrug	Phase 2, ongoing
	AP CD/LD	Prolonged gastric retention	Phase 2
	DM-1992	Combined IR/ER gastric retention	Phase 2
COMT inhibitors	Opicapone	COMT inhibition	Phase 3, ongoing
	0DM-101	Novel LD/CD/ENT combination	Phase 2, ongoing
LD delivery	LD/CD intestinal gel	Cont. jejunal delivery	Phase 3, completed
	ND0612/0650	s.c. LD/CD delivery	Phase 1/2, ongoing
	CVT-301	LD inhaler	Phase 3, planned

CD, carbidopa; *CR*, controlled release; *ENT*, entacapone; *LD*, levodopa; *R*, immediate release.
Poewe, W., & Antonini, A. (2015). Novel formulations and modes of delivery of levodopa. *Movement Disorders*, *30*, 114–120.

3.1 Treatment of Dyskinesia

Dyskinesia, being defined as involuntary, irregular, and purposeless movements of various body parts, mainly involving the lower body, was first described by Cotzias, Papavasiliou, and Gellene (1969) as early as 1969. The incidence of dyskinesias varies among the literature, being thought to affect between 40% and 50% of PD patients after 5 years of L-dopa treatment (Manson et al., 2012). The development of dyskinesias follows after L-dopa treatment and appears to be related to earlier disease onset, higher L-dopa dose, and longer duration of treatment. The underlying pathophysiology is only poorly understood, being the main mechanism of its development thought to be a pulsatile stimulation of denervated dopaminergic receptors as well as cooccurring molecular changes (Bhomraj et al., 2007). Treatment options are scarce, since the causative prevention would mean an L-dopa reduction, which would go along with an intolerable increase in Parkinsonian symptoms. The alternative of changing the treatment with L-dopa to a dopamine agonist implies other side effects, which are often not acceptable, so that the treatment options of fluctuations and dyskinesias pose an actual challenge. The currently aimed strategy is that of enhancing continuous L-dopa delivery. In this part, we will specifically focus on three of the currently developed treatments for the treatment of dyskinesia, being other listed in Table 2.

3.1.1 Amantadine HCl (ADS-5102)

ADS-5102 is an extended-release formulation of amantadine developed by Adamas Pharmaceuticals. Its efficacy is reached 12–14 h after the administration; for this reason, it is supposed to be taken once a day at bedtime. The therapeutic concentration of amantadine in the bloodstream will be reached in the morning and seems to remain high till mid-day gradually decreasing during the evening (Pahwa et al., 2015). A phase 3 trial (EASE LID) has been recently completed, using 340 mg extended-release capsules at bedtime in PD patients with troublesome L-dopa-induced dyskinesia (LID) for 25 weeks (Pahwa et al., 2015). The amount of LID (according to the Unified Dyskinesia Rating Scale, UDydRS) was significantly reduced in the patients taking ADS-5102 when compared to the ones taking placebo, and the daily "on" time without dyskinesia was increased as well. The most frequent adverse effects were hallucinations, and their incidence was higher in the group taking amantadine. Recently, the positive results of another phase 3 study (EASE LID 3) have been presented and a New Drug Application to the FDA has been submitted.

3.1.2 ASX48621-201 (Dipraglurant-IR)

Dipraglurant is a compound that inhibits the metabotropic glutamate receptor 5 and when administered together with L-dopa or dopamine agonists, has showed to reduce L-dopa-induced dyskinesias. A recent double-blind, randomized, and placebo-controlled phase 2 study on 76 PD patients showed a significant reduction of dyskinesias without worsening of motor function (Tison et al., 2016). Further phase 3 studies are planned by Addex Pharmaceuticals and the results are to be awaited.

3.1.3 Amantadine and Topiramate

Amantadine and topiramate have independently showed to reduce dyskinesia in preclinical studies (Kobylecki et al., 2011). Clinical studies on amantadine have shown beneficial effects of the drug when compared to placebo in PD patients as well (Sawada et al., 2010), but a recent study on the effect of

Table 2 Clinical Trials for the Treatment of L-Dopa-Induced Dyskinesia in PD

Pharmacological Class	Substance (References of Completed Clinical Trials)	Outcome
NMDA antagonists	Amantadine	Effective against LIDs, controversy concerning the duration of antidyskinetic effect
	ADS-5102	(Ongoing trial)
	Remacemide	No antidyskinetic effects
	Dextromethorphan	Reduced dyskinesia by 30%–40%
	AVP-923	(Ongoing trial)
	Memantine	Possibly effective against LIDs, good tolerability, and safety
	CP-101,606	Mild antidyskinetic effect, no improvement in parkinsonism, side effects
	Neu-120	(Status unknown)
mGluR antagonists	AFQ056	Reduced established LIDs, no negative effect on parkinsonism, safety, and tolerability concerns (ongoing trial)
	Dipraglurant (AX48621)	Improved parkinsonism and dyskinesia
AMPA antagonists	Talampanel	(All trials completed, but no published data available)
	Perampanel	No antidyskinetic effects
α2-Adrenergic receptor antagonists	Idazoxan	Controversial results concerning effectiveness and adverse-effect profile
	Fipamezole	Only partially effective (completed, no published data available)
Adenosine A_{2A} receptor antagonist	Preladenant (SCH 420814)	Increase in dyskinesia rates, improvement in parkinsonism
		Discontinued
	Istradefylline	Improvement in UPDRS, increased dyskinesia rates
	Tozadenant (SYN115)	No effect in dyskinesia, improvement in Parkinsonian symptoms
		Discontinued

Continued

Table 2 Clinical Trials for the Treatment of L-Dopa-Induced Dyskinesia in PD—cont'd

Pharmacological Class	Substance (References of Completed Clinical Trials)	Outcome
Nicotinic receptors agonists	Nicotine	Serious adverse effects (completed, no published data)
	SIB-1508Y	Very low tolerability
Partial dopamine agonists	Aripiprazole	Effective against LIDs, well tolerated
Pfizer D1 agonist compound	Pardoprunox	Effective against LIDs and improvement in UPDRS motor score
	Aplindore	(Completed, no published data available)
Monoamine oxidase-B inhibitors	Selegiline	Controversial results concerning efficacy against LIDs
	Rasagiline	Partially effective against LIDs
	Safinamide	Improvement of LIDs
5HT agonists	Tandospirone	No antidyskinetic effects, worsening of parkinsonism
	Sarizotane	Controversial results concerning efficacy against LIDs, probably not effective
	Piclozotan	(Completed, no published data available)
Other treatments	Valproate	No antidyskinetic effect
	Gabapentin	No antidyskinetic effect
	Zonisamide	Dose-dependent effectiveness against LIDs
	Levetiracetam	Only mild antidyskinetic effect
	Topiramate	(Early termination due to slow recruitment)
	ACR325 (odopidine)	(Completed, but no published data are available)

Simonato, M., et al. (2013) Progress in gene therapy for neurological disorders. *Nature Reviews Neurology, 9*, 277–291.

topiramate could show a significant worsening in dyskinesia and a high prevalence of adverse events, mainly being dry eyes/mouth and cognitive adverse events with hallucinations (Kobylecki et al., 2014). Recently a double-blind, placebo-controlled phase 2 study comparing add-on topiramate or add-on placebo in PD patients treated with amantadine was completed, and the results are still pending.

3.1.4 AVP-923

AVP-923 is a combination of an uncompetitive NMDA receptor antagonist and sigma-1 receptor agonist (dextromethorphan) and a CYP2D6 inhibitor (quinidine sulfate). Previous studies on NMDA receptor inhibitors had shown no effect on dyskinesias (Bara-Jimenez, Dimitrova, Sherzai, Aksu, & Chase, 2006; Parkinson Study Group, 2001); nonetheless, the compound dextromethorphan did reduce dyskinesia by 30%–40% without leading to a worsening of motor function (Jankovic, 2005; Verhagen Metman, Del Dotto, Natte, van den Munckhof, & Chase, 1998). This compound is nonetheless rapidly broken down by the hepatic cytochrome P450-2D6, so that its bioavailability is reduced. A phase 2 trial is aiming at the potential benefit of dextromethorphan on dyskinesias, overcoming its fast metabolism by blocking the corresponding liver enzyme. This phase 2, double-blind, placebo-l crossover study has recently been completed and the results are not yet available.

3.2 Treatment of Freezing of Gait

Freezing of gait (FoG) was first defined in 1992 as a brief, episodic absence or marked reduction of forward progression of the feet despite the intention to walk, and is often described by patients as if their feet are glued to the floor for a short and transient period of time (Giladi et al., 1992). Although FOG is not typical of idiopathic PD, it has only been described in association with hypokinetic, extrapyramidal movement disorders. Freezing episodes are unrelated to any weakness, flaccidity, or decreased muscle tone, and once freezing has cleared, the patient moves or performs the task at the usual pace (Yungher et al., 2014). With disease progression, FoG becomes more frequent and disabling, often leading to falls, and is much more common in the "off" state, when the effect of the L-dopa dose starts to disappear (Keating, McClellan, & Jarvis, 2001). Treatment strategies focus on avoiding wearing off increasing L-dopa therapy in frequency and dosage, but with the advancing of the disease, motor fluctuations become difficult to be controlled just by dopamine replacement therapy. Several drugs were tested over the years trying to understand the pathophysiological bases of this phenomenon (Table 3).

3.2.1 Methylphenidate (Ritaline)

Methylphenidate is an amphetamine-like psychomotor stimulant that inhibits noradrenaline/norepinephrine (NE) transporters blocking NE reuptake (Keating et al., 2001). It has been proved that in most of the PD patients, there is a loss of NE-secreting neurons (Espay, LeWitt, & Kaufmann, 2014), especially in the locus coeruleus (LC), a small cluster of brain cells in the upper dorsolateral pontine tegmentum. This seems to contribute in some way to the development of a number of PD symptoms, such as gait problems (festination and freezing of gait), autonomic disturbances, memory impairment, and sleep cycle alterations. Focusing on gait problems, several studies showed a positive effect on these symptoms after administration of methylphenidate (MPD). One of the first reported an improvement of gait speed, stride time variability, and Timed Up and Go times, 2 h after acute administration of 20 mg of MPD (Auriel, Herman, Simon, & Giladi, 2006). The first randomized, double-blinded, and placebo-controlled study testing chronic administration of MPD on gait impairment did not confirm the hypothetic efficacy of this drug (Espay et al., 2014). In this study, the patients took three doses of MPD (maximum 80 mg/day) for a period of 12 weeks and underwent several assessments during both "off" and "on" periods. Just 17 patients completed the entire 6 months of study evaluations, and despite a subjective benefit in gait, the results did not show any significant difference between the two treatment periods. Nonetheless, other results were shown in the study by Moreau et al. (2015), where the 69 recruited patients (all suffering by severe PD and undergoing subthalamic stimulation) were randomized to MPD or placebo for a period of 3 months. The freezing of gait questionnaire score was lower in the MPD-treated group than in the placebo one, and the global motor function (assessed using UPDRS part III score) was better in the MPD group. The differences between the two studies could be due to the treatment duration and the differences between the study populations (with/without concomitant subthalamic nucleus (STN) stimulation).

Table 3 The Clinical Benefit of Medications on FoG Level of Evidence

Drug	Level of Evidence (EBM Criteria)	Comments	Degree of Recommendation	References
MAO-B inhibitors				
Rasagiline	IA	FOG severity (FOG-Q) as the primary end point	B	Antonini et al. (2016); Wang et al. (2012, 2016)
Selegiline	IA	Post hoc analysis	B	Hauser et al. (2011); Schapira (2010); www.mims.co.uk; Borgohain et al. (2014); Starkstein et al. (2012)
Levodopa	IA	Secondary endpoint	A	Hauser et al. (2013); Stocchi et al. (2014); Hinson et al. (2009); Palma and Soares-da-Silva (2013); Almeida et al. (2013); Kobylecki et al. (2014); Ferreira et al. (2015)
Dopamine agonists				
Ropinirole	IA (possible worsening?)	Secondary end point	C	Almeida et al. (2013)
Pramipexole	IA (possible worsening?)	Secondary end point	C	Rocha et al. (2015)
Methylphenidate (MPD)	IV	Preliminary observation	C	Blanchet et al. (1998); Crosby et al. (2003); Bhomraj et al. (2007); Pahwa et al. (2015); Kobylecki et al. (2011); Sawada et al. (2010)
Amantadine	IV C	Retrospective data	D	Tian et al. (2013); DeLong et al. (2005)

Continued

Table 3 The Clinical Benefit of Medications on FoG Level of Evidence—cont'd

Drug	Level of Evidence (EBM Criteria)	Comments	Degree of Recommendation	References
L-Threo DOPS	Inconclusive	Conflicting results	D	Shaltiel-Karyo et al. (2016); Borkar et al. (2015); Borkar et al. (2016)
Botulinum toxin	III C	Many methodological variations	D	Playfer and Hindle (2010); Durif et al. (1991); Grosset et al. (2013b, 2013c); Shaltiel-Karyo et al. (2016)
Donepezil	IV	Preliminary observation	D	LeWitt et al. (2014)
Antidepressants/ anxiolytics	NA	Personal observation	D	

Giladi, N. (2008). Medical treatment of freezing of gait. *Movement Disorders, 23*, S482–S488.

3.3 Treatment of Motor Fluctuations

Motor fluctuations are alternations between an "on" state, in which the patient experiences a positive response to medication, and an "off" state, during which the patient experiences a recurrence of Parkinsonian symptoms. "End-of-dose wearing off" and "early morning off" are terms to describe the transition between these two states (Jankovic, 2005). With the progression of PD, these episodes tend to occur more often, needing continuous adjusting of the frequency and dosage of dopamine replacement therapy administration (Ahlskog & Muenter, 2001). The appearance of gastrointestinal issues (Baruzzi et al., 1987) along with the incorrect absorption of oral administered drugs and the resulting delayed conversion from an "off" to an "on" state lead to the necessity of new therapies, with a shorter latency between administration and absorption. COMT and monoamine oxidase (MAO) inhibitors as well as dopamine agonists are currently the most used strategies to reduce daily "off" time, even if their usage is not free from undesirable effects.

3.4 Gene Therapy

Gene therapy is aimed at supplying gene products that can replace lost or impaired functions within the cells, by means of administering deoxyribonucleic acid (DNA) or ribonucleic acid (RNA) inside vectors to the affected cells. In neurodegenerative diseases such as PD, amyotrophic lateral sclerosis, and Alzheimer's disease, the etiology of the conditions is, at least to actual knowledge, mainly idiopathic and thus not involving one specific genetic target. Therefore, the gene therapy aimed at these conditions focuses on pathways of cell repair and neuroprotection. In the case of PD, three main approaches have been discussed: induction of dopamine production, protection of neurons in the substantia nigra, and GABA-mediated inhibition of the subthalamic nucleus as seen in Fig. 4 (Simonato et al., 2013).

3.4.1 AAV2-GAD

The AAV2 vector expresses the GAD gene, which encodes glutamate decarboxylase and is intended at converting glutamate into GABA in the targeted cells. If administered to the subthalamic nucleus, it reduces excitatory output and thus improves dyskinesia and tremor (Emborg et al., 2007; Luo et al., 2002). A phase 2, double-blind, randomized,

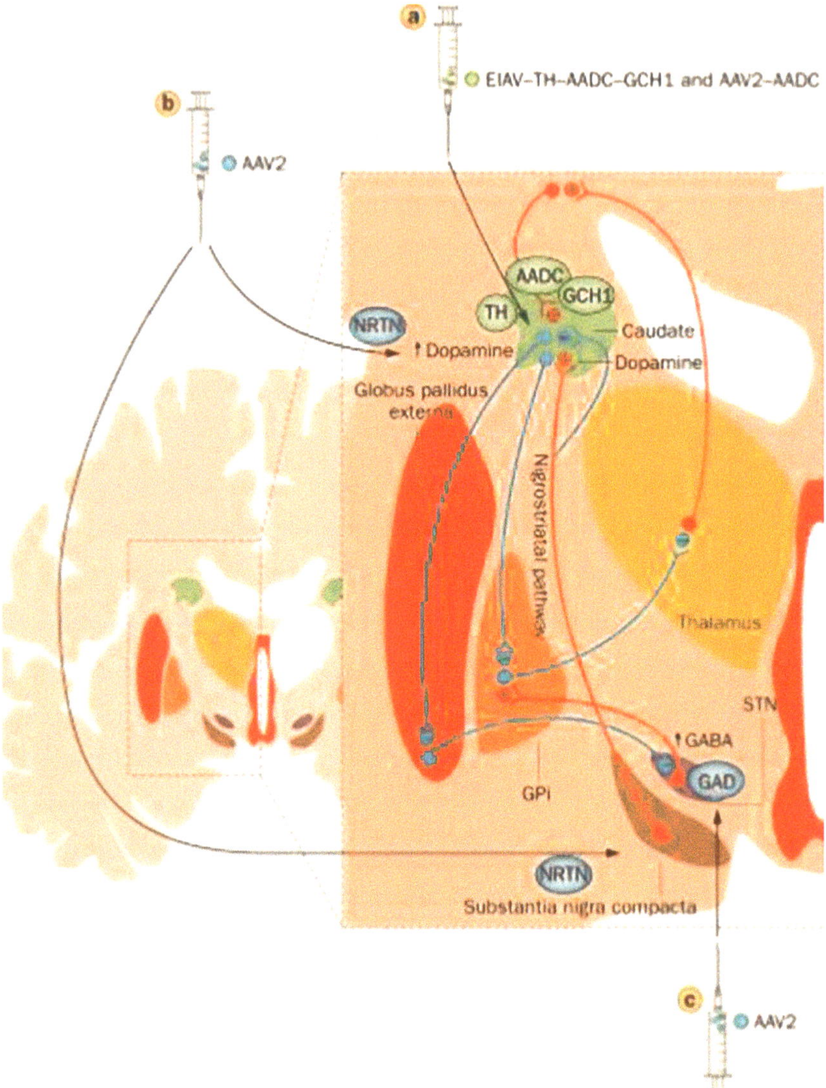

Fig. 4 Gene therapy targets and their mechanisms of action. *GABA*, gamma-aminobutyric acid; *GAD*, glutamic acid decarboxylase; *GPi*, globus pallidus internus; *NRTN*, neurturin; *STN*, subthalamic nucleus. *From Simonato, M., et al. (2013). Progress in gene therapy for neurological disorders.* Nature Reviews. Neurology, 9, *277–291.*

sham-surgery-controlled bilateral subthalamic trial by LeWitt et al. showed a significant improvement of 36% in motor function assessed by the UPDRS score when comparing the infusions of the vector with sham surgery in 66 patients (LeWitt et al., 2011).

3.4.2 AAV2-NRTN

Neurturin is a neuroprotective factor intended at preventing neurodegeneration in the nigrostriatal dopamine system. Studies analyzing its effect after intraputaminal injection compared to baseline after a 1-year period showed a significant improvement of UPDRS scores of 36% (Marks et al., 2008). Nonetheless, a further phase 2 double-blind, placebo-controlled trial with bilateral injections into the putamen could not find significant effects after 1 year (Marks et al., 2010). The postulated reason for this failure was thought to be a poor retrograde delivery of the vector, thus leading to the currently under way phase 1/2 study with bilateral injections into the putamen and substantia nigra instead of the putamen alone.

3.4.3 AAV2-hAADC

Aromatic L-amino acid decarboxylase (AADC) is an enzyme contributing to synthesis of dopamine and serotonin. Its deficiency has been described as a rare pediatric neurometabolic genetic disorder with a high prevalence among the Taiwanese population. Clinically, it imposes with early hypotonia and autonomic dysfunction, as well as features of parkinsonism, hypokinesia, oculogyric crisis, myoclonus, tremor, and athetosis. An initial assessment of administration of a vector with the precursor of this protein to eight affected patients showed an improvement in motor function in seven of the eight subjects (http://www.biotie.com/product-portfolio/syn120.aspx?sc_lang=en). Another small study on four patients showed similar promising results (Hwu et al., 2012). Furthermore, two phase-1 clinical trials on PD patients could show a safe and well-tolerated effect of delivery of this vector to the putamen (Cotzias et al., 1969; Manson et al., 2012), leading to a currently under way phase 1 open-label clinical trial on PD patients by B. Ravina, expected to be completed by December 2018 (Table 4).

3.5 Physical Amendment of Readily Existing Pharmacological Compounds

Levodopa supplementation has been the main therapeutic target ever since the early 1960s for the treatment of PD. It was first administrated to patients intravenously by Birkmayer and Hornykiewicz after discovering the loss of dopamine in brain autopsies of PD patients in 1961 as a main hallmark of the condition (Birkmayer & Hornykiewicz, 1961). Thus, complications related to its peripheral metabolism, a short half-life, long-term drug-induced dyskinesias, and motor fluctuations were observed and led to further therapeutic developments. In the early 1970s, the addition of carbidopa, a peripheral

Table 4 Summary of Gene Therapy Clinical Programs for Parkinson's Disease

Treatment (Approach)	Trial Design	Year Began	Subject Dosed[a]	Highest Total Dose (vg)	Target(s)	Largest Volume (μL)/Site	Safety Results	Efficacy Outcomes
AAV2/GAD	Ph1-uncontrolled[b]	2003	12	1×10^{12}	Subthal Nuc (unilat)	50	Acceptable	Advanced to Ph2
	Ph2-double-blind[c]	2008	22/16[d]	1×10^{12}	Subthal Nuc (Bilat)	35	Acceptable	Mixed results; program suspended
AAV2/AADC	Ph1-uncontrolled[e]	2004	10	0.3×10^{12}	Putamen (Bilat)	50	Acceptable	Program suspended; revised Ph1 recently announced
AAV2/AADC	Ph1-uncontrolled[f]	2007	6	0.3×10^{12}	Putamen (Bilat)	50	Acceptable	No further testing; revised Ph1 recently announced by the US group
AAV2/NRTN	Ph1-uncontrolled[g]	2005	12	0.54×10^{12}	Putamen (Bilat)	5(10)[h]	Acceptable	Advanced to Ph2
	Ph2A-double blind[i]	2006	38	0.54×10^{12}	Putamen (Bilat)	5(10)[h]	Acceptable	Mixed results; revised Ph1 designed
	Ph1-uncontrolled[j]	2009	6	2.4×10^{12}	Put + SN (Bilat)	50	Acceptable	Advanced to Ph2
	Ph2B-double blind[k]	2010	24	2.4×10^{12}	Put + SN (Bilat)	50	Acceptable	Program suspended
LENTI/AADC-TH-CH1	Phl/2-uncontrolled[a]	2008	15	Lentivirus dosing is not comparable to that of AAV[l]	Putamen (Bilat)		Acceptable	Program suspended; additional work to optimize vector ongoing

AAV2/ GDNF	Ph1-uncontrolled[m]	2013	Ongoing	0.7×10^{12}	Putamen (Bilat)	150	N/A	N/A
Synopsis	Total of seven phases One and three phases Two trials	2003–2013	>139	Tested up to 1×10^{12} vg AAV	Targets have included subthalamic nucleus, putamen, and SN	50 μL (most common); 150 μL (largest)	No safety issues or serious side effects noted	Efficacy outcomes generally disappointing

[a]Described as a phase 1/2 trial, this open-label (uncontrolled) study does not differ substantially from many dose-escalation phase 1 safety studies that include secondary efficacy endpoints; thus, the distinction appears to be more a semantic preference than a reflection of a substantial difference in study design.
[b]Kaplitt et al. (www.mims.co.uk).
[c]LeWitt et al. 2011 (Borgohain et al., 2014).
[d]Twenty-two subjects were dosed, but six were eliminated from efficacy analysis due to mistargeting of cannula.
[e]Christine et al. (Wang et al., 2016).
[f]Muramatsu et al. (Playfer & Hindle, 2010).
[g]Marks et al. (Crosby et al., 2003).
[h]Two 5 μL volumes infused via single needle tract ~4 mm apart.
[i]Marks et al. (Lewitt et al., 2012).
[j]Bartus et al. (LeWitt et al., 2014).
[k]Bartus et al. (http://www.fabrekramer.com/?page_id=78), Palfi et al. (Tjaden, 2008).
[l]A fivefold dose range was tested involving three dose levels (1.9×10^7 transducing units (TU); 4.0×10^7 TU; 1.0×10^8 TU).
[m]Lonser (Meltzer et al., 2010).
AAV, adeno-associated virus; *SN*, substantia nigra.
Raymond, T., et al. (2014). Parkinson's disease gene therapy: Success by design meets failure by efficacy. *Molecular Therapy, 22*, 487–497.

decarboxylase inhibitor, in order to extend the half-life availability of dopamine within the central nervous system was developed and early after the discovery of dopamine agonists was to follow, the first of them being bromocriptine (Tolosa, Marti, Valldeoriola, & Molinuevo, 1998). Currently, the administration of L-dopa together with dopa-decarboxylase inhibitors (carbidopa, benserazide) and the addition of COMT inhibitors and their development for clinical use in the 1990s (entacapone, tolcapone, or the more recently developed nebicapone and OPC) are the standard therapies in PD. Furthermore, delayed/controlled release L-dopa formulations (Madopar DR, Sinemet CR) pose another approach to tackle the above-mentioned problems by means of a physical amendment of the active compound in a matrix of insoluble substances. In the following section, the development of two newly developed compounds, the Accordion Pill and ND0611/12, will be reviewed.

3.5.1 Accordion Pill

The novel principle of this L-dopa/carbidopa containing medication has a specific physical property of being a thin layered and several times folded compound being placed in a capsule, intended to release L-dopa in a continuous way in order to enhance its bioavailability. A phase 2, randomized, open-label, crossover study on 60 PD patients comparing the Accordion pill with classical L-dopa/carbidopa showed a significant decrease of total "off" time over 24 h of 44% and 45% without significantly decreasing the "on" time, when analyzing the groups receiving 50/375 mg and 50/500 mg over 21 days, respectively, as seen in Fig. 5 (Intec Pharma; Navon, 2013).

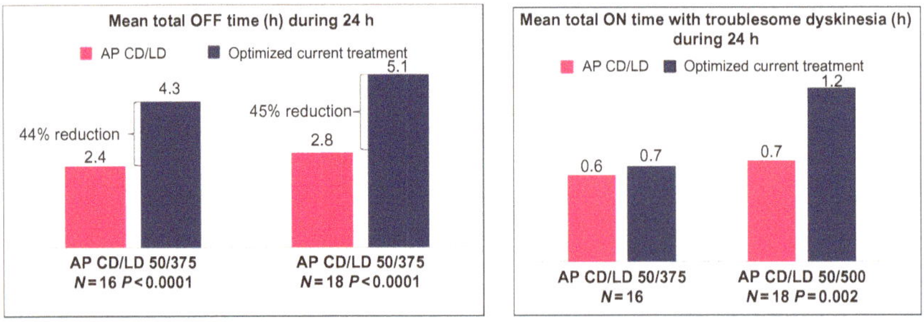

Fig. 5 Mean "off" time and mean "on" time with dyskinesia under Accordion Pill-Carbidopa–Levodopa or optimized current therapy. *AP CD/LD*, Accordion Pill-Carbidopa–Levodopa. *From Intec Pharma, The Accordion Pill™ Carbidopa/Levodopa, AP-CD/LD Phase II, Success in Phase II clinical studies with the Accordion Pill Carbidopa Levodopa product for the treatment of Parkinson's disease.*

Currently a phase 3, double-blind, active-controlled trial led by LeWitt in advanced PD patients is under way, to assess whether the Accordion pill is more effective in reducing motor fluctuations in a cohort of 328 patients; the completion of the study is expected by June 2018.

3.5.2 ND0611/0612

ND0611/0612 is a patch- or belt-pump with an L-dopa/carbidopa liquid formulation, intended to administer dopamine steadily over a 24-h period. A first clinical phase 1 study on healthy volunteers administering the patch together with Sinemet fulfilled safety and tolerability criteria positively. The preliminary clinical effectiveness was further studied in 2011 in a double-blind, placebo-controlled, crossover trial administering the patch or placebo together with Sinemet, Sinemet CR, or Stalevo in 24 advanced PD patients, showing a highly statistically significant improvement when coadministering it with the three compounds (http://neuroderm.com). In 2014 a placebo-controlled study with moderate–severe PD patients showed statistically significant reduction in plasma levodopa fluctuations as well as a reduction in "off" time, and improvement in sleep and in overall quality of life without increasing dyskinesia (Yungher et al., 2014). Further studies are led by Neuroderm and the results are to be awaited.

4. NEW THERAPEUTIC TARGETS FOR THE TREATMENT OF NONMOTOR SYMPTOMS IN PD

4.1 Cognitive Decline

Cognitive decline including the terms mild cognitive impairment (MCI) as well as dementia is one of the main burdens in an increasingly aging society. Dementia is defined by the WHO under the ICD-10 revision criteria as a chronic and progressive disease with disturbances of higher cortical function involving memory, thinking, comprehension, calculation, learning capacity, language, and judgment. The term *MCI* refers to a lesser degree of cognitive impairment, implying a concern about changes in cognition, objective impairment in one or more cognitive domains (assessed by neuropsychological testing), preservation of independence in functional abilities, and lack of diagnostic criteria fulfilling the definition of dementia (Li et al., 2015).

Readily available therapies based on agents that exert their effect by increasing cholinergic neurotransmission in the central nervous system such as rivastigmine have been studied in a placebo-controlled study by Li et al.

involving 176 PD patients assessing them with the MOCA Scale as well as measuring the number of falls as primary outcomes after a 12-month randomization, showing statistically significant higher MOCA Scores and lower amount of falls in the treated group compared to placebo (Li et al., 2015). Another study by Emre et al. (2004) analyzed the effect of rivastigmine on 410 PD patients with mild–moderate dementia, showing a moderate effect on cognition scales when compared to placebo. Another study assessing the effect of rivastigmine among PD patients with dementia with and without additional visual hallucinations showed a significant improvement among both groups when compared with placebo, being the effect on cognition larger among the PD patients who had additional hallucinations (Burn et al., 2006). Furthermore, rivastigmine is currently the only recommended therapeutic compound for dementia in PD, as published by the movement disorder society evidence-based medicine review update in 2011 (Seppi et al., 2011). Other studies studying different compounds with analogous mechanisms of action as rivastigmine like donepezil and galantamine showed similar results (Dubois et al., 2012; Litvinenko, Odinak, Mogil'naya, & Emelin, 2008) with statistically significant improvements in cognitive assessment tools. A review on the effect of the antiglutamatergic compound memantine in PD dementia could nonetheless not conclude consistent cognitive improvements in PD patients treated with it when compared to placebo (Brennan et al., 2016). This leads to the strong support for the development of novel targets to tackle this condition. In the following part, newly developed compounds that are being assessed in PD dementia will be explained.

4.1.1 Atomoxetine

Atomoxetine is a noradrenaline reuptake inhibitor, currently approved for its use in attention deficit hyperactive disorder (ADHS) in children, adolescents, and adults. Weintraub et al. performed a randomized, placebo-controlled study on 55 PD patients, to analyze whether the enhancement of noradrenaline in the central nervous system had an effect on depression and comorbid neuropsychiatric features among PD patients, with the background that multiple neurotransmitter systems might be involved in its pathophysiology and that selective serotonin reuptake inhibitors have already proven effective in treating depression in PD. The results of their study nonetheless showed no statistically significant effect of this compound with regard to depression, but an improvement in cognitive performance (minimental state examination (MMSE) scores) and daytime sleepiness (Epworth Sleepiness Scale (ESS) scores). Along with this promising result, a current phase 2 trial in a double-blind and placebo-controlled setting has been initiated by Hinson V in 2012 and is currently under way involving a total amount of 30 PD patients, randomized into a treatment and a placebo group. The results are still pending.

4.1.2 *Droxidopa*

Droxidopa is a synthetic amino acid precursor that gets transformed into the neurotransmitter noradrenaline, being able to pass the blood–brain barrier. Its use is currently approved for neurogenic orthostatic hypotension, showing a class I evidence in the treatment of orthostatic hypotension in PD (Kaufmann et al., 2014). Alongside the above-mentioned hypothesis of Atomoxetine on cognition, droxidopa is currently being assessed in its effect on cognitive function in a placebo-controlled trial involving 40 PD patients, led by LeWitt.

4.1.3 *Piribedil*

Piribedil is a dopamine agonist of the nonergotic class, working as a D2/D3 agonist and an alpha-2a antagonist. A study by Turle-Lorenzo et al. (2006) on rat models with bilateral striatal dopamine lesions analyzed the effect of piribedil on motor and nonmotor aspects and found evidence of some effect of this compound on cognitive decline, showing less attentional dysfunction in the animals receiving piribedil (Turle-Lorenzo et al., 2006). A further clinical study of piribedil in young healthy volunteers by Schuck et al. (2002) found an improvement of alertness and speed in information processing. Another study by Nagaraja et al. involving 30 patients with MCI showed a significant improvement in MMSE scores after a 90-day treatment regime comparing piribedil to placebo (Nagaraja & Jayashree, 2001). Clinical trials of this compound to assess its potential use in PD dementia have not taken place so far, so that a clinical trial to assess the effect of this compound in PD patients compared to other nonergot dopamine agonists in a randomized single-blinded setting (PIVICOG-PD) was started in 2009 under the lead of Wangemann M. The results are still to be awaited.

4.1.4 *SYN-120*

SYN-120 is a dual antagonist of the 5HT6 and 5HT2A receptors. 5-HT6 antagonists are being currently studied in humans as a potential novel target to address cognitive decline in Alzheimer's disease, with its mechanism of action believed to be via multiple modulation of various neurotransmitter systems, including the cholinergic, glutamatergic, noradrenergic, dopaminergic, and GABAergic pathways (Benhamú, Martín-Fontecha, Vázquez-Villa, Pardo, & López-Rodríguez, 2014). 5HT2A antagonists on the other hand are known to have antipsychotic effects (this receptor being the target of many of the hallucinogenic and psychotropic drugs), being of great value in PD, especially since cognitive decline and neuropsychiatric symptoms are frequently linked.

The novel compound SYN-120 combines both the procognitive and the antipsychotic mechanism of action and is being studied as a promising treatment option in a phase 2 clinical trial involving PD patients with dementia in a randomized, double-blind, multicenter, placebo-controlled setting (SYNAPSE study). The primary endpoint is the efficacy of the compound on cognition, assessed by the Cognitive Drug Research Computerized Cognition Battery (http://www.biotie.com/product-portfolio/syn120.aspx?sc_lang=en). The results are not yet available.

4.1.5 Pimavanserin

This 5HT2A receptor inverse agonist is used for the treatment of psychosis in PD. It is defined as an antagonist with negative intrinsic activity (Garay et al., 2016) and acts by modulating the serotonin receptor and its downstream Gq-G protein and PKC activation, thought to have a direct effect inhibiting pyramidal cells of the cerebral cortex (Meltzer et al., 2010). Current studies will be reviewed in Section 4.5.

4.2 Swallowing Problems and Sialorrhea

Dysphagia is defined as an inefficiency in transferring food, liquid, or saliva from the oral cavity to the stomach (Tjaden, 2008) and is a common symptom among PD patients, tending to develop after the appearance of dysarthria, which is defined as a disorder in muscular control for speech. With regard to its prevalence, literature data vary widely, with a recent published review on this topic stating a prevalence between 11% and 81% (Muller et al., 2001), thus being a little less prevalent than dysarthria, which appears in up to 90% of PD patients in the course of the disease (Takizawa, Gemmell, Kenworthy, & Speyer, 2016). The burden of dysphagia is not to be underpinned, since it can lead to malnutrition, dehydration, aspiration pneumonia, and, for instance, death due to secondary complications.

Current treatment options include rehabilitation (expiratory muscle strength training, feeding modifications, learning of swallowing techniques) as well as pharmacologic treatments with L-dopa, dopamine agonists, anticholinergic agents (glycopyrrolate, ipratropium bromide, atropine), alpha-2 receptor agonists (clonidine), alpha-1 receptor agonists (modafinil), and botulinum toxin injections into the parotid/submandibular glands. Results of a review that evaluated these different treatment approaches (Playfer & Hindle, 2010) showed some significant changes in swallowing dysfunction after L-dopa and after dopaminergic treatment, with no significant effect of botulinum toxin. The nonpharmacological interventions showed improvements in the performance of swallowing exercises, thermal-tactile stimulation, and electromagnetic stimulation, among others.

4.2.1 Tropicamide

Tropicamide is an antimuscarinic agent, which is used to produce a short lasting mydriasis over 4–8 h, being of clinical use in ophthalmology. A study on the effect of this anticholinergic drug on sialorrhea in 19 PD patients showed a significant reduction in sialorrhea symptoms and saliva amount measured by the visual analog scale and cotton rolls, respectively (Lloret, Nano, Carrosella, Gamzu, & Merello, 2011). Further studies with wider amounts of subjects have, to our knowledge, not been performed. A current clinical trial led by Gamzu et al. is therefore currently being performed, analyzing the responder rate between tropicamide and placebo-treated PD patients in a randomized, double-blind, placebo-controlled study. The results are not yet published.

4.3 Gastrointestinal Dysfunction

Gastrointestinal issues have been widely recognized in PD and constipation seems to be one of the most common nonmotor symptoms among PD patients (Edwards, Quigley, & Pfeiffer, 1992). The reduction of colon motility is thought to be due to a degeneration of the dopamine neurons sited in gut walls' plexus. It is well known that neurodegeneration in PD is related to the presence of aggregates of misfolded α-synuclein and that this aggregates seem to propagate via neural pathways following a stereotypical pattern starting from the olfactory bulb (Braak et al., 2003).

Constipation has been recognized as one of the prodromal clinical markers of PD as it can be present many years before the onset of the typical motor symptoms (Postuma & Berg, 2016).The reduced gastrointestinal motility has a big impact in quality of life as it delays the effect of oral therapies intake and reduces their efficacy. The stomach is often also involved and scintigraphy (Camilleri, Bharucha, et al., 2012) shows the presence of delayed gastric emptying (DGE) in some PD patients. Furthermore, gastroparesis, defined as DGE in the absence of mechanical obstruction and the presence of symptoms including nausea/vomiting, postprandial fullness, bloating, and epigastric pain, has been described.

Till now, constipation has been the main target of some symptomatic therapies, such as laxatives, but lately the development of stomach target therapies seem to be the main aim in order to improve oral therapies effectiveness. Domperidone has been one of the most used gastric-targeted therapies, also for its antiemetic effect. Otherwise, its use is still controversial for the high risk of cardiological side effects (Lertxundi et al., 2013). Motilin and ghrelin receptors have been discovered a long time ago, but the use of their agonists has been difficult due to the high incidence of tolerance and indesiderable effects (Deane, Fraser, & Chapman, 2009). Recently, more specific motilin and ghrelin agonists have been produced and studied in order to reduce the incidence of side effects and to provide a safe and effective enhancement of gastric motility (Sanger, 2014).

4.3.1 *Camicinal*

Camicinal (GSK962040) is a first-in-class small molecule motilin receptor agonist that can potentially accelerate gastric emptying by 30%–40% in healthy volunteers (Shaltiel-Karyo et al., 2016) and even more in critically ill patients with gastroparesis (Chapman et al., 2016). It has a high specificity for recombinant human motilin receptor and less side effects among other motilin agonist such as erythromycin that has shown to induce rapid tolerance and microbial resistance as it is first known as a macrolide antibiotic. Camicinal is now available just as an enteral formulation. A randomized, double-blind, and placebo-controlled study on critically ill patients (undergoing invasive mechanical ventilation in intensive care unit (ICU) and that developed "feed intolerance" during nasogastric feeding) (Chapman et al., 2016) has shown the efficacy of this motilin agonist, as a single dose of 50 mg, in improving gastric emptying and glucose absorption (assessed by C-octanoic acid breath test, acetaminophen absorption test, 3-OMG). Unlike erythromycin that has similar effects but seems to reduce fat absorption, camicinal seems to improve also this aspect. Adverse effects were not registered during this study, but further studies are needed.

4.3.2 *Relamorelin*

Relamorelin (RM-131) is a synthetic ghrelin agonist with similar characteristics as native ghrelin, but with a greater potency and a longer plasma half-life. As the already known ghrelin agonists, it has a potential effect in enhancing GE in patients with gastroparesis. Ulimorelin (TPZ-101), an older and similar compound as Relamorelin, has shown to have only a slight effect on gastric motility. Relamorelin has shown to have a greater effect in patients with type 1 or 2 diabetes and related gastroparesis (Shin, Camilleri, et al., 2013). In both studies, participants received a single dose of RM-131 (100 μg subcutaneously) or placebo (5% mannitol) with a gap of 7 days to ensure the complete washout. Symptoms were assessed daily using GCSI-DD (gastroparesis cardinal symptom index) and scintigraphy was used to asses GE. Both the testing methods showed a critical difference in results using placebo and relamorelin, and the latter improved GE of solids by 54.7% (Shin, Busciglio, et al., 2013) and 61% (Shin, Camilleri, et al., 2013). The drug was generally well tolerated, no side effects reported, except for hunger that seemed to be more frequent when RM-131 was administered (Fig. 6; Table 5).

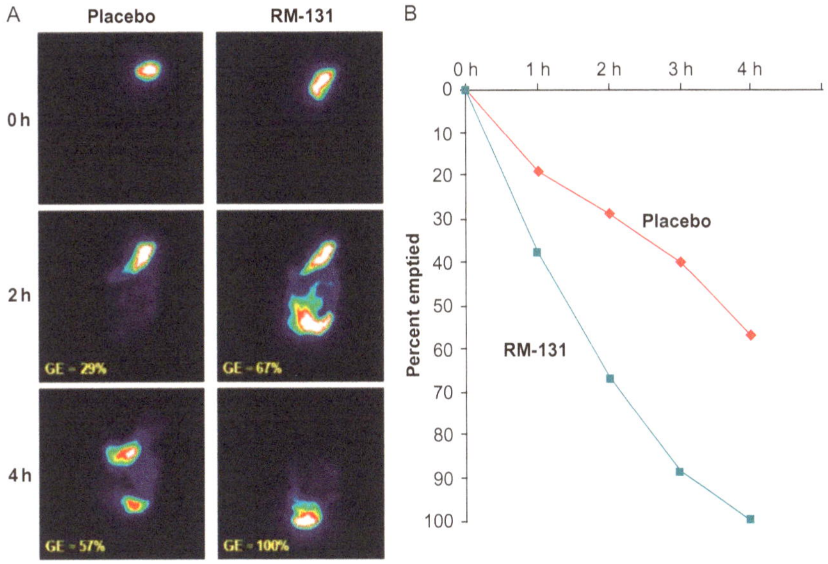

Fig. 6 Assessment of GE of solids by scintigraphy in 1 patient showing delayed GE with placebo and normal GE with RM-131 (*left panel*). GE is shown as the percentage emptied over time for placebo and RM-131 in the same individual (*right panel*). *From Shin, A., et al. (2013). The ghrelin agonist RM-131 accelerates gastric emptying of solids and reduces symptoms in patients with type 1 diabetes mellitus.* Clinical Gastroenterology and Hepatology, 11, *1453–1459.*

Table 5 Summary of Therapies for Gastrointestinal Dysfunction in PD and Their Mechanism of Action

Dopamine Agonists	Intestinal Secretagogues	Serotonin Agonists	Motilin Agonists	Ghrelin Agonists
Domperidone (D2)	Lubiprostone	Prucalopride	Ulimorelin (TPZ-101)	Relamorelin (RM-131)
Sulpiride	Linaclotide	Metoclopramide (also a D2 agonist)	Camicinal (GSK962040)	

4.4 Impulse Control Disorder

ICDs are a psychiatric complication in patients with PD and are defined as a failure to resist an impulse or temptation to perform an act that is harmful to oneself or to the others (Voon & Fox, 2007). The correction of dopamine replacement drug dose seems to be the most frequent intervention in order to resolve ICDs, but this can lead to an exacerbation of PD-related symptoms and to a possible dopamine agonist withdrawal syndrome. Also, the switch to a different dopamine therapy has shown evidence of regression or lower incidence of ICDs and an improvement of quality of life, being the switch either to prolonged-release dopamine formulations, MAO-B or COMT inhibitors or enteral infusion of levodopa–carbidopa gel (LCIG) (Catalan, Villanueva, et al., 2013) as well as continuous subcutaneous apomorphine infusion (Garcia Ruiz, Ares Pensado, et al., 2008). Nonetheless, a recent prospective study with nine de novo PD cases developed early ICDs under apomorphine pump therapy (Martinez-Martin et al., 2015). Regarding the use of dopamine agonists, rotigotine seems to be associated with a lower risk of developing ICDs compared to the others (Garcia-Ruiz et al., 2014), and cognitive behavioral therapy has shown some benefits as well (Okai et al., 2013). The use of atypical antipsychotics and antidepressants has been evaluated as a potential treatment of ICDs, but as it overlaps with PD, the worsening of motor symptoms due to dopaminergic blockade can limit their usage. Some of them, such as olanzapine and clozapine, seem not to exacerbate Parkinsonism as their effect is primarily directed toward D3 and D4 dopamine receptors (Hardwick, Ward, Hassan, Romrell, & Okun, 2013). With regard to ICDs after STN deep brain stimulation (DBS), results are controversial. Some studies showed a resolution of ICDs after the implantation of DBS and the reduction of conventional pharmaceutical treatments, and some others ended up in the development of de novo ICDs after surgery (Ramirez-Zamora, Boyd, & Biller, 2016).

The same situation has been seen for amantadine. Once again, there is a high need for further prospective studies and controlled trials to evaluate new drugs when the reduction of dopaminergic drugs fails to improve psychiatric symptoms. A group of drugs that have been recently tested in patients with ICDs as a complication of PD treatments are opioid antagonists, as shown in the following section.

4.4.1 Naltrexone

Naltrexone is a competitive, nonselective opioid receptor antagonist that has been widely used in the treatment of alcohol and opioid dependency. Numerous studies have been made for testing this drug on ICDs, especially on pathological gambling (Kim, Grant, Adson, & Shin, 2001). Naltrexone seems to be well tolerated among PD patients as it has no anti-Parkinsonian effects at the dosage of 100 mg/day. A recent randomized, double-blind, placebo-controlled study (Papay et al., 2014) has tested the effects of 50–100 mg per day of naltrexone in treating different types of ICD (compulsive gambling, buying, sexual behaviors, and eating) during a period of 8 weeks. Participants were assessed using a clinician-based rating of improvement (CGI-C) and the patient-completed impulsive–compulsive disorders in Parkinson's disease-rating scale (QUIP-RS) (Weintraub et al., 2012). The results were negative according to CGI-C, although this seemed to be due to a lack of statistical precision in excluding important differences in response rates between the two groups. Otherwise, the QUIP-RS showed a higher improvement in the naltrexone group compared to the placebo one (even if the analysis were not statistically significant). The UPDRS III part scores were reduced in both groups, confirming a good motor tolerability of naltrexone, as shown in other studies (Rascol et al., 1994). Some side effects such as nausea (without vomiting), dizziness, and headaches were reported, but all of them reported to be mild–moderate. This study, although not enough satisfactory, supports further research using naltrexone or other opioid antagonist (e.g., nalmefene) in treating ICDs in PD patients.

4.5 Psychosis

Psychosis is a common complication among PD patients. It seems to be more frequent as the disease progresses, with older age and with the development of dementia (Starkstein et al., 2012). The main features are hallucinations and delusions, these being less frequent and associated with more advanced stages of the disease. The symptoms can cause a huge distress to the patients and their caregivers. Nowadays, there are a lack of treatment options, as the mainly available antipsychotic drugs have a strong D2 dopamine receptor antagonism and can seriously worsening of the motor features of PD. Some atypical antipsychotic drugs have been tested in PD, as they seem to have more effect on D3 and D4 receptors. Quetiapine seems to be well tolerated among PD patients, but there is a lack in efficacy, as shown in studies (Rabery, Miniovitz, Dobronevsky, & Klein, 2007). Clozapine has also shown some positive results, but the risk of agranulocytosis limits its use (Pollak, Rascol, et al., 2004). The reduction of dopaminergic therapy can lead to a reduction of these symptoms, but that can be inacceptable since motor symptoms are normally at an advanced stage.

4.5.1 Pimavanserin

Pimavanserin (Nuplazid) is a selective serotonin 5-HT2A inverse agonist without dopaminergic, adrenergic, histaminergic, or muscarinic affinity (Vanover, Makhay, et al., 2006). The binding of 5-HT2A receptors seems to be mainly located in the neocortex being their increased number associated with the development of visual hallucinations (Ballanger et al., 2010). Many studies have shown the potential of this drug in improving psychotic symptoms among PD patients (Friedman, Mills, et al., 2010; Meltzer et al., 2010). A recent randomized, double-blind, parallel, placebo-controlled study (Cummings et al., 2014) tested 185 PD patients with a minimum score of six in the neuropsychiatric inventory item A (delusions) and B (hallucinations). The participants were divided into two groups, one receiving 40 mg/day of pimavanserin and the other group taking placebo. The primary outcome was the change in total Parkinson's disease-adapted scale for assessment of positive symptoms (SAPS-PD) (Voss, Cummings, Mills, Ravina, & Williams, 2013). Results showed a significant reduction in SAPS-PD score in the pimavanserin group compared with the placebo one. An improvement in quality of life and nighttime sleep was also registered. Some adverse effects such as urinary tract infections, peripheral edema, and falls were reported, but no significant difference between the two groups was found. According to previous studies, no motor worsening was noticed. This confirms the antipsychotic benefit of this new class of therapeutic agents for the potential treatment of psychosis in PD.

Readily available therapeutic options for other nonmotor aspects of PD, which have not been revised in this chapter, are shown in Table 6.

Table 6 Summary of Currently Available Therapies for Other Nonmotor Symptoms in PD

	Dopaminergic Treatment	Others
Pain	1. Rotigotine patch RECOVER study (2013) DOLORES study (2015)	Opiates 1. Naloxone 2. Oxicodone OXN PR study (2015)
Apathy	1. Piribedil Thobois et al.	Cholinesterase inhibitors 1. Rivastigmine Devos et al.
Excessive daytime sleepness	1. Piribedil	Stimulants 1. Modafinil 2. Sodium oxybate
Insomnia	1. Rotigotine patch RECOVER study (2013) 2. LCIG 3. Apomorphine 4. Pergolide	1. Melatonin
Depression	1. Rotigotine patch 2. Apomorphine infusion 3. LCIG	1. Tricyclic antidepressants 2. SSRI

REFERENCES

Ahlskog, J. E., & Muenter, M. D. (2001). Frequency of levodopa-related dyskinesias and motor fluctuations as estimated from the cumulative literature. *Movement Disorders: Official Journal of the Movement Disorder Society*, *16*(3), 448–458.

Almeida, L. R. J.-F., Falcao, A., et al. (2013). Pharmacokinetics, pharmacodynamics and tolerability of opicapone, a novel catechol-O-methyltransferase inhibitor, in healthy subjects: Prediction of slow enzyme-inhibitor complex dissociation of a short-living and very long-acting inhibitor. *Clinical Pharmacokinetics*, *52*(2), 139–151.

Antonini, A., Chaudhuri, K. R., Boroojerdi, B., Asgharnejad, M., Bauer, L., Grieger, F., et al. (2016). Impulse control disorder related behaviours during long-term rotigotine treatment: A post hoc analysis. *European Journal of Neurology*, *23*, 1556–1565.

Auriel, E., Herman, T., Simon, E. S., & Giladi, N. (2006). Effects of methylphenidate on cognitive function and gait in patients with Parkinson's disease: A pilot study. *Clinical Neuropharmacology*, *29*, 15–17.

Ballanger, B., Strafella, A. P., van Eimeren, T., Zurowski, M., Rusjan, P. M., Houle, S., et al. (2010). Serotonin 2A receptors and visual hallucinations in Parkinson disease. *Archives of Neurology*, *67*(4), 416–421.

Bara-Jimenez, W., Dimitrova, T. D., Sherzai, A., Aksu, M., & Chase, T. N. (2006). Glutamate release inhibition ineffective in levodopa-induced motor complications. *Movement Disorders: Official Journal of the Movement Disorder Society*, *21*(9), 1380–1383.

Baruzzi, A., Contin, M., Riva, R., Procaccianti, G., Albani, F., Tonello, C., et al. (1987). Influence of meal ingestion time on pharmacokinetics of orally administered levodopa in parkinsonian patients. *Clinical Neuropharmacology, 10*(6), 527–537.

Benhamú, B., Martín-Fontecha, M., Vázquez-Villa, H., Pardo, L., & López-Rodríguez, M. L. (2014). Serotonin 5-HT6 receptor antagonists for the treatment of cognitive deficiency in Alzheimer's disease. *Journal of Medicinal Chemistry, 57*(17), 7160–7181. http://dx.doi.org/10.1021/jm5003952. Epub 2014 Jun 3.

Bhomraj, T., et al. (2007). Levodopa-induced dyskinesia in Parkinson's disease: Clinical features, pathogenesis, prevention and treatment. *Postgraduate Medical Journal, 83*(980), 384–388.

Birkmayer, W., & Hornykiewicz, O. (1961). The L-3,4-dioxyphenylalanine (DOPA)-effect in Parkinson-akinesia. *Wiener Klinische Wochenschrift, 73*, 787–788.

Blanchet, P. J., Fang, J., Gillespie, M., Sabounjian, L., Locke, K. W., Gammans, R., et al. (1998). Effects of the full dopamine D1 receptor agonist dihydrexidine in Parkinson's disease. *Clinical Neuropharmacology, 21*(6), 339–343.

Bonifacio, M. J., Torrao, L., Loureiro, A. I., Palma, P. N., Wright, L. C., & Soares-da-Silva, P. (2015). Pharmacological profile of opicapone, a third-generation nitrocatechol catechol-O-methyl transferase inhibitor in the rat. *British Journal of Pharmacology, 172*(7), 1739–1752.

Borgohain, R., Szasz, J., Stanzione, P., Meshram, C., Bhatt, M., Chirilineau, D., et al. (2014). Randomized trial of safinamide add-on to levodopa in Parkinson's disease with motor fluctuations. *Movement Disorders: Official Journal of the Movement Disorder Society, 29*(2), 229–237.

Borkar, N., Holm, R., Yang, M., Mullertz, A., & Mu, H. (2016). In vivo evaluation of lipid-based formulations for oral delivery of apomorphine and its diester prodrugs. *International Journal of Pharmaceutics, 513*(1–2), 211–217.

Borkar, N., Li, B., Holm, R., Hakansson, A. E., Mullertz, A., Yang, M., et al. (2015). Lipophilic prodrugs of apomorphine I: Preparation, characterisation, and in vitro enzymatic hydrolysis in biorelevant media. *European Journal of Pharmaceutics and Biopharmaceutics: Official Journal of Arbeitsgemeinschaft fur Pharmazeutische Verfahrenstechnik eV, 89*, 216–223.

Braak, H., et al. (2003). Staging of brain pathology related to sporadic Parkinson's disease. *Neurobiology of Aging, 24*(2), 197–211.

Brennan, L., et al. (2016). Memantine and cognition in Parkinson's disease dementia/dementia with Lewy bodies: A meta-analysis. *Movement Disorders Clinical Practice, 3*(2). http://dx.doi.org/10.1002/mdc3.12264.

Burn, D., Emre, M., McKeith, I., De Deyn, P. P., Aarsland, D., Hsu, C., et al. (2006). Effects of rivastigmine in patients with and without visual hallucinations in dementia associated with Parkinson's disease. *Movement Disorders: Official Journal of the Movement Disorder Society, 21*(11), 1899–1907.

Camilleri, M., Bharucha, A. E., et al. (2012). Performance characteristics of scintigraphic measurement of gastric emptying of solids in healthy participants. *Neurogastroenterology and Motility, 24*. 1076-e562.

Catalan, M. J., Villanueva, C., et al. (2013). Levodopa infusion improves impulsivity and dopamine dysregulation syndrome in Parkinson's disease. *Movement Disorders: Official Journal of the Movement Disorder Society, 28*(14), 2007–2010.

Chapman, M. J., Deane, A. M., O'Connor, S. L., Nguyen, N. Q., Fraser, R. J., Richards, D. B., et al. (2016). The effect of camicinal (GSK962040), a motilin agonist, on gastric emptying and glucose absorption in feed-intolerant critically ill patients: A randomized, blinded, placebo-controlled, clinical trial. *Critical Care (London, England), 20*(1), 232.

Cotzias, G. C., Papavasiliou, P. S., & Gellene, R. (1969). Modification of Parkinsonism—Chronic treatment with L-dopa. *The New England Journal of Medicine, 280*(7), 337–345.

Crosby, N., Deane, K. H., & Clarke, C. E. (2003). Amantadine in Parkinson's disease. *The Cochrane Database of Systematic Reviews, 1*, Cd003468.

Cummings, J., Isaacson, S., Mills, R., Williams, H., Chi-Burris, K., Corbett, A., et al. (2014). Pimavanserin for patients with Parkinson's disease psychosis: A randomised, placebo-controlled phase 3 trial. *Lancet (London, England), 383*(9916), 533–540.

Deane, A. M., Fraser, R. J., & Chapman, M. J. (2009). Prokinetic drugs for feed intolerance in critical illness: Current and potential therapies. *Critical Care and Resuscitation: Journal of the Australasian Academy of Critical Care Medicine, 11*(2), 132–143.

DeLong, M., Wright, J., Dawson, M., Meyer, T., Sommerer, K., & Dunbar, C. (2005). Dose delivery characteristics of the AIR pulmonary delivery system over a range of inspiratory flow rates. *Journal of Aerosol Medicine: The Official Journal of the International Society for Aerosols in Medicine, 18*(4), 452–459.

Dubois, B., Tolosa, E., Katzenschlager, R., Emre, M., Lees, A. J., Schumann, G., et al. (2012). Donepezil in Parkinson's disease dementia: A randomized, double-blind efficacy and safety study. *Movement Disorders: Official Journal of the Movement Disorder Society, 27*(10), 1230–1238.

Durif, F., Jeanneau, E., Serre-Debeauvais, F., Deffond, D., Eschalier, A., & Tournilhac, M. (1991). Relation between plasma concentration and clinical efficacy after sublingual single dose apomorphine in Parkinson's disease. *European Journal of Clinical Pharmacology, 41*, 493–494.

Edwards, L. L., Quigley, E. M., & Pfeiffer, R. F. (1992). Gastrointestinal dysfunction in Parkinson's disease: Frequency and pathophysiology. *Neurology, 42*(4), 726–732.

Emborg, M. E., Carbon, M., Holden, J. E., During, M. J., Ma, Y., Tang, C., et al. (2007). Subthalamic glutamic acid decarboxylase gene therapy: Changes in motor function and cortical metabolism. *Journal of Cerebral Blood Flow and Metabolism: Official Journal of the International Society of Cerebral Blood Flow and Metabolism, 27*(3), 501–509.

Emre, M., Aarsland, D., Albanese, A., Byrne, E. J., Deuschl, G., De Deyn, P. P., et al. (2004). Rivastigmine for dementia associated with Parkinson's disease. *The New England Journal of Medicine, 351*(24), 2509–2518.

Espay, A. J., LeWitt, P. A., & Kaufmann, H. (2014). Norepinephrine deficiency in Parkinson's disease: The case for noradrenergic enhancement. *Movement Disorders: Official Journal of the Movement Disorder Society, 29*(14), 1710–1719.

Ferreira, J. J., Lees, A., Rocha, J. F., Poewe, W., Rascol, O., & Soares-da-Silva, P. (2015). Opicapone as an adjunct to levodopa in patients with Parkinson's disease and end-of-dose motor fluctuations: A randomised, double-blind, controlled trial. *The Lancet Neurology*. pii: S1474-4422(15)00336-1. doi:1016/S1474-4422(15)00336-1.

Freed, M. I., Batycky, R., DeFeo-Fraulini, T., & CVT-301-002 Study Investigators (2014). Pharmacokinetics following inhaled levodopa delivery with CVT-301: Rapid augmentation of systemic levodopa levels and improvement in motor function in PD patients with motor fluctuations. In *Poster presented at 18th international congress of Parkinson's disease and movement disorders, June 8–12, Stockholm, Sweden.*

Friedman, J. H. R. B., Mills, R., et al. (2010). A multicentre, placebo controlled, double blind trial to examine the safety and efficacy of pimavanserin in the treatment of psychosis in Parkinson's disease. *Neuropsychopharmacology, 35*(4), 881–892. http://dx.doi.org/10.1038/npp.2009.176. Epub 2009 Nov 11.

Garay, R. P., Bourin, M., de Paillette, E., Samalin, L., Hameg, A., & Llorca, P. M. (2016). Potential serotonergic agents for the treatment of schizophrenia. *Expert Opinion on Investigational Drugs, 25*(2), 159–170.

Garcia Ruiz, P. J., Ares Pensado, B., et al. (2008). Efficacy of long-term continuous subcutaneous apomorphine infusion in advanced Parkinson's disease with motor fluctuations: A multicentre study. *Movement Disorders: Official Journal of the Movement Disorder Society, 23*(8), 1130–1136.

Garcia-Ruiz, P. J., Martinez Castrillo, J. C., Alonso-Canovas, A., Herranz Barcenas, A., Vela, L., Sanchez Alonso, P., et al. (2014). Impulse control disorder in patients with Parkinson's disease under dopamine agonist therapy: A multicentre study. *Journal of Neurology, Neurosurgery, and Psychiatry*, *85*(8), 840–844.

Giladi, N., McMahon, D., Przedborski, S., Flaster, E., Guillory, S., Kostic, V., et al. (1992). Motor blocks in Parkinson's disease. *Neurology*, *42*, 333–339.

Goetz, C. G., Koller, W. C., Poewe, W., Rascol, O., Sampaio, C., Brin, M. F., et al. (2002). DA agonist–non-ergot derivatives: Apomorphine. *Movement Disorders*, *17*(Suppl. 4), S83–S89.

Grosset, K. A., Malek, N., Morgan, F., & Grosset, D. G. (2013a). Phase IIa randomized double-blind, placebo-controlled study of inhaled apomorphine as acute challenge for rescuing 'off' periods in patients with established Parkinson's disease. *European Journal of Neurology*, *20*(11), 1445–1450.

Grosset, K. A., Malek, N., Morgan, F., & Grosset, D. G. (2013b). Inhaled dry powder apomorphine (VR040) for 'off' periods in Parkinson's disease: An in-clinic double-blind dose ranging study. *Acta Neurologica Scandinavica*, *128*(3), 166–171.

Grosset, K. A., Malek, N., Morgan, F., & Grosset, D. G. (2013c). Inhaled apomorphine in patients with 'on-off' fluctuations: A randomized, double-blind, placebo-controlled, clinic and home based, parallel-group study. *Journal of Parkinson's disease*, *3*(1), 31–37.

Hardwick, A., Ward, H., Hassan, A., Romrell, J., & Okun, M. S. (2013). Clozapine as a potential treatment for refractory impulsive, compulsive, and punding behaviors in Parkinson's disease. *Neurocase*, *19*(6), 587–591.

Hauser, R. A., Ellenbogen, A. L., Metman, L. V., Hsu, A., O'Connell, M. J., Modi, N. B., et al. (2011). Crossover comparison of IPX066 and a standard levodopa formulation in advanced Parkinson's disease. *Movement Disorders: Official Journal of the Movement Disorder Society*, *26*(12), 2246–2252.

Hauser, R. A., Hsu, A., Kell, S., Espay, A. J., Sethi, K., Stacy, M., et al. (2013). Extended-release carbidopa-levodopa (IPX066) compared with immediate-release carbidopa-levodopa in patients with Parkinson's disease and motor fluctuations: A phase 3 randomised, double-blind trial. *The Lancet Neurology*, *12*(4), 346–356.

Hauser, R. A., Olanow, C. W., Dzyngel, B., Bilbault, T., Shill, H., Isaacson, S., et al. (2016). Sublingual apomorphine (APL-130277) for the acute conversion of OFF to ON in Parkinson's disease. *Movement Disorders: Official Journal of the Movement Disorder Society*, *31*(9), 1366–1372.

Hinson, V. K., Goetz, C. G., Leurgans, S., Fan, W., Nguyen, T., & Hsu, A. (2009). Reducing dosing frequency of carbidopa/levodopa: Double-blind crossover study comparing twice-daily bilayer formulation of carbidopa/levodopa (IPX054) versus 4 daily doses of standard carbidopa/levodopa in stable Parkinson disease patients. *Clinical Neuropharmacology*, *32*(4), 189–192.

Hornykiewicz, O. (2010). A brief history of levodopa. *Journal of Neurology*, *257*(Suppl. 2), S249–S252.

Hwu, W. L., Muramatsu, S., Tseng, S. H., Tzen, K. Y., Lee, N. C., Chien, Y. H., et al. (2012). Gene therapy for aromatic L-amino acid decarboxylase deficiency. *Science Translational Medicine*, *4*(134), 134ra61.

Intec Pharma, The Accordion Pill™ Carbidopa/Levodopa, AP-CD/LD Phase II, Success in Phase II clinical studies with the Accordion Pill Carbidopa Levodopa product for the treatment of Parkinson's disease.

Jankovic, J. (2005). Motor fluctuations and dyskinesias in Parkinson's disease: Clinical manifestations. *Movement Disorders*, *20*, S11–S16.

Kaufmann, H., Biaggioni, I., Low, P., Pedder, S., Hewitt, L. A., Mauney, J., et al. (2014). NOH301 Investigators. Droxidopa for neurogenic orthostatic hypotension: A randomized, placebo-controlled, phase 3 trial. *Neurology*, *83*(4), 328–335.

Keating, G. M., McClellan, K., & Jarvis, B. (2001). Methylphenidate (OROS formulation). *CNS Drugs*, *15*(6), 495–500.

Kim, S. W., Grant, J. E., Adson, D. E., & Shin, Y. C. (2001). Double-blind naltrexone and placebo comparison study in the treatment of pathological gambling. *Biological Psychiatry*, *49*(11), 914–921.

Kiss, L. E., Ferreira, H. S., Torrão, L., Bonifácio, M. J., Nuno Palma, P., Soares-da-Silva, P., et al. (2010). Discovery of a long-acting, peripherally selective inhibitor of catechol-O-methyltransferase. *Journal of Medicinal Chemistry*, *53*(8), 3396–3411.

Kobylecki, C., Burn, D. J., Kass-Iliyya, L., Kellett, M. W., Crossman, A. R., & Silverdale, M. A. (2014). Randomized clinical trial of topiramate for levodopa-induced dyskinesia in Parkinson's disease. *Parkinsonism & Related Disorders*, *20*(4), 452–455.

Kobylecki, C., et al. (2011). Synergistic antidyskinetic effects of topiramate and amantadine in animal models of Parkinson's disease. *Movement Disorders*, *26*(13), 2354–2363. http://dx.doi.org/10.1002/mds.23867. Epub 2011 Sep 23.

Lertxundi, U., Domingo-Echaburu, S., Soraluce, A., Garcia, M., Ruiz-Osante, B., & Aguirre, C. (2013). Domperidone in Parkinson's disease: A perilous arrhythmogenic or the gold standard? *Current Drug Safety*, *8*(1), 63–68.

Lewitt, P. A., Ellenbogen, A., Chen, D., Lal, R., McGuire, K., Zomorodi, K., et al. (2012). Actively transported levodopa prodrug XP21279: A study in patients with Parkinson disease who experience motor fluctuations. *Clinical Neuropharmacology*, *35*(3), 103–110.

LeWitt, P. A., Hauser, R. A., Grosset, D. G., Stocchi, F., Saint-Hilaire, M. H., Ellenbogen, A., et al. (2016). A randomized trial of inhaled levodopa (CVT-301) for motor fluctuations in Parkinson's disease. *Movement Disorders: Official Journal of the Movement Disorder Society*, *31*(9), 1356–1365.

LeWitt, P. A., Huff, F. J., Hauser, R. A., Chen, D., Lissin, D., Zomorodi, K., et al. (2014). Double-blind study of the actively transported levodopa prodrug XP21279 in Parkinson's disease. *Movement Disorders: Official Journal of the Movement Disorder Society*, *29*(1), 75–82.

LeWitt, P. A., Rezai, A. R., Leehey, M. A., Ojemann, S. G., Flaherty, A. W., Eskandar, E. N., et al. (2011). AAV2-GAD gene therapy for advanced Parkinson's disease: A double-blind, sham-surgery controlled, randomised trial. *The Lancet Neurology*, *10*(4), 309–319.

Li, Z., Yu, Z., Zhang, J., Wang, J., Sun, C., Wang, P., et al. (2015). Impact of rivastigmine on cognitive dysfunction and falling in Parkinson's disease patients. *European Neurology*, *74*(1–2), 86–91.

Litvinenko, I. V., Odinak, M. M., Mogil'naya, V. I., & Emelin, A. Y. (2008). Efficacy and safety of galantamine (reminyl) for dementia in patients with Parkinson's disease (an open controlled trial). *Neuroscience and Behavioral Physiology*, *38*(9), 937–945.

Lloret, S. P., Nano, G., Carrosella, A., Gamzu, E., & Merello, M. (2011). A double-blind, placebo-controlled, randomized, crossover pilot study of the safety and efficacy of multiple doses of intra-oral tropicamide films for the short-term relief of sialorrhea symptoms in Parkinson's disease patients. *Neurological Science*, *310*, 248–250. http://dx.doi.org/10.1016/j.jns.2011.05.021.

Luo, J., Kaplitt, M. G., Fitzsimons, H. L., Zuzga, D. S., Liu, Y., Oshinsky, M. L., et al. (2002). Subthalamic GAD gene therapy in a Parkinson's disease rat model. *Science*, *298*(5592), 425–429.

Manson, A., et al. (2012). Levodopa-induced-dyskinesias clinical features, incidence, risk factors, management and impact on quality of life. *Journal of Parkinson's Disease*, *2*(3), 189–198. http://dx.doi.org/10.3233/JPD-2012-120103.

Marks, W. J., Jr., Bartus, R. T., Siffert, J., Davis, C. S., Lozano, A., Boulis, N., et al. (2010). Gene delivery of AAV2-neurturin for Parkinson's disease: A double-blind, randomised, controlled trial. *The Lancet Neurology*, *9*(12), 1164–1172.

Marks, W. J., Jr., Ostrem, J. L., Verhagen, L., Starr, P. A., Larson, P. S., Bakay, R. A., et al. (2008). Safety and tolerability of intraputaminal delivery of CERE-120 (adeno-associated virus serotype 2-neurturin) to patients with idiopathic Parkinson's disease: An open-label, phase I trial. *The Lancet Neurology* 7(5), 400–408. http://dx.doi.org/10.1016/S1474-4422(08)70065-6. Epub 2008 Apr 2.

Martinez-Martin, P., Reddy, P., Katzenschlager, R., Antonini, A., Todorova, A., Odin, P., et al. (2015). EuroInf: A multicenter comparative observational study of apomorphine and levodopa infusion in Parkinson's disease. *Movement Disorders: Official Journal of the Movement Disorder Society*, *30*(4), 510–516.

Meltzer, H. Y., Mills, R., Revell, S., Williams, H., Johnson, A., Bahr, D., et al. (2010). Pimavanserin, a serotonin (2A) receptor inverse agonist, for the treatment of Parkinson's disease psychosis. *Neuropsychopharmacology*, *35*(4), 881–892.

Moreau, C., et al. (2015). Methylphenidate for gait hypokinesia and freezing in patients with Parkinson's disease undergoing subthalamic stimulation: A multicentre, randomised, placebo-controlled trial. *Brain*, *138*(Pt. 5), 1271–1283.

Muller, J., Wenning, G. K., Verny, M., McKee, A., Chaudhuri, K. R., Jellinger, K., et al. (2001). Progression of dysarthria and dysphagia in postmortem-confirmed parkinsonian disorders. *Archives of Neurology*, *58*(2), 259–264.

Nagaraja, D., & Jayashree, S. (2001). Randomized study of the dopamine receptor agonist piribedil in the treatment of mild cognitive impairment. *The American Journal of Psychiatry*, *158*(9), 1517–1519.

Nausieda, P. A., Hsu, A., Elmer, L., Gil, R. A., Spiegel, J., Singer, C., et al. (2015). Conversion to IPX066 from standard levodopa formulations in advanced Parkinson's disease: Experience in clinical trials. *Journal of Parkinson's Disease*, *5*(4), 837–845.

Navon, N. (2013). *Six-month oral toxicity study of the Accordion Pill™ of carbidopa/levodopa*. The Michael Fox Foundation. https://www.michaeljfox.org/foundation/grant-detail.php?grant_id=1141.

Okai, D., Askey-Jones, S., Samuel, M., O'Sullivan, S. S., Chaudhuri, K. R., Martin, A., et al. (2013). Trial of CBT for impulse control behaviors affecting Parkinson patients and their caregivers. *Neurology*, *80*(9), 792–799.

Pahwa, R., Tanner, C. M., Hauser, R. A., Sethi, K., Isaacson, S., Truong, D., et al. (2015). Amantadine extended release for levodopa-induced dyskinesia in Parkinson's disease (EASED study). *Movement Disorders: Official Journal of the Movement Disorder Society*, *30*(6), 788–795.

Palma, P. N., & Soares-da-Silva, P. (2013). Catechol-O-methyltransferase inhibitors: Present problems and relevance of the new ones. In A. Martinez & C. Gil (Eds.), *Emerging drugs and targets for Parkinson's disease: Vol. 34* (pp. 83–109). Cambridge, UK: The Royal Society of Chemistry.

Papay, K., Xie, S. X., Stern, M., Hurtig, H., Siderowf, A., Duda, J. E., et al. (2014). Naltrexone for impulse control disorders in Parkinson disease: A placebo-controlled study. *Neurology*, *83*(9), 826–833.

Parkinson Study Group. (2001). Evaluation of dyskinesias in a pilot r, placebo-controlled trial of remacemide in advanced Parkinson disease. *Archives of Neurology*, *58*(10), 1660–1668.

Pintor, L., Valldeoriola, F., Bailles, E., Marti, M. J., Muniz, A., & Tolosa, E. (2012). Ziprasidone versus clozapine in the treatment of psychotic symptoms in Parkinson disease: A randomized open clinical trial. *Clinical Neuropharmacology*, *35*(2), 61–66.

Playfer, J., & Hindle, J. (2010). Parkinson's disease in the older patient. *Nursing Older People*, *22*(5), 10.

Pollak, P. T. F., Rascol, O., et al. (2004). Clozapine in drug induced psychosis in Parkinson's disease: A randomised, placebo controlled study with open follow up. *Journal of Neurology, Neurosurgery, and Psychiatry*, *75*, 689–695.

Postuma, R. B., & Berg, D. (2016). Advances in markers of prodromal Parkinson disease. *Nature Reviews. Neurology*, *12*(11), 622–634.

Rabery, J. M., Miniovitz, A., Dobronevsky, E., & Klein, C. (2007). Effect of quetiapine in psychotic Parkinson's disease patients: A double-blind labelled study of 3 months duration. *Movement Disorders: Official Journal of the Movement Disorder Society*, *22*, 313–318.

Ramirez-Zamora, A., Boyd, J., & Biller, J. (2016). Treatment of impulse control disorders in Parkinson's disease. Practical considerations and future directions. *Expert Review of Neurotherapeutics*, *16*(4), 389–399.

Rascol, O., Fabre, N., Blin, O., Poulik, J., Sabatini, U., Senard, J. M., et al. (1994). Naltrexone, an opiate antagonist, fails to modify motor symptoms in patients with Parkinson's disease. *Movement Disorders: Official Journal of the Movement Disorder Society*, *9*(4), 437–440.

Rocha, J. F., Ferreira, J. J., Falcão, A., Santos, A., Pinto, R., Nunes, T., et al. (2015). Effect of single-dose regimens of opicapone on levodopa pharmacokinetics, catechol-O-methyltransferase activity and motor response in patients with Parkinson disease. *Clinical Pharmacology in Drug Development*, *5*(3), 232–240.

Sanger, G. J. (2014). Ghrelin and motilin receptor agonists: Time to introduce bias into drug design. *Neurogastroenterology and Motility: The Official Journal of the European Gastrointestinal Motility Society*, *26*(2), 149–155.

Sawada, H., Oeda, T., Kuno, S., Nomoto, M., Yamamoto, K., Yamamoto, M., et al. (2010). Amantadine for dyskinesias in Parkinson's disease: A randomized controlled trial. *PLoS One*, *5*(12), e15298.

Schapira, A. H. (2010). Safinamide in the treatment of Parkinson's disease. *Expert Opinion on Pharmacotherapy*, *11*(13), 2261–2268.

Schuck, S., Bentue-Ferrer, D., Kleinermans, D., Reymann, J. M., Polard, E., Gandon, J. M., et al. (2002). Psychomotor and cognitive effects of piribedil, a dopamine agonist, in young healthy volunteers. *Fundamental & Clinical Pharmacology*, *16*(1), 57–65.

Seppi, K., et al. (2011). The movement disorder society evidence-based medicine review update: Treatments for the non-motor symptoms of Parkinson's disease. *Movement Disorders: Official Journal of the Movement Disorder Society*, *26*, S42–S80.

Shaltiel-Karyo, R., Tsarfati, Y., Zawoznik, E., Weinstock, I., Nemas, M., Rubinski, A., et al. (2016). ND0701: A novel safe concentrated apomorphine formulation for continuous subcutaneous administration via a patch pump. In: *20th International Congress (abstract number: 1977).*

Shin, A., Busciglio, I., Burton, D., Smith, S. A., Vella, A., Ryks, M., et al. (2013). The ghrelin agonist RM-131 accelerates gastric emptying of solids ad reduces symptoms in patients with type 1 diabetes mellitus. *Clinical Gastroenterology and Hepatology*, *11*, 1453–1459.

Shin, A., Camilleri, M., Busciglio, I., Burton, D., Stoner, E., Noonan, P., et al. (2013). Randomized controlled phase Ib study of ghrelin agonist, RM-131, in type 2 diabetic women with delayed gastric emptying: Pharmacokinetics and pharmacodynamics. *Diabetes Care*, *36*(1), 41–48.

Simonato, M., Bennett, J., Boulis, N. M., Castro, M. G., Fink, D. J., Goins, W. F., et al. (2013). Progress in gene therapy for neurological disorders. *Nature Reviews. Neurology*, *9*(5), 277–291.

Starkstein, S. E., Brockman, S., & Hayhow, B. D. (2012). Psychiatric syndromes in Parkinson's disease. *Current Opinion in Psychiatry*, *25*(6), 468–472.

Stocchi, F., Hsu, A., Khanna, S., Ellenbogen, A., Mahler, A., Liang, G., et al. (2014). Comparison of IPX066 with carbidopa-levodopa plus entacapone in advanced PD patients. *Parkinsonism & Related Disorders*, *20*(12), 1335–1340.

Takizawa, C., Gemmell, E., Kenworthy, J., & Speyer, R. (2016). A systematic review of the prevalence of oropharyngeal dysphagia in stroke, Parkinson's disease, Alzheimer's disease, head injury, and pneumonia. *Dysphagia*, *31*(3), 434–441.

Tian, J., Du, G., Ye, L., Yu, X., Zhang, J., Wang, H., et al. (2013). Three-month subchronic intramuscular toxicity study of rotigotine-loaded microspheres in Cynomolgus monkeys. *Food and Chemical Toxicology: An International Journal Published for the British Industrial Biological Research Association*, *52*, 143–152.

Tison, F., et al. (2016). A phase 2A trial of the novel mGluR5-negative allosteric modulator dipraglurant for levodopa-induced dyskinesia in Parkinson's disease. *Movement Disorders: Official Journal of the Movement Disorder Society*, *31*(9), 1373–1380. http://dx.doi.org/10.1002/mds.26659. Epub 2016 May 23.

Tjaden, K. (2008). Speech and swallowing in Parkinson's disease. *Topics in Geriatric Rehabilitation*, *24*(2), 115–126.

Tolosa, E., Marti, M. J., Valldeoriola, F., & Molinuevo, J. L. (1998). History of levodopa and dopamine agonists in Parkinson's disease treatment. *Neurology*, *50*(6 Suppl. 6), S2–S10. discussion S44–S48.

Turle-Lorenzo, B. M., Puma, C., Chezaubernard, C., Morain, P., Baunez, C., Nieoullon, A., et al. (2006). The dopamine agonist piribedil with L-DOPA improves attentional dysfunction: Relevance for Parkinson's disease. *Journal of Pharmacology and Experimental Therapeutics*, *319*(2), 914–923.

Vanover, K. E. W. D., Makhay, M., et al. (2006). Pharmacological and behavioral profile of N-(4-fluorophenylmethyl)-N-(1-methylpiperidin-4-yl)-N'-(4-(2-methylpropyloxy) phenylmethyl) carbamide (2R,3R)-dihydroxybutanedioate (2:1) (ACP-103), a novel 5-hydroxytryptamine(2A) receptor inverse agonist. *The Journal of Pharmacology and Experimental Therapeutics*, *317*, 910–918.

Verhagen Metman, L., Del Dotto, P., Natte, R., van den Munckhof, P., & Chase, T. N. (1998). Dextromethorphan improves levodopa-induced dyskinesias in Parkinson's disease. *Neurology*, *51*(1), 203–206.

Voon, V., & Fox, S. H. (2007). Medication-related impulse control and repetitive behaviors in Parkinson disease. *Archives of Neurology*, *64*(8), 1089–1096.

Voss, T., Cummings, J., Mills, R., Ravina, B., & Williams, H. (2013). Performance of the shortened scale for assessment of positive symptoms for Parkinson's disease psychosis. *Parkinsonism & Related Disorders*, *19*, 295–299.

Wang, A., Liu, Y., Liang, R., Zhang, X., Sun, K., Wu, Z., et al. (2016). Preparation and evaluation of rotigotine-loaded implant for the treatment of Parkinson's disease and its evolution study. *Saudi Pharmaceutical Journal: SPJ: The Official Publication of the Saudi Pharmaceutical Society*, *24*(3), 363–370.

Wang, A., Wang, L., Sun, K., Liu, W., Sha, C., & Li, Y. (2012). Preparation of rotigotine-loaded microspheres and their combination use with L-DOPA to modify dyskinesias in 6-OHDA-lesioned rats. *Pharmaceutical Research*, *29*(9), 2367–2376.

Weintraub, D., Mamikonyan, E., Papay, K., Shea, J. A., Xie, S. X., & Siderowf, A. (2012). Questionnaire for impulsive-compulsive disorders in Parkinson's disease-rating scale. *Movement Disorders: Official Journal of the Movement Disorder Society*, *27*(2), 242–247.

Yungher, D. A., et al. (2014). Temporal characteristics of high-frequency lower-limb oscillation during freezing of gait in Parkinson's disease. *Parkinson's Disease*, *2014*, 606427. http://dx.doi.org/10.1155/2014/606427.

CHAPTER SIXTEEN

Device-Aided Treatment Strategies in Advanced Parkinson's Disease

Jonathan Timpka*, Bianca Nitu†, Veronika Datieva‡, Per Odin*,§, Angelo Antonini¶,1

*Faculty of Medicine, Lund University, Lund, Sweden
†Colentina Clinical Hospital, Bucharest, Romania
‡Russian Medical Academy of Postgraduate Education, Moscow, Russia
§Central Hospital, Bremerhaven, Germany
¶University of Padua, Padua, Italy
[1]Corresponding author: e-mail address: angelo3000@yahoo.com

Contents

International Review of Neurobiology, Volume 132
ISSN 0074-7742
http://dx.doi.org/10.1016/bs.irn.2017.03.001

Abstract

With peroral levodopa treatment, a majority of patients develop motor fluctuations and dyskinesia already within a few years of therapy. Device-aided Parkinson (PD) therapies refer to deep brain stimulation (DBS), levodopa–carbidopa intestinal gel infusion (LCIG), and subcutaneous infusion of the dopamine agonist apomorphine and represent effective strategies counteracting motor fluctuations and dyskinesia. These three therapy options seem to be similarly effective in reducing "time with PD symptoms (off time)" by at least 60%–65%. The use of advanced therapy also leads to a significant reduction of dyskinesia. Recent studies also indicate that these therapies can improve a number of nonmotor symptoms in advanced PD. Altogether this results in an improved health-related quality of life in most treated patients. The side effects and complications are quite different between the three; for DBS, serious adverse events include intracranial bleeding and infection, LCIG complications relate to the infusion equipment and the establishment of the percutaneous endoscopic gastrostomy, while for apomorphine infusion the most common side effect is a formation of noduli (local inflammation) at the point of infusion. The device-aided therapies are all indicated for the treatment of motor fluctuations and/or dyskinesia when peroral/transdermal PD medications cannot be further optimized. However, the choice of device-aided therapy is made on basis of indications/contraindications, but also the patients' symptom profile and his/her personal preferences. Therefore, it is important these treatments are discussed early, well before motor and nonmotor symptoms have deteriorated excessively.

1. INTRODUCTION

Levodopa therapy is the most effective treatment for Parkinson's disease (PD) medication (Olanow & Koller, 1998). However, long-term peroral levodopa intake results in clinical fluctuations and dyskinesia. Progressive loss of dopamine nerve terminals and delayed gastric emptying likely contribute to the unpredictable motor responses observed with orally dosed levodopa (LeWitt, 2014). The absorption is also compromized by other gastrointestinal abnormalities like small intestinal bacterial overgrowth and an altered gut microbiota. These abnormalities can also be responsible of nausea, early morning off and unpredictable motor and nonmotor fluctuations. Several studies show that within 2–5 year of levodopa treatment more than 50% of patients develop motor fluctuations, while the risk of dyskinesia increases by 10% per year (LeWitt, 2014; Schapira & Obeso, 2006). Three device-aided therapies constitute the main treatment strategies for advanced PD: deep brain stimulation (DBS), levodopa–carbidopa intestinal gel (LCIG), and continuous subcutaneous apomorphine infusion (CSA).

2. DEEP BRAIN STIMULATION

DBS is an established therapy for advanced PD and it has almost completely replaced ablative techniques with advantages such as reversibility, adjustability, and a lower risk of side effects (Okun, 2012). DBS is a complementary treatment option to medication with approval for several targets: the ventral intermediate nucleus of the thalamus (VIM; Zesiewicz et al., 2005), the internal globus pallidus (GPi), and the subthalamic nucleus (STN; Limousin et al., 1998; Melamed, Ziv, & Djaldetti, 2007).

2.1 DBS: Historical Review

Surgical approach in alleviating motor symptoms of PD was mentioned in the works of Bucy and even earlier as lesioning of corticospinal tract (Horsley, 1890). Early attempts were unsuccessful, but after the introduction of stereotactic head frame in the late 1940 the new era of stereotactic surgery for PD began (Spiegel, Wycis, Marks, & Lee, 1947). Modern DBS surgery for addressing tremor and PD was introduced in 1987 by Benabid (Benabid, Pollak, Louveau, Henry, & de Rougemont, 1988). Lesional procedures using radiofrequency ablation have been largely replaced by DBS, but under certain conditions, pallidotomy, thalamotomy, and even subthalamic nucleotomy remain useful alternatives, especially when DBS is economically not feasible (Metman & Slavin, 2015). More recently, MRI-guided focused ultrasound has been successfully applied for the management of tremor (Elias et al., 2016). DBS targeting VIM for tremor, and later on GPi and STN for almost all cardinal symptoms of PD, became the standard-of-care for patients with PD that is no longer adequately controlled by medications (Limousin et al., 1998).

2.2 Mechanism of Action of DBS

The exact mechanism of DBS effect is unknown. Several hypothesis have been proposed with the one most widely accepted being that high-frequency stimulation blocks the activity of the target nucleus and consequently changes activity in connected regions, consistent with a "jamming of the neuronal message transmitted through the stimulated structure and desynchronization of abnormal oscillations" (Benazzouz & Hallett, 2000).

2.3 When Is Surgery Appropriate?

As demands for mobility and QoL can be judged differentially depending on age, social integration, and disease stage, a consensus between patients, caregivers, and the treating physician should be developed over time (Krüger et al., 2015).

The response of motor symptoms to dopaminergic treatment can be considered as an important predictor of postoperative outcome. A 33% decrease in unified PD rating scale (UPDRS)-III motor score between the off-medication and on-medication states is widely considered the threshold for predicting a good outcome from DBS. Symptoms not responsive to levodopa, e.g., axial symptoms, are typically also resistant to DBS (Volkmann, Albanese, Antonini, & Chaudhuri, 2013). An exception is drug resistant tremor, which can respond well to DBS (Poewe, Kleedorfer, Wagner, Bösch, & Schelosky, 1993).

The EarlyStim study revealed that patients with a shorter disease duration (<7.5 years) and shorter duration of motor fluctuations (<1.5 years) showed similar improvements of QoL by STN DBS compared to more advanced patients and, therefore, brought up the concept of the "window of opportunity" for DBS. This window is typically limited on the long run by the emergence of doparesistant axial symptoms, which currently limit the therapeutic response of "classical" STN DBS (Mestre et al., 2014; Russmann, Ghika, Villemure, & Robert, 2004).

All patients who are candidates for DBS should be carefully neuropsychologically and psychiatrically examined in order to define cognitive functions and potential psychiatric comorbidities (especially depression), since both can aggravate after DBS (Volkmann et al., 2013).

2.4 Outcomes/Proof of Efficacy

Randomized controlled trials assessing the benefit of bilateral DBS of STN or GPi have demonstrated the efficacy of neurostimulation (Table 1).

2.5 Targets for DBS

If the main symptom is high amplitude tremor the reasonable target is VIM. Other PD-related symptoms are less responsive to thalamic stimulation.

Table 1 Deep Brain Stimulation

Study	Target/ Intervention	*N*	Follow-Up	UPDRS-III Changes
Anderson, Burchiel, and Hogarth (2005)	Bilateral STN vs bilateral GPi	20	12	48% improvement in STN group vs 39% improvement in GPi group ($P = 0.40$)
Deuschl and Schade (2006)	Bilateral STN + BMT vs BMT alone	156	6	41% improvement in DBS group vs no improvement in BMT group ($P < 0.001$)
Schüpbach, Maltete, and Houeto (2007)	Bilateral STN + BMT vs BMT alone	20	18	69% improvement in DBS group vs worsening in BMT group ($P < 0.05$)
Weaver, Follett, Stern, Hur, and Harris (2009)	Bilateral STN/ GPi BMT vs BMT alone	255	6	29% improvement in DBS group vs no improvement in BMT group ($P < 0.001$)
Okun, Fernandez, and Wu (2009)	Unilateral STN vs unilateral GPi	45	7	29.9% improvement in STN group vs 26.6% improvement in GPi group ($P = 0.64$)
Moro, Lozano, Pollak, and Agid (2010)	Bilateral STN vs bilateral GPi	51	60–72	45.4% improvement in STN group vs 20.0% improvement in GPi group ($P < 0.0001$)
Williams et al. (2010)	Bilateral surgery (STN or GPi) vs BMT	366	12	36% improvement in surgery group vs no improvement in BMT group ($P < 0.001$)
Follett, Weaver, Stern, and Hur (2010)	Bilateral STN vs bilateral GPi	299	24	25% improvement in STN group vs 28% improvement in GPi group ($P = 0.90$)
Okun et al. (2012)	Bilateral STN (OFF vs ON stimulation)	136	12	39% improvement
Weaver, Follett, Stern, Luo, and Harris (2012)	Bilateral STN vs bilateral GPi	159	36	30% improvement in STN group vs 34% improvement in GPi group ($P = 0.59$)
Odekerken et al. (2013)	Bilateral STN vs bilateral GPi	128	12	46% improvement in STN group vs 26% improvement in GPi group ($P = 0.03$)
Schuepbach, Rau, and Knudsen (2013)	Bilateral STN + BMT vs BMT alone	251	24	53% improvement in STN group vs no improvement in BMT group ($P < 0.001$)

BMT, best medical therapy; *DBS*, deep brain stimulation; *GPi*, internal globus pallidus; *STN*, subthalamic nucleus; *UPDRS*, unified Parkinson's Disease rating scale.

If also the hypokinetic-rigid symptoms must be addressed, the STN and GPi are used as targets. The most consistent difference between these targets is greater drug reduction achieved after STN DBS and direct effect of GPi DBS on reducing dyskinesia severity. Postoperative reduction in dopaminergic therapy can be effective in resolving behavioral disorders, like impulse control disorders (ICDs), dopamine dysregulation syndrome, but at the same time can provoke postoperative apathy. Excessive stimulation of the limbic portion of the STN may induce ICD and cause other behavioral problems, like mania, depression, which is not common after GPi DBS. STN DBS is more likely to produce cognitive problems, compared with GPi DBS. Due to the lower stimulation parameters STN DBS may have longer battery life compared to GPi, leading to less frequent device replacement surgeries and lower costs. However, STN DBS usually requires more follow-ups visits due to complex postoperative management. It is still not clear if either of the targets are superior to the others (Liu et al., 2014), but the most effective strategy seems to be to make the choice of target region based on individual symptoms and characteristics.

2.6 Pedunculopontine Nucleus Stimulation

The pedunculopontine nucleus (PPN) as a part of the midbrain, linked with the basal ganglia and corticospinal circuits, is suspected to play a role in the development of the axial symptoms in PD patients, such as gait disturbance, postural instability and falling (Moro, Hamani, Poon, & Al, 2010; Stefani, Lozano, Peppe, Stanzione, & Galati, 2007). The neurons of this nucleus are known to be affected in the degenerative process of PD. The PPN is currently not approved by FDA as a target. The results of studies assessing the efficacy of PPN stimulation have been rather unimpressive and inconsistent. Such an inaccuracy in results can be partially be attributed to the highly variable brainstem anatomy and the small number of patients so far investigated.

2.7 The New Phenotype of Advanced PD After DBS

Twenty-five years after the start of the DBS era, still new issues have to be addressed. There is a need for studies which could establish the optimal dopaminergic management before and after DBS. The best medical therapy after DBS might be estimated on the basis of the patients' presurgical status (Thobois, Ardouin, Lhommée, & Klinger, 2010). The problem of post-DBS dopamine withdrawal syndrome should be addressed. The neurodegenerative process continues to progress also after DBS. Axial motor problems such as freezing of gait, postural instability, and dysarthria worsen during the disease duration. Nonmotor symptoms such as dementia, autonomic dysfunction, as well as, psychiatric issues remain the main reason for a reduced quality of life. Further research is needed to identify patients who are in the group with elevated risk for developing cognitive impairment and dementia after DBS.

2.8 Complications of DBS

The perioperative complications of DBS can be classified as surgery-, hardware-, and stimulation-related issues. However, factors such as suboptimal patient selection, the lack of an intradisciplinary team to appropriately manage the patient, unrealistic patient expectations, limited access to device programming, improper programming, and medication adjustment may reduce patients' satisfaction and increase the risk for complications.

2.9 Surgery-Related Complications

The most frequently reported serious adverse events are intracerebral hemorrhage and pulmonary embolism. Intracerebral hemorrhage occurs in around 1%–5% of cases (Fenoy & Simpson, 2013; Umemura, Oka, Yamamoto, & Okita, 2011); with the risk of bleeding being 0.3%–3.6% per electrode track (Binder, Rau, & Starr, 2005; Oh, Abosch, Kim, Lang, & Lozano, 2002), and around 0.6% out of patients present permanent neurologic impairments (Binder et al., 2005; Sansur et al., 2007). Additionally, intracerebral hemorrhage may occur several hours after DBS surgery (Umemura, Jaggi, Hurtig, & Siderowf, 2003).

To prevent this complication, the patients should be screened for coagulopathy/recent use of antiplatelet agent before surgery and intraoperatively the systolic blood pressure should be less than 140 mm Hg.

Many authors report postoperative confusion (1%–36%) (Hamani, Richter, Schwalb, & Lozano, 2008; Umemura et al., 2003), cognitive problems (Pahwa, Wilkinson, Overman, & Lyons, 2003), behavioral (Pahwa et al., 2003; Woods, Fields, & Tröster, 2002), and psychiatric symptoms (De Gaspari et al., 2006).

2.10 Hardware-Related Complications

Hardware-related complications refer to problems with stimulating electrodes, extension electrodes, and implantable pulse generator (which is implanted subcutaneously in the infraclavicular region). These include DBS electrode fracture, extension wire failure, lead migration, skin erosion, IPG malfunction (for example, broken contacts of the electrode, or connector and electrode malfunction), and pain over the pulse generator (Blomstedt & Hariz, 2005; Boviatsis, Stavrinou, & Themistocleous, 2010; Hamani & Lozano, 2006).

The most feared complication after DBS surgery is infection. The postoperative incidence of infections varies between studies from 1.5% to 15% and is treated with antibiotics and often necessitate elimination of the implant (Bhatia, Zhang, Oh, Angle, & Whiting, 2010; Bjerknes, Skogseid, Sæhle, Dietrichs, & Toft, 2014; Pepper et al., 2012; Petraglia et al., 2015).

Clinically, the infections are presented as erythema, cellulitis, dehiscence, drainage, or stitch abscess and the most common pathogens are gram-positive cocci (*Staphylococcus aureus* or *Staphylococcus epidermidis*).

2.11 Stimulation-Related Complications

These are the most common problems encountered, but most of them are reversible and adjustable, with programming of the DBS system after surgery. They are often a result of the spread of the electrical current outside the target regions. Side effects depend on the site of implantation of the electrodes.

VIM DBS: dysarthria, paresthesia, and postural instability, depending on the current density delivered (Lyons, Koller, Wilkinson, & Pahwa, 2001; Obwegeser et al., 2001).

STN DBS: the most common nonbehavioral side effects are dyskinesia, worsening of axial symptoms (freezing, balance, and gait disturbance), speech disturbance (hypophonia or dysarthria), psychiatric (depression, mania, and other psychosis) (Hamani et al., 2008; Rodriguez, 2005), weight gain (Barichella, Marczewska, & Mariani, 2003; Macia, Perlemoine, Coman, & Guehl, 2004), involuntary muscle contractions, paresthesia, and ocular movements causing either monocular deviation (spread to oculomotor nucleus), conjugate gaze deviation (spread to capsule), or eyelid apraxia (Herzog et al., 2003; Machado, Deogaonkar, & Cooper, 2012).

GPi DBS: dysarthria, hypophonia, paresthesia, tonic muscle contraction (Hristova et al., 2000; Odekerken et al., 2013).

3. LEVODOPA–CARBIDOPA INTESTINAL GEL

3.1 The Basics

LCIG is a gel containing levodopa and the decarboxylase inhibitor carbidopa at concentrations of 20 and 5 mg/mL, respectively. The infusion pump can be carried in a small bag around the neck or the waist and weighs about 500 g when it is loaded with a new gel-containing cartridge. The treatment response is often evaluated during a nasoduodenal phase before initiating the full procedure. During LCIG treatment, the gel is infused continuously through the abdominal wall with the help of a percutane endoscopic gastrostomy that has been inserted during local anesthesia. The gel then passes through the ventricle and duodenum within a tube that has its distal end in the upper jejunal part of the small intestine.

The aim is often to use LCIG as a monotherapy, but it is not uncommon to use some additional dopamine agonists, catechol-*O*-methyl transferase inhibitors, or amantadine during LCIG treatment. Most patients are on 16-h regimens and only use the infusion during the waking day, but some also continue during sleep and are thus on 24-h treatment. The total daily dosage consists of three set doses: a morning bolus dose, a continuous dose, and an extra bolus dose on demand. The morning dose is used to quickly reach an effective plasma concentration and typically consists of 100–200 mg levodopa which has an effect within 10–30 min. The continuous dose consists of 20–200 mg/h levodopa that is infused throughout the day. The continuous dose is titrated in response to the clinical symptomatology; a process that is most often handled during the inpatient stay, although an outpatient titration of the maintenance dose is being used in some centers. It is appropriate to reduce the maintenance dose by around 30% during sleep if patients are on a nonstop treatment regime. The extra bolus doses consist of 10–40 mg levodopa that the patient can use when he/she feels the need for additional effect. If several extra doses are needed during the day, it may be advisable to instead increase the continuous dose and decrease the need for extra doses.

3.2 The Effect on Quality of Life

Health-related quality of life is commonly used as an outcome in studies on LCIG. The treatment has repeatedly led to significant improvements in health-related quality of life in patients with advanced PD. The instruments used for measurements of health-related quality of life are most often the disease-specific 8- or 39-item PD Questionnaire (PDQ-8/39) and the widely used five-dimension EuroQol (EQ-5D). The cause for the positive effect on health-related quality of life is probably multifactorial but is likely to be a consequence of the reduced time in off and reduction of both motor and nonmotor complications. The improvements are typically measurable at within 4 weeks of treatment (Antonini, Yegin, Preda, Bergmann, & Poewe, 2015; Fernandez et al., 2014) but are still significant at follow-up visits after 6 to 18 months (Antonini, Yegin, et al., 2015; Fernandez et al., 2014; Kwan et al., 2016; Martinez-Martin et al., 2014; Pålhagen et al., 2016; Reddy et al., 2012; Timpka et al., 2015).

3.3 The Effect on Motor Symptoms

Much like the other infusion technique that is used in the treatment of PD, i.e., CSA, LCIG has mainly been evaluated in open-label studies. Nonetheless, the results of the first randomized controlled double-blinded trial of LCIG were published in 2014 (Olanow et al., 2014). Motor symptoms improved significantly after 3 months of LCIG treatment (compared to patients on placebo intrajejunal infusion and optimized oral treatment): patients presented 4.0 h less off (controls: −2.1 h) and 4.1 h more on without troublesome dyskinesia (controls: +1.9 h). The 64% reduction of time in off reported in the randomized controlled trial corresponds well with that seen in open-label or retrospective studies, where the mean reduction of time spent in off ranges from 40% to 80% (Antonini, Odin, et al., 2013; Antonini, Yegin, et al., 2015; Fernandez et al., 2014; Kwan et al., 2016; Lopiano et al., 2016; Martinez-Martin et al., 2014; Pickut, van der Linden, Dethy, Van De Maele, & de Beyl, 2013; Reddy et al., 2012; Valldeoriola & Grandas, 2016; Volkmann et al., 2013; Zibetti, Merola, Artusi, & Rizzi, 2014).

Open-label trials also present moderate evidence for beneficial effects on UPDRS parts II, III, and/or IV, indicating effects on ADL function, motor symptoms, and improvement of motor complications (Wirdefeldt, Odin, & Nyholm, 2016). The long-term effects of LCIG are still being investigated; however, recently there have been an increasing number of long-term open-label or registry-based studies presenting satisfactory and durable effects of long-term treatment (Buongiorno et al., 2015; Pålhagen et al., 2016; Valldeoriola & Grandas, 2016; Zibetti et al., 2014).

3.4 The Effect on Nonmotor Symptoms

There is still a need for further evaluation of the nonmotor effects of LCIG treatment, but there is evidence of improvements of several nonmotor symptoms, including sleep, anxiety, depression, hallucinations, and ICD (Odin et al., 2015; Volkmann et al., 2013). There might be several different mechanisms behind these improvements, including a stronger dopaminergic stimulation and the possibility to stop or reduce other PD drugs—hence minimizing their adverse effects. The NMSS has also been used to study the nonmotor effects of LCIG treatment in a few studies with an open-label design. The effects are seen on most of the studied nonmotor symptom domains (Antonini, Yegin, et al., 2015; Martinez-Martin et al., 2014; Volkmann et al., 2013). LCIG might be superior to CSA on the domains gastrointestinal, sexual functioning, sleep/fatigue, and urinary (Martinez-Martin et al., 2014), but there was no significant difference in NMSS total score. In comparison to the effects on motor symptoms, the evidence strength for the effects on nonmotor is still weak and in need of further investigation (Wirdefeldt et al., 2016).

3.5 Safety

LCIG is efficacious and the discontinuation rate is low, but adverse events are common. Safety data from four studies on LCIG were recently merged and analyzed (Lang et al., 2016). The included patients had been treated with LCIG at a median of 911 days and the total exposure was 963 patient-years. The study made a distinction between procedure/device and non-procedure/device adverse events. Adverse events that were associated to the procedure and/or device occurred in 76% of patients and complications of device insertion and abdominal pain were the most common—occurring in 41% and 36% of patients, respectively. Most patients, i.e., 92%, had some form of nonprocedure/device adverse event–insomnia and falls being the most common as each of the two events were reported by 23% of patients. Complications to device insertion and abdominal pain were also the most common serious procedure/device adverse events at 8% and 4%, respectively. Among non/procedure/device adverse events, pneumonia and PD symptoms were the most commonly reported at 5% and 2%. Even though 8.3% of patients died during treatment, it was deemed that only 0.5% of the participants—in this case two patients—died from a cause "possibly related" to the drug or device. The most effective way of avoiding the procedure/device-related side effect seems to provide a high level of gastroenterological competence and experience.

Nerve conduction studies were not a compulsory part of the abovementioned study, but polyneuropathy was reported in 5.8% of patients. The occurrence of peripheral neuropathy during LCIG treatment has been debated recently and there is growing evidence for the need of an active monitoring of symptoms of neuropathy (Devigili, Rinaldo, Lettieri, & Eleopra, 2016; Merola et al., 2015). It is still not clear to what degree the neuropathy is a LCIG-specific phenomena, an effect of giving high doses of levodopa or an effect of the disease process itself. One of the studies included 23 patients with normal nerve conduction study results at baseline (Merola et al., 2015). After a mean follow-up of 24 months, almost half of the included patients had developed some form of peripheral neuropathy—two had developed subacute, two chronic, and seven subclinical peripheral neuropathy. The need for supplementation with vitamin B12 and folic acid should be evaluated regularly. Catechol-O-methyl transferase treatment has recently been reported to reduce the risk of polyneuropathy in levodopa-treated patients (Cossu et al., 2016).

3.6 The Indications, the Contraindications, and the "Ideal" Patient

Patients with advanced PD and severe motor fluctuations or dyskinesia despite optimized oral or transdermal treatment may be referred for LCIG. However, LCIG is less suitable for patients with a poor response to levodopa, pronounced dementia, an inability to handle the infusion pump either alone or with support from a caregiver, or contraindications for abdominal surgery. Mild cognitive impairment is not a contraindication as long as the patient has adequate support from a caregiver and does not tamper with the infusion equipment or tubing (Odin et al., 2015). There is no upper age limit for LCIG, but the subgroup of patients with advanced PD that are the most likely to benefit the most from LCIG are those that are younger, have no dementia, and experience disabling motor fluctuations.

4. CONTINUOUS SUBCUTANEOUS APOMORPHINE INFUSION

4.1 The Basics

The nonergot dopamine agonist apomorphine is a nonselective agonist for dopamine D_2 and—to a lesser extent—D_1 receptors, but also functions as an antagonist for α-adrenergic and 5-HT2 receptors. There is a need for studies investigating the effects of CSA in placebo-controlled blinded trials, but this is likely to change as a large multicenter study has recently been concluded. CSA is the least invasive of the device-aided therapies for advanced PD and it is entirely reversible. The apomorphine is infused with the help of a small infusion pump, a fine-caliber tube, and a needle that delivers the apomorphine subcutaneously, mostly on the stomach or thighs. CSA is used as a 16-h daytime treatment. It is common to try to discontinue all daytime PD medications and evaluate the effect of CSA as a daytime monotherapy, but the extent to which this is possible is subject to large interindividual differences. The majority of patients with CSA still use oral levodopa, but most often at daily doses that have been reduced with at least 50% since before the start of CSA treatment. The initiation and adjustment of CSA may be handled during an inpatient stay, but in many countries the dose titration is handled in an outpatient setting. Some centers start the procedure with an apomorphine test to evaluate the treatment response and to help increase treatment adherence due to a better understanding of the treatment among patients. The total daily dose of CSA can be divided into three subdoses: the morning dose, the maintenance dose, and the extra bolus dose. After adjustments are made, most patients end up with maintenance doses at between 4 and 7 mg/h (Trenkwalder et al., 2015). Before the start—and then continuing during the first weeks—of CSA treatment, patients may be prescribed 10 mg of the peripheral dopamine D_2 antagonist domperidone three times daily to reduce gastrointestinal side effects, orthostatic hypotension, and nausea. Due to an increased risk for development of hemolytic anemia during CSA treatment, patient should be screened for anemia before and thereafter twice yearly during treatment.

4.2 The Effect on Quality of Life

The clinical experience is that the patients' mean health-related quality of life is improved from CSA, but it is likely that patients that are able to reduce their oral medications have a greater benefit from the treatment. This is supported by one study where patients only had minor reductions in oral dosages during CSA and no significant improvements of health-related quality of life (Rambour, Moreau, Salleron, & Devos, 2014). Other studies show significant improvements of health-related quality of life after 6 months of treatment (Drapier, Eusebio, Degos, Vérin, & Durif, 2016; Martinez-Martin et al., 2014). In direct comparison with LCIG, CSA seems to be similar in its effect on health-related quality of life (Martinez-Martin et al., 2014); however, the results should be interpreted with caution.

4.3 The Effect on Motor Symptoms

As previously suggested, CSA seems to be the most effective in patients who tolerate larger dose increases and either considerable reductions or total removal of other daytime medications (Borgemeester, Drent, & van Laar, 2015; Katzenschlager, Hughes, & Evans, 2005; Rambour et al., 2014; Volkmann et al., 2013). The documented effects of CSA have first and foremost been a reduction of the time spent in off, but several other effects on motor symptoms have also been reported. The time spent in off is typically reduced by around 40% and some studies also report a corresponding increase in on time without dyskinesia. Improvements have also been seen on UPDRS parts II, III, and/or IV, indicating an improvement of ADL function and motor symptoms, while decreasing motor complications (Drapier et al., 2016; Martinez-Martin et al., 2014; Pålhagen et al., 2016; Rambour et al., 2014; Todorova et al., 2013).

4.4 The Effect on Nonmotor Symptoms

Although motor symptoms have been the focus in many of the open-label studies investigating CSA, there are documented effects also on nonmotor symptoms. At least two studies have employed the NMSS as an outcome and followed patients starting CSA in an open-label study design (Martinez-Martin et al., 2014; Todorova et al., 2013). At the end of the 6-month follow-up of the larger of the two studies, mean scores on the NMSS subscores for attention/memory, gastrointestinal, perceptual/hallucinations, sleep/fatigue, and urinary had improved together with the mean NMSS total score (Martinez-Martin et al., 2014). CSA has traditionally been used with care in patients with visual hallucinations; however, a recent review suggests that patients with visual hallucinations may indeed come in question for CSA treatment if enough attention is paid to treatment of preexisting visual hallucinations concurrent cholinergic deficits (Borgemeester, Lees, & van Laar, 2016).

4.5 Safety

Subcutaneous nodules occur in about 50% of patients with CSA and are the most common adverse event. The clinical experience is that skin nodules can be treated through a number of measures (Trenkwalder et al., 2015); however, the evidence for these methods are lacking. An expert consensus group recommend maintaining good skin hygiene at the infusion site, switching between rotation sites, using lower concentrations of apomorphine, applying ultrasound treatment, or using silicone dressings. It seems that subcutaneous nodules are more common in men than in women and the occurrence is associated with both the infusion rate and the infusion duration (Borgemeester et al., 2015). Visual hallucinations occur in about 20% of patients (Borgemeester et al., 2015). Although the hallucinations are often mild, more severe visual hallucinations also occur in about 10% of patients (Trenkwalder et al., 2015). Psychotic side effects do, however, not seem to be more common under CSA therapy compared to normal peroral/transdermal therapies. Orthostatic hypotension can often be treated with an adequate fluid/salt intake, compression socks, or careful positional changes, but sometimes pharmacological measures—such as the addition of midodrine or a mineralcorticoid—must be considered. One 6-month observational study found that 9.8% of patients with CSA reported some form of ICD during treatment (Martinez-Martin et al., 2014). Hemolytic anemia is rather uncommon but does occur in 1%–2% of patients with CSA and can be a reason for treatment discontinuation (Borgemeester et al., 2015; Trenkwalder et al., 2015). Other severe adverse events that do lead to discontinuation are, e.g., severe cases of subcutaneous nodules, visual hallucinations, or orthostatic hypotension—each being the cause for discontinuation in about 3% of patients (Borgemeester et al., 2015).

4.6 The Indications, the Contraindications, and the "Ideal" Patient

CSA is an alternative for patients with advanced PD, motor fluctuations, and dyskinesia. The treatment is not appropriate for those with dementia, a poor response to levodopa, or difficulties handling the infusion device even with support from a caregiver. For patients with a history of drug-related hallucinations or ICDs, it is advisable to consider one of the alternative treatments over CSA, although the visual hallucinations often can be handled through dose adjustments. On a group level, the patients that benefit the most from CSA are younger patients with disabling motor fluctuations and no dementia.

5. CONCLUSIONS

The safety and efficacy of device-aided therapies have been well established. In the case of DBS, the best results are achieved based on technical knowledge of the stimulation, detailed knowledge of the basal ganglia anatomy, as well as changes in the medical therapy.

Both LCIG and CSA have been studied rather thoroughly in studies with either prospective open-label or retrospective designs. With the randomized controlled double-blinded study on LCIG, the level of evidence has improved further confirming the efficacy of continuous drug delivery. The effects on nonmotor symptoms have been established in clinical practice and in open-label studies, but the overall evidence strength of these effects is still low. Long-term data of LCIG and CSA treatment are still building and will likely contribute to a future debate on the best timing for initiation of treatment.

All device-aided improve health-related quality of life in a population that is subject to great physical and physiological strain. People with PD often do not receive advanced treatment before their PD has made their working situation too difficult to manage or when they are already retired. The costs for the treatments are significant, but it is possible that the total health care costs and the rate of early retirement in the group with moderate to advanced PD could be reduced in response to an earlier initiation of advanced treatment. Similarly, the rate of return to work after initiation of treatment needs to be investigated further. It is likely that a growing number of actors will contribute to increased competition and reduced market prices; hence making the advanced treatments accessible for a larger portion of PD patients worldwide.

REFERENCES

Anderson, V. C., Burchiel, K. J., & Hogarth, P. (2005). Pallidal vs subthalamic nucleus deep brain stimulation in Parkinson disease. *Archives of Neurology*, *62*(4), 554. http://dx.doi.org/10.1001/archneur.62.4.554.

Antonini, A., Odin, P., Opiano, L., Tomantschger, V., Pacchetti, C., Pickut, B., et al. (2013). Effect and safety of duodenal levodopa infusion in advanced Parkinson's disease: A retrospective multicenter outcome assessment in patient routine care. *Journal of Neural Transmission*, *120*(11), 1553–1558. http://dx.doi.org/10.1007/s00702-013-1026-9.

Antonini, A., Yegin, A., Preda, C., Bergmann, L., & Poewe, W. (2015). Global long-term study on motor and non-motor symptoms and safety of levodopa-carbidopa intestinal gel in routine care of advanced Parkinson's disease patients; 12-month interim outcomes. *Parkinsonism & Related Disorders*, *21*(3), 231. http://dx.doi.org/10.1016/j.parkreldis.2014.12.012.

Barichella, M., Marczewska, A. M., & Mariani, C. (2003). Body weight gain rate in patients with Parkinson's disease and deep brain stimulation. *Movement Disorders*, *18*(11), 1337. http://dx.doi.org/10.1002/mds.10543.

Benabid, A. L., Pollak, P., Louveau, A., Henry, S., & de Rougemont, J. (1988). Combined (thalamotomy and stimulation) stereotactic surgery of the VIM thalamic nucleus for bilateral Parkinson disease. *Stereotactic and Functional Neurosurgery*, *50*(1–6), 344. http://dx.doi.org/10.1159/000100803.

Benazzouz, A., & Hallett, M. (2000). Mechanism of action of deep brain stimulation. *Neurology*, *55*(12, Suppl. 6), 13–16.

Bhatia, S., Zhang, K., Oh, M., Angle, C., & Whiting, D. (2010). Infections and hardware salvage after deep brain stimulation surgery: A single-center study and review of the literature. *Stereotactic and Functional Neurosurgery*, *88*(3), 147–155. http://dx.doi.org/10.1159/000303528.

Binder, D. K., Rau, G. M., & Starr, P. A. (2005). Risk factors for hemorrhage during microelectrode-guided deep brain stimulator implantation for movement disorders. *Neurosurgery*, *56*(4), 722. http://dx.doi.org/10.1227/01.neu.0000156473.57196.7e.

Bjerknes, S., Skogseid, I. M., Sæhle, T., Dietrichs, E., & Toft, M. (2014). Surgical site infections after deep brain stimulation surgery: Frequency, characteristics and management in a 10-year period. *PloS One*, *9*(8). e105288. http://dx.doi.org/10.1371/journal.pone.0105288.

Blomstedt, P., & Hariz, M. I. (2005). Hardware-related complications of deep brain stimulation: A ten year experience. *Acta Neurochirurgica*, *147*(10), 1061. http://dx.doi.org/10.1007/s00701-005-0576-5.

Borgemeester, R. W. K., Drent, M., & van Laar, T. (2015). Motor and non-motor outcomes of continuous apomorphine infusion in 125 Parkinson's disease patients. *Parkinsonism & Related Disorders*, *23*, 17–22. http://dx.doi.org/10.1016/j.parkreldis.2015.11.013.

Borgemeester, R. W. K., Lees, A. J., & van Laar, T. (2016). Parkinson's disease, visual hallucinations and apomorphine: A review of the available evidence. *Parkinsonism & Related Disorders*, *27*, 35. http://dx.doi.org/10.1016/j.parkreldis.2016.04.023.

Boviatsis, E. J., Stavrinou, L. C., & Themistocleous, M. (2010). Surgical and hardware complications of deep brain stimulation. A seven-year experience and review of the literature. *Acta Neurochirurgica*, *152*(12), 2053. http://dx.doi.org/10.1007/s00701-010-0749-8.

Buongiorno, M., Antonelli, F., Cámara, A., Puente, V., de Fabregues-Nebot, O., Hernandez-Vara, J., et al. (2015). Long-term response to continuous duodenal infusion of levodopa/carbidopa gel in patients with advanced Parkinson disease: The Barcelona registry. *Parkinsonism & Related Disorders*, *21*(8), 871. http://dx.doi.org/10.1016/j.parkreldis.2015.05.014.

Cossu, G., Ceravolo, R., Zibetti, M., Arca, R., Ricchi, V., Paribello, A., et al. (2016). Levodopa and neuropathy risk in patients with Parkinson disease: Effect of COMT inhibition. *Parkinsonism & Related Disorders*, *27*, 81–84. http://dx.doi.org/10.1016/j.parkreldis.2016.04.016.

De Gaspari, D., Siri, C., Landi, A., Cilia, R., Bonetti, A., Natuzzi, F., et al. (2006). Clinical and neuropsychological follow up at 12 months in patients with complicated Parkinson's disease treated with subcutaneous apomorphine infusion or deep brain stimulation of the subthalamic nucleus. *Journal of Neurology, Neurosurgery, and Psychiatry*, *77*(4), 450–453.

Deuschl, G., & Schade, C. (2006). A randomized trial of deep-brain stimulation for Parkinson's disease. *New England Journal of Medicine*, *355*(9), 896. http://dx.doi.org/10.1056/nejmoa060281.

Devigili, G., Rinaldo, S., Lettieri, C., & Eleopra, R. (2016). Levodopa/carbidopa intestinal gel therapy for advanced Parkinson disease: An early toxic effect for small nerve fibers? *Muscle & Nerve*, *54*(5), 970. http://dx.doi.org/10.1002/mus.25377.

Drapier, S., Eusebio, A., Degos, B., Vérin, M., & Durif, F. (2016). Quality of life in Parkinson's disease improved by apomorphine pump: The OPTIPUMP cohort study. *Journal of Neurology*, *263*(6), 1111. http://dx.doi.org/10.1007/s00415-016-8106-3.

Elias, W. J., Lipsman, N., Ondo, W. G., Ghanouni, P., Kim, Y. G., Lee, W., et al. (2016). A randomized trial of focused ultrasound thalamotomy for essential tremor. *The New England Journal of Medicine*, *375*(8), 730–739. http://dx.doi.org/10.1056/NEJMoa1600159.

Fenoy, A. J., & Simpson, R. K. (2013). Risks of common complications in deep brain stimulation surgery: Management and avoidance. *Journal of Neurosurgery*, *120*(1), 132–139. http://dx.doi.org/10.3171/2013.10.JNS131225.

Fernandez, H. H., Standaert, D. G., Hauser, R. A., Lang, A. E., Fung, V. S. C., Klostermann, F., et al. (2014). Levodopa-carbidopa intestinal gel in advanced Parkinson's disease: Final 12-month, open-label results. *Movement Disorders*, *30*(4), 500–509. http://dx.doi.org/10.1002/mds.26123.

Follett, K. A., Weaver, F. M., Stern, M., & Hur, K. (2010). Pallidal versus subthalamic deep-brain stimulation for Parkinson's disease. *New England Journal of Medicine*, *362*(22), 2077. http://dx.doi.org/10.1056/nejmoa0907083.

Hamani, C., & Lozano, A. M. (2006). Hardware-related complications of deep brain stimulation: A review of the published literature. *Stereotactic and Functional Neurosurgery*, *84*(5–6), 248–251. http://dx.doi.org/10.1159/000096499.

Hamani, C., Richter, E., Schwalb, J. M., & Lozano, A. M. (2008). Bilateral subthalamic nucleus stimulation for Parkinson's disease: A systematic review of the clinical literature. *Neurosurgery*, *62*(Suppl. 2), 863–874. http://dx.doi.org/10.1227/01.neu.0000316288.75736.1c.

Herzog, J., Volkmann, J., Krack, P., Kopper, F., Pötter, M., Lorenz, D., et al. (2003). Two-year follow-up of subthalamic deep brain stimulation in Parkinson's disease. *Movement Disorders*, *18*(11), 1332–1337. http://dx.doi.org/10.1002/mds.10518.

Horsley, V. (1890). Remarks on the surgery of the central nervous system. *BMJ*, *2*(1562), 1286. http://dx.doi.org/10.1136/bmj.2.1562.1286.

Hristova, A., Lyons, K., Tröster, A. I., Pahwa, R., Wilkinson, S. B., & Koller, W. C. (2000). Effect and time course of deep brain stimulation of the globus pallidus and subthalamus on motor features of Parkinson's disease. *Clinical Neuropharmacology*, *23*(4), 208–211. http://dx.doi.org/10.1097/00002826-200007000-00007.

Katzenschlager, R., Hughes, A., & Evans, A. (2005). Continuous subcutaneous apomorphine therapy improves dyskinesias in Parkinson's disease: A prospective study using single-dose challenges. *Movement Disorders*, *20*(2), 151. http://dx.doi.org/10.1002/mds.20276.

Krüger, R., Hilker, R., Winkler, C., Lorrain, M., Hahne, M., Redecker, C., et al. (2015). Advanced stages of PD: Interventional therapies and related patient-centered care. *Journal of Neural Transmission*, *123*(1), 31. http://dx.doi.org/10.1007/s00702-015-1418-0.

Kwan, V., van der Poorten, D., Mahant, N., Wolfe, N., Ha, A. D., Griffith, J. M., et al. (2016). Intraduodenal levodopa-carbidopa intestinal gel infusion improves both motor performance and quality of life in advanced Parkinson's disease. *Journal of Clinical Neuroscience*, *25*, 41. http://dx.doi.org/10.1016/j.jocn.2015.05.059.

Lang, A. E., Rodriguez, R. L., Boyd, J. T., Chouinard, S., Zadikoff, C., Espay, A. J., et al. (2016). Integrated safety of levodopa-carbidopa intestinal gel from prospective clinical trials. *Movement Disorders*, *31*(4), 538–546. http://dx.doi.org/10.1002/mds.26485.

LeWitt, P. A. (2014). Levodopa therapy for Parkinson's disease: Pharmacokinetics and pharmacodynamics. *Movement Disorders*, *30*(1), 64. http://dx.doi.org/10.1002/mds.26082.

Limousin, P., Krack, P., Pollak, P., Benazzouz, A., Ardouin, C., Hoffmann, D., et al. (1998). Electrical stimulation of the subthalamic nucleus in advanced Parkinson's disease. *New England Journal of Medicine*, *339*(16), 1105. http://dx.doi.org/10.1056/nejm199810153391603.

Liu, Y., Li, W., Tan, C., Liu, X., Wang, X., Gui, Y., et al. (2014). Meta-analysis comparing deep brain stimulation of the globus pallidus and subthalamic nucleus to treat advanced Parkinson disease. *Journal of Neurosurgery*, *121*(3), 709. http://dx.doi.org/10.3171/2014.4.jns131711.

Lopiano, L., Modugno, N., Sensi, M., Meco, G., Cannas, A., Gusmaroli, G., et al. (2016). Motor outcomes in patients with advanced Parkinson's disease treated with levodopa/carbidopa intestinal gel in Italy: An interim analysis from the GREEN-FIELD observational study. *Neurological Sciences*, *37*(11), 1785. http://dx.doi.org/10.1007/s10072-016-2664-0.

Lyons, K. E., Koller, W. C., Wilkinson, S. B., & Pahwa, R. (2001). Long term safety and efficacy of unilateral deep brain stimulation of the thalamus for parkinsonian tremor. *Journal of Neurology, Neurosurgery & Psychiatry*, *71*(5), 682–684. http://dx.doi.org/10.1136/jnnp.71.5.682.

Machado, A. G., Deogaonkar, M., & Cooper, S. (2012). Deep brain stimulation for movement disorders: Patient selection and technical options. *Cleveland Clinic Journal of Medicine*, *79*(Suppl. 2), S19–S24. http://dx.doi.org/10.3949/ccjm.79.s2a.04.

Macia, F., Perlemoine, C., Coman, I., & Guehl, D. (2004). Parkinson's disease patients with bilateral subthalamic deep brain stimulation gain weight. *Movement Disorders*, *19*(2), 206. http://dx.doi.org/10.1002/mds.10630.

Martinez-Martin, P., Reddy, P., Katzenschlager, R., Antonini, A., Todorova, A., Odin, P., et al. (2014). EuroInf: A multicenter comparative observational study of apomorphine and levodopa infusion in Parkinson's disease. *Movement Disorders*, *30*(4), 510–516. http://dx.doi.org/10.1002/mds.26067.

Melamed, E., Ziv, I., & Djaldetti, R. (2007). Management of motor complications in advanced Parkinson's disease. *Movement Disorders*, *22*(S17), S379. http://dx.doi.org/10.1002/mds.21680.

Merola, A., Romagnolo, A., Zibetti, M., Bernardini, A., Cocito, D., & Lopiano, L. (2015). Peripheral neuropathy associated with levodopa-carbidopa intestinal infusion: A long-term prospective assessment. *European Journal of Neurology*, *23*(3), 501. http://dx.doi.org/10.1111/ene.12846.

Mestre, T. A., Espay, A. J., Marras, C., Eckman, M. H., Pollak, P., & Lang, A. E. (2014). Subthalamic nucleus-deep brain stimulation for early motor complications in Parkinson's disease-the EARLYSTIM trial: Early is not always better. *Movement Disorders*, *29*(14), 1751. http://dx.doi.org/10.1002/mds.26024.

Metman, L. V., & Slavin, K. V. (2015). Advances in functional neurosurgery for Parkinson's disease. *Movement Disorders*, *30*(11), 1461. http://dx.doi.org/10.1002/mds.26338.

Moro, E., Hamani, C., Poon, Y. Y., & Al, T. (2010a). Unilateral pedunculopontine stimulation improves falls in Parkinson's disease. *Brain*, *133*(1), 215. http://dx.doi.org/10.1093/brain/awp261.

Moro, E., Lozano, A. M., Pollak, P., & Agid, Y. (2010b). Long-term results of a multicenter study on subthalamic and pallidal stimulation in Parkinson's disease. *Movement Disorders*, *25*(5), 578. http://dx.doi.org/10.1002/mds.22735.

Obwegeser, A. A., Uitti, R. J., Witte, R. J., Lucas, J. A., Turk, M. F., & Wharen, R. E. (2001). Quantitative and qualitative outcome measures after thalamic deep brain stimulation to treat disabling tremors. *Neurosurgery*, *48*(2), 274. http://dx.doi.org/10.1097/00006123-200102000-00004.

Odekerken, V. J., van Laar, T., Staal, M. J., Mosch, A., Hoffmann, C. F., Nijssen, P. C., et al. (2013). Subthalamic nucleus versus globus pallidus bilateral deep brain stimulation for advanced Parkinson's disease (NSTAPS study): A randomised controlled trial. *The Lancet. Neurology*, *12*(1), 37. http://dx.doi.org/10.1016/s1474-4422(12)70264-8.

Odin, P., Chaudhuri, K. R., Slevin, J. T., Volkmann, J., Dietrichs, E., Martinez-Martin, P., et al. (2015). Collective physician perspectives on non-oral medication approaches for the management of clinically relevant unresolved issues in Parkinson's disease: Consensus from an international survey and discussion program. *Parkinsonism & Related Disorders*, *21*(10), 1133. http://dx.doi.org/10.1016/j.parkreldis.2015.07.020.

Oh, M. Y., Abosch, A., Kim, S. H., Lang, A. E., & Lozano, A. M. (2002). Long-term hardware-related complications of deep brain stimulation. *Neurosurgery*, *50*(6), 1268. http://dx.doi.org/10.1097/00006123-200206000-00017.

Okun, M. S. (2012). Deep-brain stimulation for Parkinson's disease. *New England Journal of Medicine*, *367*(16), 1529. http://dx.doi.org/10.1056/nejmct1208070.

Okun, M. S., Fernandez, H. H., & Wu, S. S. (2009). Cognition and mood in Parkinson's disease in subthalamic nucleus versus globus pallidus interna deep brain stimulation: The COMPARE trial. *Annals of Neurology*, *65*(5), 586. http://dx.doi.org/10.1002/ana.21596.

Okun, M. S., Gallo, B. V., Mandybur, G., Jagid, J., Foote, K. D., Revilla, F. J., et al. (2012). Subthalamic deep brain stimulation with a constant-current device in Parkinson's disease: An open-label randomised controlled trial. *The Lancet. Neurology*, *11*(2), 140. http://dx.doi.org/10.1016/s1474-4422(11)70308-8.

Olanow, C. W., Kieburtz, K., Odin, P., Espay, A. J., Standaert, D. G., Fernandez, H. H., et al. (2014). Continuous intrajejunal infusion of levodopa-carbidopa intestinal gel for patients with advanced Parkinson's disease: A randomised, controlled, double-blind, double-dummy study. *The Lancet Neurology*, *13*(2), 141. http://dx.doi.org/10.1016/s1474-4422(13)70293-x.

Olanow, C. W., & Koller, W. C. (1998). An algorithm (decision tree) for the management of Parkinson's disease: Treatment guidelines. *Neurology*, *50*(3, Suppl. 3), S1. http://dx.doi.org/10.1212/wnl.50.3_suppl_3.s1.

Pahwa, R., Wilkinson, S. B., Overman, J., & Lyons, K. E. (2003). Bilateral subthalamic stimulation in patients with Parkinson disease: Long-term follow up. *Journal of Neurosurgery*, *99*(1), 71–77. http://dx.doi.org/10.3171/jns.2003.99.1.0071.

Pålhagen, S. E., Sydow, O., Johansson, A., Nyholm, D., Holmberg, B., Widner, H., et al. (2016). Levodopa-carbidopa intestinal gel (LCIG) treatment in routine care of patients with advanced Parkinson's disease: An open-label prospective observational study of effectiveness, tolerability and healthcare costs. *Parkinsonism & Related Disorders*, *29*, 17. http://dx.doi.org/10.1016/j.parkreldis.2016.06.002.

Pepper, J., Zrinzo, L., Mirza, B., Foltynie, T., Limousin, P., & Hariz, M. (2012). The risk of hardware infection in deep brain stimulation surgery is greater at impulse generator replacement than at the primary procedure. *Stereotactic and Functional Neurosurgery*, *91*(1), 56–65. http://dx.doi.org/10.1159/000343202.

Petraglia, F. W., Farber, S. H., Han, J. L., Verla, T., Gallis, J., Lokhnygina, Y., et al. (2015). Comparison of bilateral vs. staged unilateral deep brain stimulation (DBS) in Parkinson's disease in patients under 70 years of age. *Neuromodulation: Journal of the International Neuromodulation Society*, *19*(1), 31–37. http://dx.doi.org/10.1111/ner.12351.

Pickut, B. A., van der Linden, C., Dethy, S., Van De Maele, H., & de Beyl, D. Z. (2013). Intestinal levodopa infusion: The Belgian experience. *Neurological Sciences: Official Journal of the Italian Neurological Society and of the Italian Society of Clinical Neurophysiology*, *35*, 861–866. http://dx.doi.org/10.1007/s10072-013-1612-5.

Poewe, W., Kleedorfer, B., Wagner, M., Bösch, S., & Schelosky, L. (1993). Continuous subcutaneous apomorphine infusions for fluctuating Parkinson's disease. Long-term follow-up in 18 patients. *Advances in Neurology*, *60*, 656–659.

Rambour, M., Moreau, C., Salleron, J., & Devos, D. (2014). Continuous subcutaneous infusion of apomorphine in Parkinson's disease: Retrospective analysis of a series of 81 patients. *Revue Neurologique*, *170*(3), 205. http://dx.doi.org/10.1016/j.neurol.2013.10.012.

Reddy, P., Martinez-Martin, P., Rizos, A., Martin, A., Faye, G. C., Forgacs, I., et al. (2012). Intrajejunal levodopa versus conventional therapy in Parkinson disease: Motor and nonmotor effects. *Clinical Neuropharmacology*, *35*(5), 205–207. http://dx.doi.org/10.1097/WNF.0b013e3182613dea.

Rodriguez, M. C. (2005). Bilateral deep brain stimulation in Parkinson's disease: A multicentre study with 4 years follow-up. *Brain*, *128*(10), 2240. http://dx.doi.org/10.1093/brain/awh571.

Russmann, H., Ghika, J., Villemure, J. G., & Robert, B. (2004). Subthalamic nucleus deep brain stimulation in Parkinson disease patients over age 70 years. *Neurology*, *63*(10), 1952. http://dx.doi.org/10.1212/01.wnl.0000144198.26309.d8.

Sansur, C. A., Frysinger, R. C., Pouratian, N., Fu, K.-M., Bittl, M., Oskouian, R. J., et al. (2007). Incidence of symptomatic hemorrhage after stereotactic electrode placement. *Journal of Neurosurgery, 107*(5), 998. http://dx.doi.org/10.3171/jns.2007.107.5.998.

Schapira, A. H. V., & Obeso, J. (2006). Timing of treatment initiation in Parkinson's disease: A need for reappraisal? *Annals of Neurology, 59*(3), 559. http://dx.doi.org/10.1002/ana.20789.

Schuepbach, W., Rau, J., & Knudsen, K. (2013). Neurostimulation for Parkinson's disease with early motor complications. *New England Journal of Medicine, 368*(7), 610. http://dx.doi.org/10.1056/nejmoa1205158.

Schüpbach, W., Maltete, D., & Houeto, J. L. (2007). Neurosurgery at an earlier stage of Parkinson disease a randomized, controlled trial. *Neurology, 68*(4), 267. http://dx.doi.org/10.1212/01.wnl.0000250253.03919.fb.

Spiegel, E. A., Wycis, H. T., Marks, M., & Lee, A. J. (1947). Stereotaxic apparatus for operations on the human brain. *Science, 106*(2754), 349. http://dx.doi.org/10.1126/science.106.2754.349.

Stefani, A., Lozano, A. M., Peppe, A., Stanzione, P., & Galati, S. (2007). Bilateral deep brain stimulation of the pedunculopontine and subthalamic nuclei in severe Parkinson's disease. *Brain, 130*(6), 1596. http://dx.doi.org/10.1093/brain/awl346.

Thobois, S., Ardouin, C., Lhommée, E., & Klinger, H. (2010). Non-motor dopamine withdrawal syndrome after surgery for Parkinson's disease: Predictors and underlying mesolimbic denervation. *Brain, 133*(4), 1111. http://dx.doi.org/10.1093/brain/awq032.

Timpka, J., Fox, T., Fox, K., Honig, H., Odin, P., Martinez-Martin, P., et al. (2015). Improvement of dyskinesias with l-dopa infusion in advanced Parkinson's disease. *Acta Neurologica Scandinavica, 133*(6), 451. http://dx.doi.org/10.1111/ane.12483.

Todorova, A., Martinez-Martin, P., Martin, A., Rizos, A., Reddy, P., & Chaudhuri, K. R. (2013). Daytime apomorphine infusion combined with transdermal Rotigotine patch therapy is tolerated at 2 years: A 24-h treatment option in Parkinson's disease. *Basal Ganglia, 3*(2), 127. http://dx.doi.org/10.1016/j.baga.2013.02.002.

Trenkwalder, C., Chaudhuri, K. R., Ruiz, P. J. G., LeWitt, P., Katzenschlager, R., Sixel-Döring, F., et al. (2015). Expert consensus group report on the use of apomorphine in the treatment of Parkinson's disease—Clinical practice recommendations. *Parkinsonism & Related Disorders, 21*(9), 1023–1030. http://dx.doi.org/10.1016/j.parkreldis.2015.06.012.

Umemura, A., Jaggi, J. L., Hurtig, H. I., & Siderowf, A. D. (2003). Deep brain stimulation for movement disorders: Morbidity and mortality in 109 patients. *Journal of Neurosurgery, 98*(4), 779. http://dx.doi.org/10.3171/jns.2003.98.4.0779.

Umemura, A., Oka, Y., Yamamoto, K., & Okita, K. (2011). Complications of subthalamic nucleus stimulation in Parkinson's disease. *Neurologia Medico-Chirurgica, 51*(11), 749. http://dx.doi.org/10.2176/nmc.51.749.

Valldeoriola, F., & Grandas, F. (2016). Long-term effectiveness of levodopa-carbidopa intestinal gel in 177 Spanish patients with advanced Parkinson's disease. *Neurodegenerative Disease Management, 6*(4), 289. http://dx.doi.org/10.2217/nmt-2016-0021.

Volkmann, J., Albanese, A., Antonini, A., & Chaudhuri, K. R. (2013). Selecting deep brain stimulation or infusion therapies in advanced Parkinson's disease: An evidence-based review. *Journal of Neurology, 260*(11), 2701. http://dx.doi.org/10.1007/s00415-012-6798-6.

Weaver, F. M., Follett, K., Stern, M., Hur, K., & Harris, C. (2009). Bilateral deep brain stimulation vs best medical therapy for patients with advanced Parkinson disease: A randomized controlled trial. *JAMA, 301*(1), 63. http://dx.doi.org/10.1001/jama.2008.929.

Weaver, F. M., Follett, K. A., Stern, M., Luo, P., & Harris, C. L. (2012). Randomized trial of deep brain stimulation for Parkinson disease thirty-six-month outcomes. *Neurology, 79*(1), 55. http://dx.doi.org/10.1212/wnl.0b013e31825dcdc1.

Williams, A., Gill, S., Varma, T., Jenkinson, C., Quinn, N., Mitchell, R., et al. (2010). Deep brain stimulation plus best medical therapy versus best medical therapy alone for advanced Parkinson's disease (PD SURG trial): A randomised, open-label trial. *The Lancet Neurology*, *9*(6), 581. http://dx.doi.org/10.1016/s1474-4422(10)70093-4.

Wirdefeldt, K., Odin, P., & Nyholm, D. (2016). Levodopa–carbidopa intestinal gel in patients with Parkinson's disease: A systematic review. *CNS Drugs*, *30*(5), 381. http://dx.doi.org/10.1007/s40263-016-0336-5.

Woods, S. P., Fields, J. A., & Tröster, A. I. (2002). Neuropsychological sequelae of subthalamic nucleus deep brain stimulation in Parkinson's disease: A critical review. *Neuropsychology Review*, *12*, 111–126.

Zesiewicz, T. A., Elble, R., Louis, E. D., Hauser, R. A., Sullivan, K. L., Dewey, R. B., et al. (2005). Practice parameter: Therapies for essential tremor: Report of the quality standards Subcommittee of the American Academy of Neurology. *Neurology*, *64*(12), 2008. http://dx.doi.org/10.1212/01.wnl.0000163769.28552.cd.

Zibetti, M., Merola, A., Artusi, C. A., & Rizzi, L. (2014). Levodopa/carbidopa intestinal gel infusion in advanced Parkinson's disease: A 7-year experience. *European Journal of Neurology*, *21*(2), 312. http://dx.doi.org/10.1111/ene.12309.

CHAPTER SEVENTEEN

Palliative Care for Patients and Families With Parkinson's Disease☆

Raquel Bouça-Machado[*,†,1], Nataliya Titova[‡,1], K. Ray Chaudhuri[§,#,], Bas R. Bloem[¶], Joaquim J. Ferreira[*,†,||,2]**

[*]Clinical Pharmacology Unit, Instituto de Medicina Molecular, Lisbon, Portugal
[†]CNS-Campus Neurológico Sénior, Torres Vedras, Portugal
[‡]Federal State Budgetary Educational Institution of Higher Education "N.I. Pirogov Russian National Research Medical University" of the Ministry of Healthcare of the Russian Federation, Moscow, Russia
[§]National Parkinson Foundation International Centre of Excellence, Kings College and Kings College Hospital, London, United Kingdom
[¶]Radboud University Medical Centre, Donders Institute for Brain, Cognition and Behaviour, Nijmegen, The Netherlands
[||]Laboratory of Clinical Pharmacology and Therapeutics, Faculty of Medicine, University of Lisbon, Lisbon, Portugal
[#]Maurice Wohl Clinical Neuroscience Institute, Kings College, London, United Kingdom
[**]National Institute for Health Research (NIHR) Mental Health Biomedical Research Centre (BRC) and Dementia Unit at South London and Maudsley NHS Foundation Trust, London, United Kingdom
[2]Corresponding author: e-mail address: joaquimjferreira@gmail.com

Contents

[1] These authors contributed equally to this work.

☆ *Declaration of competing interests*: All authors declare: no support from any organization for the submitted work; no financial relationships with any organizations that might have an interest in the submitted work in the previous 3 years, no other relationships or activities that could appear to have influenced the submitted work. *Funding*: No funding was received.

International Review of Neurobiology, Volume 132
ISSN 0074-7742
http://dx.doi.org/10.1016/bs.irn.2017.02.017

Abstract

Parkinson's disease is the second most common neurodegenerative disease worldwide. There is widespread consensus that Parkinson patients, their carers, and clinicians involved in their care would benefit from a fully integrated, need-based provision of palliative care. However, the concept of palliative care in Parkinson's disease is still poorly defined and, consequently, poorly implemented into daily clinical practice. A particular challenge is the gradually progressive nature of Parkinson's disease—with insidiously increasing disability—making it challenging to clearly define the onset of palliative care needs for Parkinson patients. As people with Parkinson's disease are now living longer than in the past, future research needs to develop a more robust evidence-based approach to clarify the disease events associated with increased palliative care needs, and to examine these, prospectively, in an integrated palliative care service. The modern palliative care outlook, termed "simultaneous care,",is no longer restricted to the final stage of disease. It involves incorporating a continuity of care, effective management of the chronic-palliative interface, and a multidisciplinary network of professionals working both in the community and in specialized clinics, with active involvement of caregivers. Although promising, there is still a need to demonstrate the effectiveness of palliative care for patients with Parkinson's disease.

1. PARKINSON'S DISEASE

1.1 Epidemiology and Diagnosis

The first detailed description of Parkinson's disease (PD) was made now two centuries ago. PD is the second most common neurodegenerative disease worldwide, affecting 1%–2% of the world population above 65 years of age, and with an incidence and prevalence on the rise along with aging of the population. In Europe, the prevalence of PD for those aged 85–89 has been reported to be 3.5%, with an estimated annual cost of €13.9 billions (Kalia & Lang, 2015; Keus et al., 2014; Sveinbjornsdottir, 2016).

1.2 Clinical Features

PD is traditionally featured by its motor symptoms. More recently, it has been recognized that PD is not only characterized by motor-related features (Fig. 1). Nonmotor features, including olfactory dysfunction, cognitive impairment, psychiatric symptoms, disorders of sleep-wake cycle, autonomic dysfunction, pain, and fatigue, are also common and sometimes the chief complaint and therapeutic challenge in advanced stages of PD (Kalia & Lang, 2015; Keus et al., 2014; Williams & Litvan, 2013). These symptoms are frequently present before the onset of the classical motor symptoms and significantly affect the patient's quality of life (Kalia & Lang, 2015; Keus et al., 2014).

1.3 PD Clinical States and Progression

The classic motor features of PD typically start insidiously, are unilateral and mild, with—at least initially—an excellent response to treatment (possibly with the exception of tremor), and no changes in motor functioning across

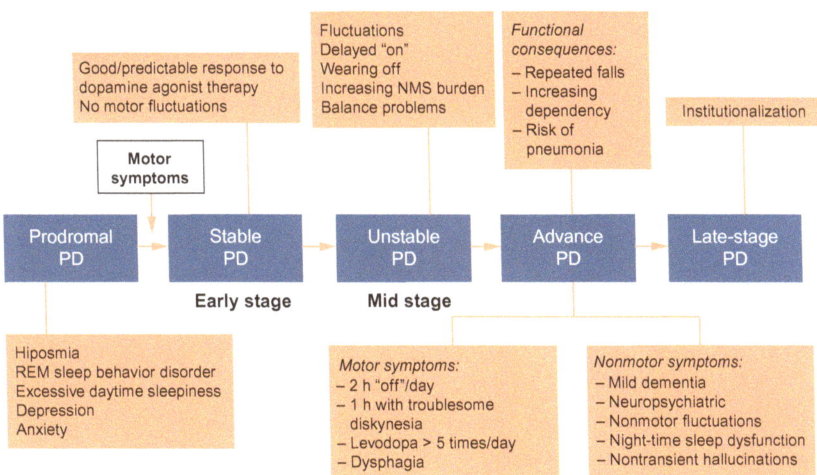

Fig. 1 A proposed "journey" pattern of a person with Parkinson's disease. *Adapted from Chaudhuri, K. R., & Fung, V. S. C. (Eds.) (2016).* Fastfacts, Parkinsonnns disease. *(4th ed.), UK: Health Press.*

the day. In this early phase, when symptoms progress and motor symptoms also appear in the contralateral side, drug response is usually reliable and patients have no major functional problems. This is often called the 'honeymoon period' (Rascol, Payoux, & Ory, 2003; Sveinbjornsdottir, 2016). After 2–5 years, with further disease progression, the majority of patients will begin to experience a shorter duration of response to individual levodopa doses (wearing-off symptoms), alternative phases with good and poor response to medication (on–off symptoms); involuntary movements of the head, trunk, or limbs (peak–dose dyskinesias); and other motor complications. Gait and balance disturbances as well as speech and swallowing difficulties commonly appear, and these generally respond poorly to treatment (Poewe, 2006; Rascol et al., 2003; Salat, Noyce, Schrag, & Tolosa, 2016; Williams & Litvan, 2013). After a prolonged disease duration of 10 or more years, most patients have developed a clearly bilateral disease, with bradykinesia having a profound impact on patients' disability, with rest tremor being less common and certainly less at the forefront. Falls and fall-related fractures or other injuries are common, the risk of fractures being aggravated by osteoporosis, which is a common comorbidity. An increasing number of patients become at least partially wheelchair-bound, particularly when in an "off" state. In this phase, dysarthria has a great impact on patient condition and hinders communication with caregivers, whereas dysphagia is a frequent cause of choking and aspiration pneumonia, sometimes necessitating tube feeding. "Off" states are on the one hand associated with high disability and dependency on caregivers, but on the other their impact on quality of life is less valued by patients once the "on" states are also not good (Coelho et al., 2010; Salat et al., 2016).

Despite the use of levodopa and other dopamine replacement therapies (DRT), PD patients have higher and earlier need for nursing home placements, higher rates of emergency hospital admissions, longer admissions, and higher in-hospital mortality than the general population (Sveinbjornsdottir, 2016). Coelho et al. (2014) assigned these differences to the greater disease severity (reflected by higher UPDRS scores), frequent falls, dementia, hallucinations, and complications associated with PD, such as urinary complaints and bone fractures. Data from the Queen Square Brain Bank suggest that the mean time from diagnosis to death is around 14 years, and the most frequent cause of death is pneumonia, followed by cardiovascular events, stroke, and cancer (Coelho et al., 2014, 2010; Poewe, 2006; Sveinbjornsdottir, 2016).

2. TRADITIONAL THERAPEUTIC APPROACHES

In spite of tremendous advances in DRT, there are still no drugs or other interventions that will halt or even slow down disease progression. However, in the past 50 years, many different treatments including drugs, surgical interventions, and nonpharmacological treatments have become available, leading to a marked improvement of motor symptoms and disability, although management of nonmotor symptoms, a key issue for palliative care, remains an unmet need (Todorova, Jenner, & Ray Chaudhuri, 2014).

2.1 Pharmacological Interventions

DRT replacement therapy in PD remains the mainstay of treatment, although modern concepts suggest that alternative nondopaminergic pharmacological strategies are also important, as PD is now recognized to be a multipeptide syndromic disorder (Jellinger, 2015; Titova, Padmakumar, Lewis, & Chaudhuri, 2016).

The timing of initiation of dopaminergic therapies depends on patient preference, degree of disability, and potential side effects of therapy. Early treatment is usually recommended. Most nonmotor symptoms, specifically cognitive impairment, autonomic dysfunction and falls, all greatly impact quality of life of patients, but cannot be resolved with dopaminergic medication.

As symptomatic control becomes more difficult to manage, advanced therapies should be considered as an option. These include deep brain stimulation or infusional therapies such as subcutaneous apomorphine or intraduodenal levodopa gel infusions. These therapies are generally reserved for patients with severe dyskinesias and wearing-off symptoms, who have failed to substantially improve on all the available oral and transdermal therapies, and for those without major cognitive or psychiatric impairment (Sveinbjornsdottir, 2016; Williams & Litvan, 2013).

2.2 Nonpharmacological Interventions

In recent years, rehabilitation has become increasingly recognized in the treatment of axial symptoms that respond poorly to drug therapy, and this includes—among others—physiotherapy, occupational therapy, and speech-language therapy (Bloem, de Vries, & Ebersbach, 2015; Ekker, Janssen, Nonnekes, Bloem, & de Vries, 2016). Its cornerstone is to maximize motor and cognitive functional abilities and to minimize secondary complications in order to optimize independence and well-being, thus enhancing quality of life (Keus et al., 2014; Rascol et al., 2003).

Physiotherapy is important as a symptomatic strategy at all stages of the disease. Some studies suggest that it may also influence the disease course, but this claim awaits actual confirmation in well-designed clinical trials (Moroz et al., 2009). The main areas of intervention are physical capacity, transfers (including posture correction), balance, and gait (including freezing). Despite this not being one of the main areas of intervention, it may also help in respiratory function and pain management. According to the latest guidelines, physiotherapy interventions in PD can be identified as: exercise, practice (motor learning and dual–task), and strategy training (cueing and complex motor sequences), each of which is supported through informing and educating the patient and their caregivers (Keus et al., 2014; Moroz et al., 2009).

Dysarthria and dysphagia can be severely limiting symptoms of PD. Speech therapy focuses on three domains: speech problems (dysarthria and communicative blocks), oropharyngeal swallowing disorders, and loss of saliva, and the limitations and participation problems that can result from this. In order to address communication problems, techniques that increase the loudness of the voice, by simultaneously activating breathing, voice quality, and articulation, are used. The most widely used techniques are the Lee Silverman Voice Treatment (LSVT) and the Pitch Limiting Voice Treatment. For swallowing disorders and loss of saliva, there are no evidence-based interventions, although the pathophysiology is becomimg more clear, offering targets for tailoired interventions (Kalf et al., 2011). The intervention largely consists of a careful evaluation of swallowing function and recommendation of modifications (Moroz et al., 2009).

Occupational therapy aims to reduce restrictions in meaningful activities, roles and tasks, all seen in each patient's individual context. Intervention can be grouped into three areas: living (personal care, housekeeping, etc.), work, and leisure (hobbies, going out, social contacts) (Sturkenboom et al., 2011). A recent RCT offered class II evidence for the merits of occupational therapy for patients with PD (Sturkenboom et al., 2014), with costs remaining about equal (despite more intensive treatment) (Sturkenboom et al., 2015). Importantly, occupational therapy and physiotherapy can often be engaged in parallel, because different and complementary strategies are used to achieve the same goals (Radder et al., 2017).

Patients and families, beginning with diagnosis, are confronted with numerous psychological problems, for which psychological intervention can provide considerable help, in particular by developing coping strategies for stressful social situations, through the use of relaxation and cognitive restructuring techniques together with situational behavioral analysis and training of social skills specifically adapted to the disease (Ellgring, Seiler, Perleth, Gasser, & Oertel, 2010; Lang & Lees, 2002). New strategies to treat cognitive and psychological problems are being developed and evaluated (Bloem et al., 2015).

3. GAPS IN THERAPEUTIC APPROACHES

Although PD is traditionally viewed as a movement disorder, in the past 10 years, the high burden of difficult-to-manage nonmotor symptoms, high caregiver distress, and a high utilization of medical services especially in the last year of life has become evident. Similarly to cancer patients, albeit for a longer duration, PD patients have considerable (and mounting) unmet physical, psychosocial and spiritual needs, and experience great problems with coordination and continuity of care (Miyasaki & Kluger, 2015; van Vliet et al., 2016).

Recently, the perspective of patients and carers about traditional therapeutic approaches has been studied. The findings can be grouped into four themes: burden of disease, access to information, support to family, and experience of healthcare services.

3.1 Burden of the Disease

PD clearly affects the lives of patients and families, not only because of the effect of motor and nonmotor symptoms on daily functioning, but also because of the unpredictability and social embarrassment that are frequently associated with it. As mentioned earlier, after the honeymoon period (which may last roughly between 2 and 5 years), the effectiveness of medication diminishes, being hampered by worsening of dopa-resistant parkinsonism and drug-induced complications, and the clinical presentation becomes frequently associated with different types of nonmotor symptoms such as pain and paraesthesia, psychiatric symptoms (anxiety, depression, paranoia, hallucinations), or autonomic symptoms (tachycardia, sweating, constipation, belching, or breathlessness). These all have a major negative impact and lead to increasing disability, they are highly correlated with a diminished self-perceived health status and are a strong predictor of the need for admission to an institution as well as a predictor of mortality (Poewe, 2006; Sveinbjornsdottir, 2016; Wilcox, 2010; Williams & Litvan, 2013).

Fatigue is the most commonly cited as the symptom which is the most difficult to cope with. Patients frequently report feeling tired all day and of not knowing how to get through the day. Others report that fatigue appears unexpectedly, leading to cancelled plans and missed important events. Associated with this, daytime somnolence is another frequent problem in PD, with many factors contributing to disturbed sleep quality and/or induced sedation in PD patients (Boersma, Jones, Carter, Bekelman, & Miyasaki, 2016; Ferreira et al., 2016; Louter, Aarden, Lion, Bloem, & Overeem, 2012). Other common symptom that patients cite as having a high negative impact on their quality of life include cognitive dysfunction associated with loss of self-awareness and changing of social roles. Patients also worry about being a burden to family and friends and losing their identity (Boersma et al., 2016; Fox et al., 2016).

3.2 Access to Information

The need of information seems a paradoxical issue. On the one hand, patients complain of a lack of information at time of diagnosis and throughout disease progression (van der Eijk et al., 2015), but on the other hand, they also fear receiving this same knowledge. It is important that the clinician tailors how the patient is informed about their diagnosis and the information they are given, to take into account the disease stage and the patient's mindset. Usually, patients report difficulties requesting information from clinicians, which leads to a sense of constant insecurity (Boersma et al., 2016; Fox et al., 2016).

There is a high emotional impact of diagnosis, which is frequently described as a traumatic moment or "death sentence," and patients often express that clinicians underestimate this impact (Boersma et al., 2016; Fox et al., 2016). Many patients describe a sense of abandonment by health professionals, due to lack of information and support, and also find the time interval too long between the disclosure of diagnosis and next follow-up appointment. Concretely, patients complain that even basic information, such as that PD is an incurable disease, are sometimes not communicated and that they have to wait at least 3 months before their next appointment (Boersma et al., 2016; Fox et al., 2016). Studies highlight that patients and their families desire more education and emotional support, particularly with regards to what they can expect in the future, that is, how will the disease progress? How can it be dealt with? And, in case of carers, how do they deal with the death of the loved one? (Boersma et al., 2016; Fox et al., 2016; van der Eijk et al., 2012). Discussing advanced directives and the support needed to deal with changing social roles and financial difficulties is also necessary. Many patients have never heard of advance care planning, and 30% of patients with advance care plans do not share these with their physicians (Boersma, Miyasaki, Kutner, & Kluger, 2014). Evidence suggests that patients' feelings of being alone and without guidance, is one of the main causes of frustration, and anger toward the healthcare team and leads to an increase in calls and visits (Miyasaki, 2013; Miyasaki & Kluger, 2015; Richfield, Jones, & Alty, 2013).

3.3 Support to Family

Caregiver burden increases with PD disease stage, with patients becoming increasingly dependent and requiring full-time care (Fox et al., 2016). Coelho et al. (2014) report that the mean time spent per week providing informal caregiving is 5 days (24 h/day). This large amount of time spent caring has a strong impact on the life and healthcare of carers, themselves often elderly or ill, and often causes of diminished socialization and increased isolation, not only from friends, but also from their children and extended family who are often unaware of the gradual increase in caregiving responsibilities. Some carers express guilt for feeling overloaded (Coelho et al., 2014; Fox et al., 2016; Miyasaki, 2013).

Miyasaki (Miyasaki and Klugerr, 2015) reports the results of a study in which, prior to death, 58% of PD patients were unable to live alone due to physical or cognitive disabilities resulting in 40% ultimately living in a skilled nursing facility. Carers sometimes experience anticipated bereavement as they grief the loss of their loved one to a nursing home, or the loss of their loved one's personality (Fox et al., 2016). Coelho (Coelho et al., 2014) reports the results of a Portuguese and Spanish cohort of 50 late-stage PD patients, where the percentage of institutionalized patients was lower than expected from independent predictors of institutionalization. The author attributes these finding to the family-centered organization of Latin societies and to financial problems (Coelho et al., 2014). According to Miyasaki, 80% of carers retired early due to PD and/or dementia, and independent living was rare, which leads to the early retirement of another family member. Until now, many societies are still not prepared to support patient care at home, which results in a heavy disease burden on caregivers and, in many instances, for the need for a paid caregiver (Coelho et al., 2014; Miyasaki & Kluger, 2015).

3.4 Experience of Healthcare Services

It is common for patients to consider the neurologist as being primarily interested in managing medication, but overlooking psychosocial and spiritual needs which often cause greater distress. When asked about who they think could help them plan for the future, patients usually do not include their doctor in the process, as they believe that he/she has no interest in discussing these issues. There are also reports that some patients withhold information about the progression of symptoms for fear of being prescribed another drug. Poor communication between healthcare professionals and ignorance of the available services is a common cause of insecurity and frustration for patients and their families (Boersma et al., 2016; Fox et al., 2016).

4. CONCEPT OF PALLIATIVE CARE

Since its first use, the concept of "palliative care" has undergone a series of transformations in how it is defined. Consequently, the area of operation and objectives has also changed. Nowadays, the concept of palliative care is no longer considered the same as "end-of-life care" (Kelley & Morrison, 2015; Pastrana, Jünger, Ostgathe, Elsner, & Radbruch, 2008; Sigurdardottir et al., 2014). The current definition of palliative care, provided by the World Health Organization (WHO), includes a broader range of aims to improve "the quality of life of patients and their families with life-threatening illness,",such as "to help patients live as actively as possible until death" and "to help the family cope during the patient's illness and in their own bereavement." It also becomes clear that it tends to benefit a broader group of chronic illnesses, which goes beyond its traditional role in cancer patients (Johnston & Abraham, 1995; Pastrana et al., 2008). In 2015, Kelley and Morrison (2015), following this definition and applying the latest models of palliative care, highlight that palliative care is the care of people and their families, of any age and who are living with a serious illness.

The WHO definition also emphasizes the use of a multidisciplinary team to "address the needs of patients and their families" and the quest to enhance "quality of life" which "may also positively influence the course of illness." In contrast to the traditional role of pain relief and alleviating distressing symptoms, palliative care "is applicable early in the course of illness, in conjunction with other therapies that are intended to prolong life… and includes those investigations needed to better understand and manage distressing clinical complications" (Johnston & Abraham, 1995; Pastrana et al., 2008). Kelley and Morrison (2015) and Campion et al. (2015) follow this definition shifting from a classic role in "end-of-life" and in the treatment of pain, to include "other symptoms, and psychological and spiritual distress, by using advanced communication skills to establish goals of care and help match treatments to those individualized goals, and by providing sophisticated care coordination, palliative care provides an added layer of support to patients, their loved ones, and treating clinicians" (Campion et al., 2015).

5. CLINICAL TRIALS IN PALLIATIVE CARE

According to a MEDLINE search, from its inception to 2005, the number of palliative care clinical trials published has quadrupled (Abernethy et al., 2010; Flemming, Adamson, & Atkin, 2008). While this may be beneficial, questions exist around the type and quality of research being undertaken. Previous reviews concluded that palliative care studies were largely descriptive, with wide variations in sample size, demographic and clinical aspects, and lacked use of recognized standard measures and consideration of key outcomes (Aoun & Nekolaichuk, 2014; Bakitas, Lyons, Dixon, & Ahles, 2006; Bouça-Machado et al., 2017; Kelley & Morrison, 2015; McIlfatrick & Murphy, 2013; Visser, Hadley, & Wee, 2015; Zimmermann, Riechelmann, Krzyzanowska, Rodin, & Tannock, 2008). Visser et al. (2015) studied the reality of evidence-based practice in palliative care and highlighted additional problems like underpowered studies, recruitment difficulties and high attrition rates, inadequate follow-up periods, difficulty defining outcomes, and avoiding the presence of performance bias (Aoun & Nekolaichuk, 2014; Hui, Glitza, Chisholm, Yennu, & Bruera, 2013; Visser et al., 2015).

6. MISCONCEPTIONS ASSOCIATED WITH PALLIATIVE CARE

On the one hand, palliative care seeks to deal with the large heterogeneity and ethical issues resulting from the expansion of its scope of intervention, while on the other hand, it appears to still be too tied into the concept of care of dying oncological patients, with a level of expertise that does not appear to have evolved to a great degree, particularly in a non-oncological setting (Bouça-Machado et al., 2017).

6.1 Palliative Care vs Terminal/Hospice Care

The most common misconception associated with palliative care is that it is synonymous to terminal or hospice care (Boersma et al., 2014). The definition of palliative care points toward a population with life-limiting disease where cure is not possible, what is frequently understood as the care of patients in their last weeks or days of life (Kelley & Morrison, 2015). However, this definition contains an additional key point that radically modifies the traditional concept of palliative care. It states that "the palliative approach is applicable during the entire course of illness, in conjunction with other disease-modifying treatments" (Provinciali et al., 2016). According to this vision, the palliative approach seeks to improve the quality of life along the entire course of the illness, from the moment of diagnosis, and regardless of the length of the illness (Provinciali et al., 2016). The lack of clarity regarding the definition of palliative care and terminal/hospice care tends to influence the view that only patients nearing the end of life are suitable candidates for palliative care (Boersma et al., 2014). Some diseases, especially chronic diseases, severely affect the quality of life of patients and family members for many years, and it is this that led to changes in how palliative care is defined (Kelley & Morrison, 2015). This change not only enables better strategies for symptom relief but also improves communication about prognosis and goals of care, as well as the support given to patients and their families in all their dimensions (physical, psychosocial, and spiritual dimensions) (Kaasa, Hjermstad, & Loge, 2006; Quest, Marco, & Derse, 2009). In the United Kingdom, the concept of palliative care is now embedded in national guidelines for PD such as the NICE guidelines.

6.2 Holistic Approach vs Symptomatic Approach

The idea that palliative care seeks to not only relieve of patient suffering in the final stages of disease but also improves the quality of life along all the course of the illness, widens the field of palliative care intervention. The palliative care approach is not confined to pain control but also deals with all the physical, psychological, and spiritual problems that worsen quality of life during the course of the disease (Provinciali et al., 2016). However, the National Institute of Health in the United States has highlighted that few publications reflect the growing needs of patients (Sleeman & Murtagh,

2014). Even in the context of symptomatic control research, important gaps in clinical evidence need to be addressed (Johnston & Abraham, 1995; Kelley & Morrison, 2015). In two systematic reviews, Albers et al. (2012) and Hui et al. (2011) pointed to the imbalance between pharmacological interventions and other interventions not related with symptom control, which represented 5% or less of the total RCTs in palliative care.

6.3 Palliative Care vs Oncology Care

Evidence shows that palliative care is still dominated by oncology (Bouça-Machado et al., 2017). If at first this looks normal due to the initial focus of palliative care on patients dying from cancer, the difference between the percentage of studies and access of patients to palliative care service in oncology and other specialties seems to show that we are now beginning to get used to the idea of palliative care in cancer, but this is far from being the case in other pathologies, specifically in neurologic diseases, and particularly when these are gradually progressive disorders with insidiously growing disability like PD (Bouça-Machado et al., 2017).

7. CONCEPT OF PALLIATIVE CARE IN NEURODEGENERATIVE DISEASES

There is growing awareness of the potential benefit of palliative care interventions, not only in oncological diseases, but also in many of the most frequent neurological diseases that are chronic, where no disease-modifying treatments are available, and that impair the patient's autonomy (Provinciali et al., 2016; van Vliet et al., 2016). Over 25% of people with long-term neurological conditions need help with activities of daily living and, in the United Kingdom, nearly one million informal carers are caring for someone with a neurological condition (Bernard, Aspinal, Gridley, & Parker, 2008; Fitzpatrick et al., 2010). Patients with a life-limiting long-term neurologic illness experience clusters of motor and nonmotor symptoms, interspersed with cognitive impairment, behavioral issues, and communication problems, which represent a significant burden to both patients and caregivers (Boersma et al., 2014; van Vliet et al., 2016). For example, on average, PD patients experience more than 10 different symptoms, and they regard the disease as something intrinsic to their person, which is similar to cancer patients, but the gradual progression of PD clearly differs from the sharp decline seen in many patients with cancer. PD patients also differ from cancer patients' perspective who see "the cancer" as something outside of themselves (Boersma et al., 2014; van Vliet et al., 2016). Furthermore, the physical and cognitive disabilities usually contribute to the patient feeling "useless" or a "burden," while the caregiver feels distressed and has a reduced quality of life, which may contribute to higher rates of depression and demoralization for both. In the case of demented patients (which is common in advanced stages of PD), caregivers also have to deal with unique psychological issues compared with cancer caregivers (e.g., losing parts of their spouse 1 day at a time, delusions of infidelity), and due to this their risk of burnout or complicated bereavement is higher (Boersma et al., 2014).

In the United Kingdom, the National Service Framework for patients with long-term neurological conditions has recommended the involvement of specialist palliative care early in the disease trajectory, and the Accreditation Council for Graduate Medical Education requires neurology residents to receive instruction in end-of-life care and palliative care. However, the traditional models of palliative care may not be the most appropriate, whereby the definition and implementation of palliative care and procedures in neurology should take into account the specific features of these conditions (Boersma et al., 2014; Provinciali et al., 2016; Saleem et al., 2013; van Vliet et al., 2016). First, there are tremendous challenges related to the long-term nature of the symptoms, their gradual development, the high variability of prognosis in the different conditions, and the difficulty in identifying the end stage of the disease (Higginson et al., 2012; Provinciali et al., 2016). Second, there is the heterogeneity and complexity of patient populations, the distinctiveness of the clinical course, and the impact of disability. Finally, the variability and peculiarity of symptoms that characterizes each condition, which significantly affect the quality of life of the patients right from the early stages of the disease and require a specific expertise in the palliative approach (Provinciali et al., 2016). Within this conceptual framework of palliative care, these differences from other diseases imply differences in symptom profile (which are beyond the treatment of pain and feeding problems), psychosocial and spiritual issues (like the difficulty in elaborating an advanced care plan due to difficulties in predicting time and features of disease evolution), and in caregiver needs. In this way, a selective approach, different goals and procedures for the implementation and different timing of intervention is indispensable (Boersma et al., 2014; Provinciali et al., 2016).

van Vliet et al. (2016) have reviewed of how integrated neurology and palliative care services are. Specifically, they report that multiple sclerosis (MS) and Parkinsonian patients seem to be the groups that have contact with a specialist palliative care. Also, the identified variations in the use of palliative care services, not only between sites but also between diseases, and noted that palliative care is related more with the trajectory of the disease than its prevalence. The authors also report improvement of PD patients' symptoms over 3 months in one Canadian palliative care service and improvements in patients' symptoms, caregiver burden, and costs after a 6-week intervention as a result of an integrated model in the United Kingdom for advanced MS in which palliative care services and neurology worked closely together (van Vliet et al., 2016).

Despite differences between disease groups, neurology patients often have limited access to palliative care services (Boersma et al., 2014; van Vliet et al., 2016). Research suggests that patients are referred to hospices too infrequently or too late (or not at all), that between 63% and 82% of all patients who passed away would have benefited from palliative care involvement, and that neurologic patients with palliative care needs are regularly hospitalized at the end-of-life, and die there (Boersma et al., 2014; van Vliet et al., 2016). There are several potential barriers preventing neurologists from appropriately referring patients to specialized palliative care services and hospices: unpredictable prognosis for specific illnesses without a clear referral cut-off point, fear of diminishing hope in patients, physicians' lack of fundamental palliative care skills due to a lack of disease-specific knowledge, palliative care experts' reluctance to take on care for noncancer patients, and, lastly, patients' reluctance due to misconception of palliative care as end-of-life care (Boersma et al., 2014; van Vliet et al., 2016).

As mentioned earlier, to accomplish an efficient palliative approach to neurological diseases, not only it is necessary for palliative care to adapt specific skills and knowledge to the particularities of these diseases, but it is also necessary that the different services collaborate by working as a multidisciplinary team where a neurologist trained in palliative care plays a central role in identifying patients' needs (Provinciali et al., 2016).

8. PALLIATIVE CARE AS PART OF THERAPEUTIC INTERVENTIONS IN PD

8.1 Concept

The new model of palliative care, termed "simultaneous care," is no longer restricted to the final stage of disease, to only includes all patients with a disabling and life-limiting disease, but instead focuses on the patient's quality of life along the entire course of disease. It is mandatory to accomplish an integration of palliative care with traditional care, in this case neurological care (Boersma et al., 2014).

Although PD might not be fatal by itself, it leads to deterioration and progression of multiple complex motor and nonmotor symptoms, with tremendous consequences for healthcare, functionality, quality of life, and personal costs that characterize the advanced PD state (Saleem et al., 2013; van Vliet et al., 2016). Palliative care potentially has an important role, and an early palliative approach seems to be largely recommended to face the appearance of symptoms leading to serious disability and loss of autonomy, such as reduced motor activity and postural impairment or autonomic disorders (Saleem et al., 2013). Unlike other progressive diseases, these symptoms appear early in the disease in PD, and worsen further in advanced stages, with the addition of motor complications and numerous nonmotor symptoms. PD patients obtain a mean score of 14 on the Palliative Outcome Scale (POS), suggesting moderate palliative care needs, with a mean of 11 physical symptoms on the POS-PD (Saleem et al., 2013). The complexity of pharmacological therapeutic intervention in PD is also related, not only with the absence of any curative or disease-modifying treatment but also because as the disease progresses, treatment targeted to one specific symptom interferes with other aspects. For example, levodopa therapy over time leads to the development of dyskinesias, or the treatment of dopa-induced psychosis (with neuroleptics) may worsen motor skills. In this way the management of Parkinsonism remains largely palliative and has to integrate pharmacological and nonpharmacological interventions (Saleem et al., 2013).

The needs of PD patients are not always identified or satisfied. Researchers have highlighted the carers perceptions of unmanaged symptoms and unmet palliative and end-of-life care provision to people with PD (Boersma et al., 2014; Saleem et al., 2013). One study with a sample of 125,242 patients who died with a diagnosis of PD reported that only 0.6% of patients used hospice services, that 43% died in hospital with only 9.7% of PD patients dying in their home, compared with 17% of the general elderly population (Boersma et al., 2014; Sleeman et al., 2013). The misconception of palliative care as cancer care could mean that carers never access the appropriate support services needed along the PD trajectory, and that their own health suffers unnecessarily as a consequence (Saleem et al., 2013). Palliative care as part of a therapeutic intervention has a threefold aim, similar to the tested approach used in the oncological field: improving health conditions through the assessment and the treatment of symptoms;

strengthening the assistance intended to enhance the patient's and the caregiver's quality of life; and searching for the suitability and efficiency of assistance actions (Provinciali et al., 2016; Saleem et al., 2013).

8.2 Models of Palliative Care Delivery in PD

Palliative care describes an approach delivered in conjunction with standard care that is not only focused on the preservation of function and prolongation of life. It also draws attention to the relief of suffering and places importance on planning for decline and death as an expected and natural outcome rather than as a failure of medical treatment, so that patients benefit from the time of diagnosis, and as they need it throughout the course of illness (Boersma et al., 2014; Richfield et al., 2013). This approach requires monitoring and recognition of unmet palliative care needs, identification of triggers for palliative care referral, and close collaboration between neurological and palliative care services. If palliative care starts as early as possible, general palliative care services and hospices, which are still more devoted to "end-of-life" care, may only be partly appropriate, as they may not be able to provide the specific complexities of treatment that PD patients require, including motor and nonmotor symptoms (Aarsland, Larsen, Tandberg, & Laake, 2000; Higginson et al., 2012).

The management of the chronic–palliative interface in PD may include both outpatient and inpatient care, based on clearly defined criteria, and also comprises a multidisciplinary team in which palliative care specialists may be incorporated. However, the best format for palliative care services for PD patients needs to be defined (Giles & Miyasaki, 2009; Hasson et al., 2010). Nowadays, ideal models of palliative care delivery in PD comprise of: hospice care (palliative care focused specifically on end of life care), inpatient or outpatient palliative care, and home palliative care delivered by a palliative care nurse (Boersma et al., 2014; Richfield et al., 2013). Specialized community-based professional healthcare networks for PD—such as the Dutch ParkinsonNet (Bloem & Munneke, 2014)—should not only include a range of nonpharmaological interventions (such as physiotherapy or occupational therapy) but also palliative care specialists (or nonpalliative care professionals with at least sufficient understanding and basic knowledge of palliative care issues). Whatever the approach, an initial thorough evaluation should be performed, that should include a close dialogue with patients and families so that the patient's wishes are understood with regards to the most disturbing symptoms and ultimately where they wish to spend the time after losing autonomy (Snell, Pennington, Lee, & Walker, 2009). Of note, although nonmotor symptoms are known to contribute to health-related quality of life (HRQoL) in PD patients, they are often not actively reported to healthcare professionals and hence the use of validated scales and questionnaires and the caregiver's cooperation is essential in recognizing the patient's full needs (Chaudhuri et al., 2010; Goy, Carter, & Ganzini, 2007; Higginson et al., 2012).

In countries where they are implemented, despite restricting eligible access criteria (the hospice guidelines for neurologic disorders in the United States (Boersma et al., 2014) are summarized in Table 1), hospice care is associated with a high overall quality of satisfaction. In the last decade, hospice community-based programs have been developed, with high potential of reducing costs and improving quality of care for those patients who were not eligible for hospice care (Boersma et al., 2014; Kelley & Morrison, 2015). Using multidisciplinary palliative care teams, these programs intend to establish clear goals of care, enhance symptom management and caregiver support in the home setting, coordinate care, and provide an extra layer of support to treating physicians (Kelley & Morrison, 2015).

Nonhospice palliative care services are frequently provided in an acute care hospital setting, either as through an interdisciplinary consultation team or inpatient units (Kelley & Morrison, 2015). In addition to these traditional models, in some countries new service-delivery models include dedicated ICU teams and comanagement, whereby a palliative care specialist joins an existing specialty team and initiates automatic palliative care referrals (Kelley & Morrison, 2015). In North America, as a consequence of the Advanced Certification for Palliative Care Programs established in 2011 by the Joint Commission, palliative care programs have grown by more than 150%, such that almost 90% of hospitals with 300 beds or more, and two-thirds of hospitals with 50 beds or more, now have palliative care programs (Kelley & Morrison, 2015).

With regards to nursing homes, there are currently three models for delivering palliative care (Kelley & Morrison, 2015). The most established model is hospice care, usually through a contract system with a hospice services agency. In the United States, the percentage of people in nursing homes who received hospice services before they died increased from 14% in 1999 to 33% in 2006 and this model is associated with lower rates of invasive therapies and hospitalizations, improvement of symptom

Table 1 Hospice Guidelines for Neurologic Disorders

Dementia	1. Stage 7C or higher on the FAST scale
	2. One or more of the following in the past year: aspiration pneumonia, pyelonephritis, septicemia, stage 3 or 4 pressure ulcers, recurrent fevers, other conditions suggesting limited prognosis, or inability to maintain sufficient fluid/caloric intake in past 6 months (10% weight loss or albumin <2.5 g/dL)
Stroke or coma	1. Palliative Performance Scale score ≤40%
	2. Poor nutritional status with inability to maintain sufficient fluid/caloric intake (10% weight loss in 6 months, 7.5% weight loss in 3 months, serum albumin <2.5 g/dL, or pulmonary aspiration resistant to speech therapy interventions)
Other neurologic disease including ALS, PD, MD, MG, or MS	1. Critically impaired breathing including dyspnea at rest, vital capacity <30%, O_2 need at rest, AND refusal of artificial ventilation, OR
	2. Rapid disease progression (to bed-bound status, unintelligible speech, need for pureed diet, and/or major assistance needed for ADLs) with either:
	A. Critical nutrition impairment in the prior year (inability to maintain sufficient fluid/caloric intake, continuing weight loss, dehydration, AND refusal of artificial feeding methods) OR
	B. Life-threatening complications in the prior year (recurrent aspiration pneumonia, pyelonephritis, sepsis, recurrent fever, OR stage 3 or 4 pressure ulcers)
Generic criteria	1. Terminal condition (can be multiple conditions) AND
	2. Rapid decline over past 3–6 months as evidenced by progression of disease signs, symptoms and test results, decline in PPS ≤ 40%, and involuntary weight loss >10%, and/or albumin <2.5 g/dL

Abbreviations: *ADL*, 5 activities of daily living; *ALS*, 5 amyotrophic lateral sclerosis; *FAST*, 5 Functional Assessment Staging Test; *MD*, 5 muscular dystro- phy; *MG*, 5 myasthenia gravis; *MS*, 5 multiple sclerosis; *PD*, 5 Parkinson disease; *PPS*, 5 Palliative Performance Scale.

management, and higher family satisfaction with care (Kelley & Morrison, 2015). Another model is palliative care consultation, in which an external palliative care physician or nurse practitioner provides recommendations to the nursing home clinicians. Finally, some nursing homes have developed internal palliative care teams or specialized units, which are focused primarily on residents with advanced dementia (Kelley & Morrison, 2015).

An outpatient regimen is often more suitable for PD patients who are still cared for at home. In this regard, it is starting to be recognized that the development of PD clinics are needed to provide the complexity of care needed in advanced-stage PD, conducted on an outpatient basis (Ghoche, 2012; Miyasaki et al., 2012). The multidisciplinary professional team in this setting would include a Movement Disorders Specialist, a palliative care physician or geriatrician, a physiotherapist, and palliative care nurses. This format would link the neurologist's expertise in managing neurological symptoms and the specialized palliative care approach to nonneurological symptoms, such as pain (Politis et al., 2010). Close monitoring by PD clinics could potentially result in a higher prevalence of advanced-PD patients living at home and would anticipate the late complications of the disease and also predict the need to shift to a more intensive modality of care, including short periods of admission in order to adjust medications or permanent care (Ghoche, 2012; Miyasaki et al., 2012). This type of outpatient regimen is already underway in leading centers, and encompasses some relevant features such as addressing the home situation and the assessment of symptom burden (Ghoche, 2012; Miyasaki et al., 2012).

In-patient palliative care is intended for patients who need specialized care or when caregivers are no longer able to attend to their needs (Lökk, 2011). A 2011 report on the outcomes of the first PD permanent care unit showed promising results, but the follow-up period was short (Lökk, 2011). The unit consisted of 30 single rooms, common areas for meals and training facilities as well as the possibility for patients to engage in daily living tasks. At admission, a multidisciplinary care plan was elaborated for each patient, not only regarding their medical care but also regarding social, emotional, cultural, and spiritual needs. Regular visits with a movement disorders specialist, geriatrician, physiotherapist, and occupational therapist were provided, and the care plan continuously reviewed. Family members actively participated in the planning of patient care. The objectives of this unit corresponded with palliative care aims, namely the preservation of the patient's quality of life and functionality, as well as alleviating their symptoms (Lökk, 2011).

8.3 Time to Referral to Specialist Palliative Care Services

Exactly how and when patients are referred and the exact intervention format is unclear (van Vliet et al., 2016). Referral varies considerably between countries. For instance, the United States have their own guidelines (Table 1), while many Canadian provinces use the Palliative Performance Scale. One criterion for admission to a hospice has been a life expectancy of 6 months or less, but this is not universal, and in the United Kingdom, a prognosis-based system is used for consideration of palliative care, with professionals encouraged to ask "would I be surprised if this patient died in the next 12 months" (Boersma et al., 2014; Miyasaki & Kluger, 2015; Richfield et al., 2013). The American Stroke Association has recently endorsed an integrated approach between neurology and palliative care services for stroke patients, where palliative care is provided in the neurologic field based on need rather than on prognosis or disease stage. According to this method, palliative care can be used as needed and neurologists are taught and expected to provide primary palliative care in less complex situations (van Vliet et al., 2016).

In general, it seems neither feasible nor desirable that palliative care be the sole concern of palliative care or that palliative care take over neurological care (Richfield et al., 2013; van Vliet et al., 2016). The majority of palliative care needs could be resolved through a palliative approach existing within neurological services. The function of specialized palliative care should be to train and support neurological services and to deal with more complex situations (Richfield et al., 2013). In a 1996 review (Boersma et al., 2014), the American Academy of Neurology Ethics and Humanities Subcommittee stated: "Many patients with neurologic disease die after long illnesses during which a neurologist acts as the principal or consulting physician. Therefore, it is imperative that neurologists understand, and learn to apply, the principles of palliative medicine." The Irish Palliative Care in Parkinson's Disease (2016) outlines three levels of palliative care provision, referring to the expertise of the staff providing the service (Table 2).

The prognosis of neurologic diseases is not always clear and the referral for specialized palliative care is frequently linked with the concern of having a depressive and demotivating effect on the patients and their families and the risk of losing the continuity of health professionals, since the integration between neurology and the specialized palliative care team is not an established reality in the majority of countries (Provinciali et al., 2016).

Table 2 Levels of Palliative Care Specialization

Level 1	Palliative care approach	All health care professionals should appropriately apply palliative care principles
Level 2	General Palliative Care	At an intermediate level, a proportion of patients and families will benefit from the expertise of health care professionals who, although not engaged full-time in palliative care, have had some additional training and experience in palliative care
Level 3	Specialist Palliative Care	Specialist palliative care services are those services whose core activity is limited to the provision of palliative care

BOX 1 Red Flags for Unmet Palliative Care Need that Should "Trigger" SPC Referral

Swallowing problems
Recurrent infections
Marked decline in physical function
First aspiration pneumonia
Cognitive difficulties
Weight loss
Significant complex symptoms

Furthermore, there is a lack of understanding by those responsible for such referrals that palliative care may be appropriate earlier in the course of the disease for incurable patients without cancer (Saleem et al., 2013). The identification of red flags for unmet palliative care need should "trigger" specialized palliative care referral (Box 1) and could aid the implementation of the aforementioned integrated model of care. These red flags include clinical features associated with causes of death or those that consistently herald the terminal phase of disease (Richfield et al., 2013).

8.4 Palliative Care Multidisciplinary Team in PD Management

Given the chronic progressive course of PD, the burden and the wide variety of symptoms, a multidisciplinary team including a neurologist, an specialized palliative care physician, a nurse, a psychiatrist, a physiotherapist, a speech therapist, an occupational therapist, a social worker, a psychologist, a dietician, family caregivers, and community resources are required to ensure successful management of the disease and improve the quality of life of patients (Fereshtehnejad, 2016; Miyasaki & Kluger, 2015).

Given the difficulty of PD assessment, the caregiver is recognized as a key member of the multidisciplinary team, and his/her input is invaluable and necessary to understanding the complex and individual experience of the patient (Miyasaki & Kluger, 2015).

Palliative care can particular provide expertise in managing some aspects of the disease for patients and caregivers, for example, symptoms that do not respond to traditional pharmacological therapies, depression, social withdrawal, existential distress, all of which have a high impact on a patient's quality of life (Provinciali et al., 2016; Saleem et al., 2013).

Communication is one of the milestones of palliative care practice and one of the most common complaints patients make about health professionals (Boersma et al., 2016; Fox et al., 2016). Nowadays, there are a number of tools that physicians can use to communicate bad news, such as SPIKES (Setting up the interview, assessing patient's Perception, obtaining patient's Invitation, giving Knowledge, address Emotions, Strategy and Summary) or the Vital Talk Web. Evidence suggests that physicians when disclosing the diagnosis focus their full attention on the patient, use open-ended questions and assess emotions and feelings to ascertain what is known about the diagnosis and how much the patient wants to know about potentially distressing information, such as prognosis (Boersma et al., 2014). It is vital that during the diagnostic disclosure meeting a follow-up is scheduled so that the patient has a chance to process the information and can raise more specific questions. In order to support the patient and minimize feelings of abandonment, physicians may try to understand important life goals, patient and caregiver fears, and discuss with both the overall goals of care (Boersma et al., 2014).

Contrary to the common clinical perception, patients want to discuss advanced directives and often cite their expectation for physicians to initiate this discussion when asked about barriers to planning for the future. Research shows that patients who discuss end-of-life issues with their doctors report greater satisfaction with their care. Advance care planning includes topics such as medical durable power of attorney, financial power of attorney, and cardiopulmonary resuscitation directives. All neurologists should have knowledge and training about discussing advance care planning with their patients, while they are cognitively able.

To instruct and provide information resources to patients and caregivers is of the utmost importance. They should have knowledge about both motor and nonmotor features of PD, course of progression, treatment approaches and complications, and the specific physical and emotional needs of PD patients. This would be facilitated if they know what to expect in the course of disease, and would allow the home environment to be better prepared to encounter difficulties resulting from the different symptoms that may manifest, and thereby likely reduce the use of emergency room services (Fereshtehnejad, 2016; Miyasaki & Kluger, 2015). For example, the awareness that cognitive function and clarity can be maximized, but frequently at the expense of motor function, allows patients to make fully informed choices (Miyasaki & Kluger, 2015).

Nonmotor symptoms are functionally among the most limiting for patients over time, and affect caregiver burden and overall quality of life more than motor symptoms (Boersma et al., 2014). These demand a careful examination by the neurologist, since proper management depends on their recognition, and also since patients often do not mention them unless when asked (Table 3). Regarding those incapacitating symptoms that are untreatable, neurologists should still closely follow the patient as additional support or advance care planning may be required (Boersma et al., 2014). Some studies show that dopaminergic medication should be continued at the end of life in cases where it may help reduce symptom load. It has been suggested that L-dopa dose be increased in those with motor complications, and for whom tremor or rigidity are the most troublesome motor symptoms (Fabbri et al., 2016; Walker et al., 2014). It is known that an acute benefit with L-dopa may not translate into long-term improvement, and drowsiness may not occur if L-dopa dose is increased slowly. However, completely stopping L-dopa therapy could slowly and severely aggravate some motor symptoms among late-stage PD patients (Fabbri et al., 2016). The use of alternative methods of drug administration, like soluble medication (e.g., dispersible madopar), apomorphine subcutaneous injections, or skin patches (e.g., rotigotine) should be considered particularly as for some patients, nonoral routes may be more effective (Walker et al., 2014).

Palliative care transcends the historical patient-physician dyad, focusing on the family as the unit of care, addressing caregiver strain, and offering supportive services to family members such as respite care and counseling (Boersma et al., 2014). Caregivers' quality of life reflects on patients' quality of life. Their support from neurologists begins by adequately assessing their needs, and this support is usually received with appreciation and may relieve

Table 3 Management Strategies to Address Key Motor and Nonmotor Symptoms

Key Symptoms	Assessments	Interventions	Therapy	Others
Pain	Kings PD Pain Scale PAINAD	Analgesia: Paracetamol Opiates Oxycodone-Naloxone (PANDA study)	Range of motion exercises and posture adjustments TENS and Manual therapy Hot and cold therapy Peripheral desensitization techniques	Botulinum toxin
Severe rigidity	POS ESAS—PD	Trial of rotigotine or apomorphine injections Liquid levodopa	Range of motion exercises Manual therapy Hot therapy	Botulinum toxin to avoid contractures
Constipation	NMSQuest NMSS ESAS—PD POS	Polyethylene glycol 1–2 capsules/day Senokot 1–4 tablets each day Lactulose	Dietary modification and use of whole grains with fibers and adequate hydration	
Sleep dysfunction	PDSS PSQI ESS	Opiates may help insomnia and pain Benzodiazepines for onset insomnia Trial of modafinil for severe EDS	Pain control	
Psychiatric disorders	ESAS—PD QUIP	Clozapine/quetiapine Reduce dopaminergic therapy	Treat underlying infection Often aspiration pneumonia	
Anxiety. Depression	BDI ESAS—PD NMSQuest	Antidepressant use	Relaxation techniques Counseling	
Swallowing problems	ESAS—PD NMSQuest Swallowing Disturbance questionnaire	Assess if off period related. If yes then trial of nonoral dopaminergic agents (rotigotine, apomporphine could be considered)	Referral to speech and language therapy Dietary modification PEG tube if required	

caregiver concerns that their only role in the patient's illness is a supportive one (Boersma et al., 2014). Caregiver assessments should include questions relating to their ability to provide adequate care and also, self-care. Assistance with providing care may include home safety evaluations, information regarding the illness and therapeutic interventions, knowing who to contact to handle complications or in case of an emergency, and to assess the need of respite or home health services. This simple approach provides an important validation of the caregiver and reduces the risk of burnout (Boersma et al., 2014).

Nowadays, e-health technology has revolutionized clinical practice by providing opportunities for improvement in quality and efficiency of care, engagement of individuals in clinical decision-making, and empowering patients' to adopt healthy behaviors, all of which could be implemented in the field of PD (Boersma et al., 2014). Personalized quantification and measurement of different features of PD, together with personalized evaluation and analysis of the most important drivers of quality of life, are the future keys for implementation of the most efficient personalized strategy to maintain quality of life in each individual with PD (Boersma et al., 2014).

8.5 New Initiatives

The OPTCARE Neuro trial (Gao et al., 2016) led by Professor Irene Higginson from London, United Kingdom, is currently the world's largest palliative care study in people with long-term neurologic conditions including PD. It recruited both patients ($N=356$) with and without capacity, as well as their carers (maximum $N=356$). This randomized, double-blind, multicenter study aims to provide key evidence on the shorter term effectiveness of Short-term Integrated Palliative Care Services which is delivered by a multidiscipline palliative care team and will be compared to standard care.

In the United States, through the initiative of the Parkinson's Disease Foundation, a first international meeting on Palliative Care and PD was held and in 2015, the Patient Centered Outcomes Research Institute funded the first comparative effectiveness trial of outpatient palliative care for PD. This novel approach addresses palliative care as a strategy to care for PD patients and their families seeking to reduce suffering through a range of spiritual, psychosocial, and medical support which begins at the time of diagnosis and continues through end-of-life care and bereavement (Boersma et al., 2014).

In the Netherlands, the ParkinsonSupport trial has just been initiated to improve knowledge about palliative care needs in PD. Specifically, this study will perform a mixed methods study to evaluate the experiences of patients (bereaved), family caregivers, and palliative care professionals. Phase 1 will retrospectively explore the views of caregivers and professionals by conducting individual interviews and focus group interviews. Phase 2 involves a prospective follow-up of PD patients and their family caregiver for up to 12 months.

The International Parkinson's and Movement Disorder Society has also set up a new initiative with a task force on palliative care in PD. The committee will address unmet needs in palliative care for PD and address its implementation at a global level.

9. ADDRESSING SYMPTOM BURDEN IN ADVANCED-PD: OUTCOMES AND MEASURES

Current concepts for palliative care in PD address behavioral and cognitive decline with pharmacologic manipulation, and are assessed using the UPDRS (Miyasaki et al., 2012). The complexity of PD symptoms is better accounted for with the use of multidimensional constructs, such as HRQoL scales that are able to provide information about the effect of an intervention from the patient perspective (Fereshtehnejad, 2016; Politis et al., 2010; Stowe et al., 2011). Furthermore, patient-reported outcome measurement also plays a significant role in palliative care, namely in the assessment of patients, evaluation of the effectiveness of interventions, or implementation of outcome measures in clinical practice (Bausewein, Le Grice, Simon, & Higginson, 2011). Therefore, the primary outcome of palliative care in PD should rely on improved HRQoL measures, emphasizing the needs of patients and families (Agar & Luckett, 2012; Stowe et al., 2011). However, studies focusing on HRQoL measures in advanced-PD are still lacking (Stowe et al., 2011).

Several HRQoL scales have been used in PD patients to assess objective functioning and subjective perception of different domains, such as physical, psychological, social well-being, and satisfaction related to health (Martinez-Martin, Rodriguez-Blazquez, Kurtis, Chaudhuri, & NMSS Validation Group, 2011). Preferably, these instruments are sensitive to change, are helpful in ascertaining the outcome of clinical interventions, and may show association with UPDRS and Hoehn and Yahr scores (Martinez-Martin, Rodriguez-Blazquez, et al., 2011).

A recent Movement Disorder Society Task Force reviewed the psychometric properties of these scales. Four generic scales, the EuroQoL (EQ5-D),

Nottingham Health Profile (NHP), Medical Outcomes Study—Short Form (SF-36), and Sickness Impact Profile (SIP); and five specific scales, the 39-item Parkinson's Disease Questionnaire (PDQ-39), Parkinson's Disease Questionnaire Short Form (PDQ-8), Parkinson's Disease Quality of Life Questionnaire (PDQL), Parkinson's Impact Scale (PIMS), and Scales for Outcomes in Parkinson Disease—Psychosocial (SCOPA-PS) reached the level of "recommended" (Martinez-Martin, Jeukens-Visser, et al., 2011).

Other widely used scales, such as the NMS questionnaire (NMSQuest, self-completed) or the POS can be useful to highlight and flag nonmotor problems, which are known to contribute to HRQoL in PD patients (Chaudhuri, Odin, Antonini, & Martinez-Martin, 2011; Chrischilles et al., 2002; Martinez-Martin, Rodriguez-Blazquez, et al., 2011; Miyasaki et al., 2012; Saleem et al., 2013). Miyasaki et al. (2012) adapted the most emblematic scale in palliative care research, The Edmonton Symptom Assessment Scale (ESAS), to address PD-specific symptoms and enable comparison with other palliative populations (Miyasaki et al., 2012). ESAS was designed as a 10-point scale for evaluation of psychological and physical domains of palliative care patients. It is a brief, useful, bedside tool and includes domains reflecting the holistic approach including tiredness and sense of well-being in addition to the traditional symptoms of pain, nausea, and shortness of breath. In order to measure PD symptoms, items related to constipation, difficulty swallowing, stiffness, and confusion were added to the scale and it was named as The Edmonton Symptom Assessment Scale-Parkinson Disease (ESAS-PD) (Miyasaki et al., 2012). Caregiver stress and burden can be addressed using the Zarit caregiver burden tool (Gort et al., 2007).

A generic tool for palliative care outcomes in people with LTNC has also been validated and is known as the IPOS Neuro-S8 (Gao et al., 2016). This is an eight-item scale for addressing the symptom burden at a palliative stage and can be applied to PD.

10. IMPLICATION FOR CLINICAL PRACTICE AND FOR RESEARCH

Some healthcare professionals see palliative care as "giving up on patients" or "no care"; however, research suggest that early palliative care interventions may positively affect both quality of life and survival. Notably, palliative care is appropriate at any age and at any stage in a serious illness, and can be provided together with symptomatic treatment (Boersma et al., 2014). There is a substantial and growing need for neurologists to increase their knowledge and apply the principles of palliative medicine to the care of patients with progressive, chronic illnesses such as PD (Boersma et al., 2014). They should also have training to improve communication skills, in particular in diagnostic disclosures, and in communicating bad news or discussing advanced care plans (Boersma et al., 2016, 2014; Fox et al., 2016). A patient survey from 2014 suggests that at least 50% of patients with PD want to discuss advanced care documents with their physician early in the disease course (Boersma et al., 2016, 2014; Fox et al., 2016). Regarding symptom management, multiple studies show that neurologists frequently fail to adequately assess and treat many nonmotor symptoms associated with quality of life, including depression, fatigue, pain, and sleep (Boersma et al., 2014).

Future research should develop brief clinical tools to aid clinicians with palliative care needs in daily practice and develop a more robust evidence base for managing terminal symptoms (Richfield et al., 2013).

The ideal timing for the implementation of palliative care in PD should also be better defined. Well-defined criteria are essential to take advantage of the different settings of care, and to promote a smooth transition between these settings, when the patient eventually progresses to later disease stages (Lanoix, 2009). Ideally, the same PD clinic should incorporate both modalities of care, permitting a less abrupt transition between settings (Lanoix, 2009).

Currently, there are no specific recommendations regarding the use of HRQoL scales in palliative care and PD. We suggest that a combination of both generic and specific instruments should be incorporated in palliative care research in PD. These instruments can provide valuable information about the effects of an intervention and thus, it would be important to include HRQoL endpoints in future clinical trials, even as the primary outcome measure (Martinez-Martin, Jeukens-Visser, et al., 2011). The comparison between the ESAS-PD scale, the POS or other palliative care scales and the recommended generic and specific scales applied to PD, is needed.

Moreover, the use of utility measures, such as the EQ-5D, which can be used for economic analysis, would also provide relevant information regarding health-related costs. This will probably influence the availability of adequate palliative services in PD. At first glance, PD units may look expensive, but they may be a way of decreasing acute complications in PD patients, such as infections and the consequences of falls, with positive implications on costs (Lökk, 2011; Martinez-Martin, Jeukens-Visser, et al., 2011).

11. CONCLUSION

Palliative care is gradually entering the lexicon of chronic disorders, and shedding its previously negative outlook. The prolonged timescales of neurological disorders, such as PD, mean that there is a broader demand for palliative medicine. The modern palliative care outlook of incorporating a continuity of care, effective management of the chronic-palliative interface, and a multidisciplinary network of professionals embedded in specialized clinics with involvement of caregivers in the process of care will contribute to palliative care becoming commonplace in the treatment of PD patients. Although promising, further research on the effectiveness of palliative care in PD is still required.

REFERENCES

Aarsland, D., Larsen, J. P., Tandberg, E., & Laake, K. (2000). Predictors of nursing home placement in Parkinson's disease: A population-based, prospective study. *Journal of the American Geriatrics Society*, *48*(8), 938–942. http://doi.org/10.1111/j.1532-5415.2000.tb06891.x.

Abernethy, A. P., Aziz, N. M., Basch, E., Bull, J., Cleeland, C. S., Currow, D. C., … Kutner, J. S. (2010). A strategy to advance the evidence base in palliative medicine: Formation of a palliative care research cooperative group. *Journal of Palliative Medicine*, *13*(12), 1407–1413. http://doi.org/10.1089/jpm.2010.0261.

Agar, M., & Luckett, T. (2012). Outcome measures for palliative care research. *Current Opinion in Supportive and Palliative Care*, *6*(4), 500–507. http://doi.org/10.1097/SPC.0b013e32835a66ca.

Albers, G., Harding, R., Pasman, H. R. W., Onwuteaka-Philipsen, B. D., Hall, S., Toscani, F., … Deliens, L. (2012). What is the methodological rigour of palliative care research in long-term care facilities in Europe? A systematic review. *Palliative Medicine*, *26*(5), 722–733. http://doi.org/10.1177/0269216311412232.

Aoun, S. M., & Nekolaichuk, C. (2014). Improving the evidence base in palliative care to inform practice and policy: Thinking outside the box. *Journal of Pain and Symptom Management*, *48*(6), 1222–1235. http://doi.org/10.1016/j.jpainsymman.2014.01.007.

Bakitas, M. A., Lyons, K. D., Dixon, J., & Ahles, T. A. (2006). Palliative care program effectiveness research: Developing rigor in sampling design, conduct, and reporting. *Journal of Pain and Symptom Management*, *31*(3), 270–284. http://doi.org/10.1016/j.jpainsymman.2005.07.011.

Bausewein, C., Le Grice, C., Simon, S., & Higginson, I. (2011). The use of two common palliative outcome measures in clinical care and research: A systematic review of POS and STAS. *Palliative Medicine*, *25*(4), 304–313. http://doi.org/10.1177/0269216310395984.

Bernard, S., Aspinal, F., Gridley, K., & Parker, G. (2008). Integrated policy making in England for adults with long-term neurological conditions (LTNCs): Some preliminary findings from a scoping study. *International Journal of Integrated Care, 8*, e60.

Bloem, B. R., de Vries, N. M., & Ebersbach, G. (2015). Nonpharmacological treatments for patients with Parkinson's disease. *Movement Disorders, 30*(11), 1504–1520. http://doi.org/10.1002/mds.26363.

Bloem, B. R., & Munneke, M. (2014). Revolutionising management of chronic disease: The ParkinsonNet approach. *BMJ (Clinical Research Ed.), 348*, g1838.

Boersma, I., Jones, J., Carter, J., Bekelman, D., & Miyasaki, J. M. (2016). Parkinson disease patient's perspectives on palliative care needs: What are they telling us? *Neurology: Clinical Practice, 6*(3), 209–219. http://doi.org/10.1212/CPJ.0000000000000233.

Boersma, I., Miyasaki, J. M., Kutner, J. S., & Kluger, B. (2014). Palliative care and neurology: Time for a paradigm shift. *Neurology, 83*(6), 561–567.

Bouça-Machado, R., Rosário, M., Alarcão, J., Correia-Guedes, L., Abreu, D., & Ferreira, J. J. (2017). Clinical trials in palliative care: A systematic review of their methodological characteristics and of the quality of their reporting. *BMC Palliative Care, 16*(1), 10. http://doi.org/10.1186/s12904-016-0181-9.

Campion, E. W., Kelley, A. S., & Morrison, R. S. (2015). Palliative care for the seriously Ill. *New England Journal of Medicine, 373*(8), 747–755. http://doi.org/10.1056/NEJMra1404684.

Chaudhuri, K. R., Odin, P., Antonini, A., & Martinez-Martin, P. (2011). Parkinson's disease: The non-motor issues. *Parkinsonism & Related Disorders, 17*(10), 717–723. http://doi.org/10.1016/j.parkreldis.2011.02.018.

Chaudhuri, K. R., Prieto-Jurcynska, C., Naidu, Y., Mitra, T., Frades-Payo, B., Tluk, S., ... Martinez-Martin, P. (2010). The nondeclaration of nonmotor symptoms of Parkinson's disease to health care professionals: An international study using the nonmotor symptoms questionnaire. *Movement Disorders, 25*(6), 704–709. http://doi.org/10.1002/mds.22868.

Chrischilles, E. A. E., Rubenstein, L. L. M. L. L., Voelker, M. M. D., Wallace, R. B., Rodnitzky, R. L. R., Hadorn, D., ... Erbaugh, J. (2002). Linking clinical variables to health-related quality of life in Parkinson's disease. *Parkinsonism & Related Disorders, 8*(3), 199–209. http://doi.org/10.1016/S1353-8020(01)00044-X.

Coelho, M., Marti, M. J., Sampaio, C., Ferreira, J. J., Valldeoriola, F., Rosa, M. M., & Tolosa, E. (2014). Dementia and severity of parkinsonism determines the handicap of patients in late-stage Parkinson's disease: The Barcelona-Lisbon cohort. *European Journal of Neurology, 22*(2), 305–312. http://doi.org/10.1111/ene.12567.

Coelho, M., Marti, M. J., Tolosa, E., Ferreira, J. J., Valldeoriola, F., Rosa, M., & Sampaio, C. (2010). Late-stage Parkinson's disease: The Barcelona and Lisbon cohort. *Journal of Neurology, 257*(9), 1524–1532. http://doi.org/10.1007/s00415-010-5566-8.

Ekker, M. S., Janssen, S., Nonnekes, J., Bloem, B. R., & de Vries, N. M. (2016). Neurorehabilitation for Parkinson's disease: Future perspectives for behavioural adaptation. *Parkinsonism & Related Disorders, 22*, S73–S77. http://doi.org/10.1016/j.parkreldis.2015.08.031.

Ellgring, J. H. J., Seiler, S., Perleth, B., Gasser, T., & Oertel, W. (2010). An integrated approach for the neurological and psychological support of Parkinson patients. *New Trends in Clinical Neuropharmacology, 4*(4), 31–34.

Fabbri, M., Coelho, M., Abreu, D., Guedes, L. C., Rosa, M. M., Costa, N., ... Ferreira, J. J. (2016). Do patients with late-stage Parkinson's disease still respond to levodopa? *Parkinsonism and Related Disorders, 26*, 10–16. http://doi.org/10.1016/j.parkreldis.2016.02.021.

Fereshtehnejad, S.-M. (2016). Strategies to maintain quality of life among people with Parkinson's disease: What works? *Neurodegenerative Disease Management, 6*, 399–415. nmt-2016-0020. http://doi.org/10.2217/nmt-2016-0020.

Ferreira, J. J., Mestre, T., Guedes, L. C., Coelho, M., Rosa, M. M., Santos, A. T., … Rascol, O. (2016). Espresso coffee for the treatment of somnolence in Parkinson's disease: Results of n-of-1 trials. *Frontiers in Neurology*, 7, 27. http://doi.org/10.3389/fneur.2016.00027.

Fitzpatrick, R., Peters, M., Doll, H., Harris, R., Jenkinson, C., Playford, D., & Ziebland, S. (2010). *The needs and experiences of services by individuals with long-term progressive neurological conditions, and their carers. A benchmarking study*. Oxford, UK: Research initiative for Long Term Neurological Conditions.

Flemming, K., Adamson, J., & Atkin, K. (2008). Improving the effectiveness of interventions in palliative care: The potential role of qualitative research in enhancing evidence from randomized controlled trials. *Palliative Medicine*, *22*(2), 123–131. http://doi.org/10.1177/0269216307087319.

Fox, S., Cashell, A., Kernohan, W. G., Lynch, M., McGlade, C., O'Brien, T., … Timmons, S. (2016). Palliative care for Parkinson's disease: Patient and carer's perspectives explored through qualitative interview. *Palliative Medicine*, 1–8. Sep 28 [Epub ahead of print], PMID: 27683476. http://doi.org/10.1177/0269216316669922.

Gao, W., Crosby, V., Wilcock, A., Burman, R., Silber, E., Hepgul, N., … Higginson, I. J. (2016). Psychometric properties of a generic, patient-centred palliative care outcome measure of symptom burden for people with progressive long term neurological conditions. *PloS One*, *11*(10), e0165379. http://doi.org/10.1371/journal.pone.0165379.

Ghoche, R. (2012). The conceptual framework of palliative care applied to advanced Parkinson's disease. *Parkinsonism & Related Disorders*, *18*, S2–S5. http://doi.org/10.1016/j.parkreldis.2012.06.012.

Giles, S., & Miyasaki, J. (2009). Palliative stage Parkinson's disease: Patient and family experiences of health-care services. *Palliative Medicine*, *23*(2), 120–125. http://doi.org/10.1177/0269216308100773.

Gort, A. M., Mingot, M., Gomez, X., Soler, T., Torres, G., Sacristán, O., … Cabau, J. (2007). Use of the Zarit scale for assessing caregiver burden and collapse in caregiving at home in dementias. *International Journal of Geriatric Psychiatry*, *22*(10), 957–962. http://doi.org/10.1002/gps.1770.

Goy, E. R., Carter, J. H., & Ganzini, L. (2007). Parkinson disease at the end of life: Caregivers perspectives. *Neurology*, *69*(6), 611–612. http://doi.org/10.1212/01.wnl.0000266665.82754.61.

Group, The Irish Palliative Care in Parkinson's Disease. (2016). In S. Fox & S. Timmons (Eds.), *Palliative care in people with Parkinson's disease: Guidelines for professional healthcare workers on the assessment and management of palliative care needs in Parkinson's disease and related Parkinsonian syndromes*. Cork: University College Cork.

Hasson, F., Kernohan, W. G., McLaughlin, M., Waldron, M., McLaughlin, D., Chambers, H., & Cochrane, B. (2010). An exploration into the palliative and end-of-life experiences of carers of people with Parkinson's disease. *Palliative Medicine*, *24*(7), 731–736. http://dx.doi.org/10.1177/0269216310371414.

Higginson, I. J., Gao, W., Saleem, T. Z., Chaudhuri, K. R., Burman, R., McCrone, P., & Leigh, P. N. (2012). Symptoms and quality of life in late stage Parkinson syndromes: A longitudinal community study of predictive factors. *PloS One*, 7(11), 1–11. http://doi.org/10.1371/journal.pone.0046327.

Hui, D., Glitza, I., Chisholm, G., Yennu, S., & Bruera, E. (2013). Attrition rates, reasons, and predictive factors in supportive care and palliative oncology clinical trials. *Cancer*, *119*(5), 1098–1105. http://doi.org/10.1002/cncr.27854.

Hui, D., Parsons, H. A., Damani, S., Fulton, S., Liu, J., Evans, A., … Bruera, E. (2011). Quantity, design, and scope of the palliative oncology literature. *The Oncologist*, *16*(5), 694–703. http://doi.org/10.1634/theoncologist.2010-0397.

Jellinger, K. A. (2015). Neuropathobiology of non-motor symptoms in Parkinson disease. *Journal of Neural Transmission (Vienna, Austria: 1996)*, *122*(10), 1429–1440. http://doi.org/10.1007/s00702-015-1405-5.

Johnston, G., & Abraham, C. (1995). The WHO objectives for palliative care: To what extent are we achieving them? *Palliative Medicine*, *9*(2), 123–137.

Kaasa, S., Hjermstad, M. J., & Loge, J. H. (2006). Methodological and structural challenges in palliative care research: How have we fared in the last decades? *Palliative Medicine*, *20*(8), 727–734. http://doi.org/10.1177/0269216306072620.

Kalf, J. G., Munneke, M., van den Engel-Hoek, L., de Swart, B. J., Borm, G. F., Bloem, B. R., & Zwarts, M. J. (2011). Pathophysiology of diurnal drooling in Parkinson's disease. *Movement Disorders*, *26*(9), 1670–1676. http://doi.org/10.1002/mds.23720.

Kalia, L. V., & Lang, A. E. (2015). Parkinson's disease. *The Lancet*, *6736*(14), 1–17. http://doi.org/10.1016/S0140-6736(14)61393-3.

Kelley, A. S., & Morrison, R. S. (2015). Palliative care for the seriously Ill. *The New England Journal of Medicine*, *373*(8), 747–755. http://doi.org/10.1056/NEJMra1404684.

Keus, S., Munneke, M., Graziano, M., Paltamaa, J., Pelosin, E., Domingos, J., … Bloem, B. (2014). In *vol.1. European physiotherapy guideline for Parkinson's disease.* (1st ed.). The Netherlands: KNGF/ParkinsonNet.

Lang, A. E., & Lees, A. J. (2002). Management of Parkinson's disease: An evidence-based-review. *Movement Disorders*, *17*(Suppl. 4), S1–S166. http://doi.org/10.1002/mds.5554.

Lanoix, M. (2009). Palliative care and Parkinson's disease: Managing the chronic-palliative interface. *Chronic Illness*, *5*(1), 46–55. http://doi.org/10.1177/1742395309102819.

Lökk, J. (2011). Parkinson's disease permanent care unit: Managing the chronic-palliative interface. *Journal of Multidisciplinary Healthcare*, *4*, 33–38. http://doi.org/10.2147/JMDH.S17713.

Louter, M., Aarden, W. C. C. A., Lion, J., Bloem, B. R., & Overeem, S. (2012). Recognition and diagnosis of sleep disorders in Parkinson's disease. *Journal of Neurology*, *259*(10), 2031–2040. http://doi.org/10.1007/s00415-012-6505-7.

Martinez-Martin, P., Jeukens-Visser, M., Lyons, K. E., Rodriguez-Blazquez, C., Selai, C., Siderowf, A., … Schrag, A. (2011). Health-related quality-of-life scales in Parkinson's disease: Critique and recommendations. *Movement Disorders*, *26*(13), 2371–2380. http://doi.org/10.1002/mds.23834.

Martinez-Martin, P., Rodriguez-Blazquez, C., Kurtis, M. M., Chaudhuri, K. R., & NMSS Validation Group (2011). The impact of non-motor symptoms on health-related quality of life of patients with Parkinson's disease. *Movement Disorders: Official Journal of the Movement Disorder Society*, *26*(3), 399–406. http://doi.org/10.1002/mds.23462.

McIlfatrick, S. J., & Murphy, T. (2013). Palliative care research on the island of Ireland over the last decade: A systematic review and thematic analysis of peer reviewed publications. *BMC Palliative Care*, *12*(1), 33. http://doi.org/10.1186/1472-684X-12-33.

Miyasaki, J. M. (2013). Palliative care in Parkinson's disease. *Current Neurology and Neuroscience Reports*, *13*(8), 1–4. http://doi.org/10.1007/s11910-013-0367-y.

Miyasaki, J. M., & Kluger, B. (2015). Palliative care for Parkinson's disease: Has the time come? *Current Neurology and Neuroscience Reports*, *15*(5), 26. http://doi.org/10.1007/s11910-015-0542-4.

Miyasaki, J. M., Long, J., Mancini, D., Moro, E., Fox, S. H. H., Lang, A. E. E., … Hui, J. (2012). Palliative care for advanced Parkinson disease: An interdisciplinary clinic and new scale, the ESAS-PD. *Parkinsonism and Related Disorders*, *18*(Suppl. 3), S6–S9. http://doi.org/10.1016/j.parkreldis.2012.06.013.

Moroz, A., Edgley, S. R., Lew, H. L., Chae, J., Lombard, L. A., Reddy, C. C., & Robinson, K. M. (2009). Rehabilitation interventions in Parkinson disease. *PM & R: The Journal of Injury, Function, and Rehabilitation*, *1*(3 Suppl.), S42–S48. http://doi.org/10.1016/j.pmrj.2009.01.018.

Pastrana, T., Jünger, S., Ostgathe, C., Elsner, F., & Radbruch, L. (2008). A matter of definition—Key elements identified in a discourse analysis of definitions of palliative care. *Palliative Medicine*, *22*, 222–232. http://doi.org/10.1177/0269216308089803.

Poewe, W. (2006). The natural history of Parkinson's disease. *Journal of Neurology, 253*(Suppl. 7), 2–6. http://doi.org/10.1007/s00415-006-7002-7.

Politis, M., Wu, K., Molloy, S., G. Bain, P., Chaudhuri, K. R., & Piccini, P. (2010). Parkinson's disease symptoms: The patient's perspective. *Movement Disorders, 25*(11), 1646–1651. http://doi.org/10.1002/mds.23135.

Provinciali, L., Carlini, G., Tarquini, D., Defanti, C. A., Veronese, S., & Pucci, E. (2016). Need for palliative care for neurological diseases. *Neurological Sciences, 37*(10), 1581–1587. http://doi.org/10.1007/s10072-016-2614-x.

Quest, T. E., Marco, C. A., & Derse, A. R. (2009). Hospice and palliative medicine: New subspecialty, new opportunities. *Annals of Emergency Medicine, 54*(1), 94–102. http://doi.org/10.1016/j.annemergmed.2008.11.019.

Radder, D. L., Sturkenboom, I. H., van Nimwegen, M., Keus, S. H., Bloem, B. R., & de Vries, N. M. (2017). Physical therapy and occupational therapy in Parkinson's disease. *International Journal of Neuroscience*, 1–14. Jan 4 [Epub ahead of print], PMID: 28007002. http://doi.org/10.1080/00207454.2016.1275617.

Rascol, O., Payoux, P., & Ory, F. (2003). Limitations of current Parkinson's disease therapy. *Annals of Neurology, 53*, 3–15. http://doi.org/10.1002/ana.10513.Address.

Richfield, E. W., Jones, E. J. S., & Alty, J. E. (2013). Palliative care for Parkinson's disease: A summary of the evidence and future directions. *Palliative Medicine, 27*, 805–810. http://doi.org/10.1177/0269216313495287.

Salat, D., Noyce, A. J., Schrag, A., & Tolosa, E. (2016). Challenges of modifying disease progression in prediagnostic Parkinson's disease. *The Lancet Neurology, 15*(6), 637–648. http://doi.org/10.1016/S1474-4422(16)00060-0.

Saleem, T. Z., Higginson, I. J., Chaudhuri, K. R., Martin, A., Burman, R., & Leigh, P. N. (2013). Symptom prevalence, severity and palliative care needs assessment using the Palliative Outcome Scale: A cross-sectional study of patients with Parkinson's disease and related neurological conditions. *Palliative Medicine, 27*(8), 722–731. http://doi.org/10.1177/0269216312465783.

Sigurdardottir, K. R., Oldervoll, L., Hjermstad, M. J., Kaasa, S., Knudsen, A. K., Løhre, E. T., … Haugen, D. F. (2014). How are palliative care cancer populations characterized in randomized controlled trials? A literature review. *Journal of Pain and Symptom Management, 47*(5) 906–914.e17. http://doi.org/10.1016/j.jpainsymman.2013.06.005.

Sleeman, K. E., Ho, Y. K., Verne, J., Glickman, M., Silber, E., Gao, W., & Higginson, I. J. (2013). Place of death, and its relation with underlying cause of death, in Parkinson's disease, motor neurone disease, and multiple sclerosis: A population-based study. *Palliative Medicine, 27*(9), 840–846. http://doi.org/10.1177/0269216313490436.

Sleeman, K. E., & Murtagh, F. E. (2014). Increasing the value of research in palliative care. *Palliative Medicine, 28*(10), 1165–1166. http://doi.org/10.1177/0269216314556718.

Snell, K., Pennington, S., Lee, M., & Walker, R. (2009). The place of death in Parkinson's disease. *Age and Ageing, 38*(5), 617–619. http://doi.org/10.1093/ageing/afp123.

Stowe, R., Ives, N., Clarke, C. E., Handley, K., Furmston, A., Deane, K., … Gray, R. (2011). Meta-analysis of the comparative efficacy and safety of adjuvant treatment to levodopa in later Parkinson's disease. *Movement Disorders, 26*(4), 587–598. http://doi.org/10.1002/mds.23517.

Sturkenboom, I., Graff, M. J. L., Hendriks, J. C. M., Veenhuizen, Y., Munneke, M., Bloem, B. R., … OTiP study group (2014). Efficacy of occupational therapy for patients with Parkinson's disease: A randomised controlled trial. *The Lancet Neurology, 13*(6), 557–566. http://doi.org/10.1016/S1474-4422(14)70055-9.

Sturkenboom, I., Hendriks, J. C. M., Graff, M. J. L., Adang, E. M. M., Munneke, M., Nijhuis-van der Sanden, M. W. G., & Bloem, B. R. (2015). Economic evaluation of occupational therapy in Parkinson's disease: A randomized controlled trial. *Movement Disorders*, *30*(8), 1059–1067. http://doi.org/10.1002/mds.26217.

Sturkenboom, I. H. W. M., Thijssen, M. C. E., Gons-van Elsacker, J. J., Jansen, I. J. H., Maasdam, A., Schulten, M., ... Munneke, M. (2011). *Guidelines for occupational therapy in Parkinson's disease rehabilitation*. Nijmegen, The Netherlands: ParkinsonNet/ National Parkinson Foundation (NPF).

Sveinbjornsdottir, S. (2016). The clinical symptoms of Parkinson's disease. *Journal of Neurochemistry*, *139*(Suppl. 1), 318–324. http://doi.org/10.1111/jnc.13691.

Titova, N., Padmakumar, C., Lewis, S. J., & Chaudhuri, K. R. (2016). Parkinson's: A syndrome rather than a disease? *Journal of Neural Transmission (Vienna, Austria: 1996)*. review [Epub ahead of print], PMID: 28028643. http://doi.org/10.1007/ s00702-016-1667-6.

Todorova, A., Jenner, P., & Ray Chaudhuri, K. (2014). Non-motor Parkinson's: Integral to motor Parkinson's, yet often neglected. *Practical Neurology*, *14*(5), 310–322. http://doi. org/10.1136/practneurol-2013-000741.

van der Eijk, M., Faber, M. J., Post, B., Okun, M. S., Schmidt, P., Munneke, M., & Bloem, B. R. (2015). Capturing patients' experiences to change Parkinson's disease care delivery: A multicenter study. *Journal of Neurology*, *262*(11), 2528–2538. http://doi.org/ 10.1007/s00415-015-7877-2.

van der Eijk, M., Faber, M. J., Ummels, I., Aarts, J. W. M., Munneke, M., & Bloem, B. R. (2012). Patient-centeredness in PD care: Development and validation of a patient experience questionnaire. *Parkinsonism & Related Disorders*, *18*(9), 1011–1016. http://doi.org/ 10.1016/j.parkreldis.2012.05.017.

van Vliet, L. M., Gao, W., DiFrancesco, D., Crosby, V., Wilcock, A., Byrne, A., ... Higginson, I. J. (2016). How integrated are neurology and palliative care services? Results of a multicentre mapping exercise. *BMC Neurology*, *16*(1), 63. http://doi.org/ 10.1186/s12883-016-0583-6.

Visser, C., Hadley, G., & Wee, B. (2015). Reality of evidence-based practice in palliative care. *Cancer Biology and Medicine*, *12*(3), 193–200. http://doi.org/10.7497/j.issn.2095-3941. 2015.0041.

Walker, R. W., Churm, D., Dewhurst, F., Samuel, M., Ramsell, A., Lawrie, C., ... Gray, W. K. (2014). Palliative care in people with idiopathic Parkinson's disease who die in hospital. *BMJ Supportive & Palliative Care*, *4*(1), 64–67. http://doi.org/10.1136/ bmjspcare-2012-000412.

Wilcox, S. K. (2010). Extending palliative care to patients with Parkinson's disease. *British Journal of Hospital Medicine (London, England: 2005)*, *71*(1), 26–30. http://doi.org/10. 12968/hmed.2010.71.1.45969.

Williams, D. R., & Litvan, I. (2013). Parkinsonian syndromes. *Continuum (Minneapolis, Minn)*, *19*(5), 1189–1212. http://doi.org/10.1212/01.CON.0000436152.24038.e0.

Zimmermann, C., Riechelmann, R., Krzyzanowska, M., Rodin, G., & Tannock, I. (2008). Effectiveness of specialized palliative care: A systematic review. *JAMA*, *299*(14), 1698–1709. http://doi.org/10.1001/jama.299.14.1698.

CHAPTER EIGHTEEN

Multidisciplinary Care in Parkinson's Disease

Mubasher A. Qamar*,†,#,1, Grace Harington*,†, Sally Trump*,†, Julia Johnson*,†, Fiona Roberts*,†, Emily Frost*,†

*National Parkinson Foundation International Centre of Excellence, Kings College and Kings College Hospital, London, United Kingdom

†National Institute for Health Research (NIHR) Mental Health Biomedical Research Centre (BRC) and Dementia Unit at South London and Maudsley NHS Foundation Trust, London, United Kingdom

#Maurice Wohl Clinical Neuroscience Institute, Kings College, London, United Kingdom

[1]Corresponding author: e-mail address: mubasher.qamar@nhs.net

Contents

Abstract

Parkinson's disease (PD) is now known to be a multisystemic and multipeptide neurodegenerative disorder, whereby patients have an array of symptoms both motor and nonmotor. Nonmotor features of PD have been shown to arise almost 15–20 years prior to motor symptoms and, as such, are also a key determinant to the quality of life of a patient. Therefore, there is increasing evidence that a PD patient's management must encompass a multidisciplinary approach to effectively manage and treat the patient's PD and also their individual symptoms. Therefore, the notion that a PD nurse specialist and a neurologist are the only key players, is no longer the case. Rather, the involvement of speech and language therapist, physiotherapists, palliative care, and others is vital for a patient's recovery and their effective management. Here we discuss a few professions who should ideally be present for each PD patient.

International Review of Neurobiology, Volume 132
ISSN 0074-7742
http://dx.doi.org/10.1016/bs.irn.2017.02.001

1. INTRODUCTION

Parkinson's disease (PD) is a multisystem, multipeptide, and heterogeneous neurodegenerative disorder (Chaudhuri, Healy, Schapira, & National Institute for Clinical Excellence, 2006; Chaudhuri, Martinez-Martin, et al., 2006), which requires a multidimensional approach to management. PD has classically been recognized as a motor syndrome; however, this has now been largely abandoned due to the identification of the prodromal period of PD characterized by a range of nonmotor symptoms (NMS) (Zis, Erro, Walton, Sauerbier, & Chaudhuri, 2015). With PD patients reporting NMS as a key determinant of their quality of life (QoL) and further impact of increased hospitalization and institutionalization, the need to manage patients holistically is vital (Chaudhuri, Healy, et al., 2006; Martinez-Martin et al., 2011). Therefore, a structured multidisciplinary team (MDT) bringing together healthcare professions from different specialities is essential to maximize patient management.

In this chapter, we explore the key stakeholders in a typical PD patient's MDT, with the aim to outline the need to provide this network in all healthcare sites dealing with PD patients. The scope of this chapter will not detail every discipline involved; Fig. 1 depicts a broad overview of the various specialities benefiting MDT.

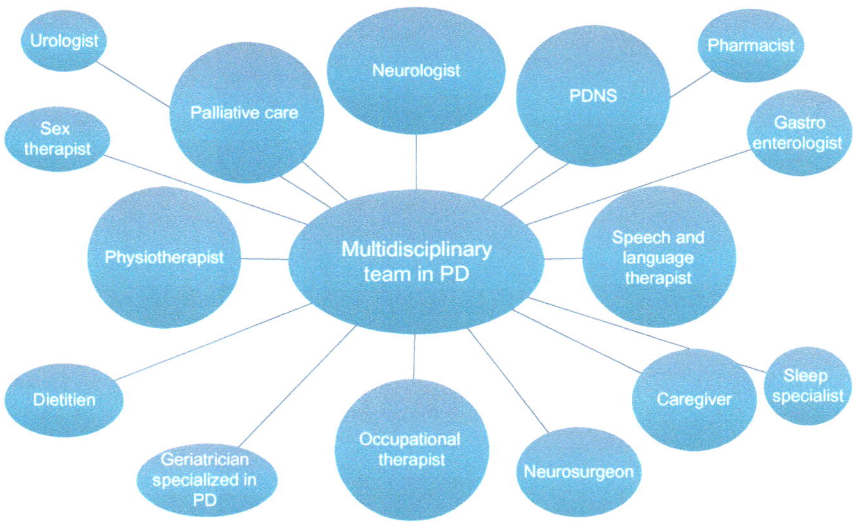

Fig. 1 Multidisciplinary team disciplines. *PD*, Parkinson's disease; *PDNS*, Parkinson's disease nurse specialist.

2. CURRENT APPROACH TO PARKINSON'S DISEASE CARE

Current PD treatment with pharmacotherapy and surgery can greatly improve many of the NMS that are so disruptive to patients. Arguably, the NMS have a higher level of burden and are known to have large impacts on the QoL for patient (Chaudhuri et al., 2015; Martinez-Martin et al., 2011; Zis et al., 2015). Furthermore, pharmacotherapies often fall short of alleviating the broad spectrum of NMS. Pharmacological treatment can also present challenges in advanced PD, with the gold standard dopamine therapy, levodopa, often leaving the patient with debilitating dyskinesia (Chaudhuri & Schapira, 2009).

An MDT approach to PD treatment is suited to address the complex nature of symptoms that PD patients suffer from (Van Der Marck et al., 2009). In combination with the physician, MDT's primary team members are specialists in nursing, physiotherapy, occupational therapy, speech and language therapy, and palliative care (Van Der Marck et al., 2013). A broader aspect of MDT care incorporates a number of other specialists including dietitians, gastroenterologists, urologists, psychologists, and more, as shown in Fig. 1 (Van Der Marck et al., 2013).

Encouraging patients to have an active role in their care and providing access to social groups and educational activities has shown to be beneficial in the management of PD (Trend, Kaye, Gage, Owen, & Wade, 2002; Van Der Eijk, Nijhuis, Faber, & Bloem, 2013). Studies have found that motivated self-care management schemes result in independent decision making and self-sufficiency, which can ultimately improve treatment compliance and an overall QoL (Van Der Eijk et al., 2013). The need to equip patients to self-manage their condition is becoming vital, which has led to the development of validated tools such as the NMS questionnaire (NMSQuest) and the King's PD Pain questionnaire (KPPQ) (Chaudhuri, Martinez-Martin, et al., 2006; Rizos et al., 2016). This has given patients the ability to identify NMS, which would otherwise be missed in a busy clinical consultation. This type of identification further assists better management by allowing clinicians to refer patients to specific healthcare professions to manage certain symptoms.

The role of the carer for the PD patient is becoming increasingly important in their treatment regime (Schrag, Hovris, Morley, Quinn, & Jahanshahi, 2006; Tod et al., 2016). The carer is fundamental in liaising with the MDT, allowing for the patient's concerns and problems to be better communicated (Giladi, Manor, Hilel, & Gurevich, 2014; Schrag et al., 2006). Conversely, a strong MDT management plan should include and address the needs and well-being of the carer as well (Schrag et al., 2006; Van Der Marck et al., 2009). Studies show that the QoL of the caregiver can greatly improve patient care and can even delay the need for nursing home placement (Schrag et al., 2006; Tod et al., 2016). The burden of PD on the caregiver can be substantial; hallucinations, confusion, and falls are among the greatest burden to carers and predicators of institutionalization (Aarsland, Larsen, Tandberg, & Laake, 2000; Carter et al., 1998). Thus, taking the carer's well-being into account can subsequently decrease institutionalization and reduce the social economic burden of PD treatment (Vossius, Nilsen, & Larsen, 2009). Recognition that PD is not a single person's disease, rather a syndrome that can have a far-reaching affect, is vital.

2.1 Parkinson's Disease Nurse Specialist

The PD nurse specialist (PDNS) plays a central role in all stages of PD, from coordinating care and offering education to providing emotional support (Axelrod et al., 2010). They fundamentally act as both an interface between primary and secondary care settings, as well as patients and their families (Chaudhuri, Martinez-Martin, et al., 2006). This ranges from community-based nurses supporting patients in their own home, to hospital-based teams, running nurse-led clinics, and supporting hospital staff with the care of PD patients during admissions.

PDNSs have been involved in patient care for several decades, particularly in the United Kingdom; their need and support is well documented. Significant benefits to a patients' perception of their care has been reported over standard care when attended by a PDNS (Jarman, Hurwitz, Cook, Bajekal, & Lee, 2002). This is partially due to the amount of time a nurse can spend with the patient in each clinic compared to clinicians whose time is increasingly in demand. Nursing clinics can also be used to supplement the typical six monthly visits to a neurologist, meaning that the patient can be seen by a professional more frequently. The PDNS is therefore able to identify any problems a patient may be having through a holistic assessment of both motor and nonmotor features of PD and refer to the appropriate specialties. This may identify any urgent physical or mental health requirements of the patient, before any acute crisis occurs. In this way, the PDNS can reduce the incidence of hospital admissions and reduce healthcare costs (Carter et al., 1998), as well as increasing the patient's confidence in their care and management of disease (Jarman et al., 2002). The role of a PDNS has been reported to be valued by other healthcare professions, as PD patients would encounter a range of nurses and other professionals who may not be well informed about PD management (Reynolds, Wilson-Barnett, & Richardson, 2000).

2.2 Speech and Language Therapists

The speech and language therapist within an MDT is responsible for working on communication and swallowing management with the patient (Parkinson's UK, 2013). It is their aim, in conjunction with other team members, to improve patient's speech, swallowing, and communication through various therapy exercises and activities.

The progressive voice difficulties and gradually less distinct articulation associated with PD are often insidious in onset and may go unrecognized by the person with PD. James Parkinson in 1817 identified speech and language problems in his original text:

> *his senses, and the powers of his mind, unimpaired; he was attentive to, and sensible of everything which was said in conversation, and shewed himself very desirous of joining in it; but was continually checked by the impediment in his speech, and the difficulty which his hearers were put to*
>
> ***Parkinson (1922)***

As outlined in his case study, the impairment of speech and articulating of language can adversely affect a patient. Problems initiating and maintaining conversations are exacerbated by bradyphrenia, a freezing of thought, and may be further complicated by cognitive decline (Mahler, Ramig, & Fox, 2015). This may lead to withdrawal from social situations and increased social isolation. Treatment programs focus on methods of speech delivery, assuming the role of an actor projecting a voice into a larger space (Mahler et al., 2015).

Swallowing assessment and management is important as swallowing difficulties may lead to problems, such as aspiration pneumonia, a primary cause of death in people with PD (Troche et al., 2009). Dribbling of saliva (or sialorrhoea) is reported to result from a reduction in the regulation of involuntary swallows which would clear saliva. Thus, failure in this action leaves saliva resting in the mouth and at risk of spillage, both anteriorly out of the lips or posteriorly into the pharynx, or open airway (Srivantichapoom, Pandey, & Hallett, 2014). Additionally, medications aimed at reducing saliva production are often contraindicated. The speech and language therapist swallowing assessment may include instrumental examinations, such as videofluoroscopy and fibreoptic nasendoscopy, to supplement clinical observations (Srivantichapoom et al., 2014; Troche et al., 2009). Swallowing efficiency and safety can be improved with changes to the texture of food and liquids and trialing techniques, such as a chin tuck posture to aid airway protection. Exercises which strengthen the vocal cords and expiratory pressure on coughing also help to protect the lungs from pneumonia.

The goal is to maintain vigilance and encourage exercise and activity for the patient throughout the course of PD. Improvements in speech and language will increase social interactions, give confidence, and subsequently improve QoL for the patients.

2.3 Physiotherapy

The role of the physiotherapist is to increase the patient's ability to perform daily functional activities throughout the course of PD (Keus, 2007; Van Der Marck et al., 2009). The physiotherapist plays a key role in PD management from early to very advanced stages of PD, especially in Hoehn and Yahr stage 3 onward, where balance is affected. Mobility, gait, balance, and strength can be improved through a variety of exercise therapies, cueing strategies, and cognitive movement therapies (Keus, 2007).

The impact of falling in PD can be hugely detrimental to the treatment of patients and is a major cause of clinical visits (Keus, 2007). Cueing strategies have shown to be particularly beneficial in improving gait, posture, fluency of walking, freezing episodes, and the confidence to carry out skills without falling (Keus, 2007; Nieuwboer et al., 2001). Exercise therapy has proved to be effective in increasing physical capacity in numerous studies, helping patients with postural impairments, and reeducating stooped walking and balance issues (Fisher et al., 2008). Cognitive movement therapy has improved success of transfers in patients, i.e., turning around in bed or rising from a chair and can be beneficial in tackling dual tasks that are often difficult or avoided completely by patients (Keus, Munneke, Nijkrake, Kwakkel, & Bloem, 2009; Van Der Marck et al., 2009).

Physiotherapy intervention has been mentioned in several trials including controlled studies. Data on its efficacy are controversial; however, exercise has emerged as a key management strategy in PD, with some suggestions of neuroprotective effects (Da Silva, Domingues, De Carvalho, Allodi, & Correa, 2016; Jang et al., 2016) and improvement in QoL (Keus, 2007). Thus, physiotherapists, alongside occupational therapists, play an integral role in encouraging physical activity. They should aim to facilitate patient independence and ultimately create the best environment and conditions for patients to maintain a level of normality.

2.4 Occupational Therapy

The occupational therapist (OT) is responsible for promoting health and well-being through occupation, with the primary goal being to enable participation in everyday activities (WFOT, 2010).

When assessing and treating individuals with PD, OTs utilize a holistic approach; focus is on an individual's skills, as well as considering what is involved in the activity itself, breaking it down into components, and the physical environment in which the activity is to be completed (Letts et al., 1994). PD patients typically have difficulty with dual tasks and problems with falls when postural reflexes are impaired. OT plays an essential role by having modifications, especially in the bathroom and kitchen areas, where falls and other such injuries can often occur. Furthermore, useful advice is often provided by OT support for special disability help with tremor, writing, walking aids, and home friendly improvements (like thermoregulation problems). To facilitate independence during tasks and reduce carer burden, an OT can incorporate different techniques, which include remedial, educational, and compensatory tasks (Fisher, 2013; Fisher et al., 2008).

Some of the most important aspects of OT support are maintaining a person's role (for example, in their family and work place), promoting independence and participation with activities of daily living, such as personal care, mobility and transfers, and consideration of the environment on safety and efficiency during these activities (NICE, 2006). Interventions can include optimizing activities, incorporating specific strategies for initiating and maintaining movements (Aragon & Kings, 2010; Parkinsons.org.uk, 2015). The OT role also includes being an educator, networker, and supporter of people with PD (Deane, Ellis-Hill, Dekker, Davies, & Clarke, 2003). Referrals to an OT facilitate intervention at an early stage of the disease, which can optimize an individual's occupational performance and QoL (NICE, 2006).

2.5 Palliative Care

Palliative care with respect to PD is not terminal end-of-life care, but palliative management of symptoms in advanced PD. The scope and role of palliative care in PD is not well defined; however, the Movement Disorder Society has set up task forces to examine the scope and delivery of palliative care (Movementdisorders.org, 2016). Typically, palliative care is reserved for people with PD for end-of-life care and refractory symptoms, largely motor and nonmotor that may occur in late PD. This includes effective management of symptoms, but also advice in relation to emotional health and distress, and practical issues such as writing a will, breaking bad news to the family, and so on. Palliative care is now an essential speciality in PD, but is already well established in other neurodegenerative conditions such as Alzheimer's disease. Recently, advances include the first placebo OCT-care neuro for PD and parkinsonism disorders (Boersma, Miyasaki, Kutner, & Kluger, 2014) (Table 1).

3. LIMITATIONS AND BARRIERS

MDT care is increasingly being adapted into the daily care of PD patients; however, there is minimal clinical evidence on the actual success of MDT care in PD (Trend et al., 2002; Van Der Marck & Bloem, 2014). The diversity of patients and a constantly changing healthcare environment create challenges in implementing MDT care (Craig et al., 2008). Furthermore, a tangible structure for integration does not currently exist at all medical sites (Van Der Marck & Bloem, 2014; Van Der Marck et al., 2013). MDT, in theory, provides the best treatment plan for each specific case; however, the logistics behind such a complex framework and its organizational structure are complicated.

First and foremost, collaboration and communication between disciplines is fundamental and the success of an MDT is predicated on an investment in coordination and resource allocation, both of which require a time commitment and financial support (Van Der Marck & Bloem, 2014; Van Der Marck et al., 2013). Expertise, availability, and accessibility also dictate the functionality of the team (Boon, Verhoef, O'Hara, & Findlay, 2004). The primary purpose of an MDT is combining individual strengths to best benefit the patient and carer. Therefore, it is crucial that MDTs work in a synergistic manner across all domains to guarantee integrative care (Boon et al., 2004). Despite similar treatment goals, there is a tendency for disciplines to work in isolation rather than with a collaborative approach (Van Der Eijk et al., 2013; Van Der Marck & Bloem, 2014),

Table 1 The Ideal Composition of a Multidisciplinary Team Members in Parkinson's Disease

Specialist	Role	References
Neurologist	Patient diagnosis, prognosis, and treatment; lead of the MDT	Giladi et al. (2014)
Parkinson's disease nurse (PDNS)	Provide information, education, and support on PD and related issues; a center point for communication between the patient and other MDT members	Trend et al. (2002)
Psychologist and neuropsychiatrist	Evaluate the mental status of the patient (anxiety, depression, psychosis, etc.); provide psychosocial support, cognitive behavior therapy, and psychotherapy medications if necessary	Chaudhuri, Healy, et al. (2006) and Giladi et al. (2014)
Speech and language therapist	Assist patients in communication, speech, and swallowing management using a variety of exercise therapies	Giladi et al. (2014) and Trend et al. (2002)
Physiotherapist	Help patients stay mobile with exercise therapies; develop physical ability and skills to perform functional daily activities of living	Giladi et al. (2014)
Occupational therapist	Promote health and well-being through occupation; enable patients to complete daily activities of living	Parkinsons.org.uk (2015)
Sleep specialist	Evaluate sleep disturbances associated with PD	Chaudhuri (2009)
Caregiver	Communicate and work with the MDT in patient management and treatment plans Provide a good level of social care for the patient and self	Schrag et al. (2006) and Tod et al. (2016)
Urologist	Evaluate and address issues with urinary retention and bladder stability	Jost (2013)
Gastroenterologists	Evaluate and treat issues that arise with entire gastric tract and gastric functioning	Chaudhuri, Healy, et al. (2006)

Continued

Table 1 The Ideal Composition of a Multidisciplinary Team Members in Parkinson's Disease—cont'd

Specialist	Role	References
Dietitian	Mediate nutrition, alleviate swallowing difficulties and constipation, and support the maintenance of a healthy weight for the patient	Parkinsons.org.uk (2016)
Pharmacist	Manage pharmacotherapy treatment	
Psychosexual therapist	Promote sexual health with counseling in sexual function and dysfunction	Giladi et al. (2014)
Neurosurgeon	Assess patients for neurosurgical treatment to potentially alleviate and control motor symptoms	Perlmutter and Mink (2006)

PD, Parkinson's disease; MDT, multidisciplinary team.

4. FUTURE OF MDTs IN PARKINSON'S DISEASE

Future directions should aim to foster a standard framework that accommodates motor and NMS, patient diversity, and the evolving healthcare system. A drive for healthcare management driven by patient requirements will best benefit the patient and the caregiver. Developing collaboration, integration, mutual respect, and communication between the healthcare team members and the patients and carers will lead to the greatest quality of disease management and ultimately improve the QoL for the patient and carer in the long term.

REFERENCES

Aarsland, D., Larsen, J. P., Tandberg, E., & Laake, K. (2000). Predictors of nursing home placement in Parkinson's disease: A population-based, prospective study. *Journal of the American Geriatrics Society*, *48*, 938–942.

Aragon, A., & Kings, K. (2010). Occupational therapy for people with Parkinson's best practice guidelines. *College of Occupational Therapists*, 3–54. Available at: https://www.cot.co.uk/sites/default/files/publications/public/OT-People-Parkinsons.pdf. [Accessed 10 Nov. 2016].

Axelrod, L., Gage, H., Kaye, J., Bryan, K., Trend, P., & Wade, D. (2010). Workloads of Parkinson's specialist nurses: Implications for implementing national service guidelines in England. *Journal of Clinical Nursing*, *19*, 3575–3580.

Boersma, I., Miyasaki, J., Kutner, J., & Kluger, B. (2014). Palliative care and neurology: Time for a paradigm shift. *Neurology, 83*, 561–567.
Boon, H., Verhoef, M., O'Hara, D., & Findlay, B. (2004). From parallel practice to integrative health care: A conceptual framework. *BMC Health Services Research, 4*, 15.
Carter, J. H., Stewart, B. J., Archbold, P. G., Inoue, I., Jaglin, J., Lannon, M., et al. (1998). Living with a person who has Parkinson's disease: The spouse's perspective by stage of disease. *Movement Disorders, 13*, 20–28.
Chaudhuri, K. R. (2009). The dopaminergic basis of sleep dysfunction and non motor symptoms of Parkinson's disease: Evidence from functional imaging. *Experimental Neurology, 216*, 247–248.
Chaudhuri, K. R., Healy, D. G., Schapira, A. H., & National Institute for Clinical Excellence (2006). Non-motor symptoms of Parkinson's disease: Diagnosis and management. *Lancet Neurology, 5*, 235–245.
Chaudhuri, K. R., Martinez-Martin, P., Schapira, A. H., Stocchi, F., Sethi, K., Odin, P., et al. (2006). International multicenter pilot study of the first comprehensive self-completed nonmotor symptoms questionnaire for Parkinson's disease: The NMSQuest study. *Movement Disorders, 21*, 916–923.
Chaudhuri, K. R., Sauerbier, A., Rojo, J. M., Sethi, K., Schapira, A. H., Brown, R. G., et al. (2015). The burden of non-motor symptoms in Parkinson's disease using a self-completed non-motor questionnaire: A simple grading system. *Parkinsonism & Related Disorders, 21*, 287–291.
Chaudhuri, K. R., & Schapira, A. H. (2009). Non-motor symptoms of Parkinson's disease: Dopaminergic pathophysiology and treatment. *Lancet Neurology, 8*, 464–474.
Craig, P., Dieppe, P., Macintyre, S., Michie, S., Nazareth, I., Petticrew, M., et al. (2008). Developing and evaluating complex interventions: The new Medical Research Council guidance. *BMJ, 337*, a1655.
Da Silva, P. G., Domingues, D. D., De Carvalho, L. A., Allodi, S., & Correa, C. L. (2016). Neurotrophic factors in Parkinson's disease are regulated by exercise: Evidence-based practice. *Journal of the Neurological Sciences, 363*, 5–15.
Deane, K. H. O., Ellis-Hill, C., Dekker, K., Davies, P., & Clarke, C. E. (2003). A survey of current occupational therapy practice for Parkinson's disease in the United Kingdom. *British Journal of Occupational Therapy, 66*(5), 193–200.
Fisher, A. G. (2013). Occupation-centred, occupation-based, occupation-focused: Same, same or different? *Scandinavian Journal of Occupational Therapy, 20*, 162–173.
Fisher, B. E., Wu, A. D., Salem, G. J., Song, J., Lin, C. H., Yip, J., et al. (2008). The effect of exercise training in improving motor performance and corticomotor excitability in people with early Parkinson's disease. *Archives of Physical Medicine and Rehabilitation, 89*, 1221–1229.
Giladi, N., Manor, Y., Hilel, A., & Gurevich, T. (2014). Interdisciplinary teamwork for the treatment of people with Parkinson's disease and their families. *Current Neurology and Neuroscience Reports, 14*, 493.
Jang, Y., Koo, J. H., Kwon, I., Kang, E. B., Um, H. S., Soya, H., et al. (2016). Neuroprotective effects of endurance exercise against neuroinflammation in MPTP-induced Parkinson's disease mice. *Brain Research, 1655*, 186–193.
Jarman, B., Hurwitz, B., Cook, A., Bajekal, M., & Lee, A. (2002). Effects of community based nurses specialising in Parkinson's disease on health outcome and costs: Randomised controlled trial. *British Medical Journal, 324*, 1072–1075.
Jost, W. H. (2013). Urological problems in Parkinson's disease: Clinical aspects. *Journal of Neural Transmission, 120*, 587–591.
Keus, S. H. J. (2007). Cueing training in the home improves mobility in Parkinson's disease. *Australian Journal of Physiotherapy, 53*, 285.

Keus, S. H. J., Munneke, M., Nijkrake, M. J., Kwakkel, G., & Bloem, B. R. (2009). Physical therapy in Parkinson's disease: Evolution and future challenges. *Movement Disorders*, *24*, 1–14.

Letts, L., Law, M., Rigby, P., Cooper, B., Stewart, D., & Strong, S. (1994). Person-environment assessments in occupational therapy. *The American Journal of Occupational Therapy*, *48*, 608–618.

Mahler, L. A., Ramig, L. O., & Fox, C. (2015). Evidence-based treatment of voice and speech disorders in Parkinson disease. *Current Opinion in Otolaryngology & Head and Neck Surgery*, *23*, 209–215.

Martinez-Martin, P., Jeukens-Visser, M., Lyons, K. E., Rodriguez-Blazquez, C., Selai, C., Siderowf, A., et al. (2011). Health-related quality-of-life scales in Parkinson's disease: Critique and recommendations. *Movement Disorders*, *26*, 2371–2380.

Movementdisorders.org. 2016. *MDS Task Forces*. [Online] Available at: http://www.movementdisorders.org/MDS/About/Committees–Other-Groups/MDS-Task-Forces.htm [Accessed 10 Nov. 2016]. https://www.parkinsons.org.uk/content/dietary-therapy. [Accessed 10 Nov. 2016].

NICE. (2006). Parkinson's Disease National Clinical Guideline for Diagnosis and Management in Primary and Secondary Care. *NICE Clinical Guidelines*. https://www.nice.org.uk/guidance/CG35. [Accessed 1 Mar. 17).

Nieuwboer, A., De Weerdt, W., Dom, R., Truyen, M., Janssens, L., & Kamsma, Y. (2001). The effect of a home physiotherapy program for persons with Parkinson's disease. *Journal of Rehabilitation Medicine*, *33*, 266–272.

Parkinson, J., (1922). An essay on the shaking palsy. *Archives of Neurology and Psychiatry*, 7, 683–710.

Parkinson's UK. Speech and language therapy information sheet. *parkinsons.org.uk*. 2013 [Online] Available at: https://www.parkinsons.org.uk/content/speech-and-language-therapy-information-sheet. [Accessed 12 Nov. 16].

Parkinsons.org.uk. 2015. *Parkinson's UK—Occupational Therapy and Parkinson's*. [Online] Available at: https://www.parkinsons.org.uk/content/occupational-therapy-and-parkinsons. [Accessed 10 Nov. 2016].

Parkinson's UK. Dietary therapy. *parkinsons.org.uk*. 2016. [Online] Available at: https://www.parkinsons.org.uk/content/dietary-therapy. [Accessed 12 Nov. 16].

Perlmutter, J. S., & Mink, J. W. (2006). Deep brain stimulation. *Annual Review of Neuroscience*, *29*, 229–257.

Reynolds, H., Wilson-Barnett, J., & Richardson, G. (2000). Evaluation of the role of the Parkinson's disease nurse specialist. *International Journal of Nursing Studies*, *37*, 337–349.

Rizos, A., Martinez-Martin, P., Pal, S., Carroll, C., Martino, D., Sophia, R., et al. (2016). The first Parkinson's Disease Pain Questionnaire (King's PD Pain Quest)—An interim analysis of a multicentre study of the patient's perspective. *Parkinsonism & Related Disorders*, *22*, e41.

Schrag, A., Hovris, A., Morley, D., Quinn, N., & Jahanshahi, M. (2006). Caregiver-burden in Parkinson's disease is closely associated with psychiatric symptoms, falls, and disability. *Parkinsonism & Related Disorders*, *12*, 35–41.

Srivantichapoom, P., Pandey, S., & Hallett, M. (2014). Drooling in Parkinson's disease: A review. *Parkinsonism & Related Disorders*, *20*, 1109–1118.

Tod, A. M., Kennedy, F., Stocks, A. J., McDonnell, A., Ramaswamy, B., Wood, B., et al. (2016). Good-quality social care for people with Parkinson's disease: A qualitative study. *BMJ Open*, *6*, e006813.

Trend, P., Kaye, J., Gage, H., Owen, C., & Wade, D. (2002). Short-term effectiveness of intensive multidisciplinary rehabilitation for people with Parkinson's disease and their carers. *Clinical Rehabilitation*, *16*, 717–725.

Troche, M. S., Okun, M. S., Rosenbek, J. C., Musson, N., Fernandez, H. H., Rodriguez, R. L., et al. (2009). Aspiration and swallowing in Parkinson's disease and rehabilitation with EMST: The ASPIRE study. *Movement Disorders*, *24*, S283–S284.

Van Der Eijk, M., Nijhuis, F. A., Faber, M. J., & Bloem, B. R. (2013). Moving from physician-centered care towards patient-centered care for Parkinson's disease patients. *Parkinsonism & Related Disorders*, *19*, 923–927.

Van Der Marck, M. A., & Bloem, B. R. (2014). How to organize multispecialty care for patients with Parkinson's disease. *Parkinsonism & Related Disorders*, *20*(Suppl. 1), S167–S173.

Van Der Marck, M. A., Kalf, J. G., Sturkenboom, I. H., Nijkrake, M. J., Munneke, M., & Bloem, B. R. (2009). Multidisciplinary care for patients with Parkinson's disease. *Parkinsonism & Related Disorders*, *15*(Suppl. 3), S219–S223.

Van Der Marck, M. A., Munneke, M., Mulleners, W., Hoogerwaard, E. M., Borm, G. F., Overeem, S., et al. (2013). Integrated multidisciplinary care in Parkinson's disease: A non-randomised, controlled trial (IMPACT). *Lancet Neurology*, *12*, 947–956.

Vossius, C., Nilsen, O. B., & Larsen, J. P. (2009). Parkinson's disease and nursing home placement: The economic impact of the need for care. *European Journal of Neurology*, *16*, 194–200.

WFOT. World Federation of Occupational Therapists: Statement on occupational therapy. *wfot.org*. 2010 [Online] Available at: http://www.wfot.org/Portals/0/PDF/STATEMENT%20ON%20OCCUPATIONAL%20THERAPY%20300811.pdf. [Accessed 12 Nov. 16].

Zis, P., Erro, R., Walton, C. C., Sauerbier, A., & Chaudhuri, K. R. (2015). The range and nature of non-motor symptoms in drug-naive Parkinson's disease patients: A state-of-the-art systematic review. *NPJ Parkinson's Disease*, *1*, 15013.